Global Surgery

Mark A. Hardy • Beth R. Hochman
Editors

Global Surgery

How to Work and Teach in Low- and Middle-Income Countries

Springer

Editors
Mark A. Hardy
General, Vascular & Abdominal Transplant Surgery
Columbia University Medical Center
New York, NY, USA

Beth R. Hochman
General Surgery & Critical Care Medicine
Columbia University Medical Center
New York, NY, USA

ISBN 978-3-031-28126-6 ISBN 978-3-031-28127-3 (eBook)
https://doi.org/10.1007/978-3-031-28127-3

This Springer imprint is published by the registered company Springer Nature Switzerland AG
The registered company address is: Gewerbestrasse 11, 6330 Cham, Switzerland

I dedicate this book to my wife, Ruth, for her support, love, and understanding, and to my children, Peter, Arthur, and Karen, and their spouses, and to my grandchildren.

Mark A. Hardy

I dedicate this book to my parents, Marcia and Harry, for their undying support and their unparalleled empathy and generosity that inspired my interest in global health.

Beth R. Hochman

Acknowledgments

We would like to thank:
Richard Lansing (Springer Editorial Director) and Richard Hurska (Springer Executive Editor) for seeing the potential in our project and accepting this undertaking on behalf of Springer, and Kristopher Spring (Springer Senior Editor) for seeing it through.

Dhanapal Palanisamy (Project Coordinator) for so patiently working with us as we navigated the process of generating and gathering content, and helping us stay organized despite our near constant attempts to embrace entropy.

Shalini Kameshwaran, Sendhilkumar Jayakumar, and Geetha Dhandapani (Project Managers) for graciously and effectively ushering us to the finish line.

Mark A. Hardy
Beth R. Hochman

Contents

1 Introduction

Mark A. Hardy and Beth R. Hochman

The idea that some lives matter less is the root of all that is wrong with the world.

– Paul Farmer

Abbreviations

ACS	American College of Surgeons
DALYs	Disability-Adjusted Life Years
HICs	High-Income Countries
LMICs	Low- and Middle-Income Countries
NGO	Non-Governmental Organization
SSA	Sub-Saharan Africa
WHO	World Health Organization

First, Do no Harm

Global surgery is defined by a commitment to achieving equitable and sustainable access to surgical care in all environments. This involves two primary challenges: first, expanding surgical capacity in areas with low surgical volume (whether due to limited population density, infrastructural resources, or clinical expertise), and second, ensuring that patients are readily able to access necessary surgical care without barriers (whether physical, socioeconomic, or political). Some of these challenges have been previously addressed by others [1–3]. In this book we focus on components of the first challenge, but it is paramount to recognize the pervasive impact of the second challenge throughout the care continuum, and at times our own potential contribution to the problem. Exposure to surgical care delivery in differently resourced environments and in the context of different cultures and lived experiences is thus an invaluable starting point for all global surgeons. However, exposure alone is inadequate; an effective global surgeon understands how one's own identity and the interplay with that of others influences both patient engagement in health care and successful clinician teamwork. The positionality of HIC partners working in surgical and anesthesia practices in LMICs can be particularly complex. Therefore, our initial chapter focuses on the ethical and decolonization aspects of collaborations between clinicians from differing cultural, medical, and economic backgrounds while another chapter explores preparatory considerations from a HIC perspective when engaging in HIC-LMIC partnership.

M. A. Hardy (✉)
Department of Surgery, Columbia University Vagelos College of Physician and Surgeons, New York, NY, USA
e-mail: mah1@columbia.edu

B. R. Hochman
Department of Surgery, Columbia University Vagelos College of Physician and Surgeons, New York, NY, USA
e-mail: brh2106@cumc.columbia.edu

M. A. Hardy, B. R. Hochman (eds.), *Global Surgery*, https://doi.org/10.1007/978-3-031-28127-3_1

The principle of "Primum non nocere" (first, do no harm) guides all of these discussions. Francis Moore, former chairman of the Department of Surgery at Peter Bent Brigham Hospital, once said, "you can't learn to play the piano by attending concerts" [4] (i.e., you have to practice somewhere), but we must emphasize another adage that, "anything is NOT usually better than nothing." All surgical practice must be firmly grounded on the standard ethical principles of beneficence, nonmaleficence, autonomy, and justice. In all environments, surgeons and surgical capacity-building must rely on informed consent, graded responsibility, close supervision for trainees, and ultimately, senior availability and gradual transfer of skills. Understanding our colleagues and our patients is the foundation for success.

Know Your Patients

In reviewing our (MAH & BH) experiences with our trainees in Ethiopia, Kenya, Vietnam, and India, we realized that our main contacts with patients occurred primarily on the operating table, and, as noted by one of our colleagues, Dr. Nishikawa, we knew little about where or how they lived (many traveled from remote rural areas or distant mountains). Our patients often had very little understanding of doctors or western medical interventions; most of their illnesses were treated by traditional healers with practices unfamiliar to us. Many of our patients were unfamiliar with what we considered commonplace – owning a pair of shoes, riding in a car, and having consistent access to electricity and running water. Some had never previously met anyone from outside their own community, and by the same token, we had not previously met anyone from their community.

Learning from and contributing to high-quality care both in and out of the operating room relies on a baseline understanding of our patients. Part of educating faculty and residents working in new environments with patients from unfamiliar backgrounds necessarily includes an introduction to their patients' languages, religions, living and working conditions, cultural practices, and beliefs about illness and medical care. As Dr. Nishikawa suggested, it is important, if possible, to visit patients in their own environment at least once to better understand how different perceptions evolve based on these fundamental aspects of our lives. Whether a patient has never interfaced with a medical establishment or visits them frequently, a surgeon's understanding of that patient's journey will enhance their ability to deliver patient-centered care, including quelling any fear or anxiety they may experience when confronted by an operating room filled with bright lights, flashing monitors, and a group of masked strangers.

Reach Your Objectives

When engaging in academic clinical partnerships, host and visiting faculty have to be clear about their goals, respectful of each other's needs, and diplomatic in their actions. The theme of "How To" build surgical capacity in resource-limited environments permeates the first half of this book. We hope this can serve as a guide for bidirectional partnership participants who are formulating their own targeted goals. Topics include "How to" efficiently and effectively organize new services and facilities, recruit and train faculty, staff, trainees, and students, and organize teams and quality improvement efforts. We also include chapters on "How To" function ethically in unfamiliar cultural environments with the support of the hospital and many other involved agencies. As is emphasized in several chapters, all activities should be done in concert with approval of the host hospital, the regional administration, and in some instances the Ministry of Health. We also review considerations for obtaining funding, gaining approval and support from the local community, and building cooperation with professional staff consisting of local doctors, nurses, technicians, and hospital administrators. We emphasize that independent and non-approved actions are not looked upon kindly, and frequently not forgiven; therefore, visitors must always tread gently and wisely.

Learn, Teach, and Serve with the Humility to Listen, Learn, and Grow

District (also called first-level, first-referral, or rural) hospitals are charged with providing essential general medical and surgical care, whereas higher-level hospitals offer increasingly specialized and complex services. Surgical educators in district hospitals area are therefore primarily concerned with teaching basic surgical skills for the treatment of common problems requiring the so-called Bellwether procedures (laparotomy, cesarean section, fracture fixation, trauma resuscitation and stabilization). This book addresses urgent and emergent problems that a general surgeon working in a district hospital must learn to manage, with a focus on pathologies seen more commonly in LMICs than in HICs (e.g., typhoid bowel perforations and extrapulmonary tuberculosis). We also highlight pathologies seen when diagnosis is delayed or neglected (e.g., breast malignancies and thyroid masses) and surgical approaches for these problems when resources are limited.

Surgical faculty and trainees participating in bidirectional partnerships have a unique opportunity to engage in a collaborative exchange of cultural beliefs, medical knowledge, and technical skills. With this in mind, we review "How To" concepts underlying educational techniques (Chaps. 15–20 in the Education section)), and we also describe experiences with building surgical capacity beyond the district level to regional care coordination and highly specialized care such as transplant surgery (Chaps. 4–13 in the Systems Strengthening section). Expansion of surgical specialty care in LMICs has historically met resistance as a consequence of limited or absent local expertise and of insufficient funding. We hope to inspire innovation with approaches to surgical training and with the recognition that investment in surgical capacity enhances population health and prosperity.

Support and Interactions

Health care around the world has long come from multiple sources guided both by community and religious traditions as well as resource availability. Many LMICs perceived to be in greatest need have been visited by missionaries and non-governmental organizations (NGOs) which made meaningful contributions. In 2015, the World Health Organization (WHO) formally resolved to strengthen essential surgical care worldwide, and the Lancet Commission and World Bank attempted to quantify the level of need. This enthusiasm has been accompanied by rapidly growing interest among professional medical societies such as the American College of Surgeons (ACS) and HIC academic medical centers and surgical training programs, which in many instances have expanded relationships created by retired or senior academic surgeons. In these instances, HIC surgeons rotate to their partner sites occasionally with trainees in tow and then try to facilitate commensurate rotations of partner surgeons to their home institutions for true bidirectional benefit. However, these relationships remain relatively uncoordinated and insufficiently focused and funded. Formal academic linking with LMICs remains very much in its nascency and should be encouraged and cultivated.

The call for closer interaction between wealthy medical institutions and LMICs to expand surgical training becomes obvious when considering that more than 5 billion of the world's 7.9 billion people live in poverty in LMICs [5], and a large portion of the global burden of disease is concentrated in LMICs. Surgical conditions precipitate the majority of the world's disability-adjusted life years (DALYs) [6, 7, 11], yet only 3.5% of the world's surgical procedures are performed in LMICs, which spend less than $100 per person on health care annually [7]. As of 2018, there were only 0.53 surgeons per 100,000 population in Sub-Saharan Africa [11] as compared to 5.2/100,000 surgeons in the United States in 2019 [8, 9]. According to a systematic analysis of the 2010 global burden of disease, 21% of the injury burden calculated in LMICs (52.3 million DALYs) could have been averted by the presence of basic surgical care [6]. Furthermore, according to the Lancet Commission in 2015, approximately 30% of the global burden of disease could be treated with surgical care. This translates not only to impaired welfare of millions of individuals, but also to stunted economic development of entire communities if not nations [10]. These numbers likely significantly underestimate common curable surgical diseases that remain poorly measured, including biliary disease, hernias, ulcers, appendicitis, correctible congenital anomalies, and cancers. In comparison to the attention given to communicable diseases such as HIV/AIDS, malaria, and TB, the relative dearth of accurate data regarding surgical needs (addressed in Chap. 8 and others) and the errant belief that surgery is prohibitively expensive have hindered progress in the development of adequate surgical care for underserved communities. As we have learned all too well from the COVID pandemic, disparity in access to health care is pervasive and may be equally poorly quantified in both LMICs and in HICs. Partnerships between HICs and LMICs at an academic level offer a major opportunity to systematically quantify these problems and help formulate and implement effective global solutions.

Specific Surgical Interventions

In addition to its "How To" segments, this book provides guidance on a variety of surgical pathologies and treatments with which a general surgeon should become familiar and be able to apply when a specialist is not available. We aim to complement material that can be readily found in standard surgical texts which largely focus on problems encountered in HICs. The surgical pathologies seen in LMICs often differ significantly from those most commonly seen in HICs as a consequence of variations in infectious disease prevalence, environmental exposures, physical access to medical care, and attitudes toward Western medicine. These differences commonly include presentation of significantly advanced disease or precipitate an entirely different set of differential diagnoses. For example, a patient with an untended traumatic open fracture may present with near-fatal systemic infection. A pediatric patient might present with a brain mass due to Echinococcus, whereas the same lesion in an HIC would more likely be a tumor. Abdominal distention in an adult male in Kenya might be more likely the result of volvulus or bezoar than the adhesions more commonly seen in HIC patients. Nevertheless, the diagnosis and management of all of these problems should be familiar to all general surgeons, including those in training.

We provide tools to manage many, but not all, urgent and emergent surgical situations in general surgery as well as in Orthopedics (Chap. 36), Urology (Chap. 38), Obstetrics and Gynecology (Chap. 37), and Neurosurgery (Chap. 21). We address pathologies encountered as a consequence of delayed diagnosis, such as advanced breast cancer (Chap. 29), and opportunities to institute cancer surveillance methods like colonoscopy (Chap. 26). We review approaches to standard surgical problems including abdominal catastrophe (Chaps. 25–27), hernia (Chap. 28), burns (Chap. 30 and 31), and wounds and soft tissue infections (Chap. 32 and 33), all with emphasis on conditions more common to LMICs.

Surgical and Anesthesia Program Initiatives

Most of the authors of the various chapters have been selected on the basis of their extensive experience working either as volunteers or as permanent staff in LMIC hospitals on several continents and in many countries. Several American surgeons have helped to organize significant initiatives in LMICs, such as Pan African Surgical Residency Programs (Haisch, C), Neurosurgical Pediatric Spina-Bifida and Hydrocephalus Programs (Koning, M), Renal Transplantation Program (Punch, J), Facing Africa Program (Lawrence & colleagues), and institutional exchange programs (Hardy, MA). Others have had input through national or international agencies such as WHO (Park, KB), Pan African Congress (Oluwole, S), or American College of Surgeons-College of Surgeons of East, Central and Southern Africa (ACS-COSESCA) Surgical Training Collaborative (Hochman, B).

Additional Challenges

Surgical knowledge and training are only small parts of the greater mission to achieve equitable and sustainable access to surgical care. Operating rooms in LMICs face challenges of inconsistent utilities (e.g., electricity and running water) and limited critical supplies (e.g., ventilators and oxygen) in addition to personnel deficits from anesthesiologists to operating room nurses to biomedical specialists. The barriers that prevent patients from arriving to the hospital such as roads and transportation compound the above limitations found in many LMIC. Many potential patients have a poor understanding of illness and medicine, many are limited by the prohibitive costs relative to their income, and yet others have no means of transportation or face threats to their own security en route. Precise quantification of surgical burden, resource need, and barriers to access are all processes that HIC partners might help facilitate. Clarity with these variables is a powerful tool in compelling local, national, and international authorities and funding sources to allocate support toward surgical care. Investment in surgical infrastructure elevates all aspects of health care systems. As Dr. Farmer previously said, "global health need not be a competitive race for scarce resources…we can build a coherent movement that comes to include surgery" [11, 12].

References

1. Meara JG, McClain CD, Mooney DP, Rogers SO Jr, editors. Global surgery and anesthesia manual: providing care in resource- limited settings. Boca Raton-London-New York: CRC Press; 2015.
2. Swaroop M, Krishnaswami S, editors. Academic global surgery, Series in academic surgery. Cham: Springer; 2016.
3. Park A, Price R, editors. Global surgery: the essentials. Cham: Springer; 2017.
4. Personnal Communication - Dr. Francis Moore -1976.
5. Organisation for Economic Co-operation and Development (OECD) 2022. https://www.investopedia.com/terms/o/oecd.asp
6. Higashi H, Barendregt JJ, Kassebaum NJ, Weiser TG, Bickler SW, Vos T. Burden of injuries avertable by a basic surgical package in low- and middle-income regions: a systematic analysis from the Global Burden of Disease 2010 Study. World J Surg. 2015; 39(1):1–9.
7. Haagsma JA, Graetz N, Bolliger I, et al. The global burden of injury: incidence, mortality, disability-adjusted life years and time trends from the Global Burden of Disease study 2013. Inj Prev. 2016;22(1):3–18.
8. https://familymedicine.uw.edu
9. https://bulletin.facs.org/2018
10. Meara JG, et al. Global surgery 2030: evidence and solutions for achieving health, welfare, and economic development. Lancet. 2015;386(9993):P569–624.
11. Farmer PE, Kim JM. Surgery and global health: a view from beyond the OR. World J Surg. 2008;32(4): 533–6.
12. Bae JY, Groen RS, Kushner AL. Surgery as a public health intervention: common misconceptions versus the truth. Bull World Health Organ. 2011;89(6):394.

Part I

System Strengthening

2 How to Prepare for Short- or Long-Term Surgical Practice in Low- and Middle-Income Countries

Mark A. Hardy, Brian A. Chang, Richard M. Smiley, Richard K. Raker, and Beth R. Hochman

A teacher affects eternity. He can never tell where his influence stops.

– Henry Adams

Abbreviations

ABS	American Board of Surgery
ACGME	Accreditation Council on Graduate Medical Education.
GME	Graduate Medical Education.
LMIC	Low- and Middle-Income Country.
PD	Program Director.
PDT	Pre-departure Training.
RCS	Royal College of Surgeons.
RRC-S	Residency Review Committee for Surgery.
WACS	West African College of Surgeons.

Scope of Medical Trainee or Practitioner in Global Health Involvement

Interest and participation in global health opportunities has increased among surgical residents, medical students, and other fully-trained health care clinicians from high-income areas. These opportunities are primarily in "underserved" countries, frequently referred to as low- and middle-income countries (LMICs). As is well known these vary significantly by their economic profiles, health and training systems, and even by their locations, especially urban as compared to rural. Even in developed countries, such as the USA, there are underserved areas, such as many Indian reservations or in countries where some district hospitals are well staffed and equipped because of provincial or political support while

M. A. Hardy (✉)
Department of Surgery, Columbia University Vagelos College of Physician and Surgeons, New York, NY, USA
e-mail: mah1@columbia.edu

B. A. Chang
Department of Anesthesia, Columbia Medical Center, NY Presbyterian Hospital, New York, NY, USA
e-mail: bac9046@nyp.org

R. M. Smiley · R. K. Raker
Department of Anesthesia, Columbia University Vagelos College of Physicians and Surgeons, New York, NY, USA
e-mail: rms7@cumc.columbia.edu; rkr1@cumc.columbia.edu

B. R. Hochman
Department of Surgery, Columbia University Vagelos College of Physicians and Surgeons, Milstein Hospital, New York, NY, USA
e-mail: brh2106@cumc.columbia.edu

M. A. Hardy, B. R. Hochman (eds.), *Global Surgery*, https://doi.org/10.1007/978-3-031-28127-3_2

others may be given inadequate budgets by the Ministry of Health. Numerous general surgery residency programs have established collaborative efforts with partner institutions in LMICs. Many clinical specialists such as anesthesiologists, plastic surgeons, otolaryngologists, or ophthalmologists provide their services in LMICs as teams which address specific health problems. This is best illustrated by the Team Face Africa described in Chaps. 34–40 specializing in reconstruction of the face for Nona. There are also other teams that specialize in cleft palate repairs, cardiac surgery, cataract and glaucoma operations, and other interventions. An anonymous survey of incoming interns revealed that >75% were interested in participating in medical mission trips, and approximately two-thirds of them were interested in incorporating global health into their long-term careers [1]. Specifically, interest and participation in global surgical programs has increased over the past two decades, as has their availability. The need for global surgery has become emphasized and more obvious [2]. This increase in interest has led to a rapid rise in the number of global health opportunities worldwide. They are now offered through numerous medical schools and residency training programs. Over the last two decades, the proportion of US medical schools offering global health opportunities has tripled [3]. More than half of both medical and surgical residency training programs offer residents the opportunities to participate either in short mission trips or in dedicated global health tracks which offer specific short (4–8 weeks) rotations, or some other intervals of several months [3–6]. These may or may not be recognized by the American Board of Surgery (ABS) depending on the degree of direct supervision and the accreditation of the foreign institution and its surgical staff as accredited trainers by the Residency Review Committee for Surgery (RRC-S). Junior and recently retired surgical faculty are major volunteers who frequently participate in LMICs on rotations from 1 to 6 months, and rarely longer. There are many reasons why individuals decide to participate in global health experiences. These include the desire to improve access to health care in low-resource settings, to improve medical knowledge or language skills), or to experience new destinations and culture [4–7]. The types and duration of global health experiences are just as heterogeneous as the reasons for participation. Some senior volunteers participate in trips where they are responsible for setting up temporary clinics and providing medical supplies. Others may engage in needs-based assessments, or develop educational instruction workshops that improve emergency care or other specialties, for example, chest tube insertions in Ethiopia, or insertion of stents for obstruction by esophageal cancer in Malawi.

The involvement of trainee and faculty volunteers has led to a call for "pre-departure" training and orientation programs. Opportunities for international volunteer work are widely available for the interested practicing or retired surgeons, surgical residents or students [3]. https://www-sciencedirect-com.ezproxy.cul.columbia.edu/science/article/pii/S0039606012000980?via%3Dihub - bib4. Adequate preparation for their experiences and responsibilities in an unfamiliar clinical and cultural environment prior to such educational visits is critical to achieve the greatest effectiveness and benefit for both the host institution and the visiting staff. This applies to both the teaching and learning efforts of all the involved individual professionals, as well as patients. Based on our own experiences in working in LMICs, we have prepared a practical guide for residents and students to adequately prepare them for such international surgical rotations [8]. Although little has been written about the need for preparation of fully-trained clinicians and health care staff, the need for rational and thorough preparation is not unique to medical students and resident trainees [8, 9].

Recognition of common problems due to lack of adequate pre-departure training (PDT) has led to a number of studies which focused on various methods to improve PTD, mostly for medical students or resident physicians, since these groups are most amenable/available for organized training [8–16]. A general consensus on topics that should be addressed has been

Table 2.1 Core themes for pre-departure training/preparation

Theme	Recommendation
Trainee specific	
Personal health and safety	• Review site-specific recommendations for vaccination and antimicrobial prophylaxis. • **Ensure health insurance/evacuation plan.** • Identify site-specific safety risks. • Emergency contact information. • Plan for who to contact and where to go in case of an emergency/need for personal medical care.
Emotional wellness	• Consider risk of "culture shock" and "reverse culture shock".
Communication	• Learn (when possible) appropriate language skills (i.e., host institution's native language and unspoken forms of communication). • Identify members of the host community to serve as liaisons between volunteers and members of the community.
Personal development	• Reflect on personal motivations for participating in global health experience. • Consider and clarify goals and expectations of both the volunteer and host institution.
Cultural competency	• Learn about local culture and customs, especially how it impacts the host community's interaction with the health care system. • Cultural humility.
Ethical considerations	• Discuss culturally appropriate communication techniques to navigate difficult situations. • Reflect on volunteer role and level of training; only engage in appropriate tasks. • Emphasize the importance of upholding same standards of care and ethics that trainees maintain at home institution (the issue of "standard of care" is a complex area that is hard to define in one sentence).
Program-specific logistics	• Identify licensure and other legal document requirements necessary for practice/taining/teaching in programs at host country/institution. • Encourage bidirectional communication prior to departure to ensure similar expectation between trainee and host institution. • Ensure appropriate supervision of trainees.

developed, and they should be applicable with some modifications, for any physician contemplating a global project [12–18]. In 2008, the Association of Faculties of Medicine of Canada published guidelines for PDT programs, which included the following domains: personal health, travel safety, cultural awareness, language competencies, and ethical considerations [17]. Since then, several studies have expanded these initial guidelines to provide a more encompassing outline of the topics that should be covered during PDT programs [5, 18–21]. These recommendations are summarized in Table 2.1. The following which has been previously published by one of us (MAH) [8] is partially based on a brief practical guide for visitors to prepare for a surgical visit, elective rotation, or mission to an underserved region.

Preparations

The first task is to **determine why, where, and for how long one can go**. This will obviously depend on the schedule, support, level of training and expertise and the need for visitor(s) as contributor, teacher, organizer, or administrator following an invitation by the host institution. The other important factors to consider are the age and obligations of the visitors and the stability of political situation in the host country. To enjoy and succeed in an international rotation/elective one has to define one's goals and objectives. Among many objectives is to see, examine, and treat a variety of cases new to the visitor, depending on the region's epidemiology. Surgical rotations tend to be more time-demanding than others. There are many cultural and language barriers, simple housing, usually without air-conditioning and sometimes no fan in the hot climates, but usually with an electric heater in cold climates. It is critical to keep an open mind and remember that as guests, the visitors ought to act graciously and not be a burden to the host hospitals and their staff.

Goals and objectives must be continually reevaluated according to the situation. There may be a smaller number of operations than expected if there is a shortage of supplies or personnel. It is judicious to bring gloves, masks, caps, scrub suits, coats, and some sutures if one can, regardless of the role that one may play. No matter what the difficulties with accreditation may be, it is important to realize at the outset that the role of an observer, rather than as a responsible physician, may be more appropriate and equally valuable for a resident or a student.

Where one wants to go is partially dictated by language abilities, cultural interests, degree of hardship one wishes to tolerate, and most importantly, the surgical or medical experience and the degree of collaboration and/or supervision that is available. The tendency to group LMICs together is misleading and the term "underserved areas" may be more appropriate. Various countries have vastly different economic profiles, health systems, and opportunities for service. Because of such striking differences among hospitals, especially those in major urban areas as compared to the district hospitals in the rural areas, first-hand accounts from previous volunteers are very helpful in choosing a site for the rotation. The host facility can provide the student/resident/attending with details on the regional safety and the epidemiology of diseases in the region, and may provide details on specialized medical skills and knowledge that is required. Others who have foreign contacts can also provide helpful information. It may be a chairman, a colleague, a senior resident, or someone that one meets at a convention. Having a close acquaintance in the host country can provide comfort and safety to the visitor. Organizations such as Surgeons OverSeas (SOS) [22], Operation Giving Back of the American College of Surgeons [23], and Global Pediatric Surgery Network [24] have facility databases that include pertinent information about each hospital or facility, such as case mix, volume, available supervision, and travel information. Information sharing with residents from other institutions who have had experience in the desired area should also be used.

The duration of a surgical rotation in an underserved region must provide enough time to gain benefit from the visit and to be tolerated, if needed, by the volunteer's partner. In addition, permissions are required from the Host Institution, visitor's PD, and from the Director of Institutional Graduate Medical Education (GME) office. Adequacy of funding will also influence the length of the rotation. The longer the rotation, the greater the possible medical contribution to the host, and the greater the educational and cultural benefit to the volunteer. The longer rotations lead to more lasting and more effective relationships with the hospital personnel and administration. They also permit greater continuity of patient care. Repeat rotations to the same hospital are encouraged throughout the visitor's lifetime.

Implementation of formal PDT programs can be hindered by inadequate time for preparation and occasionally by lack of dedication to PDT by non-global health educators [19]. In non-academic training environments, where individuals themselves are primarily responsible for their own training, it may be difficult to replicate the programs of large academic institutions. In the absence of a formal PTD program, there are many resources that can assist in the preparation of volunteers for their global health experiences. For instance, the United States State Department website (www.travel.state.gov) contains information regarding potential safety concerns in the host country. Similarly, the Centers for Disease Control and Prevention website (www.cdc.gov) provides recommendations regarding vaccinations and antimicrobial prophylaxis. The Consortium of Universities for Global Health also offers an open-source "Global Health Competencies Toolkit", which can serve as a reference for developing one's own pre-departure curricula (https://www.cugh.org/online-tools/competencies-toolkit/). There are also a number of medical societies that provide resources to help prepare for global health experiences. These include the following: 1) Society for Education in Anesthesia (www.seahq.org); 2) American Society of Anesthesiologists (https://www.asahq.org/charity); Canadian Anesthesiologists" Society International Education Foundation (https://casief.ca/); American College of Surgeons (https://www.facs.org/ogb); Lancet Commission on Global Surgery (https://www.lancetglobalsurgery.org/); World Health Organization (https://www.who.int/teams/integrated-health-services/patient-safety/research/safe-surgery); United States State Department website (www.travel.state.gov); Centers for Disease Control and Prevention website (www.cdc.gov); The Consortium of Universities for Global Health also offers an open source "Global Health Competencies Toolkit" (https://www.cugh.org/onlinetools/competencies-toolkit/).

Consultation and approval of the rotation by one's family, professional partners, department chairman and division chief, program director or medical student advisor are essential. The host facility almost always requires written confirmation of medical qualifications from the visitor's hospital or institution. There are many other requirements, depending on the site, regarding licensing and permits in some cases, travel arrangements, and establishment of contacts at the host institution to devise a specific plan for the rotation. The required documents usually need to be obtained at least 6 months in advance to permit appropriate processing at both the host's and visitor's sites. Funding which may be possible through medical schools, home hospitals or institutions, or local surgical societies and various foundations, also requires adequate advanced time for applications. Without funding, it may be necessary for the volunteers to take either unpaid leave or use their vacation times. Malpractice insurance coverage is essential and should be carried by the individual through their sponsoring institution.

To determine which items to bring along is part of the preparation. These include personal items appropriate for the climate and seasonal conditions. Appropriate clothes for rainy, cold, or hot seasons should follow cultural and medical indications for some clothes (e.g., long pants and long-sleeved shirts to decrease mosquito bites and to follow cultural mores, especially for women, while thick-soled shoes may be needed where snakes are found). Other items include personal medical equipment, some of which may be left behind, such as a portable Doppler, camping forehead battery-powered light to be used when the electricity and the generator fail, and any other items that are needed and may be left behind such as gloves, caps, medical coats for personal use, and vascular grafts, meshes, or even a donated portable ultrasound machine, if possible. Some of these items may be subject to import fees if declared as donations (the hospital may help to bypass the customs fees). They may be brought in as personal items and then "forgotten" at departure. A detailed list of necessary items to bring is available on the Surgeons OverSeas (SOS) website (http://www.surgeonsoverseas.org) under the "Resources" section. After consulting with your hosts, bring only OR equipment that has been requested or that is absolutely needed to perform specialized operations by the visiting faculty. Customs regulations are generally very strict, and advice should be sought from host institution before importing any major medical equipment, or even minor supplies. They have experience in facilitating entry of imported equipment at the lowest cost possible.

To be a smart traveler arrange visas, vaccinations, flight arrangements, living, and travel arrangements as soon as rotation plans are solidified. Some countries may require work visas and registry as a doctor which may be a prolonged process. Flight arrangements to remote locations may also require careful planning in both directions, depending on seasons. Attention to clean food and potable water (even if it has to be boiled) is critical to one's health. Living quarters, whether provided by the host hospital or a hotel, need to be protected from mosquitoes (netting and other antimalarial precautions). Windows and shutters, and a working fan in tropical climates or heater or radiator in cold climates (as in the high mountains) may be necessary. Select a comfortable season (e.g., avoid monsoons or winter in the

Himalayas). Places that are unstable or war zones are not suitable for visiting rotations. At times of local climate disasters such as aftermath of an earthquake or a tsunami, communicate with local experts on whether volunteers are needed and what precautions should be taken before offering one's services. It is wise to notify your embassy or consulate of your arrival in the country and of your location in cases of emergency (check the respective embassy's website). Provide information about local contact who has some degree of responsibility for you. It is highly recommended to keep a list of important local addresses and telephone numbers and to be familiar with a reliable evacuation route to safety, such as the embassy or consulate. Safety for oneself must remain the top priority.

Take care of your own health. It is wise to have a full medical examination with a chest X-ray, EKG, full laboratory workup, including tests and up-to-date vaccinations for major viral infections and for TB. This can serve as a baseline for any problems that may be discovered during or after the rotation. One's health is of concern not only to the volunteer but also to his colleagues, both local and visiting. Doctor's records, X-rays, EKGs, and latest laboratory data should accompany the visitor and be available for comparison if need arises. Tentative plans for evacuation to more modern or home hospital (with appropriate travel insurance) should be available if a major emergency arises that requires transfer to the nearest specialty hospital. Simple medications, such as oral rehydration solutions and anti-diarrhea medications, can reduce downtime should the volunteer fall ill. Anti-allergy medications and antibiotics, including epinephrine and steroids, should also be brought. Be aware that any pre-existing medical conditions might worsen in a different climate and with a different diet.

The Visitor's Role at the Host Facility

Interaction with Administration is critical for everyone's satisfaction. It is important to adhere to the local chain of command and not try to take shortcuts to achieve goals regardless of whether one is a senior surgeon or a junior medical student. The chain of command usually begins with the CEO of the hospital, but special requests may occasionally require approval of the regional or national Ministry of Health. If this rule is not followed not only may new projects or initiatives be stopped, but the initiator may be asked to leave the institution and not return. There are really no legal or public appeals where such decisions may be reversed. Independent initiatives by visiting faculty or by residents, without the consent by the administrative host hospital, are not only frowned upon but may lead to disciplinary actions. The role of partially trained personnel, such as surgical residents and medical students on surgical rotations or elective trips, is variable and frequently initially ill-defined. This may lead to misunderstandings which must be avoided as much as possible and corrected promptly when they occur.

Work within the local system(s) and protocols since it is important to maintain the local chain of command into which the visitors must fit and adjust themselves. This includes absolute discretion regarding the use of social media to express experiences with the patients or with the hospital, as well as criticisms of the staff, ORs, procedures, or protocols. Most improvements and corrections can be achieved if presented in collaboration with the local practitioners and approved by the senior administrators. Any press releases about innovations must be initiated by the local administrators and NOT by the visitors. Long-term changes or innovations are not likely to succeed unless they were developed and introduced in collaboration with the local staff and, most importantly, approved and introduced by the local administrators, frequently with the recommendation of the Minister of Health or his/her deputies.

Availability of Supervision

Assurance that adequate clinical supervision is available is a frequent issue regarding operative procedures performed by residents. Visiting residents should have an accredited local or visiting surgical attending within short walking distance to the operating room where the senior resident may be operating alone (junior residents should rarely be permitted to operate alone and only on appropriate cases for their level of training). It is prudent that the attending surgeon (either visiting or host) be present in the operating room for the critical parts of any major operation (both decision and technical aspects). In 2011, the American Board of Surgery (ABS) and the Residency Review Committee for Surgery (RRC-S) of the Accreditation Council on Graduate Medical Education (ACGME) approved international elective experiences for credit toward graduation requirements, under strict guidelines [25] https://www-sciencedirect-com.ezproxy.cul.columbia.edu/science/article/pii/S0039606012000980?via%3Dihub - bib11). RRC-S has determined a set of eligibility criteria to ensure that surgical residents benefit maximally from an international rotation's education potential. Although the idea of performing at a more complex level than they have been trained may seem to the residents to be very attractive, it raises serious ethical and legal issues and must be discouraged if adequate clinical supervision is not available. The popular concept that "some surgery, however inexpert, is better than none" is erroneous. To perform the surgical procedures correctly the first time and avoid a higher rate of iatrogenic morbidity and/or mortality is most important in LMICs, as it is everywhere. It is important not to place an unnecessary burden on an already stressed resource-poor health care system. To avoid and/or prevent any harm to patients it has now become a requirement from the RRC to have a faculty member on site during the international rotation before it can be approved [25]. It is best for both patients and resident/students that the supervisors be officially accredited as trained surgeons (by American, European, British, or African surgical boards), or may even be local experienced surgical practitioners. Prior to choosing a rotation, it is essential first to determine the type of hospital, the expected surgery to be encountered, the volume of surgery, and most importantly, to identify the level and quality of surgical and medical supervision that is available.

Remember that local training programs take priority. It must be clearly understood that local trainees have priority, if qualified, to perform elective and emergency surgical procedures under supervision of visiting or local faculty. The visiting trainee's learning opportunities should never supersede that of the local trainees. Collaborators on research project should include local staff and they should be included in designing and executing the project. Eventually, they should be included as co-authors on submitted manuscripts.

Record Keeping

Maintain a surgical case log (end of each day) despite the fact that in most instances the resident will NOT get credit for the rotation from the RRC-S unless all the conditions are fulfilled by the resident's program prior to the rotation (especially continuous supervision by Board certified surgeons (ABS, RCS, WACS) and many other conditions). Keeping a log is important for your own personal use and for teaching purposes, as well as recruitment of faculty and residents in the future. With the recently approved guidelines for implementation of international rotations by the ABS and RRC-S [26], the accreditation process will be evolving and developing in the coming years. At present, it is important to determine the status of the RRC-S regulations in regard to the visitor's institution and host institution, as well as the degree of accreditation of the supervising faculty. International rotation for residents and faculty should serve to broaden their clinical knowledge and improve their skills to make diagnoses with hands, eyes, and brain, at least as well, or perhaps even better and faster, than with the radiographic equipment and laboratory tests which may likely be unavailable. To maintain a diary of cases and experiences serves not only as a specific reminder of the rotations for many years, but may serve as a basis for reports, articles, and as teaching tools for future trainees. The diary should also include photographs for which consent has been obtained, so that they can be used ethically and legally in future publications. In keeping diaries and records of the visit, it is imperative to avoid any public discussion on social media of any details of the medical aspects of the hospital or its staff and administration. Regardless of whether the comments may be positive or negative, they may be misinterpreted by the readers with serious negative consequences for the visitor and discontinuation of future rotations. Communication with others regarding the rotation must be respectful and restricted only to facts with avoidance of speculations, personal opinions about staff, or criticisms.

Consider opportunities for using/establishing blogs or mass e-mail. This has to be done with great care and adherence to patient rights to privacy. Commentaries about staff or institutions, other than flattering, are not welcome by the host institutions and countries. Adverse comments may lead to dissolution of relations, as has happened previously. It is wisest to avoid any professional communications with colleagues via blogs or mass e-mails.

Activities after your return. The main goal is to encourage others to volunteer or elect similar experiences and service to the underserved. This may take the form of lectures to staff, informal discussions with colleagues, and formation of clubs or groups to encourage this type of volunteerism. Efforts should be directed to raise funds, collect professional books, and obtain surgical instruments and monitoring equipment that may be surplus or no longer needed from the hospitals and then ship it to your previous host, if it is needed and requested. One should try to maintain contacts with colleagues at host institution after thanking them appropriately soon after return to home institution. All joint publications should include a member of host staff as a co-author.

Continue communication with hosts after your experience. This is easily accomplished by e-mail or telephone. It should be maintained at scientific meetings and at any available social interactions. If at all possible financially, it is very desirable to invite the host staff members for a rotation at your hospital, even as an observer, if accreditation rules forbid anything else for medico-legal reasons. Continuous contact with the staff of the host institution will facilitate future rotations of residents, students, and faculty to the same institution.

Provide a written summary to your sponsor(s). This record is important when archived confidentially as a source of detailed information for future volunteers. This summary should comment about the staff, type of patients, available resources, living conditions, cultural environment, obstacles encountered, and other pertinent observations. These details need to remain confidential in the Residency Program Director's (PD) office and be available only on a "need to know" basis. Such material may be very useful for a future volunteer as he/she chooses a site for a rotation [25].

Volunteer as an advisor to residents and students who wish to follow. This may be accomplished via PD or Dean of Students if a distinct Global Surgery Program is not yet established. If a distinct Program exists, its leader and its members may be the best source of information for future candidates. We have highlighted a list of suggestions that are by no means complete, and are meant to be only a practical guide to a safe and productive experience. Adequate preparation for an international surgical rotation is vital to its success, its benefits to the participants, to the host institution, and to the development of meaningful and fruitful exchanges among surgeons from different backgrounds. Such exchanges will benefit patients in both the visitors' and hosts' nations.

Impact of Global Health Experiences

Volunteer-Trainee Perspective

Many studies have evaluated the impact of these experiences on volunteers and trainees and their respective host institutions. Some have reported benefits of these experiences, such as improved medical knowledge and clinical skills, exposure to a wider spectrum and stages of illnesses, increased awareness of social determinants of health, and improved understanding of cultural competencies and health care disparities.

Table 2.2 Risks and benefits of global health experiences

Medical Volunteer Perspective		Host Institution Perspective	
Benefits	Risks	Benefits	Risks
• Medical knowledge. • Communication skills. • Learn about provision of health care in low-resource settings. • Increased cultural awareness. • Provide motivation to practice in underserved communities (for trainees). Personal satisfaction.	• Exposure to health and safety dangers. • "Culture shock"/ homesickness • Exposure to ethical dilemmas. • Exposure to poor clinical outcomes. • Inability to communicate with practitioners and patients.	• Establishment of bidirectional learning opportunities. • Collaboration in academic pursuits. • Access to resources (i.e., funding and medical supplies. • Access to health care services, otherwise unavailable.	• Lack of mutual benefit. • Lack of sustainability of interventions. • Inadequate follow-up. • Increased burden of work in an already overburdened system. • Trainees practicing above level of training. • Cultural insensitivity. • Perceived devaluation of host institution/ country practitioners.

Occasionally these experiences have long-term impacts on the practice of volunteers after their return home [3, 9–11]. Additionally, in some cases, these experiences have motivated health care personnel to pursue careers which focus on LMICs [10]. However, PDT can put participants at risk (Table 2.2). Lack of knowledge regarding emergency contacts, necessary vaccinations, or prophylactic medications can put volunteers' personal health and safety at risk [12]. There are also numerous anecdotes of culturally incompetent volunteers encountering ethical dilemmas that result in inappropriate or damaging interactions with the host hospital staff, patient-doctor relationships, poorer patient outcomes, and unpleasant experiences [12, 14]. Again, while much of this literature concerns trainees embarking on short-term projects, most of the issues and problems are just as relevant to the seasoned practitioner as he/she heads off to an unfamiliar environment.

For surgical or anesthesia missions, the types of "preparation", described in detail above, can be classified as "clinical" and "personal". The "clinical" preparation involves ensuring that the appropriate equipment and surgical, nursing, and anesthesia skills and personnel are adequate at the host institution. It is also critical to ensure that the other necessary resources are available (water, light, oxygen, medications, ORs, and tables) to avoid major limitations. The "personal" preparation should include familiarity with the culture (and potentially the geography) of the foreign site and how these may affect the visitor's behavior or safety. The visitor must also have full understanding of the scope and limitations of the mission. Attention to appropriate personal medical matters (e.g., vaccines, malaria prevention, anti-diarrhea medication, post-exposure HIV prophylaxis strategy, and other necessary medications) and to desirable or required documents (health insurance, proper travel documents, licenses, etc.) is also crucial to success. When the mission is sponsored by a large international agency many of these issues are settled during formal orientation sessions or informational documents and e-mails, including checklists. For those traveling alone or with smaller organizations, these issues require careful thought and early individual attention.

Host Institution Perspective

The impact of the visitors' experiences on the local host institutions is variable and depends on the individual or group mission (e.g., direct care, teaching, joining a locally established team, or various combinations of these functions) as well as on the preparation and resultant performance and behaviors of the individuals involved. Inadequately prepared volunteers may (usually inadvertently) devalue local providers' performance (sometimes, only as a perception), alter continuity of services, promote a post-colonial narrative, and manage patients inappropriately due to lack of cultural competence [3, 8–10]. Such inappropriate interactions can overtax the host institution's infrastructure and may put patients at an increased risk for adverse outcomes [16] (Table 2.2). In the best case scenario, global health rotations and visits can lead to prolonged academic collaboration, the establishment of bidirectional educational opportunities, long-term sustainable partnerships, and improvement in patient care and local resources [15].

In summary, as has been learned in the assessment of clinical adverse events, debriefing following a visit is also both important and very useful. Post-trip reflection allows for individuals to gain a better understanding of themselves and their experiences [2, 27, 28]. It may of course provide feedback for institutions and organizations in their planning of future missions [21]. Reflection may also permit analysis of previously encountered distressing situations and outcomes which will lead to avoidance of future discouragement. The entire team, including members of the host institution, should participate in an analysis of the impact of a global health experience [18]. This bidirectional feedback can help improve partnerships between the visiting and host institutions and ensure that the relationships benefit both the hosts and the volunteers.

As the number of global health opportunities for volunteers, medical trainees, and clinicians continues to increase, it is important to develop more standardized PDT programs and following the visitors' return, implement more rigorous evaluations and debriefings to avoid repetition of problems and errors. Better-prepared volunteers and health care workers will be less likely to put themselves and members of the community they are serving at risk. Most importantly, they are more likely to provide appropriate services for the patients they will care for and improve the experience and long-term outcomes for themselves and the programs that they serve.

References

1. Birnberg JM, Lypson M, Anderson RA, Theodosis C, Kim J, Olopade OI, Arora VM. Incoming resident interest in global health: occasional travel versus a future career abroad? J Grad Med Educ. 2011;3:400–3.
2. Meara JG, Leather AJ, Hagander L, Alkire BC, Alonso N, Ameh EA, Bickler SW, Conteh L, Dare AJ, Davies J, Merisier ED, El-Halabi S, Farmer PE, Gawande A, Gillies R, Greenberg SL, Grimes CE, Gruen RL, Ismail EA, Kamara TB, Lavy C, Lundeg G, Mkandawire NC, Raykar NP, Riesel JN, Rodas E, Rose J, Roy N, Shrime MG, Sullivan R, Verguet S, Watters D, Weiser TG, Wilson IH, Yamey G, Yip W. Global Surgery 2030: evidence and solutions for achieving health, welfare, and economic development. Lancet. 2015;386:569–624.
3. Hau DK, Smart LR, DiPace JI, Peck RN. Global health training among U.S. residency specialties: a systematic literature review. Med Educ Online. 2017;22:1270020.
4. Kaeppler C, Holmberg P, Tam RP, Porada K, Stryker SD, Conway K, Schubert C, Medical Student Global Health Study Group. The impact of global health opportunities on residency selection. BMC Med Educ. 2021;21:384.
5. Chetta MD, Shakir A, Paek LS, Lee GK. Evaluating resident perspectives on international humanitarian missions. J Craniofac Surg. 2018;29:279–85.
6. Melby MK, Loh LC, Evert J, Prater C, Lin H, Khan OA. Beyond medical "missions" to impact-driven short-term experiences in Global Health (STEGHs): ethical principles to optimize community benefit and learner experience. Acad Med. 2016;91:633–8.
7. Vu MT, Johnson TR, Francois R, Simms-Cendan J. Sustained impact of short-term international medical mission trips: resident perspectives. Med Teach. 2014;36:1057–63.
8. Henry JA, Groen RS, Price RR, Nwomeh BC, Kingham TP, Hardy MA, Kushner AL. The benefits of international rotations to resource-limited sttings for U.S. surgery residents. Surgery. 2013;4:445–54.
9. Bessette J, Camden C. Pre-departure training for student Global Health experiences: a scoping review. Physiother Can. 2017;69:343–50.
10. Kaur G, Tabaie S, Brar J, Tangel V, Pryor KO. Global health education in United States anesthesiology residency programs: a survey of resident opportunities and program director attitudes. BMC Med Educ. 2017;17:215.
11. Prin M, Phelps J. International elective opportunities in United States anesthesia residency programs. J Educ Perioper Med. 2017;19:E613.
12. Imperato PJ, Bruno DM, Sweeney MM. Ensuring the health, safety and preparedness of U.S. Medical students participating in global health electives overseas. J Community Health. 2016;41:442–50.
13. Kung TH. Host physician perspectives to improve pre-departure training for global health electives. Med Educ. 2018;52:3–5.
14. Peluso MJ, Kallem S, Elansary M, Rabin TL. Ethical dilemmas during international clinical rotations in global health settings: findings from a training and debriefing program. Med Teach. 2018;40:53–61.

15. St Clair NE, Pitt MB, Bakeera-Kitaka S, McCall N, Lukolyo H, Arnold LD, Audcent T, Batra M, Chan K, Jacquet GA, Schutze GE, Butteris S, Global Health Task Force of the American Board of Pediatrics. Global health: preparation for working in resource-limited settings. Pediatrics. 2017;140
16. Ouma BD, Dimaras H. Views from the Global South: exploring how student volunteers from the Global North can achieve sustainable impact in global health. Glob Health. 2013;9:32.
17. Anderson KC, Slatnik MA, Pereira I, Cheung E, Xu K, Brewer TF. Are we there yet? Preparing Canadian medical students for global health electives. Acad Med. 2012;87:206–9.
18. Herbst de Cortina S, Arora G, Wells T, Hoffman RM. Evaluation of a structured predeparture orientation at the David Geffen School of Medicine's Global Health education programs. Am J Trop Med Hyg. 2016;94:563–7.
19. Anderson K, N. Bocking, Slatnik M, Pattani M, Breton J, Scaciragic L, Dhillon S. Preparing medical students for electives in low-resource settings: a template for national guidelines for pre-departure training. 2008.
20. Crump JA, Sugarman J, Working Group on Ethics Guidelines for Global Health Training. Ethics and best practice guidelines for training experiences in global health. Am J Trop Med Hyg. 2010;83:1178–82.
21. Purkey E, Hollaar G. Developing consensus for postgraduate global health electives: definitions, predeparture training and post-return debriefing. BMC Med Educ. 2016;16:159.
22. Surgeons OverSeas (SOS) web site; 2022. http://www.humanitariansurgery.org/
23. Operating Giving Back web site; 2022. http://www.operationgivingback.facs.org/
24. Global Pediatric Surgery Network web site; 2011. http://globalpediatricsurgery.org/
25. Residency Review Committee website. Criteria for approved international rotations; 2022. http://www.acgme.org/acWebsite/navPages/nav_440.asp
26. Mitchell KB, Tarpley MJ, Casey KM. Elective global surgery rotations for residentgs: a call for cooperation and consortium. World J Surg. 2011;35:2617–24.
27. Abedini NC, Gruppen LD, Kolars JC, Kumagai AK. Understanding the effects of short-term international service-learning trips on medical students. Acad Med. 2012;87:820–8.
28. Chang BA, Karin E, Davidson ZA, Ripp J, Soriano RP. Impact of a short-term domestic service-learning program on medical student education. Ann Glob Health. 2019:85.

How to Maintain Ethical Standards of Global Surgery Practice and Partnerships

3

Barnabas T. Alayande, Robert R. Riviello, and Abebe Bekele

The single story creates stereotypes, and the problem with stereotypes is not that they are untrue, but that they are incomplete. They make one story become the only story.

– Chimamanda Adichie

Abbreviations

HIC	High-Income Country
IRB	Institutional Review Board
LMIC	Low- and Middle-Income Country

Introduction

Global surgery is an area of study, research, practice, and advocacy that seeks to improve health outcomes and achieve health equity for all people who require surgical care, with a special emphasis on underserved populations and populations in crisis [1]. The Lancet Commission on Global Surgery estimated that 5 billion people lack access to affordable, available, adequate surgical care when needed. It is agreed that this burden tilts significantly towards low- and middle-income countries (LMICs), where over 148 million additional surgeries are needed annually to meet the global surgical need [2]. This special emphasis on underserved populations and LMICs, along with the often-colonial mindset that is associated with high-income surgical providers intervening in these contexts, many times raises a multifaceted ethical challenge. This challenge is compounded by the vulnerability of the sick and injured within an already vulnerable low-income system. Most interventions brought from a high-income country (HIC) setting comes with an intrinsic power dynamic-skin color,

B. T. Alayande (✉)
Center for Equity in Global Surgery, University of Global Health Equity, Kigali, Rwanda

Program in Global Surgery and Social Change, Harvard Medical School, Boston, MA, USA
e-mail: balayande@ughe.org

R. R. Riviello
Center for Equity in Global Surgery, University of Global Health Equity, Kigali, Rwanda

Program in Global Surgery and Social Change, Harvard Medical School, Boston, MA, USA

Center for Surgery and Public Health, Brigham and Women's Hospital, Boston, MA, USA

Department of Global Health and Social Medicine, Harvard Medical School, Boston, MA, USA
e-mail: riviello@post.harvard.edu

A. Bekele
Center for Equity in Global Surgery, University of Global Health Equity, Kigali, Rwanda

School of Medicine, Addis Ababa University, Addis Ababa, Ethiopia
e-mail: abekele@ughe.org

M. A. Hardy, B. R. Hochman (eds.), *Global Surgery*, https://doi.org/10.1007/978-3-031-28127-3_3

resource, educational advantage, exposure, institutional prestige, political power, passport and visa privilege, knowledge gradient, and money.

Ethics refers to the branch of moral philosophy concerned with the "manner people should act in a knowledge context, based on what they know, ought to know, and should know and do." It is a "value-laden judgment about actions, the rules guiding the actions, and the appropriate choices of reasonable steps to take in a context" [3]. Surgical ethics have been defined as the application of ethics to situations specific to surgical practice, considering the peculiarity that surgery literally causes harm before healing, and that it is intrinsically characterized by intense accountability [4]. Four domains have been identified in the ethics of global surgery – ethics of clinical care, research, education, and collaborations [5]. Most ethical considerations in literature are, however, skewed toward ethics of clinical practice during short-term missions, and up to 80% of this literature is from HICs, specifically academic institutions in the United States, Canada, and the UK [5]. This raises ethical questions within the development of ethics for LMIC engagement, as the recipients of most global surgery engagements are not at the table to contribute to this important subject matter. Partnerships are key to effectively engaging the problems of surgical burden, insufficient manpower, inadequate surgical infrastructure, frail surgical systems, and inadequate surgical financing. While local surgical champions provide the context, often, they do not have adequate resources to address the very real problems they are steeped in. Ethical considerations of partnerships are therefore extremely important to global surgery ethics.

Colonialism refers to the policy or practice of acquiring full or partial political control over another country, occupying it with settlers and exploiting it economically. Arguably, frank colonialism is fading, and giving way to more subtle control of country systems without open conquest, or unabashed exploitation. Neo-colonialism is associated with unfair exchange, resource exploitation and extraction, a "strings-attached" model of funding, one-sided partnerships, non-contextual interventions, and gifting of results without capacity building among other issues. This neo-colonialism might be perceived by some as more acceptable than colonialism, but still represents the same principles, with more covert practices [6]. The fact that LMIC collaborators do not speak up or comment on these issues might reflect power imbalances, post-colonial cultures, host country cultures and norms, respect to guest or the elders, perceptions of respect, fear of funding loss, lack of trust and deep engagement, or even that surgical visitors to these contexts are simply not listening. It is also not uncommon for surgical visitors to have backings of hospital and ministry leaders that intimidates local surgeons. The decolonizing global health movement (inclusive of global surgery) was born in an attempt to counter these norms, and has gained traction in the past few years, catalyzed by the COVID pandemic [7].

Decolonizing is an essential part of the journey to equity, but we must be careful to move beyond attempting to dismantle structures to constructively building partnerships focused on inclusive access to surgical care and education based on quality and on diversity. As we learn from the colonial past, our greatest focus should be on equity for the future. If decolonization is not an ending of partnerships, then we must unlearn, learn, and relearn global surgical relationships. This chapter is focused on identifying the common ethical challenges experienced in global surgery surrounding the domains of clinical delivery of health care, of education in global surgery, and also of trainee exchange, surgical research, and collaborations and partnerships [5]. We describe frameworks for ethical and equitable partnerships which intend to help readers reflect on the ethics of their current work. We also aim to bring HIC partners to terms with pervasive structural racism and suggest how to mitigate the likelihood of permitting these systems to work in global surgery. Finally, we hope that readers will learn how to initiate difficult discussions (constructively confront), ask forgiveness (humble vulnerability), and change practice (sensitive accompaniment) as they seek to be ethical in their engagements with LMIC surgery programs.

It was Pelegrini that stated that surgery is a moral practice, and every surgeon is therefore a moral agent [8]. Ethical principles are universal, but the specific details of the application of these principles are influenced by context, geography, and personal experiences. Global surgery in difficult international terrain is intrinsically complex and invites subtle and overt moral ambiguity – a literal "how to" manual effectively over-simplifies the compound reality. In addition, most literature on global surgery ethics is intrinsically biased, as 80% is written exclusively by authors from HICs [5]. Note that this is not a literal step-by-step "how to," but a general guide that must be put into action contextually, thoughtfully, and as guided by partners with whom readers will be engaging. We aim to advocate for the recognition of ethical challenges and provide principles that guide global surgeons to ethical conclusions.

Ethical Challenges in the History of Global Surgery

Investigating the roots of global health and global surgery is necessary if practitioners are to understand the original problematic frameworks that guided the engagement of privileged surgical health systems with less privileged ones. Traced back to colonial and "tropical" medicine, which was an attempt by colonial powers to protect their troops and governing officials from infectious diseases rampant in colonized territories, global health has evolved in nomenclature in an attempt to distance itself from unwholesome historical ideologies and practices. Unfortunately, the foundations of global health were not built on equity. The colonized were second or third class and were not the primary consideration in their own countries – medications were prioritized in favor of the colonizers, training of locals in healthcare was limited, health systems were neglected at basic levels by the colonizers, and under-trained caregivers worked freely in low-income settings [9].

As consciousness of the inappropriateness of the approach to Tropical Medicine spread, nomenclatures morphed to "Humanitarian Medicine," "International Health," and then "Global Health." However, many things did not change at the core, including the often prescriptive and exploitative nature of engagements with struggling health systems. White privilege, white supremacy, and systems of whiteness are still a sad reality in global health today despite the independence gained by most LMICs with their own budgetary systems. Global Surgery as a movement has inherited a number of these challenges (Table 3.1).

Humanitarian and faith-based surgical missions are some of the earliest documented global surgery efforts [10]. Ethical concerns around motives, promotion, publicity, photography, and funding of these organizations have been raised. The International Committee of the Red Cross, born of an epiphany in the 1859 Battle of Solferino, and ***Médicine Sans Frontières*** inspired in 1971 are humanitarian organizations that have contributed to global surgery efforts. Ethical critique around neutrality and impartiality versus a focus on patient's rights have been raised concerning these kinds of platforms – for example, decisions not to speak up in the face of grave violations of human rights [9]. Plastic surgery-led short-term reconstructive missions focused on cleft surgery, burns, and cancrum oris (noma) followed, and came out of HIC universities in the 1960s. The challenge with many of these efforts is that they have historically been extremely vertical and use a "hit and run" model without adequate training of the local providers. Many of these interventions did not include health systems strengthening and it is questionable that the primary focus of these organizations was informed based on locally defined priorities. Air, land, and sea-based self-contained surgical platforms were introduced in the 1970s, in part to circumvent the need for any local resources during short-term missions. Despite the convenience and efficiency introduced by this model, cost-effectiveness has been found to be sacrificed, local supply chains which are underfunded and inadequate continue to being undermined.

Table 3.1 Unethical global surgery motivations: few parallel lessons from history[a]

S/n	Motivations of historical colonialism	Motivations of global surgery neocolonialism
1.	Cheap raw materials	Cheap research papers
2.	Abundant raw materials	Abundant data, patients and pathologies
3.	Limited competition	Limited academic competition
4.	Limited regulation	Less rigorous institutional review boards: Grant money solves it all (subject to culture of bribery), permission from "higher bodies" in leadership
5.	Demand for raw materials in colonizing countries	Demand for publishing as a prerequisite for promotions; demand to include LMIC partners by funders, the pictures are demanded by funders and validate one on social media
6.	Need for stop-over ports, or locations for sightseeing	Involve low- and middle-income countries whenever convenient or usually invited for specialty knowledge
7.	Colonies as assets in the balance of power	Low- and middle-income country connections are assets in academic power although providing needed assistance and teaching (by invitation)
8.	Inequitable exchange of goods for slaves/workers[b]	Surgical donations that end up in hospital junkyards, pragmatic over-emphasis by HIC funders on bringing in huge grant funding into the LMIC setting
9.	The prestige of conquest	Pseudo-conquest (an LMIC author on the paper)

[a] Table developed from original slides by Barnabas Alayande presented at the Consortium of Universities for Global Health 2021 Global Surgery Satellite Session. Used with permission

[b] In Nigeria's Badagry port, 10 slaves were exchanged for a glass bottle of gin or a ceramic plate, 40 for an umbrella or a Dane gun, 100 for a canon, while the number exchanged for a mirror was negotiable

Specialty mission hospitals were later developed and have provided historical contrasts in sustainability, local partnerships, and training. Approval of global surgery electives in 2011 by the American Board of Surgery and the Accreditation Council for Graduate Medical Education has helped popularize existing and new global surgery electives, fellowships, and academic partnerships. This has heightened the need for equity in partnerships, and the need to focus deliberately on preventing paternalistic visits by educating both visiting and hosting organizations on equity in Global Surgery [9].

Western medical ethics though traceable to religious foundations were formalized rather reactively following Nazi war experimentation and the Nuremberg trials, written in the Nuremberg code, the Belmont report, the Helsinki Declaration, the declaration of Geneva [11]. Ethics specific to global surgery are also elucidated as a result of missions gone wrong, or in response to identified ethical challenges [12]. These western medical ethics focus on individual autonomy, as opposed to low-resource settings where the emphasis tends to be on the common good or community-centered public health ethics [13].

Frameworks for Global Surgery Ethics for Practice and Partnerships

Maintaining ethical standards of practice and partnerships requires thinking within ethical boundaries and frameworks, and not just "going with the gut." The enduring principles of beneficence, nonmaleficence, autonomy, and justice, undergirded by integrity, truthfulness, dignity, and honesty are important in considering global surgery ethics [14]. Beneficence demands that global surgeons should act in the best interest of others. Nonmaleficence as a principle demands that our work does not inflict harm or the risk of harm through negligence on others. It reflects Sir Robert Hutchison's physician's prayer, "From inability to let well alone, from too much zeal for the new and contempt for what is old, from putting knowledge before wisdom, science before art and cleverness before common sense, from treating patients as cases and from making the cure of the disease more grievous than the endurance of the same, good Lord deliver us" [15]. Autonomy speaks of self-determination based on the conditions of liberty and agency. Justice as a principle speaks to equitable distribution of limited healthcare resources, the perception of health as a human right, and respect for the patient's rights.

A number of ethical frameworks exist from the proverbial to the academically defined that cover practice, partnerships, and educational exchange. Five such useful frameworks are briefly described below.

The Ethical Fishing Principles

The often-used proverb in global health "Give a man a fish and you would have fed him for a day" versus "Teach a man to fish and you will feed him for a lifetime" are only but part of the considerations in Global Surgery. We must ask the man whether he wants to fish at all or would rather hunt or pick fruit. Then if he chooses to fish as is relevant to his context, we must fish alongside him with a non-arrogant accompaniment.

This anecdotal framework focuses on local ownership and leadership of projects, relevance of outputs and outcomes to local context, and capacity building as core ethical principles of global surgery engagement.

Projects – Guidelines for HIC Surgeons on Establishing Projects in Low-Income Countries

A series of recommendations for HIC surgeons seeking to establish projects in LICs were developed by Grimes and colleagues in collaboration with the International Development Committee, College of Surgeons of East, Central and Southern Africa, International Federation of Surgical Colleges, Association of Surgeons of Great Britain and Ireland, West African College of Surgeons and the Operation Hernia Foundation [16]. Recommendations include appropriately identifying partners, establishing local needs and resources, training local surgical teams and ensuring sustainability, using appropriate technology and skills, monitoring the quality of surgery, taking responsibility for and managing post-operative complications, considering costs and mitigating financial impact on host institutions, and working with indigenous local and regional training programs [16].

Partnerships – The Monette Principles Applicable to Global Surgery

Monette et al. carried out a scoping review of guiding principles informing "good" global health research partnerships and identified an ethical framework global surgeons would do well to embrace [17]. Themes include mutual benefit, collective agenda setting, equity in partnerships, accountability, and incorporation of capacity building. Specific principles are shown in Box 3.1 [17].

Box 3.1 Monette Principles

Reciprocity
Benefit
Mutual benefits
Shared benefits
Collective writing and publishing
Sharing of data and networks
Pooling of profits and merits
Focus
Setting baseline goals, objectives
Setting future milestones
Collective agenda setting
Equity
Responsiveness to causes of inequities
Proportionality
Accountability to partnership
Accountability to beneficiaries
Development of national research capacity
Enhance capacities
Sustainability
Commitment to the future

Investing in relationships
Sharing, assigning, and clarifying responsibilities
Interacting with stakeholders
Broad consultative process
Understanding contextual values
Critically engaging context
Ensuring research influences policy
Application of research results
Effective communication
Humility
Inclusivity and inclusion
Promotion of mutual learning
Social justice
Disclosure of financial interests
Commitment to transparency
Authentic partnerships
Adapt and respond
Leadership
National ownership
Prevention of adverse impact
Promotion of common good
Relinquishing of power by the Northern partner and acceptance of autonomy of the Southern partner
Respect
Stewardship

Education – The Fair-Trade Learning Rubric and Principles Applicable to Global Surgery [18]

Hartman and colleagues published a rubric used to generate discussion between partners and that is relatable to fair trade exchange programs or surgical visits between HICs and LMICs. Key elements considered are.

1. **Common purpose**: The global surgery exchange must be based on mutually established long-term goals.
2. **Host community program leadership**: The programs should be locally led and host community driven, with co-owned research.
3. **Host community program participation**: Local communities must embrace and participate in the program.
4. **Recognition and protection of rights of the vulnerable**: Rights of the most vulnerable must be recognized and deliberately protected. LMICs, the poor, the uneducated, women, children, and minorities must be protected both as patients and care-providers within the partnership.
5. **Resourcing:** Local sourcing of human and material resources is key. The environmental and economic impact of any visits should be discussed. The economic structure of the programs should be discussed and shared.
6. **Transparency**: Financial budgets and grant details should be available to all parties and costs equitably shared.
7. **Recruitment, publications, and social media**: Equal opportunities should undergird recruitments, and remuneration should be equitable. Decisions on whether to, who to, where to, and how to publish should be jointly taken and relevant to the context. Social media use should be guided by principles of confidentiality, and respect for persons.
8. **Clarity of commitment and evaluation of partnership success**: There should be clear metrics prior to the engagement for what success looks like and all parties should show tangible commitment to the partnership.
9. **Appropriate communication**: Lines of communication and dissemination of partnered program results should be clear.
10. **A focus on partnerships beyond a single program**: This implies a focus on system strengthening. Timelines and commitments should extend beyond a single "mission."
11. **Community and learners' theory of change**: Motivations for the partnership and the expected community outcomes are identified and welcomed by diverse community stakeholders including any learners.

Practice – Mitigating the "Seven Sins of Humanitarian Medicine" Framework [12]

Welling and colleagues provide a list of ethical pitfalls applicable to global surgery that can serve as a framework to challenge ethical engagement.

Although it focuses on failures in humanitarian (surgical) missions, it also presents the challenge for improvement. Ethical pitfalls to note using this lens include leaving a mess behind, failing to match technology to local needs and abilities, competition and failure of cooperation, failing to have a follow-up plan, politics over true service, going where one is not needed or wanted, being poor guests and doing the right thing for wrong reasons [12].

Ethical engagement in global surgery requires careful planning based on local needs and priorities. There should be mutual benefit, clarity in terms of engagement, roles, and goals. Equity is key, and these engagements must not create dependence. An ethical emphasis is capacity development – the aim is to literally "work yourself out of the job." Institutional reflections can be carried out by using the Council on Health Research for Development (COHRED), Research Fairness Initiative Reporting Guide [19].

Practical Considerations

Ethical Considerations in Trans-Border Global Surgical Care Delivery

Overview Teams must plan for long-term follow-up and continuity of care. Ensure that local human resources are not diverted from core needs to surgical missions and that local material resources are not exhausted or stretched by diversion from basic use to less urgent, elective missions [6, 12, 20]. Equity in patient choice and procedure selection is key – avoid biased selection of healthcare workers' relatives, those that can pay for services or have higher social capital. Also mitigate corrupt practices that skew patient selection. Always practice within your scope of training, avoid compromising patient's quality of care, and avoid substandard approaches [5]. For instance, an urologist performing an elective thyroidectomy is performing surgery way out of their scope of training. An extreme focus on task-shifting by engaging unqualified providers as part of the "it is for Africa" syndrome should also be avoided.

Consider that standards of care might be variable in the LMIC context based on resources. Be prepared for highest quality care in low-resource contexts; for instance, operating the patient with suspected acute appendicitis without an abdominal CT scan is not considered a compromise of quality of care where it is not available or is financially prohibitive, but is a recognized variation in standard of care. A general surgeon performing a Dunhill's modification of a subtotal thyroidectomy, rather than a total thyroidectomy for benign thyroid disease, in a village where replacement L-thyroxine is not available, follow-up is difficult, health insurance cover is poor, and out-of-pocket cost for medication is prohibitive can be considered a variation in standard of care.

The waste of the global north in single-use materials and overwhelming packaging of disposables should be avoided in all settings. Reduce, reuse, recycle. Climate considerations resulting from this waste are an often-neglected ethical consideration. Safe cleaning and adequate low-emission sterilization can allow reuse of some (not all) disposables, and repurpose materials like diathermy pencils, tubes, monitors, etc.

To maintain contextual ethics for practice, develop a firsthand cultural, religious, and social awareness of the host community, and do not transpose your own culture, biases, or assumptions. Be careful of linguistic peculiarities, and within your capacity, learn at least the basics of the communicating and medical language. Review ethical informed consent for the environment – several African contexts for example view consent as a family or communal decision. Understand that confidentiality for core family members is extremely contextual. Deal with the adult individual concerned but involve appropriately the social support system with consent and by context. Do not undermine local healthcare provision by innocent, but demeaning comparative comments to patients, health professionals, or colleagues. This reduces the confidence of locals in their health systems and increases their dependence on foreign missions and interventions.

In sync with the Plan-Do-Study-Act framework, ethics of global surgery can be elaborated using a cycle that insists on continuous improvement (Fig. 3.1). No partnership is intrinsically "perfect"; the emphasis of this framework is not as much on an ideal partnership, as on the need

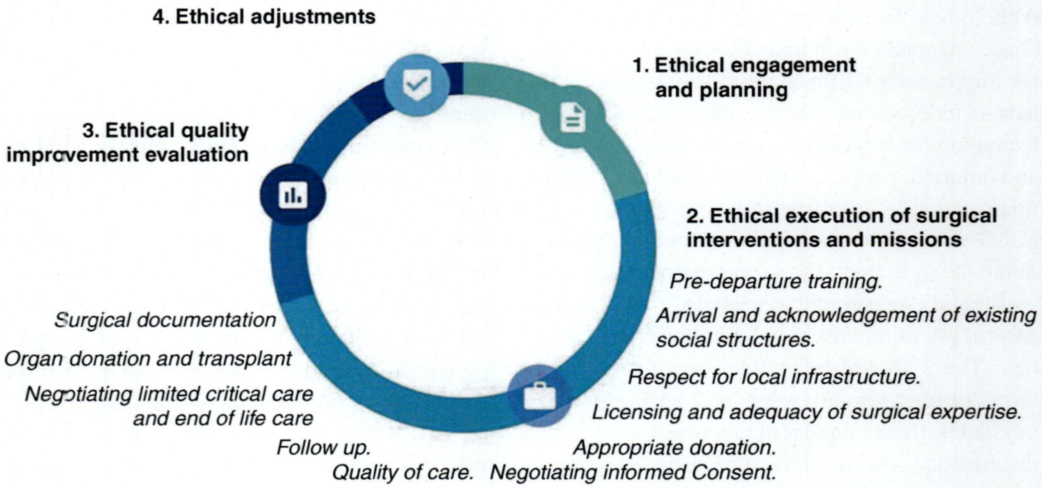

Fig. 3.1 The ethics cycle of engagement in global surgical care delivery

for partners to bear in mind the need for continuous review and improvement throughout the cycle of their engagements and to bring ethics into their quality improvement processes. Ethical challenges encountered in each phase are described below.

Ethical Engagement and Planning

Parachute missions are a constant reality, with funded HIC partners implementing global surgery projects and deciding priorities for LMIC recipients. Many times, partners providing funding for these projects exercise the right to direct them, and strings attached to resources create a neocolonialist framework for control. The ethics, value, goal, and outcome of the whole project need to be agreed to by both parties prior to the mission to avoid misunderstandings. They should not permit the creation of a social structure or power disparity in which there are debtors and creditors. Approach these global surgery engagements as equal partners or as accepted and desired mentors and mentees in an educational setting if invited to do that.

"Buy-in" in global surgery does not refer to a 1- to 2-day workshop that can be included in your final report or write up [21]. It implies jointly determining engagement priorities using frameworks, empowering partners to speak up, valuing the culture and preferences of contextual partners, sharing leadership, and deferring program leadership to LMIC partners. It also involves agreeing before sending proposals to Institutional Review Boards for review and before seeking grant funding. We term this "The grave error of sequence." A number of such projects are actually dead-on-arrival. Many surgical groups are already on a mission before they reach out to local partners. Grant funding is already obtained before contacting local partners [21]. This is unacceptable – no matter how good the idea – and leads to internal and external conflict even if LMIC institutions bend over backward to receive this funding. Funding disparities are also an ethical concern, with HIC volunteers earning much more in stipends from their HIC institutions than LMIC partners do from their governments who do more contextual work even when they reside in the same context for the duration of the project.

In planning, we must also avoid the "least effort, greatest gain" syndrome, where we identify problems that are easy to tackle, and leave the most difficult surgical challenges to the resident teams. It is best to encourage purchases using the local supply chain, and be willing to improvise using local material, if it is available and of sufficient quality to be acceptable for surgical interventions. We also need to make sure all stakeholders that contribute to the project are acknowledged.

Execution of Surgical Interventions and Missions

Stay within your certified scope of work, uphold your responsibility to local collaborators and community members, and identify, acknowledge, and mitigate your intrinsic biases and power dynamics.

Pre-Departure/Pre-Arrival Training

Inadequate pre-departure training sets up teams to fail, and this in itself is unethical. Kalbarczyk and colleagues identified culture, safety, project-specific knowledge, ethics, travel medicine, language, mentorship, professionalism, emotional wellness, language, and culture shock as minimal domains that need to be covered in a rounded pre-departure training. It is best that trainers are, at the very least, in part, true indigenous contextual experts, and that such training is evaluated [22] (see Chap. 2). Trainings in cultural sensitivity, integration, and global health ethics are very important.

Arrival On Site, and Acknowledgement of Existing Social Structures, and Community Hierarchies

Much of western culture has lost its appreciation for community hierarchy. This contrasts with many LMIC settings, where elders, local political leaders, religious leaders, chiefs, and community heads have significant influences. The influences that senior doctors, nurses, lab techs, administrators, and healthcare providers have in hospitals – even if they are not related to the specific project – should not be underestimated. Local protocols should be adhered to, and approvals must be ensured before moving in for surgical missions or system strengthening activities in any place. This should be regardless of whether the recipient system is strong enough to legislate and monitor this, or if such systems are underdeveloped.

It is unethical and arrogant to perceive oneself as the expert over a resident local professional just because one has served as visitor in the same setting for a few years [21].

Respect for Local Infrastructure

Many global surgery interventions use local operating rooms, wards, clinics, and other facilities. An ethical challenge arises when elective cleft repairs and hernia repairs, for instance, as the focus of a mission, displaces emergency laparotomies, or when booked operating room space is taken up by visiting surgeons, resulting in a disruption of the surgical eco-system for local patients and surgeons. These missions sometimes result in a backlog of deprioritized patients. Discussion with the local team and leadership is mandatory to make these arrangements, and the decisions must be left to the local administrator. After all, the mission is his/her guest.

The Question of Adequacy of Surgical Expertise

Surgical residents who have minimal or no exposure in certain interventions in their HICs often travel to LMICs to gain experience and perform more cases. In some cases, medical students who do not have appropriate licensing or exposure scrub in on highly technical cases during global surgery engagements. The ethics of this is clearly challenging as sometimes in rural and remote locations, such visitors are the only available surgical provider who can attempt an intervention. Dilemmas arise: "would you let this patient die, or try out this emergency open laparotomy, even though it is your first?" General guidance is to absolutely ensure appropriate local licensure, and to operate within the confines of the local license, all the time. Never operate above your abilities or knowledge without due supervision and avoid the assumption that local expertise (even task sharers) cannot attempt what you think you can exclusively do. Many issues have arisen from blurring of these lines in the name of compassion.

Appropriate Surgical Equipment Donations

A large proportion (70–90%) of well-intended donations from HICs end up in surgical junkyards in the global south [23]. Very often, there is a disconnect between donors and the recipient context. Inappropriate voltages, non-functional equipment, ambient temperature differences, old models of surgical gadgets for which there is no more technical support, high-cost maintenance equipment, incompatible machines, absence of battery backup for locations with inadequate electricity supply, and lack of training of recipients on the use of these donations are a few of the reasons for these equipment waste sites. This applies to anything from syringes and vacutainers to anesthesia machines, ultrasound, and CT scan machines. Up to thirty-three frameworks have been suggested to guide ethical medical donations in low-income settings [23]. It is also not unusual to hear about donations stuck in airports and ports just because the local team does not have the necessary funds to pay taxes and clearance fees or there are existing laws that prohibited entry of such equipment and resources. Donations should first start from discussion with the local team as team as to what is needed in the set up, what their priorities are. Practical things such as checking the voltage of donations against local power, including step-down voltage transformers and stabilizers, ensuring maintenance, and discussing extensively with recipient sites prior to bringing donations can help address this. Donated equipment should be discussed with the host staff and agreed on which is wanted and on the best method of importing it to avoid unnecessary costs, and mitigate against delays in transport (Box 3.2).

Box 3.2 Ethical Donations Require

1. Pre-requisite agreement from the recipient site on the need of the donated equipment.
2. Pre-import refurbishment certificates.
3. Alignment with the rules and regulations of the country regarding import permits.
4. Presence of onsite capacity in human resources to operate and maintain equipment.
5. Environmental considerations of adequate space, water, electricity, low energy consumption, and environmental safety.
6. Material resources like replacement parts and supply chains.
7. Maintenance capacity through training and sufficient financing.
8. Educational resources and manuals for ongoing training in equipment use, and interpretation of output.

Consent

Consent must be negotiated carefully and respectfully particularly in the presence of a language barrier. Mutilating surgeries such as amputations, mastectomies, colostomies, ileostomies, hysterectomies, tubal ligations, and orchiectomies are particularly ethically distressing given the often irreversible and psychologically significant nature of these interventions. Local healthcare workers should lead or help guide this process, and patient's families, caretakers, or an elder member of the family should be involved in the decision (as per the existing cultural norms). Independent translators should be employed if they are available.

Quality of Care

There is often a tension about the quality of surgical care delivered at LMIC sites compared to the home institution. Making a diagnosis of acute appendicitis, without a CT scan, or operating on a toxic goiter without a thyroid scan for example, is rather a norm than unethical. The pragmatic ethical standpoint will be to give the best possible care, within the context of available resources, while improving the quality of care as you are able. Various diagnostic tests are not available in many of these contexts, and emphasis should be placed on visitor's clinical acumen, basic available investigations, and local experience to make diagnoses. Given the above, however, quality of care should not be compromised.

Follow-Up of Surgical Patients

A very important ethical consideration is the follow-up of operated patients. Some vertical interventions focus more on the short-term outcomes than long-term results. Overtly, few-day short-term missions without provision for follow-up may be dangerous since numerous complications including surgical site infections or hemorrhage are missed. The need for re-operation is also a potential threat. To mitigate this catastrophe, the local physicians must be included as co-surgeons and trained to care for the patients when the mission departs.

Covertly, surgeries with long-term, late-onset complications are also missed when there is no provision for longer term follow-up. This should be done by trained local surgeons who preferably, if possible, participate in the original operation. These include cancer recurrences, long-term complications such as adhesions after laparotomy and hypothyroidism after thyroidectomy. All global surgical engagements and local health authorities should focus on strengthening systems that leave continuing care for native recipients of interventions.

Surgical Documentation

Many surgical missions done outside hospital sites have the challenge of under-documentation. Quite often, patients presenting in LMIC facilities following global surgical interventions have little to no documentation of their surgeries or surgical findings. This can be challenging if there is need for repeat surgeries or further evaluation. Records should never be extracted or completely taken away by the visiting team. In addition, patients must understand clearly, and possibly have personal documentation of the interventions in adequate detail for future reference. Documentation given to the patient should best be not only a description of the procedure, but include a simple drawing of the operation. Given experts are involved in the treatment, plan on further management would also be very productive.

End of Life Care, Physician-Assisted Suicide, and Limited Critical Care Ventilation

Although this remains a subject of debate in Western countries, the ethics of the concept of DALYs in favor of youth is perhaps contestable in many African, Asian, or Middle Eastern cultures. Religious and socio-cultural beliefs many times also do not approve the hastening of death, and hold the sanctity of life over the quality of life. We must ensure that a "western perspective" of "death with dignity" versus "life prolongation at any cost" of these ethics is not forced on non-western cultures. Decisions on end-of-life care are best taken by a contextual expert, based on contextual laws, taking full cognizance of autonomy, beneficence, non-maleficence, and justice. Death is a personal experience, but some more religious societies that believe in an afterlife are more at rest with the non-finality of demise. These cultures may be more accepting of death and dying. Family decisions may also be more nuanced, with decisions taken to stop treatment when expenditure is catastrophic, and lands and property have been sold with little or no improvements seen. Families may take decisions to remove severely ill patients from orthodox medical care or hospital to traditional or spiritual healers or refuse disfiguring surgeries on behalf of their patient.

Ethical dilemmas around critical care are accentuated by a lack of resources. With 1 bed in an ICU serving two million people, who gets the bed following a mass casualty? The decision for or against putting a patient on a ventilator or using other limited critical care resources has often been taken by default in low-resource countries. Where these are scarce, and expert intensivists are unavailable, those needing serious ICU care are automatically not likely to live. This is an inequity in and of itself, but the ethics around who gets what is strongly locally driven by considerations of futility, patient's wishes and sadly, costs. The ethics in this sort of dilemma will need to be formulated in the context of individual cultural, social, religious, socio-economic and legal backgrounds, and is best left to a local expert in context.

Organ Donation and Transplantation

All countries do not take the same approach to organ donation. In Iran for example, a transplant patient association controls the process of organ donation and allocation through the government health authority. Teams must be aware of the peculiar ethics behind this.

Issues of the "red/black" market also arise in LMICs as many illegally harvested organs make their way into the transplant market. The illegal market knows no ethical boundaries [24]. Visiting surgeons should be careful to verify the source of donated organs and the veracity of consent by donors. "On-table" and under anesthesia donors should raise a red flag. Trace, and avoid non-system-based purchases. Purchase of organs from any living donor (even friends and distant family members) is now forbidden by both law and all Transplant Societies and Agencies in almost all Western and Asian countries, even China now. The law is still sometimes broken and punishable by imprisonment and by large fines of doctors and donors, recipients, and those who have been paid. As a foreigner that is not as conversant with the intricacies of the local organ donation system, private unethical sourcing, and black-market organs can find its way to your operating room when you work through loose systems that need to be tightened. The local hospitals that permit these illegal practices should be exposed, penalized appropriately by the regional and federal health authorities, and reported to the International Transplantation Society which can take appropriate actions to limit and eliminate such practices.

Ethical Quality Improvement Assessment

To close the loop of the ethics cycle of global surgery engagement, evaluation of every intervention, visit, and mission is necessary. Quantitative and qualitative methods should be used to assess the local practitioner's and host's perception of the ethics of the visitor's practice with a view to improvement [25]. There are suggestions that some hosts will hold back negative information so as not to hinder subsequent donations, funding, or visits, as a result of power imbalance, or simply out of respect as these partnerships are valued. Reports by visitors of unethical or illegal practices of the host hospital administrations and/or physicians should also be reported to appropriate authorities, even at the cost of not being allowed to return. Trust is essential to permit open discussion that can be used for ethical quality improvement. Schoenbrunner et al. designed a useful tool to review ethics of scope of practice and standard of care (nonmaleficence and beneficence), impact on local system (justice), informed consent and photography (autonomy) [25].

Ethical Adjustments

Utilizing feedback in an ethical manner is important to improve global surgery practice. Open and honest discussions should be held from the place of vulnerability with a willingness to apologize and correct unethical behavior going forward. Partners should be able to safely and constructively confront, ask forgiveness, and change practice as appropriate.

Ethical Considerations in Trans-Border Global Surgery Education

Visiting global surgeons should seek to include an educational or training aspect to encounters for clinical, research, or other skills transfer; but also realize that this should be bidirectional [6]. Remember that even when not overtly expressed by hosts, visitors might not be appropriately qualified to teach, and content taught might be inappropriate for the host's curriculum. Ensure that skills transferred are relevant to the LMIC context. It is ethical to ensure that resources required to implement knowledge or skills transferred are available, and that visiting trainees are supervised appropriately both by their mentors and by the local host surgeons based on their level of training. Refuse assumptions that coming from a HIC makes one a global expert. Visitors should also resist the temptation to "lecture about something" even when the content is not suitable to the available audience.

Ensure that visiting trainees are conversant with relevant contextual pathologies, presentations, and management and are taught appropriately by the host faculty. The saying that "when you hear hooves, think horses, not zebras" can easily be reversed in East Africa. Depend heavily on those working in context to guide in navigating clinical challenges – never assume.

Teams should ensure that training opportunities for residents in the host community are not usurped by visiting surgical trainees. They should be given priority in patient care and in the ORs. Promote reciprocity. "What is good for the goose is good for the gander." Exchange programs should not be one-sided, with HIC trainees getting opportunities to operate freely in LMIC contexts and LMIC trainees less likely to visit the HIC, and when they do manage to secure funding for travel and subsistence, are restricted to hands-off shadowing or observerships, almost always due to legal licensing demands and malpractice demands in some countries. While medical emigration is an individual choice influenced by stick, stay, push, and pull factors, it is unethical to promote brain drain from human resource-limited environments through global surgical exchanges. This needs to be corrected by an appropriate increase in salaries in LMICs as compared to those for staff in HICs.

Ethical Considerations in Trans-Border Global Surgery Research

Academic global surgery focuses on teaching and research in LMIC contexts, as over 1000 articles are produced per year from global surgery partnerships, and there are numerous ethical landmines to consider [26]. However, it should be noted that research by internist teams, not surgeons, is more frequently funded. Testing of any drugs, vaccines, and evaluation of treatments by internists must be done jointly with the local physicians. Be sure to appropriately involve and adequately credit LMIC surgical researchers [27]. Ethical clearance is best obtained from both the local and the international collaborating institutions. Never assume you do not need ethical approval for any study. It is best to ask and receive a waiver from the responsible committee, without payment and without artificial delays, than to proceed without regard to local standards. Where such a committee does not exist, helping in the building local capacity for this function is essential to maintain ethical standards. Excessive emphasis on "generalizability" and "transferability" to the detriment of work that is beneficial to the local community should be avoided as research should primarily benefit them. In addition, any populations that can be exploited for financial, or academic gain must be identified and protected. Informed consent must be true informed consent – in a familiar language, and with a dynamic that does not coerce the uneducated, poor, or ill with no alternatives for treatment or withhold permission to stop or drop out of a study at any point without any consequences, other than not receiving the experimental intervention or control drug.

Surgical outcomes including complications must be evaluated and documented. Surgical problems (post-operative complications left to the hosts' care, ill feelings by both hosts and visitors, and lack of trust by both sides) should not be left behind [12]. Clearly, this may lead to no repeat invitation and/or no wish to return.

Ethics of Involvement of Partners in Research

Generally speaking, human resources for health and research are constrained in LMIC contexts. Many surgical staff are over extended and busy in their practice, and may not have the time, and perhaps expertise to facilitate research projects. As much of the surgical research concerns evaluation of surgical needs or outcome studies, rather than testing of new equipment, or novel operations, collaboration is mandatory to execute the study properly. The ethical dilemma of wanting to "get things done" rather than wait for local engagement or to complete the work by the HIC partners and getting a rubber stamp by the low-income setting partners is real. Grants often have deadlines, and reporting requirements that focus on getting the work done, over developing capacity in partners. The ethical approach is to aim to grow local partners' capacity for research rather than externally sourcing human resources for the project.

Ethics of Authorship

The question of authorship often arises in global surgery engagements, and ethical pitfalls exist on both sides of the road. On one side, there are guest and gift authorship – adding in a known and influential name in a paper for the sake of publicity and sprinkling of local authors to tick the boxes to avoid taking the flak on twitter. On the other side, excluding local contributors because we determine that they do not meet authorship criteria because they only "collected the data" and did not have the expertise to do the analysis is not rare [21]. The expertise of LMIC global surgery contributors is key to global surgery research, and they need to be genuinely included. Hedt-Gauthier et al raised the issue of authorship order, showing that most LMIC contributors are "Stuck in the middle," with first and last author positions predominantly filled by HIC authors, especially when HIC contributors are from top US institutions [28]. In some cases, LMIC authors and partners have been circumvented because results are slow, or approvals are difficult. If studies are designed and carried out by local surgeons, as in many outcome studies, the local investigator must be first or last author and the visitors that he/she recruits for statistical analysis or to help interpret the results, who meet authorship criteria should be appropriately placed. Authorship order should be clearly and equitably decided after a transparent discussion among the team members, not by the initiator or funds holder of the study.

Institutional Review Boards (IRB) and Permissions for Research

Those that have been involved in IRB applications in some more bureaucratic LMIC contexts understand that it is easy to follow the path of least resistance. Some ethics committees sit once a month and have 3–6-months turnovers of applications. It is tempting to circumvent the intellectual and emotional stress of delays and depend on a HIC ethical clearance from a home academic institution to do work in such contexts. This temptation should be refused, as it underscores a colonial approach and is questionable. Advance planning and strong local partnerships can help to mitigate this. Due process integrates you into context and legally covers you to carry out research in these contexts. Extortion should not be permitted on the part of local partners in the form of exorbitant differential IRB payments for visitors. Time to review should also not be cost-dependent.

Data Management and Publishing

The question of where to publish global surgery research is primarily practical in terms of probability of acceptance and satisfactory dissemination of the information, but it can also be an ethical one. Data obtained from LMICs resulting in publications that should benefit LMIC surgeons are often published in foreign "high impact" journals inaccessible to them. Publishing these articles behind paywalls (driven by the often-exorbitant price of open access publishing) is another dilemma that can be considered unethical, as the knowledge taken from a context is not accessible to those from whom the knowledge is obtained. HIC researchers should be committed – to the best of their abilities – to open access publishing. Some major journals now have open access preprints, or on-line publications prior to appearance in the journal. This may help local physicians have access through libraries or their institutions.

Photography, Publicity, and Social Media

Thought has gone into the ethics around photography in global surgery (for clinical education, education, publication, advertising, and marketing) more recently. Treating global surgery like medical tourism with patient selfies, and unsolicited pictures with patients in difficult circumstances to be used to score narcissistic points on Instagram or Twitter is considered unethical, unacceptable, and may be illegal [6, 29]. This becomes even worse when patients are identifiable in the pictures. Informed consent must be considered while visiting in low-resource contexts, as it does in their own countries, and the ethics of privacy, confidentiality, image storage, image distribution, and social media use must be respected. Equitable use of medical photography involves standardization of the photographic method, and environment. The intended uses of the photographs and the potential risks and benefits should be made clear to the patients. Storage of these images, masked to avoid identification, must be confidential, and dissemination appropriate to maintain patient's privacy. One ethical challenge of posting these pictures on social media is that consent cannot be withdrawn once published [29]. When specimens, intra-operative images, and findings are photographed without the potential of identifying patients, discussion with the local team should be conducted in regard to acceptability of using such images on social media or for teaching.

Ethical Considerations in Trans-Border Global Surgery Partnerships and Collaborations

Capacity building should be at the core of collaborations. Partners should discourage perpetual dependence on financial or external material aid in the partnership and encourage production of needed materials that meet standards within the country perhaps utilizing governmental subsidies. Box 3.3 shows practices that reflect poor and unethical collaborations.

Box 3.3 Practices in Global Surgery that Reflect Poor Collaborations

Undermining of local surgical providers and surgical systems
Neglecting the local team in patient selection
Neglecting the local team in the planning phase
Neglecting patient follow-up in the planning and execution
Diversion of local resources
Lack of local capacity development/knowledge exchange
Inadequate prior notice for site visits
Sub-standard surgical approaches
Disruption and cancellation of local scheduled procedures
"Savior mentality" and paternalistic attitudes/"global health arrogance"
Prescriptive, one-sided partnerships with inequitable exchanges
Lack of program integration
Partnerships and programs not focused on local needs
Gift and guest authorship (naming authors on articles who have not contributed to research)
Unhelpful equipment donations
Non-reciprocity
Data collection and research malpractice

Conclusions

Focus on ethics in global surgery must begin with a willingness to acknowledge the power dynamics in the field of global health irrespective of its idealistic roots. HIC institutions and individuals generate income through their national grants and enhance profiles through international work. On the other hand, some HIC surgeons provide services for free, covering their own living expenses and salaries. One-sided partnerships sometimes occur, with trainees from the global north benefiting disproportionately from exchanges, even though local trainees benefit from training opportunities by HIC specialists. Organizations and individuals return from a short-term mission trip with pictures to market themselves and their work on social media to raise funds for more missions, generally not supported by local hospitals or health authorities. Vertical missions (dumping cash into programs, outreaches, and intervention events) with narcissistic African poster-child photographs and touching social media posts may make many local patients receive sometime unattainable operations and make donors and visiting healthcare workers feel good. However, this is not enough to grow a sustainable health system if thought is not given to long-term surgical systems strengthening, and local government or private funding is not available or dedicated to growth of healthcare facilities and their maintenance. The misuse of funds by local governments, issues of corruption that dictate distribution of national budgets, with minimal funding for health and surgery contribute to the ethical dilemma. All this is in a setting of poor, vulnerable patients, and surgical providers struggling with an under resourced, inadequate health system, who are not well positioned by history, ability, or power to determine agenda or benefit sustainably from these arrangements [30]. These are significant contributors to an ethical quagmire.

The focus of this chapter has been largely on ethics pertinent to HIC visitors in a cross-border location. It must be emphasized that hosts also have an obligation to high ethical standards. Concerns about payment (to the point of "price gouging"), and sudden changes in costs demanded from visitors for services they provide for free to the hospital is unethical. Partners must be careful that bribery and corruption do not influence donations in cash or kind, even when it is perceived as the norm for doing business in the context. It must be said that several countries experience pervasive corruption at many levels, particularly with medical purchases, licenses, patient selection for special care or for rehabilitation, and staffing of hospitals. This should not be encouraged even if it would cost the loss of future projects in the context. An insistence on integrity should be considered as part of overall surgical and healthcare systems strengthening. Host organizations should adhere to contractual obligations and keep their word, as ethical obligations are bilateral.

Visiting surgeons must listen carefully to local surgical providers. Maintaining an HIC pose and gaze in an LMIC is an ethical disadvantage [25]. Visiting surgeons optimize their ethical advantage by keenly listening to, and understanding, the perspectives of their local partners (Box 3.4).

Box 3.4 Recommendations

- Operate within an established ethical framework, and do not just "trust your gut."
- Listen to and work closely with the host global surgery community and be led by a true contextual expert.
- Study, study, study – The people, the practice, and the power dynamics. Never impose your constructs on host communities.
- Recognize and mitigate your intrinsic biases. Do not find others from your context and talk about how "slow, resource deprived, untimely, inefficient or corrupt" hosting systems are in such a way as to put down those working hard to effect system change within such systems.
- Acknowledge your position and privilege in the new setting and think deeply about how you fit in the foreign context. Appropriately hand over, or share your privilege, and do not abuse it.
- Remember: This is also an opportunity to learn, create friendships, and long-lasting professional partnership.
- Though the tensions will perpetually exist in low resource settings, always err on the side of maintaining high standards of practice over "just doing something."

References

1. Dare AJ, Grimes CE, Gillies R, Greenberg SL, Hagander L, Meara JG, Leather AJ. Global surgery: defining an emerging global health field. Lancet. 2014;384(9961):2245–7. https://doi.org/10.1016/S0140-6736(14)60237-3. Epub 2014 May 19
2. Meara JG, Leather AJ, Hagander L, Alkire BC, Alonso N, Ameh EA, Bickler SW, Conteh L, Dare AJ, Davies J, Mérisier ED, El-Halabi S, Farmer PE, Gawande A, Gillies R, Greenberg SL, Grimes CE, Gruen RL, Ismail EA, Kamara TB, Lavy C, Lundeg G, Mkandawire NC, Raykar NP, Riesel JN, Rodas E, Rose J, Roy N, Shrime MG, Sullivan R, Verguet S, Watters D, Weiser TG, Wilson IH, Yamey G, Yip W. Global Surgery 2030: evidence and solutions for achieving health, welfare, and economic development. Lancet. 2015;386(9993):569–624. https://doi.org/10.1016/S0140-6736(15)60160-X. Epub 2015 Apr 26
3. Agunloye OA. Ethics in academic research and scholarship: an elucidation of the principles and applications. Glob Educ Res. 2019;3(2):168–80. https://doi.org/10.5038/2577-509X.3.2.1036.
4. Little M. The fivefold root of an ethics of surgery. Bioethics. 2002 Jun;16(3):183–201. https://doi.org/10.1111/1467-8519.00281.
5. Grant CL, Robinson T, Al Hinai A, Mack C, Guilfoyle R, Saleh A. Ethical considerations in global surgery: a scoping review. BMJ Glob Health. 2020;5(4):e002319. https://doi.org/10.1136/bmjgh-2020-002319.
6. Scheiner A, Rickard JL, Nwomeh B, Jawa RS, Ginzburg E, Fitzgerald TN, Charles A, Bekele A. Global surgery pro-con debate: a pathway to bilateral academic success or the bold new face of colonialism? J Surg Res. 2020;252:272–80. https://doi.org/10.1016/j.jss.2020.01.032.
7. Chawla B, Lindert J, Sharma D. Post-decolonisation: global health and global surgery's coming of age. Indian J Surg. 2022;84(2):259–61. https://doi.org/10.1007/s12262-022-03330-6.
8. Pellegrini CA, Ferreres A. Surgical ethics symposium "ethical dilemmas in surgical practice". World J Surg. 2014;38(7):1565–6. https://doi.org/10.1007/s00268-014-2563-6.
9. Bowder AN, Alayande B, Fowler Z. History of global surgery. In: Kpodonu J, editor. Global cardiac surgery capacity development in low and middle income countries. Sustainable development goals series. Springer International Publishing; 2021. p. 3–15. https://doi.org/10.1007/978-3-030-83864-5_1.
10. Ellis DI, Nakayama DK, Fitzgerald TN. Missions, humanitarianism, and the evolution of modern global surgery. Am Surg. 2021;87(5):681–5. https://doi.org/10.1177/0003134820979181.
11. Baker R, McCullough L. What is the history of medical ethics? In: Baker RB, McCullough LB, editors. The Cambridge world history of medical ethics. Cambridge: Cambridge University Press; 2008. p. 1–15.
12. Welling DR, Ryan JM, Burris DG, Rich NM. Seven sins of humanitarian medicine. World J Surg. 2010;34(3):466–70. https://doi.org/10.1007/s00268-009-0373-z.
13. Schwartz L, Hunt M, Sinding C, Elit L, Redwood-Campbell L, Adelson N, de Laat S. Models for

humanitarian health care ethics. Public Health Ethics. 2012;5:81–90.
14. Beauchamp TL, James FC. Principles of biomedical ethics. 8th ed. New York: Oxford University Press; 2019.
15. The physician's prayer. BMJ. 1998;317(7174):1687A. PMID: 9857128; PMCID: PMC1114481.
16. Grimes CE, Maraka J, Kingsnorth AN, Darko R, Samkange CA, Lane RH. Guidelines for surgeons on establishing projects in low-income countries. World J Surg. 2013;37(6):1203–7. https://doi.org/10.1007/s00268-013-1999-4.
17. Monette EM, McHugh D, Smith MJ, Canas E, Jabo N, Henley P, Nouvet E. Informing 'good' global health research partnerships: a scoping review of guiding principles. Glob Health Action. 2021;14(1):1892308. https://doi.org/10.1080/16549716.2021.1892308.
18. Hartman E, Paris CM, Blache-Cohen B. Fair trade learning: ethical standards for community-engaged international volunteer tourism. Tour Hosp Res. 2014;14(1-2):108–16. https://doi.org/10.1177/1467358414529443.
19. Council on Health Research for Development (COHRED). Research fairness initiative research fairness initiative reporting guide. https://rfi.cohred.org/wp-content/uploads/RFI_Reporting_Guide_2.pdf. Accessed 3 June 2022.
20. Velin L, Lantz A, Ameh EA, Roy N, Jumbam DT, Williams O, Elobu A, Seyi-Olajide J, Hagander L. Systematic review of low-income and middle-income country perceptions of visiting surgical teams from high-income countries. BMJ Glob Health. 2022 Apr;7(4):e008791. https://doi.org/10.1136/bmjgh-2022-008791.
21. Jumbam DT. How (not) to write about global health. BMJ Glob Health. 2020;5(7):e003164. https://doi.org/10.1136/bmjgh-2020-003164.
22. Kalbarczyk A, Nagourney E, Martin NA, Chen V, Hansoti B. Are you ready? A systematic review of pre-departure resources for global health electives. BMC Med Educ. 2019;19(1):166. https://doi.org/10.1186/s12909-019-1586-y.
23. Marks IH, Thomas H, Bakhet M, Fitzgerald E. Medical equipment donation in low-resource settings: a review of the literature and guidelines for surgery and anaesthesia in low-income and middle-income countries. BMJ Glob Health. 2019;4(5):e001785. https://doi.org/10.1136/bmjgh-2019-001785.
24. Bianchino AL. The international illegal trade of organs on the "red" market: how the will to live can become the recipe to die by invoking ethical, criminal and property implications around the globe. J Int Bus Law. 2021;20(2):197–221.
25. Schoenbrunner AR, McIntyre JK, Nthumba P, Muchemwa FC, Sigler A, Gosman AA. Ethical dilemmas in global plastic surgery: divergent perspectives of local and visiting surgeons. Plast Reconstr Surg. 2022;149(4):789e–99e. https://doi.org/10.1097/PRS.0000000000008957.
26. Baison GN, Maine R, Chu K, Gillies R, Ntakiyuruta G, Meara JG. Authorship equity in global surgery research from low and middle-income countries (LMICs). Ann Glob Health. 2014;80(3):240. https://doi.org/10.1016/j.aogh.2014.08.205.
27. Miles S, Renedo A, Marston C. Reimagining authorship guidelines to promote equity in co-produced academic collaborations. Glob Public Health. 2021:1–13. https://doi.org/10.1080/17441692.2021.1971277.
28. Hedt-Gauthier BL, Jeufack HM, Neufeld NH, Alem A, Sauer S, Odhiambo J, Boum Y, Shuchman M, Volmink J. Stuck in the middle: a systematic review of authorship in collaborative health research in Africa, 2014–2016. BMJ Glob Health. 2019;4(5):e001853. https://doi.org/10.1136/bmjgh-2019-001853.
29. Teven CM, Goldman JJ, Rebecca AM. Ethical considerations in clinical photography: an updated perspective. Plast Reconstr Surg. 2021;147(2):366e–8e. https://doi.org/10.1097/PRS.0000000000007577.
30. Biehl J, Petryna A. When people come first: critical studies in global health. Princeton, NJ: Princeton University Press; 2013.

How to Develop Bidirectional Partnerships

4

Rondi M. Kauffmann and Carl E. Haisch

With rare exceptions, all of your most important achievements on this planet will come from working with others – or in a word, partnership.

– Paul Farmer

Abbreviations

COSECSA	College of Surgery of Central, East and Southern Africa
HICs	High-Income Country
LMIC	Low- and Middle-Income Country
PAACS	Pan-African Academy of Christian Surgeons
VUMC	Vanderbilt University Medical Center
WACS	West African College of Surgeons

Introduction

The concept of "bidirectional partnership" to describe global surgical efforts involving stakeholders from high-income countries (HICs) and low-middle income countries (LMICs) is a commonly used buzzword. Increasing interest in addressing global health disparities among medical students, surgical trainees and surgical faculty, identification of surgery as a key component of public health, and the inclusion of access to safe surgical care in the World Bank's Disease Priorities has led to a steep growth in the field of academic global surgery [1–3]. Many Departments of Surgery and surgical residency programs have responded by creating opportunities for clinical rotations, surgical education initiatives, and research projects in an LMIC [4]. While not all such partnerships are formal, many rely on the "twinning" of an academic institution in a HIC and an institution in an LMIC. Inherent power imbalances in these partnerships can lead to unequal benefits, with emphasis placed on advancing the careers of faculty and trainees from the HIC over those in the LMIC. The imbalanced, unilateral nature of many global surgical initiatives is far-reaching and includes failure to include LMIC authors on publications, funding streams that prioritize HIC initiatives over the stated needs of the LMIC population, unequal access to clinical trials in LMICs, HIC trainees providing care that is outside their scope of practice while in an LMIC, and HIC trainees rotating

R. M. Kauffmann (✉)
Division of Oncologic and Endocrine Surgery, General Surgery Residency, Vanderbilt University Medical Center, Nashville, TN, USA
e-mail: rondi.kauffmann@vumc.org

C. E. Haisch
Surgery, Division of Surgical Immunology and Transplantation, Surgical Education and Faculty Development, Brody School of Medicine, East Carolina University, Greenville, NC, USA
e-mail: haisch@ecu.edu

M. A. Hardy, B. R. Hochman (eds.), *Global Surgery*, https://doi.org/10.1007/978-3-031-28127-3_4

at LMIC sites without reciprocal opportunities for LMIC trainees to rotate at HIC sites [5, 6]. Responsible engagement in global surgical partnership requires intentional work to minimize inequity between the partners and active effort over time to ensure that both parties benefit from the collaborative relationship. In this chapter, we present two successful frameworks for bidirectional partnership – one at the level of a surgical accreditation program and the other at an individual institutional level. These are not intended to represent the only possible frameworks for bidirectional partnerships, but to serve as examples of successful programs.

The Pan-African Academy of Christian Surgeons Experience

Both Vanderbilt University Medical Center (VUMC) and the Pan-African Academy of Christian Surgeons (PAACS) have a presence at AIC Kijabe Hospital outside of Nairobi, Kenya. In this section, we examine the history and interactions of PAACS with Kijabe Hospital. It is the policy of PAACS that an individual hospital must approach PAACS to establish a relationship. This can be initiated by an individual clinician or administrator at the hospital on behalf of the institution and begins a process of close communication between hospital personnel and the administration of PAACS to establish a surgical training program at that hospital. The presence of a formal residency training program benefits both the hospital and its patients, increasing the number of patients served and elevating the hospital's prestige in the region. PAACS provides oversight, accreditation, and financial support. PAACS ensures that the hospital meets specified clinical standards in the operating room (both surgical and anesthetic), laboratory support, surgical beds, and nursing staff, as well as educational standard including conference rooms, medical library, internet, and access to an adequate number of cases to train residents. Most hospitals also provide housing for residents and their families. A team from PAACS visits the hospital prior to acceptance to review the hospital facilities, speaks with the administration, and assists with making necessary changes to meet standards. The number of residents that can be trained at that location is determined and PAACS partners with the hospital to provide funding for resident salaries. This is a particularly important component of attracting high-quality residents to train at PAACS hospitals, as many training programs in the region do not provide salary support for trainees. A memorandum of understanding between PAACS and the hospital is signed and reviewed regularly.

PAACS is a faith-based non-governmental organization founded in 1996 by a group of missionary surgeons who desired to train African nationals who would remain in Africa to address the immense burden of surgical needs on the continent. It is financed entirely by philanthropic gifts. The administration and support staff in the United States (U.S.) are paid and PAACS pays a large percentage of the resident salaries while they are in training. The faculty and program directors are paid by their own mission organization and the hospitals are frequently administered by a third organization. This structure calls for open and careful communication among all parties involved [7].

The goal of PAACS is to train African nationals in mostly rural mission hospitals that are equipped with at least three surgeons that are board-certified by a recognized national or international organization who act as faculty and program directors. The curriculum is designed to provide graded responsibility in which the residents train in the full breadth of general surgery and the surgical sub-specialties with the aim of equipping them to work in either a rural or metropolitan area within Africa. The curriculum is five years and covers general surgery, orthopedics, urology, obstetrics/gynecology, neurosurgery, and pediatric surgery. Prior to the COVID pandemic, up to 200 board-certified surgeons per year volunteered their time and visited PAACS sites to help train residents. Most of these surgeons were from the U.S. and represented a variety of surgical sub-specialties to increase the breadth of expertise to which the PAACS residents were exposed. With the COVID pandemic and political unrest in some of the countries, this number has decreased markedly.

Early in the development of PAACs, the leadership recognized the importance of an affiliation with a U.S.-based university to give PAACS academic credibility in the eyes of African governments and African surgical societies. A number of universities were considered, and Loma Linda University agreed to evaluate hospitals and their training programs on a regular basis. Upon satisfactory completion of the five-year program, a resident receives a certificate from Loma Linda University in addition to the PAACS certificate. Loma Linda University has continued in this role and reviews programs every five years with an in-person visit. The team is comprised of surgeons who have educational expertise and experience in evaluating surgical training programs. Based on the findings, the visitation team makes recommendations to strengthen and improve each program. The recommendations are sent to both the central administration of PAACS and the hospital administrator.

PAACS also has a relationship with the West African College of Surgeons (WACS) and the College of Surgery of Central, East and Southern Africa (COSECSA). COSECSA has granted certification to most of the PAACS training sites with WACS certifying a few. If a resident has trained in the appropriately certified training site, they may seek fellowship in the respective organization. Most of the residents have been certified by COSECSA, first at the Membership level and then three years later at the Fellowship level. PAACS has trained over 130 residents since its founding, and all have stayed in Africa and are working in over thirty African Countries. Thirteen percent of the teaching faculty are African nationals who have been trained by PAACS.

In 2006, AIC Kijabe Hospital opened a pediatric unit called Bethany Kids. A Canadian board-certified pediatric surgeon developed a pediatric surgery rotation for general surgery residents which could be from two to twelve months in length. Most of the residents needed some exposure to pediatric surgery and this was deemed to be the optimal place for this to be carried out. The residents were exposed to the operative, perioperative, and outpatient management of children with neurosurgical conditions such as spina bifida, hydrocephalus, anorectal anomalies, Hirschsprung's disease, hypospadias, plastic surgery, cleft lip and cleft palate, skin grafting, and burn contractures. Subsequently, in 2007, Kijabe started a formal two-year pediatric surgery fellowship, offered after the completion of a five-year general surgery residency training program. This fellowship has continued to the present and has trained twelve pediatric surgeons who are practicing in eight African countries. These surgeons are practicing in rural settings, government agencies, and urban centers.

In 2007, Kijabe hospital was also approved to train PAACS residents. This approval was granted by PAACS after the hospital requested to be a training center for general surgery residents. The hospital agreed with the Memorandum of Understanding and easily met the criteria for PAACS approval. Over the years PAACS has learned that the minimum number of faculty in general surgery needs to be three. Faculty members rotate out for furlough, vacation, illness, and meeting attendance. Three full-time faculty members are needed to fulfill the training needs of the residents. Programs not meeting this requirement are placed on probation, with re-review six months later. Subsequent to PAACS approval, COSECSA approved Kijabe Hospital for training at the MCS level and then approval at the FCS level, making it a fully accredited surgical training program. Since that time, Kijabe Hospital has trained a number of general surgery residents and has expanded to train pediatric surgeons and orthopedic surgeons. The program has also started an anesthesia residency program to train anesthesiologists.

The Vanderbilt-Kijabe, Kenya Experience

In 2011, VUMC's Department of Surgery established a formal partnership with AIC Kijabe Hospital in Kijabe, Kenya. PAACS had established a general surgery residency training program at Kijabe in 2007 and VUMC already had an anesthesia faculty member living in Kijabe who hosted anesthesia residents yearly. A surgical faculty member from VUMC with 15 years of experience living in West Africa began discussions with VUMC and Kijabe leadership regarding the possibility of establishing a formal global surgery partnership between the two institutions. Discussions began with leadership from VUMC traveling to Kenya to meet with leaders of Kijabe Hospital. The primary goals of those meetings were to conduct a "needs assessment" to define priorities of the partnership as stated by Kijabe leadership, set "ground rules" to ensure that the presence of VUMC surgical residents would not jeopardize the education and experience of Kijabe's surgical residents, specify expectations of each party's responsibilities in the partnership, identify strategies to ensure benefit to Kijabe's residents and faculty, and create the framework for a longitudinal collaboration including anticipated deliverables and joint ownership of the partnership [8].

The initial priority identified by leadership at Kijabe was capacity-building through surgical education initiatives. Because Kijabe already had their own surgical residency training program, VUMC residents were asked to be willing to assume any role on the surgical team that was needed at the time of the rotation in Kijabe. During times when Kijabe's residents were rotating elsewhere on the continent, on vacation, or out of town for exams, VUMC residents would be the senior resident on the service. When Kijabe's resident complement was complete, VUMC residents would act in a junior resident role and double-scrub cases. Not taking cases from Kijabe's residents was emphasized repeatedly during pre-travel orientation for VUMC residents. In addition, grant and philanthropic funding was secured to establish a center for surgical and anesthesia simulation training in Kijabe. Finally, VUMC granted adjunct professor status to faculty in Kijabe who were actively involved in resident education in order to facilitate access to key resources such as the VUMC digital biomedical library, Redcap, and statistical support.

As the partnership has matured, re-assessment of the needs of each partner has been conducted at regular intervals, both formally and informally. When a faculty member from Kijabe approached a faculty member from VUMC about creating an open-access digital surgical atlas for resource-constrained settings, the two collaborated on the project and VUMC hosted the atlas on their web server [9]. After a VUMC resident returned from Kijabe and mentioned that the senior residents in Kijabe had expressed an interest in mock oral board practice, the weekly joint Kijabe-Vanderbilt mock oral board training sessions with VUMC faculty and PGY 4 and PGY 5 residents from both institutions via zoom was started. Upon notification that PAACS began requiring completion of a research project by all residents prior to graduation, faculty members from both institutions partnered to create and direct the Kijabe-Vanderbilt Research Methodology for Healthcare Providers Course held weekly every spring via virtual conferencing. All projects (abstracts posters, manuscripts) from that course have their principal investigator (PI) and first/senior authors from Kijabe, with any VUMC faculty and residents listed in secondary authorship positions. As Kijabe's need for capacity building in surgical research has increased, the focus of the partnership has turned to expanding collaboration in that aspect of global surgical care. Keeping in mind the importance of ensuring equality in benefit for both partners, subsequent applications for grant funding have included a PI from both institutions, funding for both institutions, and emphasis on the research priorities identified by researchers in Kijabe (Table 4.1).

Table 4.1 Summary of key components of bidirectional partnership and how programs discussed in this article addressed them

	Prioritizing local needs	Clarity of roles	Resources	Capacity building	Sustaining relationships
PAACS	Hospital approaches PAACS to start relationship	PAACS provides oversight, authority to enforce standards, accreditation. Hospital responsible for adhering to standards and adjusting as needed	Hospital funds part of resident salaries, provides housing for faculty and residents. PAACS funds remainder of resident salaries	Accreditation of surgical training programs with goal of retaining surgeons within Africa	Formal relationship between PAACS, WACS, COSECSA. Loma Linda to provide in-person evaluation of training programs and conferring of certificates to residency graduates. Frequent in-person visits by PAACS personnel, PAACS volunteer surgeons assist with training of PAACS residents
Vanderbilt-Kijabe	Face-to-face needs assessment prior to creation of memorandum of understanding, frequent re-evaluation of needs of trainees and faculty in Kijabe, VUMC grants adjuvant faculty status to faculty in Kijabe, publications all with joint authorship	VUMC to prepare residents prior to rotation in Kijabe. Kijabe to provide housing and assistance with obtaining temporary licensure. VUMC residents to ensure that they are not taking cases from Kijabe's residents.	VUMC to fund all expenses for their residents. VUMC to provide access to online biomedical resources for adjunct faculty in Kijabe.	Joint educational programs, mock oral programs, research training programs. Advocacy to create new licensure category in Tennessee to allow residents from Kijabe to rotate at VUMC.	Regular involvement by VUMC faculty in Kijabe's research and educational initiatives. Frequent check-ins regarding additional areas of partnership to ensure needs of both parties are met. In-person visits by VUMC faculty.

Barriers to Bidirectional Partnership and a Call to Action

Focused efforts to address needs of the LMIC partner, mentor LMIC faculty and trainees, and ensure equity in benefit for both partners engaged in a global surgery collaboration minimizes the risk that global surgery programs between HICs and LMICs are just the "bold new face of neocolonialism" [10]. However, the inequity of sending HIC trainees to LMICs without reciprocity of LMIC trainees coming to HICs should not be ignored [11]. Licensing restrictions in the U.S. limit trainees from abroad to observerships only in most cases. This reality severely hampers efforts at true bidirectionality and must be addressed if global surgery is to move toward equity of benefit for both partners. Furthermore, these "equitable exchanges in global health education" are vital to "support international goals for health, improve the long-term stability of global health training, and to ensure that strong health care systems exist everywhere" [5]. Very few states provide a pathway for a foreign medical graduate (FMG) to spend time participating in patient care for any amount of time. VUMC is located in Tennessee where no licensure category existed to facilitate an FMG partner from Kenya to come to VUMC for anything other than an observership. While each state's licensing rules and categories differ, in Tennessee the power to create a new licensure category rests with the state legislature. After identifying this imbalance in the partnership, VUMC sponsored a bill to propose a new temporary licensure category for FMGs to spend time at an institution within the state of Tennessee, for purposes of clinical care, research training, and surgical education in a supervised setting, with the goal of expanding surgical capacity in LMICs. This bill was signed into law in May 2022 [12]. This form of advocacy on behalf of our global surgical LMIC partners, replicated in all states, is needed to move academic global surgery toward true bidirectional, equitable, sustainable collaborations.

References

1. Merson MH. University engagement in global health. N Engl J Med. 2014;370:1676–8.
2. Meara JG, Leather AJ, Hagandar L, et al. Global Surgery 2030: evidence and solutions for achieving health, welfare, and economic development. Lancet. 2015;386:569–624.
3. Debas HT, Donkor P, Gawande A, et al. Essential surgery; disease control priorities, vol. Vol 1. 3rd ed. Washington, DC: The World Bank; 2015.
4. Abraham PJ, Abraham MN, Corey BL, et al. Cross-sectional analysis of global surgery opportunities among general surgery residency programs. J Surg Educ. 2020;77(5):1179–85.
5. Hudspeth JC, Rabin TL, Dreifuss BA, et al. Reconfiguring a one-way street: a position paper on why and how to improve equity in global physician training. Acad Med. 2019;94:482–9.
6. Taylor-Robinson SD, Spearman CW, Suliman AAA. Why is there a paucity of clinical trials in Africa? QJM. 2021;114(6):357–8.
7. Thompson, D, Steffes, B. God's surgeons for Africa. Personal communication.
8. Tarpley M, Hansen E, Tarpley JL. Early experience in establishing and evaluating an ACGME-approved international general surgery rotation. J Surg Educ. 2013;70(6):709–13.
9. https://www.vumc.org/global-surgical-atlas/. Accessed 3 June 2022.
10. Scheiner A, Rickard JL, Nwomeh B, et al. Global surgery pro/con debate: a pathway to bilateral academic success or the bold new face of colonialism? J Surg Res. 2020;252:272–e280.
11. Debas H, Olusegun A, Balch CM, et al. Academic partnerships in global surgery: an overview of the American Surgical Association Working Group on Academic Global Surgery. Ann Surg. 2020;271(3):460–9.
12. https://wapp.capitol.tn.gov/apps/BillInfo/Default.aspx?BillNumber=SB1902. Accessed 3 June 2022.

How to Strengthen Surgical Systems in Low- and Middle-Income Countries

5

Rennie X. Qin, Belain Eyob, Emmanuel Makasa, and Kee B. Park

Perhaps no sin so easily besets us as a sense of self-satisfied superiority to others.

– William Osler

Abbreviations

HICs	high-income countries
HPSR	health policy and systems research
LCoGS	the Lancet Commission on Global Surgery
LMICs	low- and middle-income countries
NSOAP	National Surgical, Obstetric, and Anesthesia Plan
PGSSC	Program in Global Surgery and Social Change
SAT	surgical assessment tool
SDG	Sustainable Development Goal
SOA	surgical, obstetric, and anesthesia
UHC	universal health coverage
WHA	World Health Assembly
WHO	World Health Organization

R. X. Qin (✉) · B. Eyob
Program in Global Surgery and Social Change, The Department of Global Health and Social Medicine, Harvard Medical School, Boston, MA, USA
e-mail: be2256@cumc.columbia.edu; belain_eyob@hsph.harvard.edu

E. Makasa
Orthopedics, Witwatersand University, SADC Regional Collaboration Center for Surgical Healthcare, University of Witwatersrand, Johannesburg, South Africa

K. B. Park
Program in Global Surgery and Social Change, The Department of Global Health and Social Medicine, Harvard Medical School, Boston, MA, USA

Program in Global Surgery and Social Change, Harvard Medical School, Boston, MA, USA

Introduction

Surgical system strengthening is an increasingly used term in global surgery. Surgical system strengthening looks beyond clinical service provision and teaching by individual surgeons toward improving the broader health system around surgical, obstetric, and anesthesia (SOA) care. Improving outcomes from surgically treated diseases requires much more than the performance of surgery inside the operating theatre. For example, the survival of a patient with abdominal hemorrhage following a road traffic accident requires not only a surgeon and an operating theatre but also roads, a functioning emergency transport system, a referral system, blood bank, sterilization services, radiology, physiotherapy, rehabilitation, and health information system, among other components.

The publication of the Lancet Commission on Global Surgery (LCoGS) in 2015 redefined the field of global surgery and shifted its focus from merely supporting health systems to strengthen-

M. A. Hardy, B. R. Hochman (eds.), *Global Surgery*, https://doi.org/10.1007/978-3-031-28127-3_5

ing them [1]. Beyond the delivery of clinical care and teaching to fill health system gaps in low- and middle-income countries (LMICs), global surgery must improve the system's capacity to deliver surgical services in the long term. Although surgical system strengthening is not traditionally within the purview of the academic surgeon or textbooks on Global Surgery, it is the next necessary step to improve the outcome of surgical care. Surgical system strengthening also has implications for other services far beyond surgical care that require similar health system elements, such as emergency care, and critical care.

Surgical system strengthening requires an understanding of health systems, the development of policy and advocacy skills, and the knowledge of disciplines beyond medicine and epidemiology, such as economics, political science, sociology, and anthropology.

In this chapter, we define surgical system strengthening, explore its history, and discuss how to conduct surgical system strengthening and acquire the necessary knowledge and skills to do it. In doing so, we are targeting practitioners from both HICs and LMICs, as surgical system strengthening efforts must ultimately be driven by and led from within countries.

What Is Surgical System Strengthening?

The concept of surgical system strengthening arose from that of health system strengthening. In order to understand surgical system strengthening, we must start by exploring the concept of health system strengthening and delving into the field of health policy and systems research (HPSR).

What Are Health Systems?

The World Health Organization (WHO) defines health systems as the ensemble of "all organizations, institutions, resources, and people whose primary purpose is to promote, restore or maintain health" [2]. The WHO building blocks framework is commonly used to conceptualize health systems [2]. It describes the health system to consist of six components or "building blocks": service delivery, workforce, health information system, essential medicines, finance, and leadership/governance (Fig. 5.1). A health system converts inputs, such as workforce and essential medicines and technologies, into the immediate output of service delivery, which can be measured in terms of its coverage, access, quality, and safety, and ultimately into the outcomes and goals of improving health outcomes, equity, and financial risk protection.

One critique of this framework is that health systems do not only consist of a laundry list of individual components but also the dynamic interaction between the components to improve health outcomes. Another flaw of the framework is that it conceives the health system as a "black box". Inputs are automatically converted to outputs, and the process that occurs in between is

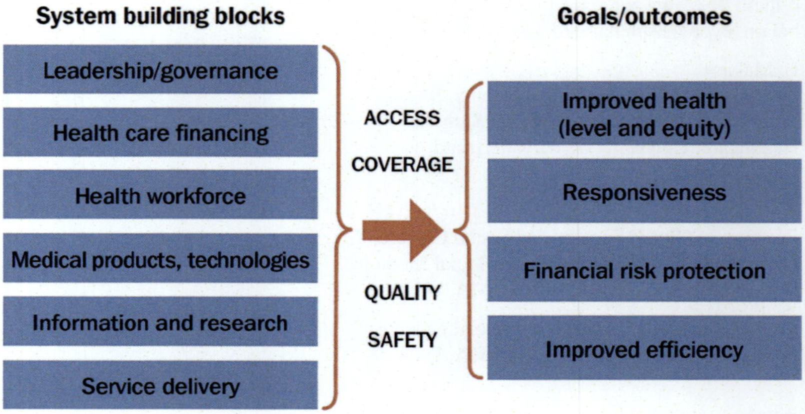

Fig. 5.1 The World Health Organization building blocks framework, adapted from WHO (2010) [2]

assumed to be opaque [3]. However, the process that translates inputs to outputs can and must be understood and studied. There is increasing attention within health system research to do so.

In recent years, there has been a shift to view health systems as complex adaptive systems. They are dynamic, interconnected, dependent on history and context, socially constructed, and shaped by power [4]. The field of HPSR is dedicated to the study of health systems. It draws on economics, political science, sociology, anthropology as well as public health and epidemiology [4].

Box 5.1 Definitions of Key Terms

Health policy and systems research (HPSR) is an emerging field that seeks to understand and improve how societies organize themselves in achieving collective health goals, and how different actors interact in the policy and implementation processes to contribute to policy outcomes. By nature, it is inter-disciplinary, a blend of economics, sociology, anthropology, political science, public health and epidemiology that together draw a comprehensive picture of how health systems respond and adapt to health policies, and how health policies can shape – and be shaped by – health systems and the broader determinants of health.

Health systems consists of all the organizations, institutions, resources, and people whose primary purpose is to promote, restore or maintain health.

Health system strengthening is any array of initiatives and strategies that improve one or more of the functions of the health system and that leads to better health through improvements in access, coverage, quality, or efficiency.

Surgical care is an overarching term used to denote care for adults and children delivered by anesthetists, obstetricians and gynecologists, and surgeons from various backgrounds including, but not limited to, adult and pediatric general surgery, orthopedics, neurosurgery, urology, ophthalmology, otorhinolaryngology, and vascular surgery, as well as nursing, midwifery, and all allied health professionals.

Surgical system strengthening is strengthening of health system components that are required to deliver surgical, obstetric, and anesthesia care to improve the outcome of diseases requiring treatment by surgical, obstetric, and anesthesia care.

What Is Health System Strengthening?

Despite being an increasingly popular concept in global health, health system strengthening remains misused and misunderstood. Health system strengthening represents a new direction in global health that arose in reaction to vertical, disease-focused programs that dominated global health for much of the twentieth century. In contrast to vertical programs focusing on ensuring the necessary inputs for the delivery of single interventions, health system strengthening takes a horizontal approach and improves the overall functioning of the health system to tackle multiple diseases. The WHO defines health system strengthening as "any array of initiatives and strategies that improve one or more of the functions of the health system and that leads to better health through improvements in access, coverage, quality, or efficiency" [5]. This definition requires the interaction between the building blocks to create improvement across health services and health outcomes.

Chee et al. distinguished health system strengthening from health system support activities [6]. While health system support activities fill health system gaps to improve short-term outcomes, health system strengthening makes the system permanently function better in the long term. There is concern that health system strengthening is broad and vaguely defined. Several sets of criteria for health system strengthening activities have been developed to address this [6, 7]. In order for interventions to qualify as "health system strengthening", they must:

1. Yield benefits for more than one disease area.
2. Address constraints that cause sub-optimal health system performance or improve the interaction between health system components.
3. Create long-term sustainable impact beyond the duration of the intervention.
4. Improve the goals of the health system: health outcomes, equity, and financial risk protection.

Many activities labeled as health system strengthening remain vertical and disease-focused, risking undermining rather than improving the functioning of health systems. Ultimately, health system strengthening activities must not only improve health system functioning but also improve the health outcomes for the population. The diagonal approach is increasingly used, which combines the vertical and horizontal approach to improve health system functioning through targeting several health services or disease areas.

Why Is Global Surgery Health System Strengthening Important?

For decades, global surgery activities predominantly constituted of health system support activities that were based in a single facility, focused on service delivery to fill gaps, and lacked sustainable impact beyond the duration of their implementation. Health system strengthening marks a new era in global surgery. The shift from short-term clinical service delivery by visiting specialists toward teaching, capacity building, and longer-term workforce development mark some of the first steps toward health system strengthening in global surgery.

Improving surgical care delivery in LMICs has the potential to fulfill many criteria for health system strengthening.

- Firstly, surgical care is **cross-cutting**. It encompasses multiple interventions for multiple disease areas. Up to a third of the global burden of disease is estimated to require surgical care [1]. Surgical care is an example of a service delivery platform, which can provide a range of services that require common health system components. For example, the provision of Caesarean sections, appendicectomy, and open fracture management all require the common inputs of operating theatres, surgical instruments, anesthesia services, central sterilization, blood bank, radiology, and laboratory, among other components. For this reason, "surgical care" in global surgery often refers to not only surgical specialties but also obstetric and anesthesia care, bundled together as "SOA care".
- Secondly, improving surgical outcomes requires not only individual hospitals but the entire health system at the **national and subnational levels**. It requires functioning interconnection between facilities at the different levels, such as pre-hospital transport, referral systems, and telecommunication systems.
- Thirdly, scaling up safe and affordable surgical care has enormous potential to **improve health outcomes** and **financial risk protection**. Surgical care is critical to achieving the Sustainable Development Goals (SDG), particularly SDG target 3.1 of reducing the global maternal mortality ratio to less than 70 per 100,000 live births [8]. 3.7 billion people are estimated to be at risk of catastrophic expenditure due to surgical care. Improving the access and affordability of surgical care could reduce the financial risk incurred in seeking surgical care [1].
- Lastly, improving health system components involved in delivering surgical care could address **health system operational constraints**. Curative hospital-based care has traditionally been underdeveloped in LMICs due to the focus on infectious diseases and vertical programs on the global health agenda. As such, strengthening health services for surgical care could improve the outcome of a range of services beyond surgical care, such as emergency care and intensive care.

The indispensable role of surgical care in health system strengthening toward achieving universal health coverage (UHC) has been recognized by World Health Assembly (WHA) resolution 68.15 [9]. More recently, during the COVID-19 pandemic, the versatility of surgical systems has become apparent as surgical operating theatres, human resources, and supply chains provided critical surge capacity for pandemic preparedness not only in LMICs, but also in HICs.

Improving surgical services could contribute significantly to health system strengthening. Therefore, we defined surgical system strengthening as the strengthening of health system components required to deliver SOA care, which in turn, should improve the outcome of diseases requiring treatment by SOA care.

Key Steps in Surgical System Strengthening

Similar to health system strengthening, surgical system strengthening has become a buzzword in recent years. Some initiatives labeled as surgical system strengthening are, in fact, vertical, based in single facilities, and target micro-level behavioral changes of individual clinicians without taking a system-based approach. Prior to the advent of the field of global surgery, health system support activities for individual building blocks, such as equipment donation and teaching, have already been occurring through surgical missions for decades. Efforts that truly strengthen and not just support surgical systems must have sustainable, long-term impact. Despite increasing recognition of the importance of surgical system strengthening, its optimal method remains undefined [10]. There is a need for more studies to evaluate the impact of surgical system strengthening initiatives. As the focus of global surgery shifts from health system support activities delivered by visiting surgeons to strengthening surgical care systems in LMICs, it must be led by LMICs. A criticism of health system strengthening is that it can remain donor-led and donor-defined, similar to the vertical infectious disease-focused programs from which it is trying to distinguish itself [11]. In this vein, health system strengthening reflects a mere shift in donor agenda rather than a fundamental shift in the power of priority-setting from external parties to the countries. Surgical system strengthening interventions must be locally contextualized to address the most critical health system constraint in each country or sub-national region.

We highlight several steps to consider in surgical system strengthening. This provides a **guidance** rather than a prescription and should be tailored to country-specific contexts.

Securing Political Commitment

Securing political commitment is a prerequisite for surgical system strengthening due to the historically low priority of surgery on the global health agenda. While surgical system support activities have occurred in decentralized settings around the world through surgical missions, charity hospitals, and humanitarian assistance, surgery has been the "neglected stepchild of global health" on the agenda of the WHO and major global health funder [12].

In recent years, advocacy and diplomacy by the global surgery community have elevated the position of surgery on the global health agenda. Globally, the WHA resolution 68.15 recognized emergency and essential surgery as a critical component of UHC in 2015 [9]. Similar regional resolutions were passed by the Southern African Development Community in 2018 and at the Pacific Health Ministers Meeting in 2019 [13]. In 2020, Member States of WHO Western Pacific Region unanimously endorsed the ***Action Framework for Safe and Affordable Surgery in the Western Pacific Region (2021–2030)*** at the seventy-first Regional Committee Meeting [14]. Nationally, nine countries have made political commitments through developing national strategic plans for SOA care, and many more countries are in the process of doing so.

Political commitment at the national level has been generated through a mixture of international diffusion of global and regional commitments, top-down leadership, and bottom-up mobilization. The leadership of surgeons who hold key positions in governments and Ministries of Health has resulted in high-level political commitments by a number of countries. In other countries, the mobilization and advocacy of SOA providers and non-government organizations have exerted bottom-up pressure on governments leading to the agenda adoption of surgical system strengthening.

Conducting Health System Assessments

Once the political commitment has been secured, surgical system strengthening could begin with an analysis of health system capacity, gaps, and opportunities for SOA care provision. This could include a literature review, quantitative facility assessment, and qualitative stakeholder interviews. Chapter 7 is devoted to the summary of the various approaches and to the methodologies of conducting such assessments.

A quantitative surgical assessment tool (SAT) has been developed by the WHO in conjunction with the Program in Global Surgery and Social Change (PGSSC) at Harvard Medical School [15]. This covers all six building blocks of the health system. Data is collected through a hospital walkthrough, a review of operating room logbooks, and admission and discharge records. A criticism of this tool is that it is focused on inputs and outputs without paying attention to the interaction between building blocks, critical points of operational constraint, population health needs, and the outcome of surgical care. More in-depth facility assessments could be developed to suit country-specific contexts (see Chap. 7).

Qualitative stakeholder interviews could supplement the quantitative SAT. These could qualitatively explore the dynamic interaction between inputs, critical system constraints, and the process that converts inputs to outputs and outcomes in more depth. Not only do the interviews serve as a means of obtaining information, but they also provide an opportunity to engage and mobilize stakeholders.

A review of the literature could shed light on the population's health needs in terms of the burden of surgically treated diseases and the country's social, political, economic, and cultural context. In addition to the academic literature, a review of the grey literature and policy documents could provide information on existing initiatives, upon which surgical system strengthening interventions can build.

Priority Setting and Planning

A comprehensive national strategic plan for surgical system strengthening could be developed within which individual surgical system strengthening activities nestle. Strategic planning is useful for surgical system strengthening for a number of reasons. A plan could (1) secure ongoing political commitment, (2) guide coordinated resource allocation to reduce fragmentation, and (3) provide a long-term vision for sustainable impact.

Several frameworks could guide strategic planning for surgical system strengthening, including the National Surgical, Obstetric, and Anesthesia Plan (NSOAP) framework developed by the PGSSC and the WHO ***Regional Action Framework for Safe and Affordable Surgery***, tailored to the Western Pacific context [14, 16].

The planning process involves several components.

1. A policy direction: vision- and priority-setting of the package of SOA care that should be available at different levels of health facility on a five- to ten-year time scale.
2. A strategic plan: the development of a set of strategies based on the analysis of key health system gaps and opportunities for improvement to realize the broad policy direction.
3. An operational plan: in conjunction with a long-term national strategic plan, an operational plan should be developed in order to translate the long-term strategy into shorter-term implementation.

Having a strategic plan does not automatically result in the strengthening of surgical systems. The plan must be translated into action. Strategic plans are at risk of isomorphic mimicry. A country might mimic other successful countries and devise a plan that looks good on the shelf but does not translate well into action [17]. Attention is paid to appearance rather than function. "Looks like" substitutes for "does". Two strategies are essential in countering the risk of isomorphic mimicry: developing a short-term operational plan and bottom-up, inclusive, and genuine stakeholder engagement. The strategic plan must be co-created with the people who will implement it [18]. A deliberative priority-setting process is critical in ensuring that the priorities reflect the needs of the population and have the buy-in of stakeholders.

Designing and Implementing Locally Contextualized Interventions

The strategic plan must be supplemented with short-term actions. According to Kotter's eight-step model for leading change, the generation of short-term wins could (1) aid plan implementation, (2) mobilize and empower stakeholders, and (3) make changes stick [19] (Fig. 5.2). As a part of the strategic planning process, two to five areas of critical health system constraint could be selected for targeted short- to medium-term interventions.

Table 5.1 lists some examples of existing and possible interventions by health system component. This list is by no means exhaustive and should not be interpreted as a laundry list. It merely provides ideas for possible surgical system strengthening interventions. Many initiatives introduced by visiting HIC surgeons default to teaching and checklist use, as these health system gaps tend to be the most visible to them. However, these interventions target individual clinician behavior at the micro-level and do not address system-level deficits. Longer-term workforce development initiatives that have evolved from short-term teaching constitute some of the earliest surgical system strengthening efforts. Health system gaps, such as biomedical engineering, sterilization services, or waste management, might not be as familiar to visiting surgeons who are used to operating in health systems where these components are well-functioning. However, these components can be equally deserving of

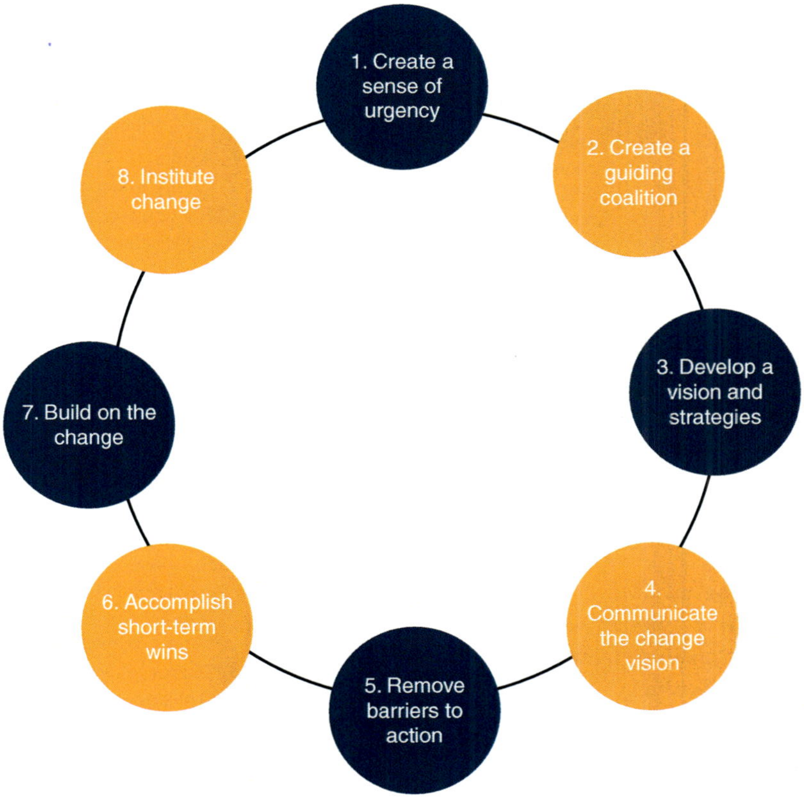

Fig. 5.2 The Kotter eight-step model for leading change [20]

Table 5.1 Surgical system strengthening interventions by health system building block

Health system building block	Surgical system strengthening interventions
Infrastructure	Refurbishing operating room, recovery room, and critical care space and patient flow Strengthening surgical equipment and consumable procurement Streamlining supply chains Improving central sterilization services Strengthening biomedical engineering Surgical instrument innovation and development by LMICs
Workforce	Workforce training and planning Task-shifting
Service delivery	Telemedicine Early diagnosis and screening (e.g., cervical and breast cancer screening) Service delivery redesign (e.g., outreach, regionalization of services) Strengthening emergency and mass casualty response Improving referral pathways
Information management	Registry development Research capacity building Incorporation of LCoGS indicators into routine health indicators
Finance	Developing a social insurance scheme with coverage of surgical care Improving the efficiency of surgical care delivery to reduce cost Developing a mechanism to assist patients with financial recovery post-surgery
Governance	Guidelines and accreditation standards for surgical care Creation of ministerial advisory committees or focal persons for surgical care

attention as workforce development in LMICs. Therefore, global surgery practitioners should stretch our imagination and heed close attention to local health system needs to identify the most critical intervention. Ultimately, the optimal intervention should be selected and designed with the country-specific context in mind.

This categorization in Table 5.1 merely indicates the predominant health system component under which interventions fall. It does not intend to unnecessarily fragment the health system and underplay the interaction between components. In fact, each intervention requires the coordination of several health system components. For example, task-shifting would require not only workforce training but also sound policy and guideline development to delineate the scope of practice of healthcare professionals of different cadres.

Monitoring and Evaluation

Lastly, the impact of surgical system interventions should be monitored and evaluated. At the system level, the LCoGS indicators on timely access, surgical workforce density, surgical volume, perioperative mortality rate, and financial risk protection should be incorporated into routinely reported national health indicators (Table 5.2). In addition, other indicators may be

Table 5.2 Lancet commission on global surgery indicators [1]

Indicator	Target by 2030
1. Access to timely essential surgery – The percentage of the population that can access, within 2 hours, a facility capable of providing bellwether procedures (caesarean section, laparotomy, and open fracture management)	80%
2. Specialist surgical workforce density – Number of surgical, anesthesia, and obstetric specialists per 100,000 people	20
3. Surgical volume – Procedures performed in an operating theatre per 100,000 population per year	5000
4. Perioperative mortality – All-cause death rate before discharge in patients who have undergone a procedure in an operating theatre	Monitored
5. **% risk of** ***catastrophic out-of-pocket expenditure**** on surgical care	0%
6. **% risk of** ***impoverishment due to out-of-pocket expenditure***** on surgical care	0%

required to track the performance of specific surgical system interventions, such as surgical consumable stockout rate or surgical site infection rate, and the outcome of key surgically treated conditions, such as maternal mortality and cervical cancer mortality.

Developing a Toolkit for Surgical System Strengthening

Health system strengthening has not been traditionally covered by medical education and surgical residency. How can surgeons equip themselves with the knowledge and skills necessary to strengthen surgical systems?

Although surgeons from HICs have played a leading role in visiting teams and teaching, surgical system strengthening activities must be led by practitioners from LMICs. Therefore, this chapter is intended as much for LMIC practitioners as it is for HIC practitioners. HIC practitioners should play a supportive role in surgical system strengthening in LMICs. However, attention must be paid to protecting local ownership and autonomy and to ensuring this supporting role does not transform into a leading one. For example, if HIC partners were to assist with health system assessment, they must be careful to use the data collected to assist LMIC stakeholders to set priorities rather than to do so on their behalf. In carrying out surgical system strengthening activities, explicit attention should be paid to enhancing local capacity for implementation rather than to creating parallel systems that drain from it.

Health system strengthening is new to HIC and LMIC surgeons alike. Although HIC visiting surgeons may be the expert in teaching and performing specialized operations, they are not necessarily experts in surgical system strengthening. HIC surgeons are used to operating in well-functioning health systems where they might not have an appreciation of all the components that go into surgical care beyond the operating theatre, such as equipment innovation and design, sterilization, and biomedical engineering. LMIC surgeons, urged by their resource constraint environment, often have a much more expansive view of health systems than HIC surgeons.

Surgical systems in LMICs, though under-equipped compared to surgical systems in HICs, should not be a direct translation of HIC surgical systems. The flaws of some HIC surgical systems should also be recognized. For example, the health system in the United States is known to be fragmented, inefficient, and high cost, with inadequate focus on community and primary care, compared to some other HICs. Therefore, a critical awareness of the limitations of one's knowledge and experience and constant self-reflection are essential to surgical system strengthening.

Surgical system strengthening requires the knowledge of health systems and health policy, skills in advocacy and diplomacy, an understanding of local context, and the building of coalitions. In order for surgeons to gain an understanding of **health systems and health policy**, they must expand their training beyond the traditional academic surgery disciplines of epidemiology and biostatics into economics, political science, sociology, and anthropology. This knowledge could be developed through formal postgraduate training, such as a Masters of Public Health with health policy or health system as concentrations. Outside formal degree programs, there are many opportunities to develop an understanding of health systems by attending short courses and reading key publications. Health systems and policy publications could be introduced to the journal club of academic surgery units, in addition to clinical epidemiology studies that are commonly discussed.

Skills in advocacy, policy, and diplomacy are best learned by practice rather than from textbooks. Although these skills are relatively new to global surgery, fortunately, there is much that the global surgery community could learn from advocacy efforts towards other global health priorities, such as HIV/AIDS, tobacco control, and climate change. Advocacy and policy workshops of even a few hours in duration could be highly effective. One could start small and practice honing these skills by setting up meetings with political representatives, organizing a public rally for surgical care, and writing press releases.

An understanding of local **political, social, economic, cultural, and historical context** is implicit for LMIC practitioners leading surgical system strengthening efforts in their countries. However, the same cannot be assumed for HIC practitioners who may be invited to play a supportive role in these activities. HIC practitioners must develop a nuanced understanding of the context of the country and the health system by dedicating time to background reading and research. They need to always maintain a supportive, and not a leading position in discussions and negotiations.

Surgeons in HIC often work within the siloes of their specialty. However, **coalition building** is essential to surgical system strengthening. Coalitions should be built with other existing global health agendas, such as maternal and child health and cancer control. Although surgeons in HICs are frequently only exposed to secondary and tertiary care settings, strengthening the interface with primary and community care to build systems for early screening and detection, referral and follow-up, and the performance of minor procedures is critical in global health.

Future Directions for Surgical System Strengthening

Despite the exciting momentum that has been built for surgical system strengthening in the last decade, it is still a relatively new and underdeveloped field. The global surgery movement so far has been largely driven by the passion of individual clinicians. Going forward, there should be greater collaborative organization and engagement with communities and patients as co-producers of health. Surgical system strengthening needs to look beyond the health sector and build inter-sectoral collaboration with entities such as transport infrastructure, water engineering, waste management, and pandemic and disaster response, to list only a few examples.

There needs to be research to document and share innovations from around the world for surgical system strengthening from LMICs and to generate an inventory of evidence-based surgical system strengthening interventions to serve as examples and teaching tools.

Ultimately, surgical system strengthening must improve not only the health system capacity for surgical care but also the outcome of surgically treated diseases. As surgical care rises in prominence in the global health agenda, not only surgical care must be upheld, but all neglected areas of services that contribute to the treatment of surgically treated diseases.

Conclusion

Surgical system strengthening looks beyond clinical service provision and teaching by individual surgeons toward making permanent improvements in the health system that delivers surgical care. Surgical system strengthening activities must cross-cut disease areas and health system components, have a scope beyond a single facility, and create sustainable, long-term impact. Steps involved in surgical system strengthening may include obtaining political commitment, conducting health system assessment, developing priorities and plans, designing and implementing targeted interventions, and monitoring and evaluation. Surgical system strengthening requires not only clinical operative and teaching skills but also a knowledge of health systems, health policy, and local social, political, economic, and cultural context, as well as skills in advocacy, policy, diplomacy, and coalition building. Efforts to strengthen surgical care capacity in LMICs must be led by in-country global surgery practitioners. Surgical system strengthening is the next necessary step in global surgery going forward and has a major and significant potential to create equitable, sustainable, long-term impact in improving the outcome of surgically treated diseases.

References

1. Meara JG, Leather AJM, Hagander L, Alkire BC, Alonso N, Ameh EA, et al. Global Surgery 2030: evidence and solutions for achieving health, welfare, and economic development. Lancet. 2015;386(9993):569–624.

2. World Health Organization. Monitoring the building blocks of health systems: a handbook of indicators and their measurement strategies. Geneva: World Health Organization; 2010.
3. Frenk J. The global health system: strengthening national health systems as the next step for global progress. PLoS Med. 2010;7(1):e1000089.
4. Sheikh K, Gilson L, Agyepong IA, Hanson K, Ssengooba F, Bennett S. Building the field of health policy and systems research: framing the questions. PLoS Med. 2011;8(8):e1001073.
5. World Health Organization. Everybody's business - strengthening health systems to improve health outcomes: WHO's framework for action. Geneva: World Health Organization; 2007.
6. Chee G, Pielemeier N, Lion A, Connor C. Why differentiating between health system support and health system strengthening is needed. Int J Health Plann Manage. 2013;28(1):85–94.
7. Witter S, Palmer N, Balabanova D, Mounier-Jack S, Martineau T, Klicpera A, et al. Health system strengthening—Reflections on its meaning, assessment, and our state of knowledge. Int J Health Plann Manage. 2019;34(4):e1980–9.
8. Roa L, Jumbam DT, Makasa E, Meara JG. Global surgery and the sustainable development goals. Br J Surg. 2019;106(2):e44–52.
9. WHO. WHA 68.15: strengthening emergency and essential surgical care and anaesthesia as a component of universal health coverage. Geneva: World Health Organization; 2015.
10. deVries CR, Rosenberg JS. Global surgical ecosystems: a need for systems strengthening. Ann Glob Health. 2016;82(4):605–13.
11. Swanson RC, Atun R, Best A, Betigeri A, de Campos F, Chunharas S, et al. Strengthening health systems in low-income countries by enhancing organizational capacities and improving institutions. Glob Health. 2015;11(1):5.
12. Farmer PE, Kim JY. Surgery and global health: a view from beyond the OR. World J Surg. 2008;32(4):533–6.
13. WHO. Outcomes of the thirteenth pacific health ministers meeting. Tahiti: World Health Organization; 2019.
14. World Health Organization regional office for the Western Pacific. Action framework for safe and affordable surgery in the Western Pacific region: 2021–2030. Manila; 2021. Report No.: CC BY-NC-SA 3.0 IGO.
15. Lin Y, Raykar NP, Saluja S, Mukhopadhyay S, Sharma S, Frett B, et al. Identifying essential components of surgical care delivery through quality improvement: an updated surgical assessment tool. Int J Surg. 2020;1(82):103–7.
16. UNITAR. National surgical, obstetric, and anesthesia planning manual. Geneva. United Nations Institute for Training and Research (UNITAR); 2020.
17. Andrews M, Pritchett L, Woolcock M. Looking like a state: the seduction of isomorphic mimicry. In: Building state capability. Oxford: Oxford University Press; 2017. [cited 2022 Mar 16]. https://oxford.universitypressscholarship.com/10.1093/acprof:oso/9780198747482.001.0001/acprof-9780198747482-chapter-3.
18. World Health Organization. Strategizing national health in the twenty-first century: a handbook. Geneva: World Health Organization; 2016.
19. Kotter JP. Leading change, with a new preface by the author. 1R ed. Boston, MA: Harvard Business Review Press; 2012. p. 208.
20. The 8-step process for leading change | Dr. John Kotter [Internet]. Kotter. [cited 2022 Jun 25]. https://www.kotterinc.com/8-step-process-for-leading-change/

How to Do Surgical Needs Assessments: Where to Start, How to Do It, and What to Keep in Mind

6

Reinou S. Groen, K. Gianaris, and M. Lamine Gueye

We are here to add what we can to life, not to get what we can from life.

– William Osler

Abbreviations

DALYs	Disability-Adjusted Life Years
EaCC	Emergency and Critical Care
ERQI	Education/Research/Quality Improvement
GT-SET	Global Trauma System Evaluation Tool
INTACT	International Assessment of Capacity for Trauma
LMICs	Low- and Middle-Income Countries
MoH	Ministry of Health
NGO	Non-Governmental Organization
NPCs	Non-Physician Clinicians
NTDs	Neural Tube Defects
PIPES	Personnel, Infrastructure, Procedures, Equipment, and Supplies
SOS	Surgeons OverSeas
SOSAS	Surgeon OverSeas Assessment of Surgical Needs
TSAAEESC	Tool Situational Analysis to Assess Emergency and Essential Surgical Care

R. S. Groen (✉)
Department of Gynecology and Obstetrics, Johns Hopkins Hospital, Baltimore, MD, USA

Department of Obstetrics and Gynecology, Alaska Native Medical Center, Anchorage, AK, USA
e-mail: rgroen@southcentralfoundation.com

K. Gianaris
Indiana University School of Medicine, Indianapolis, IN, USA
e-mail: kgianari@iu.edu

M. L. Gueye
Department of Surgery, Cheikh Anta Diop University, Aristide Le Dantec Teaching Hospital, Dakar, Senegal

Introduction

Initiation of a surgical program starts with a **surgical needs assessment**: what is already available, what is additionally required, and what is optimally desired by the stakeholders of the surgical program. There are a variety of ways to approach this, and different methods to achieve it. The type of assessment will depend on the mission, goals, and opportunities of the investigators. Many types of research strategies can be used to conduct surgical needs assessments and to study surgical epidemiology. In this chapter we discuss which frameworks to use for surgical needs assessment, the research methodologies for stud-

M. A. Hardy, B. R. Hochman (eds.), *Global Surgery*, https://doi.org/10.1007/978-3-031-28127-3_6

ies of surgical epidemiology, and the quality assurance of surgical programs.

What Is Surgical Care? What Is "Surgical Need"?

Surgery can be defined as the branch of medical practice that treats or diagnoses injuries, diseases, and deformities by physical removal, repair, or adjustment of organs and tissues, often involving incisions in the body.

At the simplest level, the surgical need is the requirement by the patients for operative interventions minus the access that the patients have to such surgical interventions. Surgical needs are determined by the prevalence of surgically treatable conditions in a specific population and vary according to its demographics. These include age, sex, genetics, and environmental exposures. The access to surgical care is generally influenced by the ease and ability to reach it and to receive it and is also determined by many factors discussed in detail later in this chapter.

Initiation of Surgical Needs Research

Local Leadership and Expertise

The initiation of a surgical needs assessment should begin by discussions with the local medical professionals and by optimal awareness of the existing issues. It is critical for the assessors to thoroughly understand the local medical and socio-cultural situation, to avoid duplicating previous work or to pursue projects which are impossible to achieve in that setting. The local medical professionals have the greatest experience and expertise to assist in the most effective assessment of the surgical needs in the area.

Open Mind – An Approach Beyond the Operating Room

While investigating surgical needs, it is important to approach the situation with an open mind. Limiting factors for access to surgical care may include both surgical staff limitations and also limitations of access to the operating rooms.

Assessment and data collection tools are needed to obtain data-driven responses. Most often, a mixed-methods approach which combines both qualitative and quantitative data may be most effective to evaluate the intended programs. Quantitative and qualitative research have a symbiotic relationship where the progress of one drives the studies on the other. To develop quantitative tools for a given population, precedent qualitative research may be needed to formulate the questions and to better design the quantitative tools. For example, focus group discussions on healthcare costs may facilitate the development of a more relevant quantitative survey on how people in a specific community pay for their health care. Once a quantitative tool is developed and employed, qualitative research can help to emphasize pertinent findings and provide appropriate conclusions. An example of this is when through a quantitative study it is found that few men undergo vasectomies while qualitative studies indicate that many wish to no longer father children. A follow-up qualitative study could then explain why this effective surgery is not accepted more widely. The combination of these two methods and continued monitoring can create the most powerful data for decision-making.

Beyond Treatment

Finding ways to avoid operations and initiate early non-operative treatment may be more challenging and effective than implementing complicated surgical interventions. To maintain an open mind permits one to avoid a limited impact due to unrecognized external factors. An example of an open-minded approach which led to innovative solutions is the effort to reduce the global incidence of neural tube defects. When neurosurgeons noticed that increased folic acid intake by women in reproductive age groups prevented neural tube defects (NTDs) in 92% of newborns, it was found that the operation was no longer needed [1]. Most developed countries have now adopted mandatory folic acid fortification of many processed foods to reduce the incidence of NTDs. In this case, prevention is relatively simple and effective for most patients while surgical treatment is now rare except in some lower and middle-income countries (LMICs). It is the prerogative of neurosurgeons to advocate for systemic change to target the prevention of a surgical disease and free resources for other neurosurgical interventions.

Similar efforts have been undertaken in the field of road traffic accidents. Charles Mock and others argue that targeting preventative safety measures for the massive burden of road traffic incidents is critical to reduce death, disability, and healthcare burdens [2]. Unintentional injuries comprise a massive number of deaths worldwide, and these injuries disproportionately affect LMICs when accounting for age-standardization. Many of these risk factors can be targeted, especially in the realm of road traffic accidents, to reduce the burden of trauma surgery and to reduce death and disability. It has become clear that enforcement of specific road traffic laws, like seatbelts and motorcycle helmet requirements, have lower or equal costs per disability-adjusted life years (DALY) than many treatments for infectious diseases that are widely accepted and funded. Again, surgeons can use the power of data and advocacy to make greater impacts outside of the OR.

Biases

As with any research, surgical needs assessments can be highly influenced by cognitive biases. Biases can affect the internal and external validity of a study and must be minimized as much as possible. These biases can affect research at every level: planning, conduct, and analysis [3]. For example, when focusing on the design portion of a study, susceptibility bias must be minimized. Susceptibility bias refers to the fact that certain factors cause patients to be more susceptible to specific disease progressions or to receiving specific treatment options. In study design, this can manifest itself in either selection bias, channeling bias, or chronology bias. For surgical needs assessments, it is important to focus on the most common disease progressions and on treatment availabilities in the studied region. For example, one study in rural Bangladesh found that pregnant women were more likely to use the available health facilities for delivery if there was a complication [4]. Data used from these facilities about Caesarean delivery rates in the community could potentially lead to an overestimation because of susceptibility bias. Randomization, stratification, and controlling for more variables can help minimize such biases.

When conducting a study, information, transfer, and performance biases are most important. Performance bias refers to the differences in the proposed procedures or interventions. Such bias is especially pertinent in surgery where there are variations among surgeons and even among various procedures. When measuring surgical outcomes in a research study, enforcing uniform standards on subjects and on procedures among the comparison groups is necessary to limit skewing of data. This rule extends to all phases of surgical care, both pre-operative and post-discharge. Since there may be dramatic differences in performance among different institutions, it is important to enforce standard protocols or to acknowledge differences when conducting multicenter studies.

To minimize the information bias, uniform procedures and factors of comparison are necessary when conducting any research study. Information bias describes issues causing data inconsistencies which arise from corrupted information or mismatched comparisons. When initiating the Surgeon's OverSeas Assessment of Surgical Needs (SOSAS) survey tool that is discussed later in this chapter, the enumerators conducting the survey were thoroughly trained about the survey and the randomization strategies to minimize the information bias [5]. Information from the pilot study was used in the training and remained available each day to ensure that the randomization and survey tools were used correctly and to troubleshoot as needed. These actions minimized any information bias.

Table 6.1 Pertinent biases in surgical needs assessments

Bias	Description	Ways to limit
Susceptibility	Uncontrolled factors leading a patient to be more susceptible to certain diseases or to receive treatments	Randomization, stratification, increased variable controls
Performance	Differences in the procedure or intervention undertaken	Enforce protocols, control for differences in performance, acknowledge differences
Information	Information is corrupted leading to data inconsistencies	Training research staff to conduct the study uniformly
Optimism	Believing new interventions are superior to old ones leading to distorted analysis	Double blinding
Citation	Citing and referring to sources preferred by the authors	Examining a wide breadth of sources in a systematic way

In the analysis phase, there are two main biases: optimism bias and citation bias. Optimism bias which refers to the idea that new interventions are superior to old ones can influence both participants and researchers. This bias can be prevented by double blinding. Citation bias can take many forms, but it often results from reference to studies that are preferred by the author. This can lead to a distortion of existing facts and can influence the analysis of collected new data to misdirect in a specific direction. Citation bias can be minimized by interfacing with a wide variety of sources in a systematic way that may fit the data in the existing paradigm. This section is summarized in Table 6.1.

Frameworks

This section will discuss several frameworks required for discussion and design of surgical needs assessment and for surgical epidemiological research.

Framework 1: Surgical Measurements and Phases of Surgical Care

Research on surgical needs can be structured along the five phases of surgical care which can all impact the quality of continuum of care given [6]. The five phases consist of the following: (1) Pre-operative; (2) Peri-operative; (3) Intra-operative; (4) Post-operative; and 5) Post-discharge.

The first phase, pre-operative, designates the beginning of the patient's encounter with the surgical team. Depending on the local environment the pre-operative period may begin with the primary care physician's referral or with the local self-referral possibilities. Needs assessments which target this initial phase can examine factors such as patient's understanding when to search for a surgical consultation, referral patterns for surgeons in low resource settings [7], as well as being sufficiently fit to undergo surgery.

The peri-operative phase 2 will start once the need for surgery has been established by the physician and the patient. This includes pre-operative preparation of the patient including optimization of co-morbidities, and logistical preparations including transport and scheduling of surgery. Improvement in this aspect of care can not only facilitate the surgery but can also improve outcomes. Undernutrition in LMICs prior to surgery needs to be corrected prior to operation [8].

The intra-operative phase 3 begins with the initiation of anesthesia and ends with termination of anesthesia and extubation. This phase can be assessed for surgical needs by measuring the following: (1) the operating room set-up; (2) staff (nurses, assistants) availability; (3) instrument availability; (4) anesthesia medication and gases availability, including oxygen: (5) lights, electricity, and water; (6) ventilators. To conduct this line of surgical needs assessment, it is imperative to have an appreciation of different methods of doing similar surgeries. Foreign visitors, some with limited training, may quickly and falsely conclude that specific equipment is missing, since evaluated procedures are performed well by local standards with different instruments (e.g., anastomoses with sutures rather than staples). Deficiencies in medical equipment may be characterized not by lack of availability, but rather by no access to biomedical engineering personnel to maintain it or by lack of parts or specific supplies for their repair [3].

The post-operative phase 4 includes monitoring of the recovery of the patient after surgery, initially in the post-anesthesia care unit (Recovery Room), and afterward in the hospital if indicated. Studies in this area can look into post-operative patient progress, including, for example, wound infection or post-operative fever. Origins of such complications may be system problems that require corrections and should be included in the assessment. These may include locally adapted post-operative provisions, such as mosquito-netting, to prevent postoperative malaria.

In the post-discharge phase 5, the surgeon ideally should follow the patient and treat any complications that may arise. This is not always practical because of distances and lack of roads and transport in LMICs. As many as 50% of the surgical site infections may occur post-discharge [4]. Some can be diagnosed with the use of telemedicine, but the tools for this may not be available [9]. For hand and limb surgery, physical therapy must be an integrated part of improving outcomes. If any significant alteration of diet is indicated after surgery, the post-discharge phase should include follow-up to ensure adherence to instructions. Research in this area could look at readmission rates and long-term outcomes.

Framework 2: The 5As of Access to Health Care

The 5As of access to health care explores the factors that permit patients to participate in the local healthcare system. The concept was pioneered by Penchansky and Thomas in 1981 and includes affordability, availability, accessibility, accommodation, and acceptability [10]. Since its structured approach has evaluated the access from the patient's perspective, a broader idea will also include the 5As from the supply side (Table 6.2).

The first A, Affordability, acknowledges the inherent cost of providing health care and stimulates discussion about the potential ways to decrease these costs. It considers the cost of services for both the provider and for the patient, including the latter's ability and willingness to pay. This has been recently one of the hottest issues of debate in global surgery, although there is ample evidence that surgery is not only essential but can be very cost-effective [11]. However, it requires special planning to ensure that surgery can be performed at a price that the local population can afford and is willing to pay. It is important to ensure that local

Table 6.2 Five A's of access to surgical care (modified from Ref. [10])

Demand side		Supply side
Cost for procedure	Affordability	Reimbursement for work
Volume and type of physicians, facilities, and specialized services that the patient may access	Availability	Number of surgical staff available, cost of specialized equipment or building more centers
Patient can physically reach the healthcare services, including the transportation and transportation costs	Accessibility	Maximal catchment areas for healthcare services, convenience of transportation for the staff
Patient can receive surgery at convenient times with minimal barriers, includes walk-in clinics, telephone services	Accommodation	Surgical staff has structure to their work life and is not overbooked/overworked
Patient accepts the type of care proposed and accepts the intangible qualities of the provider including race, gender, age	Acceptability	Provider accepts the type of procedures that need to be performed and the intangible qualities of the patient, including race, gender, age, etc.

surgical care is more affordable than traveling to obtain equal or superior surgical care in a different area or country. To achieve the best affordability, it may require collaboration among the hospital, the administrators, and the community to either reduce costs at the healthcare level or increase the payment capacity at the community level.

The second A, Availability, describes the ability of the health system to provide to the patient the necessary components of health care in a timely fashion. Availability is heavily contingent on personnel, infrastructure, procedures, equipment, supplies, and established standards for pre-hospital, intra-hospital, and post-hospital settings. To facilitate this aspect of organizing surgical care, a matrix called the personnel, infrastructure, procedures, equipment, supplies, and standards (PIPESS) tool was developed to assess surgical capacity based on 108 variables [12]. This tool is designed to evaluate and compare the differences in care being provided by both local and international organizations. This tool facilitates planning by delineating the complexity and magnitude of needs contextually in relation to specific points in time, location, and scope. When conducting a surgical needs assessment with the goal of establishing a surgical partnership, a cogent place to start is to first examine the current availability and then to define goals for the desired level of availability.

The third A, Accessibility, differs from availability by defining the location of the medical services in relation to the local population base. Surgical care should be imminently accessible to the local population. A state-of-the-art healthcare facility that is impossible to access for the majority of the population does not meet surgical needs. Climate changes and transportation are important considerations in this regard. It is critical to understand these issues in the local context to provide adequate accessibility. Geospatial mapping and determination of updated population estimates will further clarify these problems, especially in countries with highly displaced populations or with new populations of refugees.

The fourth A, Accommodation, refers to the opportunities for patients to stay close to the hospital during their treatments and focuses on patient housing or on affordable hotel accommodations. This also focuses on the local population's understanding of technology. The potential use of tech integration with tele-health depends on the extent of web networks or on reliability of telephone networks.

The fifth A and final, Acceptability, describes the patient's acceptance of the procedure proposed by the surgical team. The patient may differ with the physician regarding the proposed procedure. This view may be based on prior experiences (historical), trauma, cultural beliefs, and family values. These considerations should be respected when surgical procedures are declined by the patient. Acceptability also relates to the more intangible relationships between the patient and the healthcare provider. This may be based on similarities and/or differences between the provider and the patient in their characteristics which may include racial, ethnic, social, gender, and age differences. Research topics in this area include qualitative feedback from a population that receives health care as was required by The United Nations South Sudan Health Cluster for anybody starting healthcare programs [13].

The Levels of Surgical Needs Assessments

As mentioned previously surgical assessments go beyond the operating room. Better understanding of where the assessment falls within the healthcare level provides opportunity for reflection about the means and goals for the assessment. Not all levels need to be addressed in each assessment; however, the different levels provide opportunities for the dissemination of research results and for improvement in the success of the implementation of the surgical program. Table 6.3 outlines the definitions of different levels.

Level 1: The Population (Fig. 6.1)

It may be initially considered counterintuitive to investigate surgical care on the basis of popula-

Table 6.3 Levels of surgical care needs.

I Population level / Public health level:

A. Qualitative research with Focus Group Discussion
B. Public health assessment/household surveys
C. Modelling strategies from HIC to LMICs or modelling procedure ratio
D. Geo-spatial assessment of access to care

II Hospital administration level

A. Personnel
B. Infrastructure
C. Procedures being done (what types and what number)
D. Equipment
E. Supplies

III Capability of surgical procedures

A. Surgeons qualitative feedback
B. Observations of surgical procedures
C. Outcome of surgical procedures
D. Continuing medical education needs and desires
E. OR support staff capabilities

IV Ministry of Health

A. Extrapolation of data
B. Rural vs. Urban health centers
C. Density of Healthcare Staff
D. Disparities in Access within a country

V Global access to surgical care

tion level. General surgery has not been part of a public health issue in the past; however, this viewpoint has been questioned and diminished on the basis of a large body of published population data.

The main goal of population-level healthcare data is to link conglomerated individual needs to to healthcare systems and to the Ministry of Health (MoH), so that appropriate allocation of resources can be given to the surgical components of health care in a timely fashion and without favoritism. This is illustrated in Fig. 6.1.

Qualitative Research

Data from population-level studies can be retrieved in a qualitative or quantitative way with each study method potentiating the understanding of the other (Fig. 6.1).

A qualitative approach allows the researcher to understand the surgical services from the aspects of the 5As and of specific cultural taboos. Collaboration with anthropologists and with other qualitative researchers can enhance the quality of such research. It is however, most

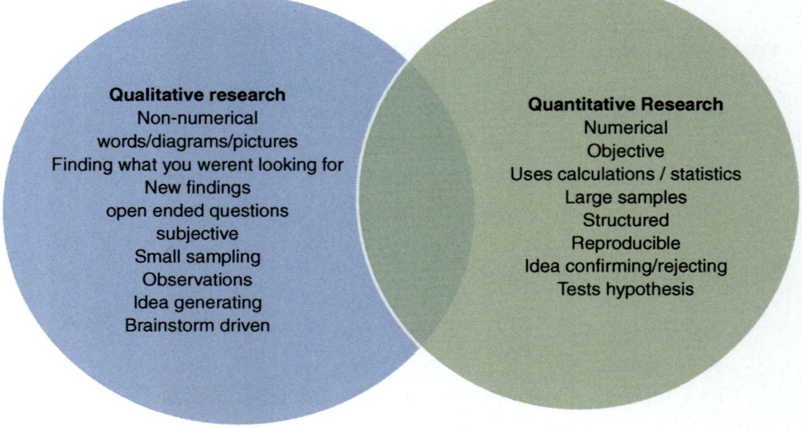

Fig. 6.1 Qualitative vs. quantitative

important that such research be performed impartially and non-judgmentally. Tools for such studies include focus group discussions, interviews, and observations in cities and villages [14], but full explanation of qualitative research is beyond the scope of this chapter.

Qualitative research is used to obtain a more granular understanding of the local population's attitudes and perceptions of health care. While time consuming and work intensive, such research is invaluable in capturing detailed and complex ideas from potential and current beneficiaries of health care. One example of successful qualitative research efforts is to understand local needs via the use of Village Health Committees. Such Committees provide a method of gathering the population in a healthcare catchment area to conduct formal or informal discussions to evaluate how to improve the local health care. To develop a Humanitarian Response Plan for the cluster system in countries where there is a humanitarian disaster, United Nations Office of the Coordination of Humanitarian Affairs (UN OCHA) and the World Health Organization (WHO) recommend performing qualitative research at the population level to ensure that health services are being received by the local community [13]. While this structure has long been recommended for primary health care, the model can be easily applied to the improvement of surgical care. It is best executed when there is local investment in the health services and a long-term relationship with the local community. This is especially critical in rural areas where perceptions of health care may not be easily obtained.

Quantitative Research

Quantitative research on population level will assist to (1) measure the prevalence of diseases that may potentially be treated with surgery, (2) measure and characterize objective barriers to access to surgical care (distance to health care or cost for transportation, etc.).

Sampling Strategies

Population data collection starts with a 5-step process (Fig. 6.2). Each step offers choices and directions, and each step is important for the final statistical analysis and interpretation of the results. Time, monetary, and personnel constraints may be leading factors in the choices that are made.

Qualitative population-based research will depend on sampling methodology since it is not feasible to sample the whole population. The common samplings methods are indicated in Table 6.4.

Probability and non-probability sampling both have their advantages and disadvantages, and the choice of one over the other depends on the question that is raised. Non-probability sampling is more cost-effective and less time-consuming. This is particularly helpful in low-resource set-

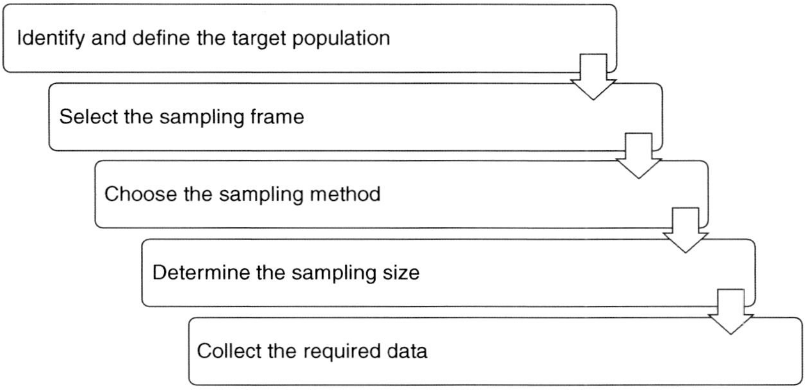

Fig. 6.2 Population data collection process [15]

Table 6.4 Sampling strategies

Probability sampling	Non-probability sampling
Simple/random	Convenience
Systematic	Quota
Stratified	Judgment
Clustered	Snowball

tings where staff and finances are already limited. However, it is important to acknowledge the biases and pitfalls that come with non-probability sampling. Though it may lead to larger sample size and greater validity, it may also introduce substantial selection bias that compromises internal validity. Efforts can be made to minimize this bias by controlling for as many variables as possible, but consequently, the ability to randomize will be limited.

Probability sampling can provide the best randomized and valid data, but it has potential negative effects which include an increased use of resources and longer time while it may lead to a smaller sample size. Ideally, a study which uses probability sampling should obtain a large, random, and representative sample. Selection bias also may occur with probability sampling if subjects that choose to participate differ from those who do not, even if there is random sampling. Probability sampling may be best to gauge the general understanding of the problems or to be able to further extrapolate the data, while non-probability sampling may permit the researchers to reach more specific conclusions and deeper understandings.

Barriers in Population-Based Research

There are many barriers to collecting valid information through population-based research. Time constraints and limited budgets may result in a less thorough sampling strategy. In addition, there are other barriers which may include all the 5As as mentioned above: geographical access to remote or displaced populations, road and weather conditions, cultural barriers or taboos on topics of interest, language barriers, or distrust in enumerators or of people outside of a specific group.

Many barriers can be overcome with thoughtful planning and collaboration with all the stakeholders in the project. Combining the quantitative method development with ongoing qualitative evaluations (expert opinions, focus group discussions, and cognitive interviewing) can also help to overcome the barriers, as can thorough testing of the tools prior to addressing the fully determined sample.

Pre-testing of the survey tool consists of asking the questions or measuring the planned observations on subjects who may not necessarily be part of the target study population. For example, one may try an in-preparation survey on college students rather than on the elderly who are the target study population. This assumes that if college students cannot reply to the questions, it is not likely that the elders will be able to answer them.

After pre-testing and adjusting the tool, a pilot-test needs to be done within the community of interest. This is highly recommended and considered mandatory by the professionals. As indicated in the bible of survey methods: "if you don't have the resources to pilot-test your questionnaire or study, don't do the study" [15].

Level 1: Population-Based Survey Tools

World Health Organization guidelines for conducting community surveys on injuries and violence outlined important considerations for household surveys to gain data on injuries for 2004 [16]. These focus on achieving better estimates of injury burden by looking directly at the population where injuries occur which may not result in hospitalization or a recorded death. In the initial planning of a study local leadership should be involved from the start and an ideal timeline and target population must be identified. The guidelines should include a checklist for the planning of the household surveys. The WHO Guidelines further explain the important aspects of how to design the questionnaire, how to conduct the survey, and how to analyze the data. The importance of quality assurance in fieldwork where the data is collected is emphasized. At this stage, the surveyors must be trained, and each area should have designated supervisors to manage any difficulties that inevitably arise. The guidelines also describe ethical concerns when household surveys are conducted.

These are guidelines rather than defined rules and should be adapted to the surgical questions that the survey tries to answer. They provide a strong framework for a particular topic which requires a measured investment.

Surgeons OverSeas Assessment of Surgical Needs (SOSAS) survey tool developed by their research team [5] was conceived to measure the prevalence of surgical conditions among the population in lower and middle-income settings. The tool initially combined elements from the World Health Organization guidelines for conducting community surveys on injuries and violence with demographic health surveys. It also used elements from other surveys on road traffic incidents, and from questionnaires on maternal, congenital, neoplastic, and infectious surgically treatable disease states. The tool was validated by cognitive interviews of recent African immigrants in the United States and of individuals in Sierra Leone and in the Netherlands. Categories of the survey included demographic data, access, cost, family history, barriers, facilitators, and past medical history of the household.

The initial pilot study was conducted in Sierra Leone by training local medical students to use iPads and go to 5 clusters of 10 households and to interview 100 people using this tool. The high response rate and ease with which the survey was conducted via iPad demonstrated its high usefulness. Part of the success of this initial assessment was due to the use of local students to conduct the door-to-door surveys and gather direct population-level data. Later larger scale uses of the tool were applied in Sierra Leone and then in Nepal, Nigeria, Malawi, Mexico, and several other nations to conduct various studies other than surgical [7]. Further validation has been the finding in Nepal that 94.6% of self-reported conditions were confirmed by physical examination. The tool has been successful in characterizing the unmet surgical needs in many different settings and has helped researchers and surgeons to understand the specifics of the barriers and to overcome them.

Local translators and staff are needed to ensure that there is sensitivity to the local culture when conducting qualitative research, such as focus group discussions or semi-structured interviews. Depending on the context, members from different tribes may not be comfortable speaking candidly with members of other tribes. Similarly, tribal leaders may be disturbed if they feel their voice is not represented. Therefore, it can be helpful to separate groups to obtain the most candid responses. For example, interviewing a women-only group led by a female facilitator may be necessary to properly characterize OBGYN needs among the local women. When interviews are done at the population level, Village Health Committees can be included along with the use of a tool like the SOSAS to gain a granular understanding of population barriers which will unveil novel perceptions of how care is received by the local population.

Extrapolation is done by analysis of a proportion of a small subset of population and expanding it to the larger population of interest. This can be done for a country or an area to estimate the surgical needs globally and to calculate surgical deaths that could have been prevented. It is possible to extrapolate from one population base to another population base. Many times, the data from countries with robust data on surgical procedures could be applied with appropriate modifications to populations who have limited data collection opportunity or expertise. This serves to obtain a global estimation of surgical needs, as described in the introduction of this chapter. This can also be used in reverse, as done in a study which estimated the surgical needs of displaced persons by using the 21 Global Burden of Disease data [17].

Extrapolated studies do not allow for the unique characteristics of subjects in specific clusters. A global approach to a surgical problem also may not allow for a granular local understanding of the issues, nor will it lead to workable solutions. A local approach is necessary to a better understanding of the community and in turn to assist in improvement of a surgical program.

Level 2: Hospital Level

At the hospital level, several tools have been developed and tested [18]. One of the basic tools is the WHO Guidelines for Essential Trauma Care that was developed in 2004 to outline the 11 essential trauma care services that should be available to every injured person worldwide [19]. These guidelines have been used extensively in several LMICs and serve as a useful basic tool for evaluating initial capacity [20]. To further examine trauma surgical care and expand on the WHO Guidelines tool, the Emergency and Critical Care tool (EaCC) was developed and piloted in Tanzania and Sierra Leone [21]. The EaCC tool examined 8 categories that were necessary for emergency and critical care services: infrastructure, human resources, training, drugs, equipment, routines, guidelines, and support services. WHO's Global Initiative for Emergency and Essential Trauma Care developed the tool in 2007 for Situational Analysis to Assess Emergency and Essential Surgical Care (TSAAEESC) [22]. This tool looked at four categories: infrastructure, human resources, interventions, and emergency equipment and supplies and has been piloted in many LMICs. This assessment tool focused on hospital capacity assessments needs improvement and needs to be more streamlined to be manageable.

Surgeons OverSeas (SOS) modified the TSAAEESC tool to create the Personnel, Infrastructure, Procedures, Equipment, and Supplies (PIPES) tool. This tool reduced the number of categories in the survey and simplified the responses [12]. It was piloted in Sierra Leone and since then has been used in many different contexts, including local, whole country, and multi-country assessments. PIPES allows for a delineation of needs based on location, time, and scope allowing for a granular assessment. The PIPES tool has been further modified into a pediatric version, PediPIPES [23].

The Harvard Humanitarian Initiative developed a surgical capacity tool by modifying the TSAAEESC. This tool examines eight aspects of surgical care: access and availability, access to human resources, infrastructure, operating room information, procedures (removed in modification), outcomes, equipment, nongovernmental organization (NGO) involvement, and pharmaceuticals [24]. This tool has been used in a wide variety of contexts as well.

There have been other capacity tools to more specifically examine trauma surgical care. The Global Trauma System Evaluation Tool (GT-SET) was piloted in South Sudan to help establish a military trauma system [25]. GT-SET looks at System Leadership, Access to Care, Initial Resuscitative Care, Acute Injury Care, Rehabilitation, Prevention, and Education/Research/Quality Improvement (ERQI). It goes beyond the hospital level to look at referrals and community-level health care. The International Assessment of Capacity for Trauma (INTACT) tool also examines a system for trauma surgical care and focuses on the surgical capacity of healthcare facilities. It was piloted in Sierra Leone and was compared to the PIPES assessment tool [26]. It was designed to be a simple tool applicable to many settings and useful for assessing trauma surgical capacity from the first patient contact until their discharge.

The hospital-level surgical capacity is one of the rate-limiting steps for surgery and is a necessary target for surgical assessment. Further assessment, reassessment, and progress reports within a system allow for a longitudinal development of clear goals for a surgical system. While the tools referenced above represent some of the most cited hospital surgical capacity tools, they do not include all. There remains a need for more specialty tools as health systems grow in complexity and volume.

Level 3: Availability and Quality of Surgical Procedures

The availability and quality of surgical procedures may appear difficult to evaluate in a systematic way. Many causes can contribute to the outcomes of surgeries, including patients' baseline health, surgical equipment availability, and surgeons training. Specifically for countries where there are no surgical programs, surgeons may have been trained with equipment that is not available to them in their home country [27, 28]. To develop strong surgical programs, improvement of this aspect of surgical assessment is necessary. If a department is large enough for a peer-reviewed quality assurance program this would be preferred. Through such a program, surgical outcomes can be reviewed in a non-punitive way and improvements suggested based on pre-operative management of the patients, renewal of equipment, or surgical continuing medical education. If a department is not large enough to form a robust quality improvement group one must find other options. One method is to qualitatively observe surgical procedures and to qualitatively interview patients as to their satisfaction. This can provide valuable insight into the day-to-day operation of the program and detect deficiencies. A qualitative approach may provide objective insights not previously anticipated or included in a survey. One example of this is an ethnographic case study in Norway at different centers where researchers qualitatively observed surgical procedures followed by in-depth interviews. This was used along with the WHO surgical safety checklist [29]. This study demonstrated the redundancy of certain aspects of the WHO surgical safety checklist and its usefulness. By transferring this framework to LMICs, researchers can gain a greater understanding of the deficiencies. The advantages of WHO safety checklist will complement its use in the conduct of assessment studies [30]. By qualitative interviews of the local surgical teams, this could also be used to minimize performance bias in data collection and to standardize surgical care.

On a quantitative level, researchers can measure verified outcomes that reflect the capability of surgical teams. This comes with advantages and disadvantages as surgical procedures are all different and vary by patient risk factors. Measures such as rate of surgical site infection or 90-day mortality may be useful, but it is important to note that these measures can reflect broader issues such as medication adherence, hospital cleanliness, and patient risk factors. These measures can be non-specific or may reflect problems elsewhere, as in the pharmacy or on the hospital wards, rather than being surgical issues. It is paramount to obtain the greatest internal validity possible when measuring these parameters. The various non-specific data combined with more specific tools can lead to better understanding and improvement in surgical outcomes and safety.

The success of any program is ultimately limited by the capability and education of the involved staff. A survey of surgeons from 22 different countries identified which procedures require greatest surgical proficiency in conditions of a disaster [31]. This shows that to have effective implementation, there need to be effective training programs for the local surgeons. This may focus on systematic training of one procedure such as an inguinal hernia repair. This was done in 16 countries over two years [32]. It started with an initial training assessment and with interval proficiency assessments prior to individual surgeons being paired with regional trainers. Technical proficiency was then rated on a scale of effectiveness. A video assessment 6 months later was evaluated for technical proficiency. Local trainees were given incentives to document surgical outcomes independently. This provides a strong framework for the successful training of surgeons and monitoring of outcomes.

Innovative measures need to be developed to train an adequate surgical workforce. The training of non-physician clinicians (NPCs) to provide perioperative and intraoperative services may offer an opportunity to fill this gap. This has been shown to result in quality care and improved access in sub-Saharan Africa, where this model is widely implemented [33]. Almost half of sub-Saharan African countries use NPCs to perform minor surgical procedures including the majority of Caesarean sections. This model can also be used to fulfill anesthetic and nursing needs. This approach with appropriate evaluation of outcomes permits better and more rapid growth and development of high-quality surgical care which may lead to greater access.

Level 4: Ministry of Health (MOH)

At the level of the MOH, it is important to note that there are various disparities in attitudes, including political, to organization of surgical care within a country. To do this effectively, assessments must be done at many different healthcare centers in different areas, rural and urban, to provide a more granular view of care. To most accurately extrapolate needs and capacity in a country one must examine hospitals at the rural community level, the district level, and the referral center level in different large areas, depending on the size of the country. Because of natural time and resource constraints, it is often impossible to evaluate every healthcare center. Using extrapolation can help the MOH make informed decisions about resource allocation and management as long as racial, economic, and political bias can be avoided.

Level 5: Global Estimations

There have been attempts to broadly estimate surgical need globally. One study in 2010 estimated minimum surgical rate per 100,000 by extrapolating surgical rates of countries with high life expectancies [34]. An estimated 310 million surgical procedures are currently performed globally each year with most being done in North America and in Western Europe. The study concluded that a proposed minimum rate of surgery varies from about 3500 to 6000 per 100,000 people and that the unmet surgical need varies dramatically by region. Direct evaluation by household sampling with physical exams in Rwanda recently found a prevalence of surgical need closer to 12,000 per 100,000, almost twice the 6145 per 100,000 estimated by modeling for East Africa [35]. To achieve more accurate broad estimates to unravel surgical need globally, more accurate local data collection and reporting are needed.

Surgical need can further be assessed from the perspective of DALYs. This has been used to assess the lives saved, however with disabilities rather than only patient survival. This metric measures years lost due to death by a disease or accident, and years lived limited by disability. Using DALYs allows comparison of treatments that result in death to treatments that result in disability. Looking specifically at surgery, Disease Control Priorities for Developing Countries can estimate the DALYs lost due to surgical conditions, such as injury, malignancy, congenital disorders, etc. [36] They estimate that surgically treatable conditions conservatively account for 11.2% of total DALYs lost globally primarily to injuries, congenital malformations, malignancies, obstetric complications, and other surgical conditions. While much of the research has shifted to local needs assessments, these estimations can provide a useful framework for understanding the gaps that continue to exist in surgical access.

Conclusions

Surgical needs assessments can be explored by a variety of approaches and methods. The greater the effort that is invested at the start into the design of a study, the better the data generated by the tools used. It is then more likely such studies will reflect the real issues faced by a population or by a situation and thus suggest most promising solutions. Various tools summarized above can provide powerful data which will lead to greater insights and then to improvement in accessibility and in quality of surgical care. Although there remain many challenges, it is expected that the readers, by following principles outlined in this chapter, can effectively assess surgical care and contribute to the improvements in surgical care world wide.

References

1. Estevez-Ordonez D, Davis MC, Hopson B, et al. Reducing inequities in preventable neural tube defects: the critical and underutilized role of neurosurgical advocacy for folate fortification. Neurosurg Focus. 2018;45(4):E20. https://doi.org/10.3171/2018.7.FOCUS18231.
2. Mock CN, Smith KR, Kobusingye O, et al. Injury prevention and environmental health: key messages from *disease control priorities*. In: Mock CN, Nugent R, Kobusingye O, Smith KR, editors. Injury prevention and environmental health. 3rd ed. Washington, DC: The International Bank for Reconstruction and Development/The World Bank; 2017.
3. Oosting RM, Wauben LSGL, Groen RS, et al. Equipment for essential surgical care in 9 countries across Africa: availability, barriers and need for novel design. Health Technol. 2019;9:269–75. https://doi.org/10.1007/s12553-018-0275-x.
4. McIntyre LK, Warner KJ, Nester TA, Nathens AB. The incidence of post-discharge surgical site infection in the injured patient. J Trauma. 2009;66(2):407–10. https://doi.org/10.1097/TA.0b013e318173f833.
5. Groen RS, Samai M, Petroze RT, Kamara TB, Yambasu SE, Calland JF, Kingham TP, Guterbock TM, Choo B, Kushner AL. Pilot testing of a population-based surgical survey tool in Sierra Leone. World J Surg. 2012;36(4):771–4. https://doi.org/10.1007/s00268-012-1448-9.
6. New approach to surgical measurement: phases of surgical care. American College of Surgeons, American College of Surgeons, https://www.facs.org/advocacy/quality/phases
7. Pittalis C, Brugha R, Gajewski J. Surgical referral systems in low- and middle-income countries: a review of the evidence. PLoS One. 2019;14(9):e0223328. https://doi.org/10.1371/journal.pone.0223328.
8. Sowerbutts AM, Knight SR, Lapitan MCM, et al. A qualitative exploration of nutrition screening, assessment and oral support used in patients undergoing cancer surgery in low- and middle-income countries. Nutrients. 2022;14(4):863. https://doi.org/10.3390/nu14040863.
9. Sandberg CEJ, Knight SR, Qureshi AU, Pathak S. Using telemedicine to diagnose surgical site infections in low- and middle-income countries: systematic review. JMIR Mhealth Uhealth. 2019;7(8):e13309. https://doi.org/10.2196/13309.
10. Penchansky R, Thomas JW. The concept of access: definition and relationship to consumer satisfaction. Med Care. 1981;19(2):127–40. https://doi.org/10.1097/00005650-198102000-00001.
11. Chao TE, Sharma K, Mandigo M, et al. Cost-effectiveness of surgery and its policy implications for global health: a systematic review and analysis. Lancet Glob Health. 2014;2(6):e334–45. https://doi.org/10.1016/S2214-109X(14)70213-X.
12. Groen RS, Kamara TB, Dixon-Cole R, Kwon S, Kingham TP, Kushner AL. A tool and index to assess surgical capacity in low income countries: an initial implementation in Sierra Leone. World J Surg. 2012;36(8):1970–7. https://doi.org/10.1007/s00268-012-1591-3.
13. 2022 Humanitarian Response Plan Guidance. *2022 Humanitarian Response Plan Guidance | Assessment & Analysis Knowledge Management Platform*, UN OCHA, 29 May 2021. https://kmp.hpc.tools/km/2022-humanitarian-response-plan-guidance
14. Groen RS, Sriram VM, Kamara TB, Kushner AL, Blok L. Individual and community perceptions of surgical care in Sierra Leone. Tropical Med Int Health. 2014;19(1):107–16. https://doi.org/10.1111/tmi.12215.
15. Survey methods in multinational, multiregional, and multicultural contexts. Janet Harkness et al. 2010. Jonh Wiley & Sons.
16. World Health Organization guidelines for conducting community surveys on injuries and violence. WHO. 2004. IBSN: ISBN 92 4 154648 4.
17. Gupta S, Groen RS, Kyamanywa P, Ameh EA, Labib M, Clarke DL, Donkor P, Derbew M, Sani R, Kamara TB, Shrestha S, Nwomeh BC, Wren SM, Price RR, Kushner AL. Surgical care needs of low-resource populations: an estimate of the prevalence of surgically treatable conditions and avoidable deaths in 48 countries. Lancet. 2015;385(Suppl 2):S1. https://doi.org/10.1016/S0140-6736(15)60796-6.
18. Zha Y, Stewart B, Lee E, et al. Global estimation of surgical procedures needed for forcibly displaced persons. World J Surg. 2016;40(11):2628–34. https://doi.org/10.1007/s00268-016-3579-x.
19. Mock C, editor. Guidelines for essential trauma care. World Health Organization; 2004.

20. Blair KJ, Paladino L, Shaw PL, Shapiro MB, Nwomeh BC, Swaroop M. Surgical and trauma care in low- and middle-income countries: a review of capacity assessments. J Surg Res. 2017;210:139–51. https://doi.org/10.1016/j.jss.2016.11.005.
21. Baker T, Lugazia E, Eriksen J, Mwafongo V, Irestedt L, Konrad D. Emergency and critical care services in Tanzania: a survey of ten hospitals. BMC Health Serv Res. 2013;13:140. https://doi.org/10.1186/1472-6963-13-140.
22. World Health Organization. Tool for situational analysis to assess emergency and essential surgical care. Geneva: WHO; 2007.
23. Okoye MT, Ameh EA, Kushner AL, Nwomeh BC. A pilot survey of pediatric surgical capacity in West Africa. World J Surg. 2015;39(3):669–76. https://doi.org/10.1007/s00268-014-2868-5.
24. Chao TE, Burdic M, Ganjawalla K, et al. Survey of surgery and anesthesia infrastructure in Ethiopia. World J Surg. 2012;36(11):2545–53. https://doi.org/10.1007/s00268-012-1729-3.
25. Remick KN, Wong EG, Chuot Chep C, et al. Development of a novel global trauma system evaluation tool and initial results of implementation in the Republic of South Sudan. Injury. 2014;45(11):1731–5. https://doi.org/10.1016/j.injury.2014.08.004.
26. Wong EG, Gupta S, Deckelbaum DL, et al. The International Assessment of Capacity for Trauma (INTACT): an index for trauma capacity in low-income countries. J Surg Res. 2014;190(2):522–7. https://doi.org/10.1016/j.jss.2014.01.060.
27. Choy I, Kitto S, Adu-Aryee N, Okrainec A. Barriers to the uptake of laparoscopic surgery in a lower-middle-income country. Surg Endosc. 2013;27(11):4009–15. https://doi.org/10.1007/s00464-013-3019-z.
28. Adamou H, Amadou Magagi I, Adakal O, Doutchi M, Habou O, Boukari M, James Didier L, Sani R. Perioperative management of gastrointestinal surgery in a resource-limited hospital in Niger: cross-sectional study. Ann Med Surg. 2020;13(54):10–5. https://doi.org/10.1016/j.amsu.2020.03.009.
29. Wæhle HV, Haugen AS, Wiig S, Søfteland E, Sevdalis N, Harthug S. How does the WHO surgical safety checklist fit with existing perioperative risk management strategies? An ethnographic study across surgical specialties. BMC Health Serv Res. 2020;20(1):111. https://doi.org/10.1186/s12913-020-4965-5.
30. Eyob B, Boeck MA, FaSiOen P, Cawich S, Kluger MD. Ensuring safe surgical care across resource settings via surgical outcomes data & quality improvement initiatives. Int J Surg. 2019;72S:27–32. https://doi.org/10.1016/j.ijsu.2019.07.036.
31. Wong EG, Razek T, Elsharkawi H, et al. Promoting quality of care in disaster response: a survey of core surgical competencies. Surgery. 2015;158(1):78–84. https://doi.org/10.1016/j.surg.2015.02.011.
32. Wagner JP, Schroeder AD, Espinoza JC, et al. Global outreach using a systematic, competency-based training paradigm for inguinal Hernioplasty. JAMA Surg. 2017;152(1):66–73. https://doi.org/10.1001/jamasurg.2016.3323.
33. Chu K, Rosseel P, Gielis P, Ford N. Surgical task shifting in Sub-Saharan Africa. PLoS Med. 2009;6(5):e1000078. https://doi.org/10.1371/journal.pmed.1000078.
34. Esquivel MM, Molina G, Uribe-Leitz T, et al. Proposed minimum rates of surgery to support desirable health outcomes: an observational study based on three strategies. World J Surg. 2015;39(9):2126–31. https://doi.org/10.1007/s00268-015-3092-7.
35. Maine RG, Linden AF, Riviello R, et al. Prevalence of untreated surgical conditions in rural Rwanda: a population-based cross-sectional study in Burera District. JAMA Surg. 2017;152(12):e174013. https://doi.org/10.1001/jamasurg.2017.4013.
36. Jamison DT, Breman JG, Measham AR, et al., editors. Disease control priorities in developing countries. 2nd ed. Washington, DC: The International Bank for Reconstruction and Development/The World Bank; 2006. https://www.ncbi.nlm.nih.gov/books/NBK11728/. Co-published by Oxford University Press, New York.

How to Build Pediatric Neurosurgical Capacity Practice in Low- and Middle-Income Countries and How to Focus on Treatment of a Neurosurgical Disease

7

Marinus Koning, Jan Koning, and Patricia O'Neill

Nothing great or new can be done without enthusiasm.

– Harvey Cushing

Abbreviations

ANC	antenatal care
ATL	Advance Trauma Life Support
CIC	Clean Intermittent Catheterization
DALYs	disability-adjusted life years
ETV	endoscopic third ventriculostomy
FA	Folic Acid
FIENS	Foundation for International Education in Neurological Surgery
GAPSBiF	Global Alliance for Prevention of Spina Bifida-F (F = folate)
HEW	Health Extension Workers
IFGlobal	International Federation for Spina Bifida and Hydrocephalus
LMICs	low- and middle-income countries
MCM	Myungsung Christian Medical Center
NS	Neurosurgery
NTDs	neural tube defects
RAF	ReachAnother Foundation
SB	spina bifida
SBH	spina bifida and hydrocephalus
VPS	ventriculoperitoneal shunt

Marinus Koning was deceased

M. Koning · P. O'Neill (✉)
ReachAnother Foundation, Bend, OR, USA
e-mail: mkoning@reachanother.org; poneill@reachanother.org

J. Koning
ReachAnother Foundation, Workum, The Netherlands
e-mail: jkoning@reachanother.nl

Background

Spina bifida is a congenital anomaly that is often used as a non-specific term to refer to neural tube defects which are the most common and severe birth defects to affect the human nervous system. As such, they are a significant cause of childhood mortality and disability-adjusted life years (DALYs) globally. Worldwide, it is estimated that there are approximately 300,000 babies born each year with spina bifida (SB) and related defects, resulting in approximately 100,000 deaths and 8.6 million DALYs. Spina bifida and hydrocephalus (SBH), largely caused by *folic acid famine,* is a major public health burden, disproportionally impacting low- and middle-income countries (LMICs). Mortality of

M. A. Hardy, B. R. Hochman (eds.), *Global Surgery*, https://doi.org/10.1007/978-3-031-28127-3_7

children affected by SBH is ten-fold higher than in non-affected children and is highest in LMICs due to limitations in specialized medical and surgical care and, in some, folate deficiency in the diet.

There is an exceptionally high incidence of SBH in Ethiopia. Neurosurgical capacity for treatment is a relatively new development. Exact quantification of the prevalence of SBH is still debated and uncertain, but Dixon estimated that 40,000 pregnancies are affected each year with 10,500 live-born cases [1]. Until 2018, despite knowledge that the problems with SBH were highly significant, there was no information about the actual prevalence of SBH in Ethiopia. Studies published in 2015 and 2018 by Sorri [2], Berihu [3], and Gedafaw [4] determined that SB occurs in 130/10,000 births in Ethiopia which is 26 times the rate seen in the USA where there is universal folic acid food fortification. In Ethiopia the condition contributes 4.5% to neonatal mortality and 6.8% to under age 5 mortality [1]. The 2018 findings led to concern by the WHO, which grew with time, but it was not until 2021 that, for the first time, the word 'epidemic' was used in the context of SB [5].

ReachAnother Foundation (RAF) was organized by the author (MK) and his brother (JK) and started to work in Ethiopia in 2009, after MK noted an extraordinarily high number of cases of infant hydrocephalus. It has since been instrumental in the development of clinical services, both for training neurosurgeons and for improving treatment of SBH. It has also become the focal point and a critical force in development of a national Ethiopian program for food fortification with folic acid in an effort to prevent SBH.

For many years, experience has taught that SBH is not compatible with life in LMICs. As a result, these newborns, and those with disability in general, were seen as cursed by God and ways were sought to "give the baby back to the river god". Even today terminating the baby by active or passive means is considered acceptable, almost regardless of the level of defect.

In the past, SBH has not been on a high priority list for the health care needs in Ethiopia. For example, during a visit, the immediate need at a regional hospital serving 750.000 people was a water well, and an ambulance to transport women with obstructed labor to the hospital. The approach to health care in Ethiopia requires a different way of evaluating needs. Solutions that seem obvious to a visitor frequently do not fit the clinical circumstance, and are not always welcomed by local or regional authorities. However, sustained, close interaction between the interested and innovative visitor and local health care facilities and their leaders eventually results in a satisfactory functional solution.

The Medical Landscape in 2009

To build a new surgical program requires knowledge, dedication, persistence, collaboration, diplomacy, local health care, financial and government support. After obtaining all this and more, such initiatives frequently require much time to achieve their goals.

In 2009 Ethiopia was a very different place compared to 2022.

It was the era when infectious disease, malnutrition, and other maladies consumed the majority of already very scarce health care resources in Ethiopia.

Spending on health care was $16 per person per year (vs $8000 in the US), but by 2019 this was $26 (in 2019 dollars) [6]. There were few physicians of any kind; 1/40.000 pop when in 2004 the Government decided to expand medical education by opening more medical schools. It started 13 new medical schools and, although by 2009 the results had not yet materialized, the strategy was visible and improved markedly by 2021 as evidenced in the Global Surgery report, published in 2015 in the Lancet [7].

Early Experience – 2009 – SBH simply was "not on the radar"

There was no prevalence data and no reliable statistics about SBH in 2009. There was little neurosurgical experience in Ethiopia in 2009 except in the capital city, Addis Ababa, at the Black Lion

University Hospital where a neurosurgical training program was started as a cooperative project between Bergen University in Norway, funded by the Norwegian Peace Corps, and staffed with cooperation of the World Federation for Education in Neurological Surgery (FIENS) [8]. The program was extended to the private Korean Myungsung Christian Medical Center (MCM). The latter had a surgical service which consisted of two Norwegian and three Ethiopian staff surgeons, supplemented by many rotating visiting foreign surgeons in various specialties, including neurosurgeons who operated daily. They also partly supervised the newly developed neurosurgical residency training.

The Birth of an Idea

The environment at MCM was stimulating and cooperative. It welcomed innovation by the visiting surgeons and encouraged them to train the MCM residents. One of the brilliant strategic steps of the Director of MCM was the building of a guest house along with the hospital. This offered free accommodations and was equipped with a wholesome Korean kitchen serving three free meals per day. MCM attracted a worldwide variety of visiting faculty, residents, and students from distinguished academic centers. This stimulating environment permitted and encouraged an exchange of experiences and ideas. Participation in hospital and mobile clinics became an important learning experience for visiting attending and resident surgeons. It encouraged them to better understand the surgical needs of the community within the existing cultural setting. For many, this became a discovery phase which could be then followed by an action plan to intervene in planning of surgical health care delivery in deficient areas such as treatment and follow-up of children with SBH. A parade of young mothers with babies with heads the size of watermelons was a striking picture of profound suffering. Knowing that successful treatment was possible, and realizing that of the few who were operated on, many were too late, one visiting general surgeon (MK) was stimulated to action which eventually led to the first Ethiopian Pediatric Neurosurgical Program. This program is still expanding throughout Ethiopia as Pediatric Neurosurgical Centers of Excellence.

Steps in Establishing the Pediatric Neurosurgical Program

1. *Feasibility of the intervention* is the first step in the process of establishing a new surgical program. At MCM it was obvious that drainage of the hydrocephalus could be accomplished not only by the visiting neurosurgeons, but also by residents and general surgeons. The skill was easily transferable and taught successfully to the local neurosurgical residents. The obvious difficulties were that transport of children with SBH was markedly delayed because of the uninformed parents (and some doctors) who did not think that any help was possible. The delay was compounded by inadequate roads and lack of ambulances or any transportation to bring the children urgently in a timely fashion to the specialists at the hospital.
2. *Consultation with the Government and Regional Health Bureaus*
   SBH was untreatable until the start of the neurosurgery training program. Close cooperation with the neurosurgeons resulted in appropriate surgical services to this very sick pediatric population. Because of financial constraints of the Federal budget, foreign NGO subsidies were and may still be required to make such a program successful. Expansion of the program to other universities has also required this cooperation. The lesson learned is that once collaboration is established, the government should be asked to gradually increase support for the patients, the hospital, and for the staff. Developing these relationships is essential to effectively educate the leaders and involve them in the development process. It is also important to realize that besides the Ministry of Health, many more agencies are required to support proposals for improvement of health care. Patience, collab-

orative effort, and networking are particularly needed if a defect as rare as SBH is. Another obstacle to initiation of treatment for a catastrophic disease like SBH is the fatalism that leads to the mistaken conviction that they "all die". Demonstration that appropriate surgical treatment leads to many satisfactory outcomes will reverse such impressions over time. The idea that surgery for the condition in question is impossible in the designated LMIC is obviously not acceptable. Persistence must dominate all efforts. Appeal to other health departments must dominate the strategic planning. Sometimes all that is needed is one department or hospital leader to advocate for the development of the project; this will then become a model for others. A minimal voluntary effort may already be in place, as there already was for SBH at Addis Ababa University and MCM. This was facilitated by the local Rotary Club (RC), by the International Federation for Spina Bifida and Hydrocephalus (IFGlobal), and by a donor from Norway, all of whom were able to periodically provide the needed shunts to the neurosurgeons. Support from an NGO can improve such efforts.

3. *Initiation of a Hospital Base* for neurosurgical interventions for SBH, required cooperation between the leadership and founders of a hospital that was willing to offer all needed personnel and facilities. Neurosurgery involves many complex procedures, but in Ethiopia, SBH and neurosurgical trauma were the most commonly performed neurosurgical operations [9] and, therefore, the initial focus was on neurosurgery. Educating neurosurgeons was a slow process that was the first major rate-limiting step in creating an SBH program. Once neurosurgical capacity was expanded, other aspects of care needed increased attention. These included more neurosurgeons, pediatricians, anesthesiologists, operating rooms with trained staff, recovery rooms with ventilator support and rehabilitation service. MCM, a private hospital, had both the personnel and the facilities needed and this significantly contributed to the initial effort.
   There was no previous estimate of the prevalence of SBH in Ethiopia. The Norwegian Neurosurgery Residency Director and the author (MK) estimated that each year approximately 2500 Ethiopian babies with hydrocephalus would require operative drainage. The program started with drainage of hydrocephalus on a few babies per week. As more babies with hydrocephalus were shunted (ventriculo-peritoneal (VP)), with the help of visiting neurosurgeons from around the world, and the news spread about the availability of neurosurgical intervention, more cases flooded in. Significant problems with acquisition of VP shunts and surgical equipment reemphasized a clear need for program expansion. In discussions with the senior visiting and local neurosurgeons, it became obvious to the author (MK) that this SBH Program needed a more focused and intense organization and execution and that it needed not only the support of the Ministry of Health, but also a dedicated site with ORs, recovery room and a rehabilitation service, as well as a well-trained neurosurgical and nursing staff. All this was a tall order that required significant financial support and public approval.

4. *How to Focus an Effort on a Sub-Specialty and on Specialists?*
   The first thing that needed to be done after obtaining cooperation from the hospital and the regional health authorities was to initiate an effort focused on the specialty and specialists. This involved contacting any national or international organizations whose interest coincided with the interest in SBH. For shunts, the effort began by contacting the Secretary General of the International Federation for Spina Bifida and Hydrocephalus (IFGlobal) which led to a long-lasting productive cooperation.
   At the same time, a small fundraising video was created by one of the authors (MK) entitled "Ethiopia, the silent tsunami" which was self-explanatory, provoked public interest,

and equated SBH to a tsunami. That led to the establishment of the ReachAnother Foundation (RAF) by the author (MK), his wife and his twin brother (JK), a vascular surgeon in the Netherlands, who has been an active partner in the SBH effort for the last 12 years, to the present time. The Ethiopian neurosurgeons were all motivated to build a new medical specialty in Ethiopia: pediatric neurosurgery. The group collaborated with RAF with its focus on SBH to make the defect much more visible within the medical community, and especially to the government in Ethiopia so as to attract support and new patients. The trainee neurosurgeons embraced the possibility of helping infants with SBH. The neurosurgeons looked to RAF to provide direct financial, administrative, and educational support for SBH treatment and indirect support for their neurosurgical training.

The Early Days of Neurosurgery in Ethiopia

1. *Recruitment of Personnel*
   Since the training program in Neurosurgery was encouraged by regional authorities and initially was based at MCM and Black Lion Hospitals, recruitment on a rotational basis of visiting neurosurgery professors was facilitated by FIENS. RAF was instrumental in bringing other specialist nurses, physicians, and educators. During the next decade, untill 2020, RAF brought more than 200 specialists from 17 different specialties. Among the first recruits were two Dutch physical therapists who helped design an in-service training for hospital nurses that was received with great enthusiasm. All these visitors brought new ideas and solutions that were welcomed by the neurosurgeons as they helped to solve their personnel, equipment, and educational problems. It became apparent that "good ideas" are readily accepted by the Ethiopian partners when they ~~understand and~~ themselves are passionate about a problem, such as SBH in infants, for which they wanted a solution.
2. *Empowering Nurses*
   To make the program functional, it was insufficient to focus only on the neurosurgeons and administrators. The nurses constitute a critical part of a team organized to treat a defect like SBH, or to programmatically treat any other surgical disease. The RAF team organized structured courses for the nurses, such as ATLS, and individual training in intensive care and conscious sedation for endoscopy. The brothers introduced instructions regarding the use of the Ambo bag and of oxygen, and improved postoperative hypothermia by installing space heaters. The nurses learned better and safer techniques of independent patient management and their monitoring, thus assuming their responsibilities with confidence. This empowerment of the nurses helped to make the hospital safer and more welcome to the new SBH program.
3. *Development of Pediatric Neurosurgery*
   As stated above, the neurosurgery training program was started in 2006 by a cooperative agreement between Addis Ababa University and Bergen University in Norway and funded by the Norwegian Peace Corps. FIENS became an active partner in recruiting faculty. The program development has been described by Lund-Johansen [7] and has been evaluated in the African context by Aswfaw [10]. Neurosurgeon density has increased >20-fold from 0.0022 to 0.045 neurosurgeons per 100,000 population between 2006 and 2020. Despite recent progress, the availability of neuroimaging equipment remains inadequate. There are in Ethiopia only 38 computed tomography scanners and 11 magnetic resonance imaging machines for a population of 112.07 million. The geographic distribution of neurosurgical facilities is limited to 12 urban centers [10].
   As Pediatric Neurosurgery developed in the context of the General Neurosurgery Program, it was quickly realized that operations for SBH represented more than 30%of the neurosurgical caseload [11, 12], and when the first

three neurosurgeons had graduated from their residencies in 2012 the Ministry of Health designated Zewditu Memorial Hospital as the new Pediatric Neurosciences facility. It became the site for pediatric neurosurgery training, consistent with RAF's goal of "surgery by Ethiopians for Ethiopians". This specialty designation permitted initiation of surgery "Campaigns" allowing performance of operations during the weekends. That initiative increased utilization of the operating rooms and prompted operative interventions for an additional 10–15 cases per weekend. The partnership between RAF and the hospital has had a far-reaching effect. RAF provided financial support for operating teams as well as equipment and supplies. Shunts for hydrocephalus were provided by Child Help. In 2011 ETV (endoscopic third ventriculostomy) training for one of the neurosurgeons was provided by CURE Neuro in Uganda which also donated an operating endoscope and care coordination assistance. ETV/CPC (Chorionic Plexus Cauterization) was then taught to all residents. The program was evolving thanks to many contributors, mobilized by RAF and by the newly designated pediatric neurosurgery hospital. At first, the operating mortality was 10% using only mask anesthesia. After adding an anesthesiologist, and with continuous process improvement, mortality improved. In 2016, with dedication and experience, a single neurosurgeon operated on 220 patients with SBH with less than 1% mortality. It was soon demonstrated that surgery was possible for patients from even the most remote areas of the country which was one of the original goals of the program.

Paradigm Shift

Since follow-up after surgery was originally inadequate, the neurosurgeons remained pessimistic about the outcomes of their operations for SBH. Since the patients returned only when there was a problem, the surgeons rarely saw those who were doing well, reinforcing their negative attitude. To address this, the ReachAnother Team started a program to make home visits and brought back video footage of children thriving after surgery. This created a paradigm shift among the neurosurgeons. They now visualized their contributions as progress by their young patients from an expectation of near certain death to the possibility of healthy and productive lives.

1. *The Hydrocephalus Campaign.*
   By 2015 the program had operated on 460 patients. At that point the Team made an ambitious 5-year plan to have each of the 25 graduating residents perform approximately 200 SBH surgeries by 2019. This "Hydrocephalus Campaign" calculated a need for 5000 operations for the 25 trainees. This seemingly impossible goal was reached during the next 5 years. To accomplish this RAF raised $250,000 for the Campaign and $750,000 for equipment and supplies to support such progress. As new neurosurgeons populated other university hospitals throughout Ethiopia, RAF continued to support them with supplies and instruments.
2. *Center of Excellence Programs*
   In 2019, with SBH surgical care well established, RAF shifted its focus from training neurosurgeons to improving aftercare and follow-up of post-operative patients.
   The SBH Program, led by the Director of St. Peter's Hospital, in collaboration with RAF, launched the first Center of Excellence Program to get rid of the waiting list. The needs of an SBH multi-specialty care team and the requirements of the training programs were described by RAF in a Memorandum of Understanding between the university and RAF. The goal was to help to develop Programs in 5 Centers of Excellence. It is projected that each of these will provide pediatric neurosurgery for 1,000 children each year. The Center of Excellence programs were expanded and approved for 5 universities by 2022.
3. *Focus on Multi-specialty Aftercare.*
   RAF further expanded the program in 2020 with an extensive Training Program for Pediatric Neurosurgery Medical Professionals. Drawing from many resources,

and in close collaboration with the Children's Hospital of Alabama University SBH Team, RAF created the Ethiopian SBH Team Training Curriculum for pediatric neurosurgery. The program is based on the Spina Bifida Guidelines [13, 14] of the US Spina Bifida Association and is also accepted by IF Global. The training is focused on developing cohesive expert teams that are needed to provide the lifelong care spina bifida patients require. Since late 2020 the training program has been taught at three universities in Ethiopia with very positive results. It is slated to be presented and initiated at 2 more universities in 2022. One of the neurosurgeons commented that "when the nurses know the information presented, they will know more about SBH than anybody else but the neurosurgeons". This is indeed the goal, so that the SBH Team functions as "physician extenders" and can address most of the problems that occur during the follow-up period.

In Ethiopia's Centers of Excellence Programs the caseloads are between 250 and 700 children per year. Management of complications, such as bladder dysfunction, inherent to spina bifida, requires early diagnosis and prompt treatment. This treatment consists of Clean Intermittent Catheterization (CIC) which aims to avoid renal failure and death [15].

Therefore, an important part of the training is focused on CIC and on establishing responsible aftercare to prevent and/or detect urological complications. Most universities have Pediatric Surgeons, who, as part of their specialty, perform the needed urologic procedures.

In the multi-specialty clinics care is patient-centered and value-based; the patients are seen during one hospital visit in the clinic by all needed specialists. To have all specialists come together in the outpatient clinic is a major step forward in program development. Fortunately, as there are now more pediatric surgeons, pediatric orthopedists, and physical therapists, staffing has become more available.

4. *The Need for Pediatric Rehabilitation Service.*

Lack of intensive rehabilitation to address the paralysis attendant to SBH is a major problem for the patients and their families after successful surgery. RAF was fully aware of the pediatric orthopedic disabilities of children with SBH. The CURE Hospital in Ethiopia, which had an orthopedic service with national outreach for many years, has a woefully limited treatment capacity and long waiting lists. Another group, Light of the World, an NGO that works in Ethiopia, also focused on community-based rehabilitation. Both were available in a limited fashion because of the enormous demand on their services and long waiting lists. RAF was eager to help develop additional rehabilitation services dedicated primarily to children with SBH to try to increase access. Through one of its founders (JK), RAF worked with one of the principal Dutch leaders from Nijmegen University who developed a strong Physical Therapy program at Gondar University. In this way RAF helped to develop a master's degree training project for pediatric disability, of which SBH is a major component. The program helped to train a significant number of therapists over the next two years and continues to do so. The physical therapy team has become one of the most important components in one designated specialty hospital and is now expanding to other regions and hospitals.

The brief outline provided above demonstrates a methodical approach on "How to" organize a specific service for a specific problem in a specific relatively small, but very important, population of children. This required hospital, medical, governmental, and popular support in addition to a supervising, organizing, recruiting, and partially funding entity like RAF in collaboration with dedicated leaders.

The program also led to the development of a training program for community health workers in pediatric disability described below.

The Ethiopian government decided to emphasize Rehabilitation as a priority specialty in 2021 and several facilities will come online in the foreseeable future.

Other Significant Considerations in Establishing a Multi-Specialty Treatment Program for SBH

1. *The Problem of the Waiting List.*
   As neurosurgery residents graduated and moved to other regional universities, RAF helped them to establish their practices and to continue their work on SBH. RAF provided equipment and supplies so that they could immediately begin regional SBH programs; these programs promptly acquired a waiting list for babies with SBH which sometimes grew to 500 patients. As expected, this raised many surgical issues and also many critical ethical issues,these concerned fairness in connection with who should get treated first – those waiting the longest or those who were sickest? Should those babies unlikely to survive precede those who had a much better prognosis and who might deteriorate while waiting? Should those who return and needed a second operation have to wait again? Should the rich who could pay precede those who could not? Finally, the biggest question was who should make such life and death decisions. Should it be the doctor, the parents, the government, or the SBH Team? Many of these questions have remained unanswered. As new neurosurgeons populated other university hospitals throughout Ethiopia, RAF continued to support them with supplies and instruments and in discussing these ethical issues.
2. *The Difficulties and the Resistance That Needed To Be Overcome*
   Spina bifida and hydrocephalus are complex conditions that require problem solving at a very high level. The mortality and complications compound the stress. Follow-up calls made by nurses prior to their focused training accentuated the problems and discouraged the nurses. Lack of capacity delayed the needed return to the hospital. As a result of such admission delays, the infants could deteriorate, either at home, or even in the emergency room. This was demoralizing for the patients and for the caregivers. Imparting only strong professional technical knowledge to care for the patients is important, but by itself it proved inadequate for success. It quickly became evident to RAF that to maintain a strong Team that protects its members, the Team must be provided with counseling and crisis intervention.
3. *Health Extension Workers (Also Known as Community Health Workers).*
   Health Extension Workers (HEW) are the de facto primary care providers in Ethiopia. Each HEW cares for approximately 500 families. The Community Health Workers are directed by Regional Health Bureaus.
   While the first SBH program was focused on the Addis Ababa region, the second one was conducted in Bahir Dar in the Northwest of Ethiopia. Focused on public education, it raised awareness of SBH. Besides educating the general population, the training focused on HEW teaching awareness, treatment, and referral of infants with SBH.
   The program also led to the development of a training program for community health workers in pediatric disability, of which spina bifida is a major component. This "module 18" was presented to the Ministry of Health as "Training Module 18" and in 2019 it was added to the national training program for these health workers, vastly increasing access to knowledge.
4. *Patient Education.*
   The extraordinary suffering caused by spina bifida and hydrocephalus is primarily experienced by the families. As a result, the parents have an insatiable hunger for information and treatment plans. Parent organizations perform a critical role in SBH care. RAF helped start such a parent organization in Ethiopia in 2016: HOPE SBH. In response to the need for parent education, RAF created the HOPE SBH Parent Handbook. The handbook is printed in English/Amharic and English/Oromifa. Now in its third printing, it is the unchallenged "bestseller" for SBH care in Ethiopia. Making such tools available will markedly strengthen any new surgical program.

5. *Parent Organization HOPE SBH.*
   Another method to increase visibility and support is to directly utilize patient families as ambassadors. In 2017, RAF helped a mother of an infant with corrected SBH to start the HOPE SBH parent organization and she also created a public and professional awareness of neural tube defects (NTD). The new organization now provides parent support and health education, as well as counseling by experienced parents and professionals. It already provides, and plans to expand, accommodations for patients from distant locations during the process of admission, after surgery, and during follow-up if necessary. The organization now represents 3,000 member families. It is establishing a House of Hope where families can get information and training to better care for their children.

Building Public Awareness of SBH

1. *Working with the Ministry of Health and with Rotary Clubs.*
   In 2016 RAF was introduced to the Director of the St. Peter Specialized Hospital in Addis Ababa. This led to a national campaign for SBH, assisted by the government, and was the serendipitous beginning of a very productive relationship, outlined briefly above, which proved to be pivotal for this first national awareness program of SBH. It also resulted in the advocacy for the use of folic acid as the preventive agent for spina bifida.
2. *Continuing to build public awareness* RAF began working with Rotary Clubs in Addis Ababa and in Oregon in 2017 to implement two Rotary Global Grants for public education, training of HEW, and support for surgical treatment of SBH. The launch of the program brought the interest of the press and other media, including TV, which facilitated recruitment of patients and increased general awareness of SBH, and gradually reduced the stigma associated. After training hundreds of HEW, working with the neurosurgeons, and creating a "buzz" with Radio and TV spots, a needed national discussion about spina bifida and hydrocephalus was generated.
3. *Rotary Clubs* have been a consistent and influential presence in Ethiopia as they are in many other countries. One of the important attributes of Rotary Clubs is their ability to provide access to government and political leadership as well as to other decision makers. Some Rotary members may have a worldwide reach and influence. RAF is working Rotary Clubs worldwide toward *Creating a World Free of Spina Bifida*. It is this type of international effort that can only come after first laying the groundwork for action in a small area, in one country. Once that is achieved, progress can be made more effective by mobilizing and motivating other stakeholders, eventually on an international scale. Ethiopian Rotarians are a valued and indispensable partner.

The Present Urgency for Prevention and Treatment of SBH is Worldwide

Since the initiation of the SBH Program nearly 10,000 children have had operations for SBH. Since then (COVID era of 2 years excluded) public interest in SBH in Ethiopia has exploded and resulted in increased awareness of neurosurgical interventions and greater demand for them. This has most recently resulted in early investment in prevention of SBH with folate (folic acid) and thus avoiding the need for operations in the future.

1. *How to Prevent SBH?*
   The question of prevention always has been foremost in the mind of the scientific community. It was felt that this was fundamentally a public health problem that defied the budgetary capacity of LMICs and of small foundations like RAF.
   In 2013 there was little awareness of the importance of folic acid in the general population [16]. Folic acid (FA) was not new in Ethiopia. In 2004 The World Bank financed distribution of FA, together with iron, to all pregnant women to prevent anemia of preg-

nancy. As many as 76% of women in main cities receive antenatal care (ANC) and most are prescribed folic acid with iron, with an overall compliance of 43% [17], In outlying rural regions this number was much lower. The number of unattended deliveries at home was estimated to be approximately 50% of all deliveries [18]. The fact that folic acid is needed *before* the mother knows she is pregnant is still largely unknown to the general population [19]. Preconceptual use of folic acid in one study was seen to be 1% [20].

To raise awareness of the critical importance of FA for the well being of the Ethiopian population on a national level, RAF provided training sessions to several hundred midwives through the Ethiopian Midwives Association, the primary delivery engine of the country. The neurosurgeons routinely provide prescriptions for FA to all young women during clinic visits, and advise them to take it for the rest of their reproductive years. The compliance with this advice is not known, but likely very low.

2. *A Blood Test to Determine a Woman's Risk of Having a SB Pregnancy?*

A randomized controlled trial in the UK 30 years ago showed that spina bifida is caused by lack of dietary folic acid (FA) [20]. Since then, food fortification by dietary FA in 56 countries worldwide has confirmed that spina bifida can be largely prevented [21]. In 2015 the WHO published blood levels of FA which are required to prevent spina bifida [22].

Red blood cell folate concentration distributions alone can be used to predict prevalence of neural tube defects and a change in prevalence reflects FA food fortification. A folate concentration above 1000 nmol/L is consistent with optimal reduction in risk of folate-sensitive neural tube defects [23]. A 2016 national nutrition survey by Ethiopian Public Health Institute [24] had shown that 83% of all women in Ethiopia do not have enough folate in their blood to prevent spina bifida. The report clearly showed a general folate deficiency among young women that needed to be addressed in order to reduce and/or prevent the high occurrence of SBH in Ethiopia.

3. *"Bring Me a Workable Solution"*

In formulating a plan of action to treat a specific disease such as SBH the ultimate goal is to eliminate the disease. In cases of infections such as malaria, it may be through vaccines as is being tried now. In case of SBH, since it was already known that it can be prevented by getting folic acid into the diet of women of reproductive age prior to any of their pregnancies RAF was invited by the Ministry of Health of Ethiopia in 2018 to "provide a workable solution to bring folic acid to all women of childbearing age in Ethiopia". In collaboration with the Center for Spina Bifida Prevention at the Rollins School of Public Health at Emory University and the most prominent spina bifida expert in the US, Dr. Godfrey Oakley, RAF took up the challenge.

Which food is universally used and fortifiable with folic acid was the central question. The Team found that the only fortifiable food eaten by everyone in Ethiopia is salt and, like in most countries in the world, salt is already being fortified with iodine (to prevent goiter and mental retardation). New research from the University of Toronto established that fortification of this salt with folic acid is possible, increasing the pH to 9 by adding baking soda [25]. This presented an ideal solution, because the vehicle is universally used and adding folic acid is relatively simple and inexpensive.

Following a meeting of a worldwide coalition of experts convened by RAF, in 2019, the Ministry of Health, in conjunction with the Ethiopian Neurosurgical Society (SENSP) and the Ethiopian Public Health Institute, presented a Policy Brief [26] which recommended food fortification with folic acid. This was accepted by the Ministry of Health. Shortly after that the Team presented a proposal for a solution to the Bill and Melinda Gates Foundation.

4. *Funding*

Anticipating delays in procuring funds, RAF, with the help of a significant contributor, provided funding for several preliminary studies to be done.

These consisted of procurement of needed folic acid, making the doubly fortified salt and evaluating its shelf-life stability. It also led to the evaluation of the supply chain and performance of an organoleptic study, making sure that women will accept the salt. The salt is now produced and is stable in Ethiopian conditions. The supply chain has been charted and evaluated, and the salt has been found acceptable by consumers.

In April of 2022 the Gates Foundation announced a major implementation grant to address National Food Fortification in Ethiopia.

The Impact of Food Fortification on Neurosurgical Manpower in Ethiopia

In 2020 RAF and the Center for Spina Bifida Prevention looked at the impact of food fortification on the need for neurosurgical manpower [27]. Although the results of the major neurosurgical effort to treat SBH have been effective, it has still been insufficient [28] At the current rate of graduating neurosurgeons, it may not be until 2040 that all patients born alive with spina bifida will receive surgery. In contrast, food fortification is expected to show its positive effect within one year of implementation. The authors show that at least 38 FTE neurosurgeons will be spared with implementation of folic acid food fortification. This estimate is low as the literature and experience shows that spina bifida and hydrocephalus for many patients requires many more than 2 operations.

The neurosurgeons are acutely aware of the tremendous cost of SBH. They have recently formed the Global Alliance for Prevention of Spina Bifida-F [GAPSiF]. The F stands for folic acid preventable. With the worldwide prevalence of grains and rice fortified with folic acid currently to be 23%, the addition of fortification of salt which is already iodized, would mean a 90% prevention will be achievable.

The economic burden of the disease is not really known, but any estimates likely greatly underestimate the true cost, let alone the tremendous personal burden of the families affected. The authors believe that worldwide elimination of 90% of spina bifida before the end of 2030 would have a profound global impact.

Conclusion

Spina bifida is a complex disease which requires more than a dozen specialists and a well-organized multi-specialty Team. Just to define the necessary team itself was a major undertaking. To teach them to interact closely and efficiently, with as little overlap as possible required patience, diplomacy, specific education, and much support from many interested parties, starting with government and hospital leadership. The goal and mission of this undertaking was, and remains, patient-centered care which is of high-quality, comprehensive, with "one stop shopping", and which serves all the needs of both the patient and the family. To do that part of the Program's mission is to save patients and their caregivers money and frequent travel, while improving access to care and careful follow up of patients. It is predicted that food fortification will result in a dramatic-almost 90% drop of SB births in about two years [15]. This will be helped significantly by a grant of five million dollars for implementation of fortification of iodized salt with folic acid provided by the Gates foundation in 2022, The authors project that this can start in Ethiopia in 2025, and that nearly all babies that would have been born with SB will be born healthy by 2029.

There is now an increased global drive to make folic acid fortification of grains and salt mandatory around the world [29]. With the important work of GAPSBiF with the WHO resolution for mandatory food fortification with folic acid, and with the new Rotary support for a World Free of Spina Bifida, such a world is possible by the end of this decade.

References

1. Dixon M, Kancherla V, Magana T, Mulugeta A, Oakley GP Jr. High potential for reducing folic acid-preventable spina bifida and anencephaly, and related stillbirth and child mortality, in Ethiopia. Birth Defects Res. 2019;111(19):1513–9.
2. Sorri G, Mesfin E. Patterns of neural tube defects at two teaching hospitals in Addis Ababa, Ethiopia, a three years retrospective study. Ethiop Med J. 2015;53(3):119–26.
3. Berihu BA, Welderufael AL, Berhe Y, et al. High burden of neural tube defects in Tigray, northern Ethiopia: hospital-based study. PLoS One. 2018;13(11):e0206212. https://doi.org/10.1371/journal.pone.0206212.
4. Gedefaw A, Teklu S, Tilahun Tadesse B. Magnitude of neural tube defects and associated risk factors at three teaching hospitals in Addis Ababa, Ethiopia. BioMed Res Int. 2018, 10 pages; https://doi.org/10.1155/2018/4829023.
5. Mekkonen H, Berhe Y. A silent epidemic of major congenital malformations in Tigray, northern Ethiopia, a hospital based study. Nature Portfolio Sci Rep. 2021;11:21–35.
6. Healthcare spending Eth 2099. https://data.worldbank.org/indicator/SH.XPD.CHEX.PC.CD?locations=ET
7. Meara J, Greenberg S. Lancet commission on global surgery, global surgery 2030 evidence and solutions for achieving health, welfare and economic development. Lancet Surg. 2015;157(5):834–5.
8. Johansen M, Leake T, Tirsti A, Munie T, Abebe M, Sahlu A, Biluts H, Wester K. An Ethiopian training program in neurosurgery with Norwegian support. World Neurosurg. 2017;99:403–8.
9. Mersha A, Abat S, Temesgen T, Nebyou A. Outcome of chronic subdural hematoma treated with single Burr hole under local anesthesia. Ethiop J Health Sci. 2020;30(1):101–6.
10. Asfaw Z, Tirsit A, Laeke T, Park K. Neurosurgery in Ethiopia: a new chapter and future prospects. World J Neurosurg. 2021;152:e175–83. https://doi.org/10.1016/j.wneu.2021.05.071.
11. Bitew Z, Worku T, Alebel A, Alemu A. Magnitude and associated factors of neural tube defects in Ethiopia: a systematic review and meta-analysis. Glob Pediatr Health. 2020;7:1–14.
12. Oakley GP Jr. Classifying by cause and preventing the many causes of spina bifida and anencephaly. Pediatr Res. 2020;87(2):183–4.
13. Guidelines for the Care of People with Spina Bifida; Spina Bifida Association of America. https://www.spinabifidaassociation.org/guidelines/
14. Kancherla V, Wagh K, Johnson Q, Oakley GP Jr. A 2017 global update on folic acid-preventable spina bifida and anencephaly. Birth Defects Res. 2018;110(14):1139–47.
15. Gethun S, Mesresha S, Zenebe E, Leke T, Tirsit A. Four-year treatment outcomes of children operated for neural tube defect in Addis Ababa, Ethiopia: a retrospective study. J World Neurosurg. 2021;148:e695–702.
16. Yunus E, Abdurahman H, Assefa D, Fitsum W. Neural tube defects and associated factors among neonates admitted to the neonatal intensive care units in Hiwot Fana Specialized University Hospital, Harar, Ethiopia. Glob Pediatr Health. 2000;7:1–9.
17. Mohammed M, Bushra A, Aljadhey H, et al. Supplement use among pregnant women in Ethiopia: prevalence and predictors. Ther Innov Regul Sci. 2013;47:416–23.
18. Sendeku FW, Azeze GG, Fenta SL. Adherence to iron-folic acid supplementation among pregnant women in Ethiopia: a systematic review and meta-analysis. BMC Pregnancy Childbirth. 2020;20:138.
19. Child health and mortality prevention surveillance: a deeper dive into CHAMPS 31 March 2022. https://champshealth.org/wp-content/uploads/2022/04/20220331-CHAMPS-Data-Webinar-Slides.pdf
20. Dessie M, Zeleke E, Workie S. Folic acid usage and associated factors in the prevention of neural tube defects among pregnant women in Ethiopia: cross-sectional study. BMC Pregnancy Childbirth. 2017;17:313.
21. Prevention of neural tube defects: results of the Medical Research Council Vitamin Study. Ethiop J Health Sci. 2020;30(1):101–6.
22. Blencowe H, Kancherla V, Moorthie S, Darlison MW, Modell B. Estimates of global and regional prevalence of neural tube defects for 2015: a systematic analysis: worldwide neural tube defects: estimates for 2015. Ann N Y Acad Sci. 2018;1414(1):31–46.
23. Cordero AM, Crider KS, Rogers LM, Cannon MJ, Berry RJ. Optimal serum and red blood cell folate concentrations in women of reproductive age for prevention of neural tube defects: World Health Organization guidelines. MMWR Morb Mortal Wkly Rep. 2015;64(15):421–3.
24. Crider K, Devine O, Dowling N, Li Z, Berry R, et al. Population red blood cell folate concentrations for prevention of neural tube defects: Bayesian model. BMJ. 2014;349:g4554.
25. Ethiopian Public Health Institute- Demographic and health survey, Central Statistical Agency Addis Ababa, Ethiopia; 2016. p. 123–126.
26. McGee E, Sangakkra A, Diosady L. Double fortification of salt with folic acid and iodine. J Food Eng. 2017;198:72e80. published online
27. Ethiopian Public Health Institute - PHI Policy Brief 2019. Nutrition International. https://www.nutritionintl.org/learning-resource/policy-briefpreventing-neural-tube-defects-in-ethiopia-large-scale-mandatory-food-fortification-urgently-needed/

28. Kancherla V, Koning J, Biluts H, et al. Projected impact of mandatoryfoodfortificationwith folic acid on neurosurgical capacity needed for treating spina bifida in Ethiopia. Birth Defects Res. 2020;113:393. https://doi.org/10.1002/bdr2.1857.
29. Kancherla V, Tsang B, Wagh K, Dixon M, Oakley GP Jr. Modeling shows high potential of folic acid-fortified salt to accelerate global prevention of major neural tube defects. Birth Defects Res. 2020:1–14. https://doi.org/10.1002/bdr2.1769.
30. Caceras A, Blount J, Messing-Junger M, Chatterjee S, Fieggen G, Salomao J. The International Society for Pediatric Neurosurgery resolution on mandatory folic acid fortification of staple foods for prevention of spina bifida and anencephaly and associated disability and child mortality. Childs Nerv Syst. 2021;37(6):1809–12.

How to Train Surgical Subspecialists in Sub-Saharan Africa

8

Jeffrey Punch

It is not enough to know what is good: you must be able to do it.

– George Bernard Shaw

Abbreviations

FMHACA	Food, Medicine, and Healthcare Administration and Control Authority
LMICs	low- and middle-income countries
NCDs	non-communicable diseases
PFSA	Pharmaceutical Fund and Supply Agency

Introduction

Surgeons have traditionally volunteered their time and expertise around the world by traveling to low- and middle-income countries (LMICs) in order to provide needed surgical care to desperate patients. Many countries have fledgling health care systems. The traditional paradigm in many successful ventures has involved highly trained teams of surgeons and nurses that travel as missions for 2–4 weeks to areas where patients are unable to access needed specialized surgical services. Frequently other specialists including Anesthesiologists and Medical Specialists accompany the team. Supplies and sometimes devices are brought by the team from the home country to the destination in order to accomplish the complex missions that are planned. While laudable, and clearly providing valuable life-saving and life-enhancing therapies, as described in the following chaps. 34–40 focused on charity missions by Facing Africa. These surgical mission trips usually impart minimal, if any expertise on the local community. In fact, such efforts can actually undermine local efforts to develop such capacities since the locals cannot compete with a free service, provided by a well-respected organization. Finally, such efforts are not sustainable because inevitably funding dries up, interest wanes after leadership retires from active operating, and disruptions like pandemics bring a halt to the activity.

In the 1980s, Dr. Tim Johnson and colleagues began the process of creating a training program for desperately needed OB/GYN specialists in Ghana [1]. This program was successful, in that the specialists that it produced stayed in Ghana and provided needed care. The program was also sustainable, in that Ghana soon developed the expertise to train more specialists without outside help. Herein is described a similar effort to bring

J. Punch (✉)
University of Michigan School of Medicine, Ann Arbor, MI, USA
e-mail: jpunch@med.umich.edu

M. A. Hardy, B. R. Hochman (eds.), *Global Surgery*, https://doi.org/10.1007/978-3-031-28127-3_8

kidney transplant services to a public hospital in Addis Ababa, Ethiopia. By training specialists in their own country, it was hoped that specialists would remain in their homeland to serve the local need and to train future specialists.

Background – Ethiopia

Ethiopia is considered the birthplace of humanity, since Lucy, the oldest fossil of the human species was discovered there. Ethiopia is the second most populous African country after Nigeria, with a population in excess of 100 Million. It is located in East Africa and is the largest landlocked country by population. The lack of a seaport increases the cost of most imports, since duties must be paid to the port of entry. Ethiopia is bordered by Somalia to the East, Kenya to the South, Sudan and South Sudan to the West, and Eritrea and Djibouti to the North. Recent estimates put the per capita income of Ethiopia at $2400, less than 4% of that in the U.S. One of the oldest continuously inhabited areas in the world, Ethiopia is notable for having never been formally colonized, although Mussolini's Italy occupied the country for five years from 1936 to 1941. After World War II Ethiopia was ruled by emperor Haile Selassie from 1941 to 1974 before being under communist rule until 1991. In 1991 the country had a revolution, ending communist rule. A constitution was written and the current Federal Democratic Republic of Ethiopia was established. The Africa Union was founded in Ethiopia in 2002. According to UNICEF Budget Brief, the per capita spending on health care in Ethiopia was approximately 8.8% in recent years. Spending is slowly increasing toward the 15% target set out in the Abuja Declaration by the African Member States.

Ethiopia Declares the Desire to Offer Kidney Transplant Services

The Health Minister of Ethiopia from 2005 to 2012 was Tedros Adhanom Ghebreyes. In order to meet the needs of the rapidly growing population, Dr. Tedros, a physician and infectious disease expert, markedly increased the number of doctors trained in Ethiopia by increasing the number of medical schools in Ethiopia during his tenure [2]. These efforts were successful because Ethiopian medical school enrolls directly from secondary school, can quickly get candidates, and can then graduate new physicians in six years. After they graduate, the newly minted doctors are required to spend about two-to-four years practicing as primary care physicians as part of national service before they can begin residency training. While highly successful, the task of bringing modern specialty care to Ethiopia was more challenging. Nevertheless, with encouragement from the legislature and the Prime Minister, Dr. Tedros made it a national goal to initiate kidney transplant services in order to provide for patients with chronic renal failure in a humane, and cost-effective way which has not been previously available in the whole country.

A physician from the University of Michigan, Dr. Senait Fisseha had grown up in Ethiopia and trained in Obstetrics and Gynecology as well as Reproductive Endocrinology in the United States. She connected with Dr. Tedros while visiting the country and evaluating opportunities to improve local health care. Through this effort, Dr. Senait became engaged with the Ethiopian Ministry of Health's desire to improve capacity. She obtained funding to expand capacities and was heavily involved in establishing training programs in many specialties at St Paul's Hospital and Millennium Medical School in Addis Ababa, including OB/GYN, General Surgery, and Pediatrics. These programs were developed using the model that Dr. Johnson, her department chairman, had demonstrated to be successful in Ghana.

St Paul's, a public hospital, was built in 1969 under the leadership of Emporer Haile Salessie. The Millennium Medical School was established in 2007, the Ethiopian millennium. At that time, the 369 beds at St Paul's provided indigent care to the community in Addis Ababa, including more than 700 outpatient visits per day. Since then, capacity at the medical school complex has grown dramatically and now includes more than 700 beds and more than 2000 outpatient visits per day.

Dr. Senait approached the kidney transplant program leadership at the University of Michigan on behalf of the Health Ministry and invited the author (JP) to visit the hospital. This first visit happened in March 2013. The hospital appeared to be staffed by enthusiastic and skilled surgical and medical clinicians. Both inpatient and outpatient facilities were co-located, along with modern surgical operating theaters where elective operations happened six days a week and emergency operations happened 24 hours a day. Basic radiology and laboratory services were available. During this visit, it was revealed that more than 100 Ethiopians were being followed by a local Nephrologist after successful kidney transplants performed in other countries. These patients appeared to be doing as well as their counterparts in Western Countries. There was also a new 15-bed hemodialysis unit, one of the few in Addis Ababa, being formed at a private Korean (MCM) hospital. JP and Senait met personally with the Minister of Health at the time, Dr. Kessetebirhan Admasu who expressed willingness to firmly commit whatever resources were necessary to successfully launch kidney transplant services at St. Paul's. It was made clear that University of Michigan's role would be collaborative and facilitative, with the goal of creating a kidney transplant center at St Paul's that could function without outside help. The goal from the outset was sustainability. On the basis of the enthusiasm observed, the strong and unwavering governmental support, and the observation that transplant recipients can thrive in the Addis Ababa environs, the plan to develop kidney transplantation services at St. Paul's became a common goal.

Background – Renal Failure Care in Addis Ababa in 2013

Hemodialysis had existed in Ethiopia since approximately 1980 [3]. When the team arrived in Ethiopia, renal hemodialysis was only occurring in approximately 20 dialysis chairs located in several private hospitals around Addis Ababa, a city of over three million inhabitants. St. Paul's Hospital did not offer chronic hemodialysis care due to the prohibitive cost. Patients paid out of pocket for dialysis services at a cost of US$ 30-50 per run, largely because of the cost of purchasing hemodialysis membranes. The high cost relative to the average income of residents meant that most patients were under-dialyzed, some profoundly so. Some could afford hemodialysis only once per week. Statistics for survival were not known at the time, but it appeared to be very uncommon for a patient to live beyond a year. More modern data still show dismal survival for patients on renal replacement therapy [4].

Background – Is Kidney Transplant Appropriate for LMIC?

The true incidence of renal failure in Ethiopia, like in Sub-Saharan Africa as a whole, is not known. However, estimates indicate that 12-23% of adults have chronic kidney disease and are at risk of developing renal failure [5]. While traditional efforts at improving lifespan in Africa have focused on infectious disease and nutrition, more recently attention has turned to non-communicable diseases (NCD). The World Health Organization has been championing the growing importance of NCD in LMIC for over ten years, pointing out that 71% of deaths globally can be attributed to NCD. Given that kidney failure can affect individuals in the prime of life, and that kidney transplantation offers a life-extending treatment that allows individuals to resume productive lives, it appears to be an appropriate option. In addition, kidney transplantation can be surprisingly cost-effective in low-resource settings, as demonstrated by the public-private partnership at the Sindh Institute of Urology and Transplantation in Pakistan [6]. Chronic hemodialysis, on the other hand, is almost certainly cost-prohibitive in LMICs.

Steps to Initiate a Kidney Transplantation Program

Program Planning and Team Selection

The team from St Paul's was selected by St. Paul's leadership with guidance from the Health Ministry. A kidney transplant committee was created, led by the Vice-Provost in charge of the Medical School and St Paul's hospital. The committee members included the St Paul's Nephrologist who was selected to lead the program, along with the chairs of Medicine and Surgery, as well as representation from St Paul's Laboratory service, procurement service, and from Radiology. Surgeons that would be training to do kidney transplantation were selected by the Medical School authorities, after an internal application process. A nurse with experience implementing new programs within the Ethiopian Health system was assigned to the project, as was a physician project manager who worked for the Health Ministry. This last individual would prove invaluable, since he was accustomed to working with various governmental entities on projects. He reported directly to the Ministry of Health's Chief of Staff.

The team of individuals from the U.S. was selected by polling colleagues at the University of Michigan Medical Center, for interest. Dr. Alan Leichtman, a senior clinical transplant nephrologist, agreed to do a site visit. Once the program was underway, Dr. Leichtman enlisted other interested transplant nephrologists from around the country. In addition, one nephrologist with U.S. training who worked abroad volunteered to participate. Two nurses with transplant coordinator experience, one of whom also had ICU experience, and an operating room nursing supervisor in charge of the transplant service line all volunteered to participate in planning and organization. Two social workers with kidney donor and recipient experience were also interested in being involved. Site visits were planned by these teams. Dr. Senait was able to fund this work initially. Travel and expenses were later supported financially by the Ethiopian Health Ministry.

The team program planning began with the creation of a list of items required for transplantation. This list was created by obtaining pick lists for the operating room for donor nephrectomy and kidney transplantation at the University of Michigan. Other supplies that would be needed, including immunosuppressants, prophylactic anti-infectives, and reagents for needed lab tests, were added to the list. The list was created in a spreadsheet and each item was color-coded based on priority. Red items were those deemed to be absolutely required in order to initiate transplantation, such as vascular instruments, methylprednisone, and tacrolimus-level kits. Medium priority items that should be available but would not be absolutely required, such as loupes for the surgeons were coded orange. Items that should be planned for in the future, such as on site histocompatibility capability, were coded as yellow.

The transplant committee met in person at St Paul's approximately every two months over a period of 30 months planning the first renal transplant operation. Additional items were added to the list over time. The list itself was helpful to keep the project organized and as a tangible goal for the team and for the Ministry of Health to fund. In addition, given how long it take for the project to come to fruition, the items on the list that were completed served as a reminder of what progress had been made over time. This kept the team engaged and enthusiastic. Experience with the recent Covid-19 pandemic, and improvements in information technology infrastructure have taught us that some of these meetings could have been done virtually. However, meetings in person helped the team to form personal bonds and to get to know each other better which was of great benefit when the program finally started.

Establishment of Legal Framework

It is critical that a legal framework for living donation is in place to protect all of the participants, as well as to be able to demonstrate to observers that ethical measures are in place to preclude exploitation of living donors. In addition, if possible, it is prudent to establish a legal framework for deceased donation as well. A bill pertaining to organ donation in Ethiopia was passed by the legislature during the first year of planning. The Ministry of Health and the transplant committee were involved with reviewing initial drafts and providing feedback. The Ministry of Health also officially designated St Paul's as a transplant hospital and added a requirement that candidate donor and recipient pairs were to be presented to an independent committee overseen by the Ministry of Health for final approval to proceed.

Establishment of Formal Training Protocols

At the outset of the program, team members were invited to the U.S. in order to observe at the University of Michigan, a busy transplant program. This included members of the transplant committee, as well as the clinicians that would be involved in patient care. This included three general surgeons, a urologist, a nephrologist, an anesthesiologist, a CRNA, and a radiologist. Obtaining visas was an initial obstacle that was overcome with the help of the Health Ministry. Professional leadership, including that of the Vice-Provost of the Medical School, on these visits turned out to be extremely valuable. While hospital policy and State laws prevented surgeons from scrubbing on any cases, they were able to witness more than a dozen transplant procedures over their month-long observership. In addition, they made rounds with the teams, shadowed clinicians in pre-transplant and post-transplant clinics, attended selection committee meetings and conferences pertaining to Transplant and Nephrology topics. In addition to the observership at the University of Michigan, the surgeons and nephrologists visited a program in Egypt that was lower volume, but where they could be permitted to have hands-on involvement. The surgeons were also invited to spend a month each at Hospital do Rim in Sao Paulo, Brazil. This hospital is solely dedicated to kidney transplantation and has the highest annual kidney transplant volume in the world at more than 750 transplants annually. This attachment was extremely valuable to the surgeons because of the opportunity to observe multi-disciplinary teams at work, and because they were exposed to a broad array of transplant complications due to the high volume of transplants.

A training curriculum was developed along with graduation criteria, modeled after the requirements set forth for kidney transplantation by the American Society of Transplant Surgeons. The curriculum was approved by the Ministry of Health, the University of Addis Ababa, and by the Food, Medicine, and Healthcare Administration and Control Authority (FMHACA) in Addis Ababa.

"The Team, The Team, The Team"

The Famous University of Michigan Football Coach Bo Schembechler was often quoted widely that success is all about teamwork. Transplant is very much a team sport. In addition to qualified surgeons and nephrologists, it is critical that nurses with the necessary skill to manage post-transplant and post-nephrectomy patients are available. Social workers and psychiatrists are also an integral part of the team that functions to assist in the selection of recipients capable of managing the rigorous post-transplant follow-up and care that will be required and of donors to assure their volunteerism and motivations, as well as their predicted response to donation. Team members made site visits to provide recommendations and developed professional relationships with their counterparts. These site visits were extremely valuable and resulted in numerous additions to the list of items required. For example, nursing noted that sinks, soap, and towels were not available in every patient room and patient care area. Since kidney transplants would be treated with immunosuppression, this was an important observation. In addition, crash carts were not available. These items were added to the list. The operating room appeared well run and utilized safe practices for sterility, but it was noted that additional storage space for consumable supplies would be required. It was strongly advised that a basic electronic medical record be instituted in order to keep track of important elements of the patients' evaluations and for efficient post-transplant care and monitoring.

It was noted that laboratory services were not available at night. The availability of 24 h a day, 7 days a week laboratory testing was added to the list as a critical item. Other upgrades needed included the ability to do flexible cystoscopy to remove ureteral stents. Given the lack of skilled interventional radiologists, it was reasoned that routinely utilizing stents would reduce the likelihood of difficult-to-manage ureteral complications. Radiology needed to be enhanced in order to provide contrast-enhanced spiral CT scans for donor screening and to provide doppler ultrasound exams of kidney grafts with calculation of resistive indices.

A dialysis unit was needed to support the program. It was felt that to ensure optimal outcomes, patients should be well dialyzed prior to transplantation. Only patients with approved donors that were accepted as transplant candidates would be able to have chronic dialysis at this facility to conserve resources. The availability of acute dialysis was also deemed to be important in the case of delayed graft function or severe acute kidney injury in a post-transplant patient at a later point in time.

Pharmacy services needed to be expanded. In particular, there was insufficient storage space to store the valuable immunosuppressant and anti-infective medications. A method of recording inventory was also needed to avoid running out of a critical drug.

Establishment of a Transplant Protocol

It was imperative for the team members to create a written protocol for the selection of recipients and donors, and for the care of patients following transplantation and donation. This process began with reviewing protocols in use in similar settings. Unfortunately, given the paucity of kidney transplantation in LMIC, few protocols in this setting existed. Fortunately, colleagues in South Africa were willing to share protocols and give advice. For example, it was advised that given the endemic nature of tuberculosis in the region, and the risk this poses to immunosuppressed patients, all recipients receive prophylaxis with isoniazid. In addition, all patients would receive anti-helminthic treatment to deworm prior to donation and transplant. To avoid the risks of over-immunosuppression, it was decided to avoid induction immunosuppression therapies that result in lymphocyte depletion.

After consideration, the team elected to pursue low-risk transplant candidates. High BMI patients, patients with known severe coronary disease or depressed ejection fraction were excluded. Because plasmapheresis would not be an option in the case of antibody-mediated rejection, donor/recipient pairs with known donor-specific antibody, even if at modest titers, were excluded. Cytomegalovirus and Pneumocystis jirovici chemoprophylaxis were deemed to be important.

Operatively, the initial plan was to proceed with hand-assisted laparoscopic donor nephrectomy, since minimally invasive nephrectomy was felt to be the state of the art. Fixed retractors were planned for the recipient operation in order to simulate the way the procedure was performed at high-volume centers.

Creation of a Transplant Center

The initial plan was to perform the donor nephrectomy and kidney transplant operations at St. Paul's hospital and care for them in a dedicated ward. This was felt to be less than optimal given the number of patients being treated for infection. While patients with tuberculosis were housed in a dedicated ward, the lack of ventilation in the facility was concerning. During a visit to the University of Michigan the Vice-Provost from St. Paul's toured the transplant ward and transplant clinic. When he returned to Addis Ababa, he was inspired to rent a facility very near the St Paul's hospital and renovate it into a dedicated transplant unit. This facility, formerly used by an Information Technology firm and later as classrooms, was located about 100 meters from the entrance to St Paul's and was on the same side of the street. This would prove to be highly efficient. The facility comprised the intensive care unit, the dialysis unit, pharmacy, laboratory, offices, and outpatient clinic area on the first floor. The second floor was dedicated to wards with private rooms for the recipients and semi-private rooms for the donors, an operating theater area with adjoining donor and recipient operating rooms as well as storage areas and lounges for physicians and nurses. Physician and nursing staff could be easily shared with St Paul's because of the close proximity.

The main drawback of the dedicated transplant center arrangement was that patients had to travel to St Paul's for imaging studies other than ultrasound. An unexpected benefit was that those individuals that worked at the dedicated transplant unit developed a sense of pride and camaraderie.

Procurement – The Biggest Challenge

Procurement of needed supplies turned out to be very difficult. Initially, it was estimated that six months would be required for planning and collecting the needed instruments, supplies, and equipment required for transplantation. This turned out to be wildly optimistic. It took two and a half years after the first visit before the first live donor kidney transplant was possible. The longest process was obtaining needed supplies. The system in Ethiopia for purchases by the government involves a mandatory bid process. If insufficient numbers of bids were received, the process had to be repeated from the beginning. The agency in charge of purchasing of health care products is called PFSA, Pharmaceutical Fund and Supply Agency; it appeared to be quite bureaucratic. In several instances the bid process resulted in the substitution of items that were not truly interchangeable, prolonging the process. For example, hand-held staplers were procured, rather than endo-staplers.

Dress Rehearsal: Porcine Transplants

The delays caused by the difficulty with procuring supplies were frustrating, but the Ethiopian surgeons had an idea. They had visited the laboratory at the University of Michigan where porcine transplants were being performed as part of experiments. They suggested that porcine transplants would be a way to test the readiness of the entire system for an attempt at human transplants [6]. This proved to be an excellent idea. Five different porcine transplants were attempted. The final transplant was successful. A number of important observations were made. At one point the power went out. This was a relatively frequent occurrence in Addis Ababa, and operations can usually proceed with back up batteries for anesthesia monitors, manual bag ventilation, and ambient light. However, during laparoscopy, one cannot proceed at all without power. While the medical complex at St Paul's had a backup generator, it clearly was not up to the task. It was also discovered that many of the very low-cost vascular instruments that had been procured were not functional and needed to be replaced with high-quality products that would actually grasp and cut tissue. It was also discovered that parts for the fixed retractor had been purchased from multiple suppliers. As a result, the ratchets and blades did not fit on the ring. The retractor was virtually worthless until the correct pieces were obtained.

Transplants Begin – The Team Learns by Doing

After two and a half years of planning, the first live donor kidney transplant in Ethiopia went off without a hitch in November of 2015. Two more transplants were performed in the following days. All six patients did well. Over the next four years more than twenty visits were made. At least one surgeon and one nephrologist were always part of the visiting team. Social workers accompanied the team every few visits. Initially, a nurse accompanied the team for every visit. A skilled nurse was initially critically important to assist and teach the St Paul's nursing team with postoperative care since they were initially not adept at many of the necessary skills needed to care for the patients. Such skills as calculating and administering intravenous boluses and how to replace urine output with IV fluid were beyond their previous experience. In addition, the nursing culture in existence did not encourage nurses to bring problems such as falling urine output or hypertension outside of expected parameters to the attention of the physician team. Over the course of the next two years the nurse always accompanied the team whenever transplants would occur and was always available at the bedside in the ICU, which also functioned as a recovery room. In addition to teaching at the bedside she gave lectures on various topics relating to transplant nursing and the use of medications. The St Paul's nursing team became competent at managing these challenging patients and the visiting nurse was no longer needed for bedside care.

Between three and five live donor nephrectomy procedures and kidney transplants were done on each visit. Typically the team left the U.S. Saturday evening and arrived late Sunday or early Monday. On Monday afternoon a team meeting was held where each donor/recipient pair was presented and the donor CT scan images were reviewed. In addition, any post-transplant patients from previous visits having complications or requiring readmission were discussed. On Tuesday through Friday one nephrectomy and one transplant was performed each day. As the team got more efficient and the backlog of patients waiting for transplant got larger, the team decided to try to do two donors and two transplants on a single day in order to do more than 4 transplants in a week. This was doable, but it stressed the four bed ICU capacity to its limit, and the team discontinued this practice, returning to a comfortable four transplants per week.

The first 48 donor nephrectomy operations were performed with hand-assisted laparoscopy. Unfortunately, at this point some critically important supplies such as endostaplers and harmon scalpel handpieces were depleted. The Ethiopia surgeons suggested flank nephrectomy as an alternative. They had witnessed this operative technique at Hospital do Rim where flank nephrectomy was the standard approach because of the increased cost of laparoscopy. From that point on, all donor operations were done through flank incisions. The patients, almost invariably thin, did remarkably well postoperatively.

After four years, the surgeons had done a sufficient number of nephrectomies and transplant operations and mastered the knowledge necessary to select appropriate candidates and manage them through their operations and recovery to become independent. A graduation ceremony was held and they were each pronounced qualified kidney transplant surgeons. The visiting team also learned much during the training process. For example, narcotic analgesia is not used at St Paul's for postoperative pain control. The patients did remarkably well with acetaminophen analgesia. There was initial concern over how thin many of the patients were. Many times the BMI was less than 15, despite excellent functional status and nutritional laboratory parameters that suggested the patient was not malnourished. These patients did very well, with no observed increased incidence of infection or surgical complications. Initially, the team was also concerned by the very high BUN on some of the patients having pre-emptive kidney transplantation. BUNs as high as 250 did not result in any particular postoperative problem such as disequilibrium or oozing that has been described for very uremic patients that suddenly are provided with rapid solute clearance. Overall, the clinical outcome at St. Paul's would be considered excellent at any transplant center in the world. The program was halted in March of 2020 due to the Covid-19 pandemic. However, the program resumed in September 2022. Despite the hiatus, the Ethiopian group was able to resume succeful living donor kidney transplants, and the program continues. The major ongoing difficulty is obtaining consumeable supplies such as ureteral stentsm, polypropyline sutures, and kits to monitor immunosuppression levels.

Summary

The experience described in this chapter is a model for sustainability of improved surgical capacity in LMIC. It proves that complex surgical and medical care is possible in low-resource settings. The key to success begins with a group of highly motivated individuals willing to dedicate themselves to a goal that may take years to reach. Equally important is the requirement for committed and supportive leadership at the institution and at the Health Ministry levels. The end result has the potential to advance health care in LMIC to a level of sophistication previously only available in the wealthy countries.

References

1. Klufio CA, Kwawukume EY, Danso KA, Sciarra JJ, Johnson T, American Journal of Obstetrics & Gynecology. Ghana postgraduate obstetrics/gynecology collaborative residency training program: success story and model for Africa. Am J Obstet Gynecol. 2003;189(3):692–6.
2. Derbew M, Animut N, Talib ZM, Mehtsun S, Hamburger EK. Ethiopian medical schools' rapid scale-up to support the government's goal of universal coverage. Acad Med. 2014;89(Supplement):S40–4.
3. Rizvi SA, Naqvi SA, Zafar MN, et al. Living related renal transplants with lifelong follow-up. A model for the developing world. Clin Nephrol. 2010;74(Suppl 1):S142.
4. Workie SG, Zewale TA, Wassie GT, Belew MA, Abeje ED. Survival and predictors of mortality among chronic kidney disease patients on hemodialysis in Amara region, Ethiopia 2021. BMC Nephrol. 2022;23(1):193; Mahteme BM et al. Milestones of Renal Replacment Therapy in Ethiopia Ethiop Med J, 2020, Supp. 1.
5. Ene-Iordache B, Perico P, Bikbov B, et al. Chronic kidney disease and cardiovascular risk in six regions of the world (ISN-KDDC): a cross-sectional study. Lancet Glob Health. 2016;4:e307–19.
6. Abebe, E. et al.. On site porcine kidney transplant simulation to prepare a novice transplant center for human living kidney transplant: the Ethiopian experience. 2020, Ethiopian Medical Journal. https://emjema.org/index.php/EMJ/article/view/1533

How to Develop a Sustainable Program for Volunteer Medical Care in Low- and Middle-Income Countries

9

Sidney B. Eisig, Roberto Fajardo, and David Hoffman

Success is not the key to happiness. Happiness is the key to success. If you love what you are doing, you will be successful.

– Albert Schweitzer

Abbreviations

CRNA certified registered nurse anesthetists
IRB Institutional Review Board
LMICs low- and middle-income countries

Introduction

Volunteer medical missions provide necessary care to underserved populations in low and middle income countries [1]. Our overarching goal is to provide the same level of care in Neiva as we do in our hospitals in the United States. Patients born with a cleft lip and palate have a high burden of care (Table 9.1). We endeavored to provide this care from birth through young adulthood. In coordination with our hosts, we expanded our team to include orthodontists, pediatric dentists, geneticists, and speech and language pathologists. Local specialists were recruited and trained if necessary to continue to provide care after we left. An ongoing IRB-approved genetics research project in collaboration with Dr. Wendy Chung of Columbia University in New York and Dr. Henry Ostos of Surcolombiana has resulted in two peer-reviewed articles. Bone grafting of the alveolar cleft around age seven and then midface advancement around age sixteen is coordinated with local orthodontists. Our bilingual speech pathologists from Teachers College in New York provide speech camp for the children and their families and continuing education for local/regional therapists, educational videos available on YouTube, and remote consultations for their local counterparts via the internet.

This past year, we utilized 10 operating rooms and provided surgical care for approximately 170 patients. Our areas of concentration have been expanded; our team provides treatment for children with congenital hip dysplasia and club feet, cleft lip and palate, microtia, burn scar contracture releases, syndactyly, polydactyly, congenital and

S. B. Eisig (✉)
Columbia University College of Dental Medicine and New York Presbyterian/Columbia University Irving Medical Center and Morgan Stanley Children's Hospital of New York, New York, NY, USA
e-mail: sbe2002@cumc.columbia.edu

R. Fajardo
Clinically Applied Science Education (CASE), University of the Incarnate Word, School of Osteopathic Medicine, San Antonio, TX, USA
e-mail: rfajardo@uiwtx.edu

D. Hoffman
Division of Oral and Maxillofacial Surgery, Staten Island University Hospital/Northwell Health System, Staten Island, NY, USA

M. A. Hardy, B. R. Hochman (eds.), *Global Surgery*, https://doi.org/10.1007/978-3-031-28127-3_9

Table 9.1 Sequence of care for the cleft lip and palate patient

Age	Procedure	Comment
3–6 months	Lip repair	
7–12 months	Palate repair, myringotomies	
4–5 years old	Speech evaluation	May require additional palatal/ pharyngeal surgery
6–9 years old	Alveolar bone graft	Phase 1 orthodontic therapy
Adolescence	Mid-face advancement	Phase 2 orthodontic therapy
Adolescence	Nose/lip revision	

traumatic hand injuries and a variety of other facial deformities.

We have also developed an electronic medical program with a fingerprint identification system. In 2020 we introduced a nutrition program taught by a well-known Colombian chef for our postoperative patients.

This chapter will discuss the requirements to developing sustainable care in low and middle-income countries (LMICs) based on our experiences in Neiva, Colombia.

Mission Statement and Guiding Principles of Care

It is important that the team develops a mission statement with a set of guiding principles in coordination with the host hospital. This will define expectations, allow the team to be focused, and will set boundaries to patient care. Treatment should be defined by assessing the local needs of the community, the resources of the hospital, and understand what restrictions and role you play in the local healthcare system. Guidelines should be established for teaching local doctors and residents

Site Selection and Developing Partnerships

It is imperative that a clinician become part of an existing team and make several trips before leading a new team. A thorough understanding of planning, logistics, transportation, fundraising, leadership, and how to execute the mission is essential. It is critical to abide by all rules and regulations related to entrance to, and exit from, the host country.

A pre-trip site visit, approximately one year in advance, is critical. A local champion is crucial to the continuing success of the partnership. The goals of this visit are to develop relationships, to meet the local leadership of the city, the hospital and chamber of commerce, to perform a needs assessment for the population, and to evaluate the standards of care and equipment in the host hospital. The expectations of the hospital must match what the team can provide. The development of a close working relationship with local healthcare providers is critical. During this visit a medical liaison is identified and local surgeons are invited to participate. Agreement is reached as to who will care for the patients when the team leaves. Emergency planning is also discussed and agreed upon during this site visit.

The anticipated patient volume, the number of operating rooms, the size of the recovery room, presence of an intensive care unit, hospital bed availability, and where the patients are being housed prior to surgery and after discharge from the hospital are ascertained.

The team administrator will assist your host in credentialling the members of the team who will be treating patients.

Security, housing, and transportation for the team must be arranged in advance. Housing for the team should be visited at the site visit.

Funding

The team needs a source of funding for travel, lodging, local transportation, meals, and medical supplies. This can be done with grants, fundraisers, or donations. One can also establish a 501C foundation and solicit donations. The local Chamber of Commerce may have the resources to assist with fundraising or provide gifts in kind such as housing, meals, and transportation.

Although medical care is provided free of charge, the hospital may need additional financial support to pay salaries of hospital employees caring for the patients and for meals for both patients, their families, and the visiting team.

Team Development

The team administrator plays an important role in planning the trip, arranging all the legal documents to practice, and logistics. The administrator must be fluent in the host country's language to ensure a smooth logistical operation of the team. The administrator serves as the direct liaison with the hospital administration and language fluency will help avoid misunderstandings and miscommunications. The administrator, along with the medical director of the Team, ensures that all supplies, equipment, and luggage arrive. The administrator also arranges the hotel and meals, transportation to and from the airport, and to and from the hospital each day. Well-structured programs are productive and may be intense. The administrator and other team leaders should remember the importance of team camaraderie. These leaders should plan team activities to alleviate the stress of work days and promote engagement among team members and the host community.

The number of OR tables, hospital capacity, and the anticipated scope of services determines the size and skill set of the team. The host hospital may provide operating room nurses and technicians. In Neiva, our host hospital provides the scrub nurse and circulator. However, we also bring one circulator per room as well.

Team members are often dropped because of their inability to work under sometimes adverse circumstances, to get along well with others, or their level of care does not meet the standards that are expected.

Anesthesia

The delivery of safe anesthesia continues to be a challenge in LMICs [2]. An anesthesia team experienced in the care of infants and children needs to be developed. This can be a combination of anesthesiologists, certified registered nurse anesthetists (CRNA), and anesthesia technicians. All applicable laws in the host country as to who can deliver anesthesia must be followed. Resident anesthesiologists need to be supervised at the same level as in their residency program. Additional anesthesiologists not assigned to an operating room are needed to provide relief, to assist in case starts, and to provide emergency care.

The visiting anesthesia team must develop a good relationship with the hospital anesthesiologists and to include them in the day-to-day operations of the mission. The local anesthesiologists are critical to help in difficult airways, emergencies, anesthesia machine maintenance, and overall care of the patient.

Anesthetic agents and supplies need to be obtained in advance and the type of anesthesia machines and monitoring equipment should be evaluated at a pre-mission site visit. The anesthesia team must investigate in advance all host country's Customs regulations regarding travel into the country with anesthetic agents and other medications.

One rule that we have followed is it only takes one healthcare provider, at any level, to cancel a patient. This is not open for debate other than for academic discussion. This avoids placing our patients at undue risk. These patients are given preference when we return the following year if they are not treated by the local surgeon.

Surgical Team

The surgical team should include a combination of skilled surgeons and residents; the resident serves as first assistant and not as the surgeon. It is important to avoid having a surgeon operating in a situation where they are not competent. In addition, there should be a designated surgical team leader that can oversee the program, scheduling, and assignments. In high-volume surgical missions, it is imperative that the surgical scheduler (typically the administrator or one on his/her team) work closely with the medical director and all attendings, discussing the creation of the schedule often. The pace of the work is intense, cases are often either included in case load for that year or are postponed a year, so this close communication helps create a smoother process that benefits the patients, surgeon, and success of the campaign.

Nursing

Nursing care is key to many medical teams. Nurses provide a variety of services on these trips from assisting in the operating room to administering pre- and postoperative care. The number of nurses is dependent on the number of patients and the availability and skill of local nurses.

Pediatricians

All patients are evaluated by our pediatricians prior to and after surgery. We prefer pediatricians with critical care training. Our pediatricians interact daily with the hospital's pediatricians and nursing staff and one of our pediatricians takes call in the hospital each night.

Comprehensive Care

Surgical teams that provide cleft lip and palate surgery are often criticized for not providing the comprehensive care these children require as they grow into adulthood. Providing comprehensive care for the cleft lip and palate patient in an under-resourced region is a challenge. Partnerships with local specialists take time to develop. These clinicians may need to be trained. All our patients are offered orthodontic care by local orthodontists so we may provide bone grafting to the alveolar cleft and maxillary advancement (if needed) when age appropriate. We incentivize the orthodontist by providing supplies through our fundraising. The children are also provided with speech therapy by local clinicians.

When you consider other specialties such as orthopedics or other types of facial reconstructive surgery, the same also holds true; postoperative therapy and long-term care (follow-ups and interim care between mission trips) have to be considered and a method to provide that should be ascertained before surgery is performed.

Emergency Planning and Postoperative Care

It is important to have a plan for medical and surgical emergencies for both patients and team members established prior to the visit. This is formulated at the time of the initial site visit and reviewed once the team has arrived. Team members must have health insurance that provides coverage for care and medical evacuation when outside the United States.

Postoperative care at nighttime needs to be decided in advance. Remember that a visiting doctor or nurse may not be fluent in the local language or familiar with how to write orders and who is available in case there was a problem developing. Including a local pediatrician, fluent in the team's primary language, can help to bridge this gap between the visiting surgical team and the hospital-based staff that will provide postoperative care. This person can then help plan who is available at night to care for patients. It is important to provide the contact information of the other team members to those on call at the hospital. Surgeons must round on their patients while the patient is in the hospital.

Medical Records

In addition to entering into the hospital's medical record, the team should maintain its own records to allow for continuity of care. Data can also drive fundraising by demonstrating good surgical outcomes and helping to develop patient stories.

Designated personnel are assigned to do this. It is helpful to have a medical student or resident from the host hospital serve in this role.

For security reasons, the mission team may not have direct access to the hospital's electronic medical record system. The mission team will be responsible for creating paper records and sharing them with the hospital. The details of these processes should be discussed before the mission to avoid logistical problems during or after the mission.

Care After the Team Leaves

Visiting teams are often given the disparaging term "weekend warriors." The team operates and leaves the problems to be taken care of by the local doctors. It is prudent to have local doctors who are willing to assume the postoperative care of the patients that you are treating included in your care of the patients. Obviously, for specific surgeries, postoperative care has its own requirements. These discussions begin at the initial site visit and are revisited when the team arrives. Unusual procedures that may require a planned or unplanned return to the operating room are discussed with the local surgeons prior to surgery. Remember, the clinicians that will provide the extended care after the team leaves do so in addition to their regular patient load. Take the time to establish close bonds with these local team members and consider ways to incentivize their participation.

Availability of Patients

We use the local media, churches, and surgeons to inform the local population of our impending visit. Our expansion into comprehensive care to include orthodontists and speech pathologists has greatly increased the number of patients we evaluate. We are now examining approximately 700 patients (from all over Colombia) on our screening day and operate on approximately 150–170 patients per trip. It is important to ensure you are not competing with a well-established program. Your hosts should be able to assist with this. Check the internet for schedules of other medical volunteer groups that might be providing care to your proposed site. An excellent working relationship with the host hospital can frequently prevent this issue from occurring.

Local Diplomacy

The visiting medical group must never upstage the local doctors. Do not create a situation where the patients and their families are made to believe that their local doctors are incompetent. It is important that every attempt be made to engage local doctors, nurses, and hospital administrators and make sure that they are given the credit for making this care possible. Mutual respect and friendships that are developed will be sustaining and rewarding.

One complication can overwhelm all the good intentions and services provided by your team. It is important to think very carefully about what could go wrong and try to avoid those situations and minimize the surgical risks. Having local doctors as part of your team will minimize the effects of the complication and avoid casting a shadow on your team. Beware and avoid any self-aggrandizing or criticisms on the social media at the expense of the local staff, administrators, or local authorities. Such irresponsible action by any member of the team may quickly lead to rupture of all relations and irrevocable termination of the program. This must be avoided at all cost.

Conclusion

Participation in a volunteer medical mission is extremely rewarding. This discussion is meant as a guideline to provide medical and surgical care in LMICs. Additional information can be gleaned from Butler et al. [3]. When people are often asked why they do this, there is no specific answer other than it is "a calling." Having spent a professional lifetime volunteering several times a year, these trips have a unique meaning that can only be understood by the individual. Whatever reasons motivate you to participate, understand that you are part of a team and that the goal is to provide medical care for people in need of your services. Two favorite quotes that epitomize volunteer work are: "You make a living by what you get; you make a life by what you give" and to "save a life is to save the world."

References

1. Meara JG, Leather AJ, Hagander L, Alkire BC, Alonso N, Ameh EA, Bickler SW, Conteh L, Dare AJ, Davies J, Mérisier ED, El-Halabi S, Farmer PE, Gawande A, Gillies R, Greenberg SL, Grimes CE, Gruen RL, Ismail EA, Kamara TB, Lavy C, Lundeg G, Mkandawire NC, Raykar NP, Riesel JN, Rodas E, Rose J, Roy N, Shrime MG, Sullivan R, Verguet S, Watters D, Weiser TG, Wilson IH, Yamey G, Yip W. Global Surgery 2030: evidence and solutions for achieving health, welfare, and economic development. Lancet. 2015;386(9993):569–624. https://doi.org/10.1016/S0140-6736(15)60160-X.
2. Hodges SC. Anaesthesia and global health initiatives for children in a low-resource environment. Curr Opin Anaesthesiol. 2016;29(3):367–71. https://doi.org/10.1097/ACO.0000000000000319.
3. Butler M, Drum E, Evans FM, Fitzgerald T, Fraser J, Holterman AX, Jen H, Kynes JM, Kreiss J, McClain CD, Newton M, Nwomeh B, O'Neill J, Ozgediz D, Politis G, Rice H, Rothstein D, Sanchez J, Singleton M, Yudkowitz FS. Guidelines and checklists for short-term missions in global pediatric surgery: Recommendations from the American Academy of Pediatrics Delivery of Surgical Care Global Health Subcommittee, American Pediatric Surgical Association Global Pediatric Surgery Committee, Society for Pediatric Anesthesia Committee on International Education and Service, and American Pediatric Surgical Nurses Association, Inc. Global Health Special Interest Group. J Pediatr Surg. 2018;53(4):828–36. https://doi.org/10.1016/j.jpedsurg.2017.11.037.

10 How to Organize a Colon Cancer Screening Program in a Low- and Middle-Income Country

Spencer E. Amory

Kindness is the language which the deaf can hear and the blind can see.

– Mark Twain

Abbreviations

ACLS	Advanced Cardiovascular Life Support
HICs	high-income countries
LMICs	low- and middle-income countries

Introduction

Colon cancer screening with colonoscopy is well established as a technique for prevention and early detection of colon cancer in the population of developed countries. However, there are many communities worldwide, such as low- and middle-income countries (LMICs), that do not have access and would benefit from this evaluation. Before offering your services, it is important to establish whether the target community perceives such a need or is receptive to considering screening. This can be achieved by contacting residents, providers, or health officials in the target community. These people can be a source of information about the burden of colon cancer in the community, the current screening options available, and the likelihood that the community will accept screening. They can also provide information about support services needed such as anesthesia, pathology, and surgery.

Establish Connection with Provider

I have found it essential when working temporarily in a distant community to establish a strong relationship with a local provider. In addition to providing valuable information about a variety of local issues, this provider can assist with evaluation and preparation of patients, follow-up of pathology reports, and referrals for surgery. This individual is often motivated to assist since they are connected to the community and would like to improve their care. Also being part of such an effort improves their continuing education and prominence on the local scene. Ideally, they would be inspired to acquire the skills to provide the service locally on an ongoing basis.

S. E. Amory (✉)
Columbia University Vagelos College of Physicians and Surgeons, New York, NY, USA
e-mail: sea99@cumc.columbia.edu

M. A. Hardy, B. R. Hochman (eds.), *Global Surgery*, https://doi.org/10.1007/978-3-031-28127-3_10

Site Visit

A preparatory visit to a proposed screening site serves many functions. One can meet with key local personnel and initiate the process of publicizing the effort. Another important task is to evaluate the local health facility for a suitable space for conducting patient interviews, performing procedures, processing of endoscopes, and storing supplies. I have found that space in or close to the operating room will usually have adequate security, and the utilities like electrical power, water, and oxygen. Also, there may be monitoring equipment necessary for endoscopic procedures. One can also assess the potential for power failures and the availability of portable generators.

Assemble a Team

Colonoscopy is a team effort. A technician skilled in cleaning and maintaining the equipment is essential especially when functioning away from the usual services of your home hospital and equipment company representative. An experienced endoscopy nurse who can administer sedation, monitor patients, and assist with procedures is also vital. An anesthesiology member on the team is ideal but often local practitioners can be utilized instead since in LMICs there is frequently a shortage of trained anesthesiologists. The members of the team should also be comfortable sharing their knowledge and skill with local counterparts in keeping with the ultimate goal of a sustainable screening program.

Acquire Equipment

Colonoscopy equipment is expensive, and this hurdle can be challenging in LMICs. Fortunately, many home facilities in high-income countries (HICs) routinely update and trade in old equipment for a nominal discount. Your home institution may be willing to donate or highly discount older but highly functional equipment to your effort. Alternatively, previously owned equipment can be obtained from the supplier at a deep discount.

Equipment List

Instrument tower (processor, light source, monitor, printer).
Colonoscopes.
Electrocautery generator, pedal activated
Pump irrigator, pedal-activated.
Disinfecting tubs for endoscopes.
Pump irrigator for endoscope cleaning.

Funding

The expenses associated with conducting screening at a distant location in LMICs include equipment mentioned previously, disposable supplies, travel, and local accommodations and transportation. There may also be expenses for medications acquired locally or for the services of anesthesia personnel. There are many variables here since donated supplies are sometimes available and some team members may choose to pay for their own travel. In any event one needs to carefully budget the expected and unanticipated expenses. I found it useful to establish a non-profit organization as a vehicle for fundraising and financing of this effort. Grateful patients are often aware of your charitable activities and willing to support these efforts, as may be charitable institutions and foundations.

Supplies

A large volume of unused supplies from the "supply packs" opened for each patient in our endoscopy suites are often discarded. Unopened packages of lubricant and gauze can be collected and stored for later use. There are organizations that routinely collect unexpired supplies from hospitals and provide them free of cost to legitimate charitable efforts. Lastly, some supplies may need to be purchased from suppliers. If these supplies can be sourced at the destination, they are often less expensive. The colon cleansing regimens to which one is accustomed may not be available. Advanced knowledge will guide the decision to obtain and ship or transport these supplies.

Endoscope disinfectant solution.
Masks 10.
Needles, sharp.
Needles, blunt.
Oxygen cannulas.
Protective eyewear.
Simethicone.
Snares, endoscopic.
Specimen containers.
Specimen bags.
Specimen traps.
Suction tubing 10.
Syringes 6, 12, 60 mL.
Underpads.
Wash brushes.
IV dressings.

Supply List

Adhesive strips.
Alcohol pads.
Angiocaths.
Baskets, endoscopic.
Biopsy forceps.
Cautery cable, snare.
Disinfecting wipes.
Enzyme cleaner.
Formalin.
Gauze.
Gloves, non-sterile.
Gloves, fitted.
Gowns, procedure.
Grounding pads.
Hand sanitizing solution.
IV tubing 16.

Raising Awareness

Wide dissemination of the advantages of colon cancer screening has not penetrated every community around the world, especially in LMICs. Some communities are focused on the challenges of daily life and others are resistant to screening for asymptomatic conditions. Some persons, especially males, may be reluctant to undergo examination via the anus. A method to communicate with the target population is essential to overcome these barriers. Interviews on local radio and television shows is one option, preferably conducted with one or more local health care providers or officials. Another approach is to target community groups and religious organizations. Ideally, a partnership with the local public health system can facilitate the dissemination of information about the value and availability of colon cancer screening. After the initial experience, word-of-mouth dissemination about the experience and benefits is a potent method of raising awareness and recruiting additional patients.

Navigating Local Authorities and Systems

Not all authorities and medical communities in LMICs welcome activities by groups perceived as outsiders. Leaders may be concerned that the care of conditions discovered by screening will place additional stress on the resources of the health care system. Physicians may feel threatened financially or be made to feel irrelevant. A local physician champion can help to persuade officials that the care of patients with advanced colon cancer is more resource intensive than the care of early disease. They can also be persuaded that efforts to improve the health of the population benefit them as leaders. The local champion can also point out to his/her colleagues that offering a new service to patients enhances their practice. Encouraging the participation and training of local physicians and nurses mitigates resistance in addition to promoting sustainability which ought to be a critical goal of the effort.

Pathology Services

The availability and quality of pathology services varies considerably in LMICs. Even the terminology used to label specimens and describe findings may be different. Advanced knowledge of this helps guide planning as well as data recording. Specimens may need to be transported to a regional laboratory. Most regional options are preferable over home-based options because of cost and the benefit of developing local and regional capabilities.

Licensing

Virtually all destinations, whether LMICs or HICs, have requirements to practice medicine. This can be as simple as submitting home documentation of training and certification. In other situations, a longer bureaucratic process is required including endorsements by local health personnel and fees. Begin early, like 6 months prior to the visit, to assess and complete the process.

Shipping/Transporting Supplies

The equipment tower with video processor, light source, and monitor will need to be partially dissembled for transport and reassembled on site. Label the connections, take pictures, and rehearse the process before traveling. The company representative can be helpful in packing the equipment safely for transport. The valuable colonoscopes should be carried onto the airplane in their protective briefcases. Airport security will often inspect but are quite accommodating of medical equipment. When practicing away from home a detailed knowledge of the equipment and how to troubleshoot is critical. Having a spare and the ability to change a blown bulb or fuse have saved the day more than once.

Setting Up Space

On arrival at your destination, budget time to set up the endoscopy space. By this time you will have already evaluated the procedure and endoscope processing space, determined how it should be arranged, and acquired all the necessary extension cords, cables, hoses, and voltage transformers. Plan to this no later the day before starting procedures. After setting up and testing the equipment in advance you will be prepared to start the procedures fresh and focused on the care of the patient.

Pre-Procedural Assessment

The well-established practice of preprocedural assessment of patient's suitability to undergo screening is even more important in populations that do not receive routine preventative care. While much of this can be accomplished by a local health care provider, I recommend reviewing that assessment and the patient's understanding of the procedure in a brief encounter prior to the procedure.

Sedation/Drugs

It is now commonplace to perform colonoscopy under deep sedation with an anesthetist using propofol. These resources may not be available in many settings in LMICs, and it is useful to be comfortable performing the procedure under moderate sedation with analgesia and a short-acting benzodiazepine. I have found that most patients are comfortable with this level of sedation. I would rather err on the side of under sedation during colonoscopy. Despite careful technique over-sedation remains a risk. In addition to Advanced Cardiovascular Life Support (ACLS) certification, the team should be well-practiced and equipped to monitor and manage airway and cardiovascular emergencies, rare as they should be.

Technique

CO_2 insufflation has become commonplace to minimize post-procedure discomfort and expedite recovery. Supplies of medical grade CO_2 are often limited or a costly option in limited resource settings. Insufflation with room air remains a satisfactory and readily available option in LMICs. Similarly, a foot-activated electrical irrigation pump may not be available. A 60 cc Luer lock syringe and blunt needle is a workable solution.

Endoscope washing machines routinely used in endoscopic suites at one's home endoscopy suite are not available in many LMICs. An endoscopy technician well versed in the manual cleaning and disinfection of endoscopes is therefore essential and can teach local nurse or technician to do this reliably. Specific information on recommended practice is available from the endoscope manufacturer or from their institutional representative.

Local Accommodations

The advent of online services to rent homes for a limited period has greatly facilitated local accommodations. One has access not only to the size and services of the housing but also to the reviews of previous users. With the vagaries of transportation, it is preferable to be housed close to the service location but the team's needs for safety, rest, and recreation should also be considered.

Entertainment

What is frequently forgotten is that volunteer health professionals who are employed at home often use paid time off to participate in voluntary health care activities. Incorporating some time for relaxation and recreation serves to keep the team refreshed and motivated. This time can also be used to explore interesting sites near the locale and learn more about the community and its needs. Interaction in a social setting enhances bonding and teamwork, especially when volunteers are drawn from different institutions, regions, or countries.

Data Recording

The demand for procedures can be overwhelming and can consume the full energy of the team. An efficient database to record important demographic information and outcome of procedures is essential if only to facilitate assessment and continuous improvement. It also serves as an important source of information for scholarly activity. It is important to gain IRB approval from the home institution and also from local authorities if research is planned. This aspect of screening is an ideal activity for medical students who wish to be involved in volunteer activities and scholarship and when there are medical school resources to fund their participation.

Follow-Up Care

Colonoscopy has a low rate of complications, and most patients feel normal by the following day. Whenever possible, schedule most procedures at the beginning of the screening interval to allow time for follow-up care and concerns. Pathology reports are often not complete by the time the team departs. Plan to have those reports forwarded preferably via the internet. An addressed prepaid envelope in the hands of a local contact serves the same purpose if regular mail is the only option. As mentioned earlier, the local team members can facilitate follow-up for those patients whose pathology dictates a need for further care. Usually, these patients are identified based on gross findings and can be counseled and referred at the end of the procedure. I have found it useful to print a copy of colonoscopy findings and recommended follow-up and provide it to the patient with post-procedure instructions. I also send a copy to the physician or clinic where the patient receives care.

Surgical Care

Some patients with pathology discovered at screening require surgical care. In most settings, local surgeons are willing to accept referred patients. Having a prearranged referral surgeon in LMICs is mandatory for rare complications such as perforation. I recommend referring patients for elective surgery who might otherwise require advanced endoscopic techniques. This approach minimizes the risk of emergency surgery in limited resource settings.

Results Review and Continuous Improvement

Age-based screening guidelines are well established in many HICs but not so in all LMICs communities. In resource-limited settings where volunteer activity is focused, one may need to adjust these guidelines to prioritize groups at highest risk. Reviewing a robust database can help to focus and practice. For example, one may choose a lower age cutoff in LMICs if life expectancy is significantly lower than the norm. Symptomatic patients will inevitably present to screening programs, skewing outcomes if these patients are not properly identified and recorded in the database.

Develop Local Resources

Colon cancer screening is usually not a single event in a patient's life. To achieve maximal benefit, follow-up procedures at prescribed intervals are necessary. From the outset, one should envision a sustainable program. Involving and training local providers is the ideal solution for sustainability. The initial success of a program can be valuable in attracting necessary investments from the local authorities or private sources. A sustainable program can proceed indefinitely with progressively less input from those who initiated it, while attention and effort shift to the next community in need.

Conclusion

This is a brief summary of a complex organization of a new medical effort in an underserved country, challenged by a foreign environment, culture, and health care system. Whether the effort is highly focused, as the one described above or one that encompasses a broader program, as described in previous Chaps. (9 and 10) undertaking, the most important factors contributing to success include collaboration with local health care providers, institutions, and regulatory bodies and major emphasis on education by involving local professionals in the development of the new effort so as to make it a permanent independent service operated by local providers. The effort must be based on mutual respect, planning, discussions, and decisions guided throughout by the interests and dedication of the community and the local health care providers and hospitals. The involvement and support of the health care authorities and independent funding agencies can be both supportive and sometimes, necessary to make colon cancer screening by creating a colonoscopy service both successful and effective.

How to Establish and Expand an Intensive Care Unit in a Low- and Middle-Income Country

11

Emnet Tesfaye Shimber

Experience is not what happens to you, it's what you do with what happens to you.

– Aldous Huxley

Abbreviations

BP	Blood pressure
CCU	Critical care unit
CVP	Central venous pressure
ETT	Endotracheal tube
GCS	Glasgow Coma Scale
ICU	Intensive care unit
IPC	Infection Prevention and Control
ITU	Intensive treatment unit
IV	Intravenous
LMICs	Low- and middle-income countries
NGT	Nasogastric tube
NICU	Neonatal intensive care unit

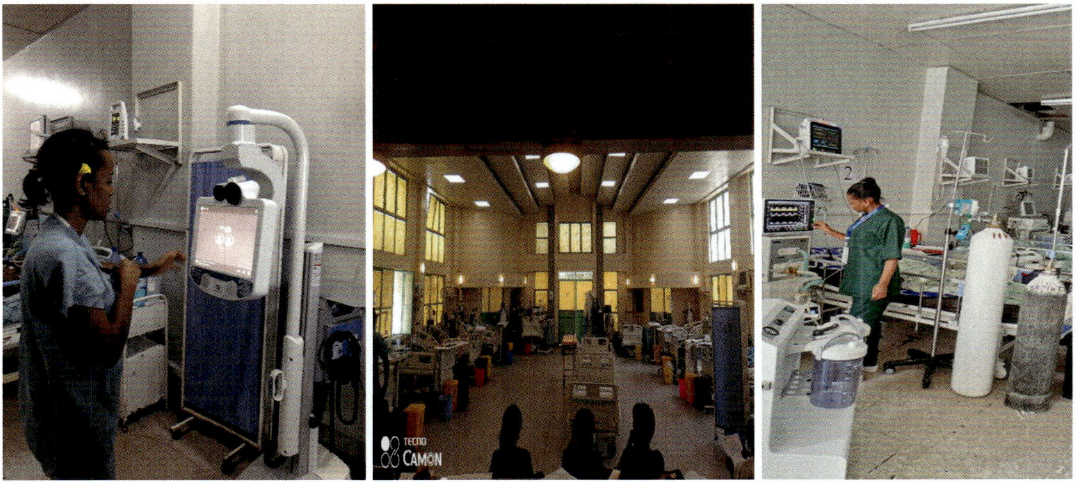

E. T. Shimber (✉)
Hawassa University College of Health Sciences and Medicine, Hawassa, Ethiopia

M. A. Hardy, B. R. Hochman (eds.), *Global Surgery*, https://doi.org/10.1007/978-3-031-28127-3_11

Introduction

An intensive care unit (ICU), also known as an intensive therapy unit or intensive treatment unit (ITU) or critical care unit (CCU), is a special department of a hospital or health care facility that provides intensive medical care. ICUs provide continuous care and monitoring for patients with severe or life-threatening illnesses and injuries with the help of life support equipment and medications until the failed organ or system improve. Critical care is a holistic care delivered to severely ill persons; otherwise, the situation may proceed to life-threatening conditions [1]. It is the delivery of a more advanced care with frequent follow-up and precise monitoring. It can be delivered at any site if the expertise and necessary resources are available.

ICUs are staffed by physicians, nurses, and respiratory and physio-therapists who received training in caring for critically ill patients. The units need and have a higher staff-to-patient ratio than regular units, despite general shortage of professional staffs. Advanced organ support medications and equipment is required which may not be available in routine wards. In low- to middle-income countries (LMICs) the commonest causes of admission to an ICU are Acute Respiratory Distress Syndrome, Sepsis and Septic shock, Heart failure, and Severe trauma. Sources of admission include emergency department, operation theatre, ward, and high dependency units. There are also specialized types of ICUs for disease-specific treatments including surgical, medical, neuro, cardiac, pediatric, neonatal and obstetrics. Most of the ICUs in Africa are general ICUs which provide services for all types of critical illnesses [2].

Africa is facing a triple burden of disease. Though epidemiologic transition studies have shifted disease burden from highly infectious and fatal to non-communicable ones, primarily surgical, both remain a large and inadequately served burden. Trauma remains a major cause of mortality which outweighs age-matched chronic illness mortality. Injury is the current epidemic in most of the LMICs in relation to urbanization, increased utilization of vehicles, poor legal enforcement, and inadequate infrastructure which results in ineffective transport from the site of injury to an appropriate health facility [3].

Most of the health care systems in LMICs are immature, especially in the delivery of intensive care. Since priority has been given to maternal and child health, neonatal care, and STDs, the advancement of critical care has been hindered. Intensive care is delivered mostly by professionals untrained in ICU techniques and at sites with low resources. The cumulative effect of low standards and inadequate personnel contributes to the observed high mortality and morbidity of critically ill patients [4].

Critical care is a relatively new concept in LMICs. Short- and long-term trainings are now available in this specialty. Majority of trainees prefer short-term skill-based training and since the demand is very high, professionals with any kind of training, or even without any specific training, can be employed in ICUs in LMICs. Most of the knowledge transfers are through informal interaction with trained colleagues. Nurses often take one- or two-week training courses in basic ICU care prior to employment and continue training on the job. Only very recently, higher level Master of Science in critical care programs are being recognized in a few institutes in LMICs. There are only few physicians with advanced critical care specialty training and most of them are concentrated in capital cities. Other ICUs are led by non-specialty trained physicians or by remote consultation with experts in large centers. Consultation process is initiated by the primary physician before transfer of the patient from their initial location which might be an ER, an OR, or a ward. After the ICU team evaluates the patient and decides on admission, critical care begins on site and continues through transfer and admission to the ICU [5].

Continent-wide critical care capacity assessment survey was done in Africa in 2020 and showed that the rate of ICU beds and mechanical ventilators were 3.1 and 0.97 respectively, per 100,000 people. This range may vary from 0.53 to 8.59 beds and 0.14 to 2.49 ventilators. There was an average of 2.42 total anesthesia providers (physician and non-physician) per 100,000 people ranging from 1.24 to 0.66 in LMICs and in the Middle African region [6, 7].

Access to critical care is a crucial component of healthcare systems in LMICs, but the capacity to provide such care in ICUs is limited. Patients with physiologic disasters (shock, sepsis, arrhythmias) are forced to stay and be managed for days in emergency departments resulting in high mortality rates. Neither the emergency departments nor wards are adequately staffed or equipped with the necessary equipment, supplies, and personnel. Most of the ICUs in resource-limited areas have too few beds and ventilator machines to accommodate the overflow of critically ill patients. Establishment of new ICU centers and expanding the existing ones is of paramount importance to improving health care quality in LMICs [7–9].

Most healthcare providers in LMICs have little experience in designing, organizing, and operating an intensive care unit. This chapter aims to guide the reader in how to either establish a new ICU or how to renovate or expand an already existing one.

The ICU Design

The developed world follows "Evidence-based design" procedure which focuses on collective knowledge from researches and benchmarking of best practices. Optimal design facilitates better patient outcome with appropriate cost and guaranteed staff satisfaction. It should create natural environment incorporating both outside views and painting over the wall as well as ceiling. Since ICU design is completely different from other hospital areas, a multi-disciplinary team of health professionals and non-clinicians should be recruited for both planning and execution of such a task. Because of complexity of the design, different needs of the clients, and significant cost of the infrastructure, composition of a team of such a diverse group is critical. All efforts must ensure the satisfaction and well-being of patients, the staff, and of all involved in the creation of a new ICU [10–12].

Project team members and their primary roles likely include:

1. *Hospital management*: this team is responsible for the overall generation of ideas and allocating the necessary budget. Also, the team supervises the progress of the project until it is completed.
2. *The clinical team*: a multidisciplinary group, including physicians, nurses, infection control specialists, pharmacists, therapists, and ancillary staff; decides on the capacity of the ICU with respect to size, sterility, non-clinical areas, and other clinically focused areas.
3. *The design team*: this team includes architects, engineers, and technology planners. They design the plan with focus on general structure, electricity and water supply, and on installation of information technology. All this is based on the input acquired from other teams. The overall design should incorporate the creation of a healing natural environment which facilitates rapid physiologic, social, behavioral, and psychologic response.
4. *Other hospital service representatives*: (facility management, environmental services, food service, and others), this team is mainly involved in supporting the overall service by facilitating safe and secured environment.

Common Design Elements

ICUs are often placed in an area adjacent to emergency rooms, operation theaters, and delivery units. The outside environment should have a waiting area for visitors with cafeteria service. Access to entrance should be limited to only allowed visitors and authorized staff. This can be controlled by security personnel with the help of camera monitoring. Assigning a porter may help in connecting staff with families especially in need of outsourced laboratory investigations and medications. A guard assigned at the entrance of an ICU needs to control the entry and exit of family, visitors, and guests. Telephone communication with the waiting room can be established for specialized ICUs between family and staff.

Visitor's policy and information contact number should be placed clearly at the entry. After the first door a green zone can be designated for change of ICU dress codes, lockers, and family-staff information exchange area. Next, a yellow zone can be designed for staff to be able to review charts, conduct brief discussions, and to maintain central patient monitoring. The final red area is the patient care zone where strict entry and management policy is applied. Each unit should have an identification marker.

Communication Infrastructure

Broadband internet and telecom device installation must be part of the initial plan. Both internal and external communication is vital for effective patient care. Internal communication between staff on duty and on call personnel is essential for patient care. External communication includes interaction with families, laboratory units, blood banks, liaison units, consultants, and other hospitals.

Patient Transportation

ICU design must consider both vertical and horizontal transport paths. Patient elevators should be near the ICU and be deep and wide enough to accommodate patient beds, support equipment, and transportation staff. Some elevators should have electrical power supplies for emergency use. Separate elevators for service traffic are recommended. Other considerations include corridor widths, door-swing directions, and timed hold-open hardware. Emergency power sources should be available in the event of medical equipment battery depletion during patient transport.

The Critical Care Unit Zones

The critical care unit design consists of four major zones:

1. The Patient Care Zone: its primary function is direct patient care equipped with appropriate monitoring devices and sources for suction, and gases for ventilation.
2. The Clinical Support Zone consists of an area which subserves functions closely related to direct patient care; not only in inpatient rooms but also in other areas of the unit, including areas for storage of supplies, locked area for pharmaceutical agents (refrigerator), Laboratory for "quick" tests (centrifuge and microscope) and storage of cultures and fluids for future analysis.
3. The Unit Support Zone: overall administrative issues and staff support space which includes communication and rest space.
4. The Family Support Zone is intended to give comfort to family and visitors.

Patient Care Zone

The Patient Care Zone refers to areas for direct patient care and is equipped with appropriate monitoring devices and sources for suction, and gases for ventilation along with space to accommodate visits by family members. Single rooms or isolated cubicles are preferable for privacy. Such rooms should resemble home arrangements to create familiarity. Children's units especially should arrange sufficient room for close family to care for the children. Multi-bed rooms should have shields and isolation curtains between beds when care and counseling is given. Bed arrangements should consider adequate space for multiple procedures and devices on all sides of the bed. Windows that can open at each bedside create views of natural environment which accelerate recovery. Electronic Medical Recording system with central monitoring is necessary for effective follow-up. Alternatives include glass walls for direct observation and frequent checks. Other considerations include sound and light control. Most of ICU equipment produce sounds which put patients under stressful condition and interfere with rest and sleep. Being able to adjust light and sound to an optimal level is important knowing that day and night illumination change facilitates normal physiologic responses.

Each room must have the following elements:

Clear Floor Area

Clear floor space is an area occupied by neither a patient nor equipment. The head of the bed should be placed at least 1 m away from the wall and the sides of the bed should be at least 2 m apart from adjacent beds. Beside privacy, this area is needed for staff activities and for portable imaging, echocardiography, transcranial Doppler examination equipment, electrocardiogram, dialysis equipment, and more. A separate room which serves all these purposes on a preset schedule is recommended and more desirable.

Medical Utility Distribution System

This system includes electronic equipment and supplies, medical gas supply, and a suction system. The medical utility outlets can be designed in one of the following ways: a flat headwall system, fixed column, suspended column, and boom configurations forms. Grounding is critical in any electric system as is a generator backup that can be promptly activated when need arises.

Medical gas, vacuum, and electrical outlets should be available for each bed. The power supply can be directly accessible from the main power source of the hospital. In case of absence of the routine electric system, automatic generator should be on standby. The oxygen system is usually accessible from a cylinder in developing countries. The storage and protection as well as inspection of the tanks on a scheduled basis is mandatory and needs to be recorded. Wall oxygen, suction, and vacuum air systems should be planned for the future, if they cannot be established immediately.

Intravenous Pumps are needed since most of ICU drugs need infusion pumps. This may require space and electric source.

Medications Cabinets for frequently needed medications should be placed by the side of the patient with the appropriate dose and clearly written order of administration.

Bedside Cabinet for food and drinks, clothes, sanitary materials, water and personal protective materials depending on the patient's need may be placed here.

Supplies' storage is needed for all other supplies which are necessary for routine care, infection prevention, and control hygiene accessories; fire extinguishers and electronic devices should also be stored in a room inside ICU with the necessary inventory and combination lock protection to prevent theft or misuse. Bedside dialysis requirement should include water treatment or an alternative.

Doors and Windows

The door should accommodate the largest ICU bed together with portable equipment and caregivers and transporters. Single entry is recommended. The room should get adequate natural light and ventilation. Ground floor ICUs should have the environmental view of a garden, if possible. Upstair rooms should provide a mirror image of nature. This helps to relieve anxiety and fastens recovery.

Walls and Ceilings

Green and blue paints have been previously shown to be favorable for tranquility. Most of the bedridden patients stare at the ceiling so that the interior design should consider non-abstract drawings and neutral lighting system. Pediatric units should have conducive wall arts with appropriate fairy tale figures.

Furniture

Bedside chair for both patients and family, waste containers, television, wall images, and clocks can be considered to create conducive environment.

Family Accommodations

Allowing families inside a patient's room should have a time limit to allow the patient to rest and the staff to deliver care in a timely manner. Considering the strong social bond and an extended family, early morning and late evening assignment of visitor hour is mandatory. For conscious patients who need frequent family support, allowing one family member extended stay might be warranted. ICU dressing code for IPC should always be in place.

Temperature Control

Depending on weather conditions air cooling and warming system should be available. In pediatric ICUs external temperature control is mandatory.

Hygiene and Sanitation

Hand hygiene should follow the WHO protocol. Water, soap, and alcohol should be readily available. There should be two sinks at entry to a room and near disposal system. A separate toilet for staff and mobile patients should be available inside the ICU. Caregivers can use bedpans or containers (for males) for fluid and urine collection for bedridden patients.

Waste Disposal System

All used equipment should be segregated in categories and disposed appropriately. Reusable materials, especially airway and mechanical ventilator equipment, should have a separate place for cleaning and storage. Sharp materials and needles should have a separate container than other wastes. All types of body fluids should be disposed of in a separate room. Strict follow-up of IPC protocol ensures appropriate waste management.

Isolation

Isolation rooms are mandatory for infected patients, patients who are prone to acquire infection, and patients who have phono- or photophobias. Creating negative pressure helps in preventing the spread of airborne pathogens but is very costly and not mandatory but ideal.

Clinical Support Zone

This area functions as storage space for equipment and supplies which are related to diagnosis and treatment of patients. Some of these may be located inside the ICU, while others may be located in more remote sites.

Team Work Areas

There is a need for sites for discussions among the members of the care team or with consultants, as well as a site for regular rounds in a separate and quiet environment. This is especially important in teaching hospitals. This should also be the location for maintenance of ICU guidelines, protocols, activity schedules, staff rosters, and standard manuals for everyone's use.

Centralized Monitoring: for electronic point of care, ICUs may have remote site centralized monitoring system. For others, documentations and order carryout can be done on site in the ICU.

Tele-ICU: For ICUs with few trained physicians, a single critical care physician can oversee several ICUs via digital supervision and continuous consultation. Such remote site consultation is also possible with direct patient visualization. It may also serve as an important tool for teaching new staff.

Pharmacy Services

There should be a separate ICU pharmacy inside an ICU with appropriate security and accountability. This permits rapid access to emergency drugs in urgent situations. Many of ICU medications need further preparation according to the prescription. A discrete sterile area in the pharmacy should be reserved for this activity and contain a refrigerator, laboratory scale, and centrifuge, and, if possible, a fume hood. After preparing the medication it should be clearly labeled with the name of the patient, hospital number, date, time, and duration of administration.

Laboratory Services

ICUs must have access to 24-h clinical laboratory services. Simple tests can be done in a satellite laboratory near or in the ICU equipped with a centrifuge, a microscope, and an incubator. There must be easy access for blood gas analysis, chemistry, hematology, fluid analysis, and cultures, while more extensive investigations should be performed in a central laboratory.

Imaging Services

Portable ultrasound and X-ray should be available in the ICU. Since transportation of critically ill patients attached to multiple devices is often a challenge, other services like CT and MRI should be easily accessible, preferably on the same floor. The equipment should be inspected on a regular basis as proscribed by the manufacturer and repaired promptly when needed.

Respiratory Therapy

A respiratory support area with storage space for mechanical ventilators, circuits, tubes, airway equipment, and oxygen tanks should be separate from the main storage area. Since a respiratory therapist may not always be available, a trained professional physician or nurse should be in charge of this unit. The team should include nurses, physicians, and biomedical technicians.

Specialized Procedure Areas
One designated patient room in the ICU should be equipped to accommodate imaging or invasive procedures. Areas for specialized medical procedures, such as biopsies, or line insertions, must be available adjacent to or near the ICU (e.g., a cardiac catheterization laboratory adjacent to a cardiac ICU).

The functional requirements for the unit will dictate the need for specialized procedure rooms. Due to equipment and staffing costs, a cost-benefit analysis should assess the probable number of cases requiring these highly specialized rooms over the lifespan of the unit.

Emergency Equipment and Supplies
Crash cart filled with emergency life-support equipment and supplies should be always available and be inspected on a regular basis, and be replenished after each use. Charge nurse should check that it is properly resupplied at least once a day. There should be written hand-over protocol confirmation of its inventory between shifts.

Nutrition Preparation Area
Kitchen appliances should be available to prepare food for patients based on their dietary need.

Unit Support Zone

The unit support zone encompasses areas where administrative, logistic, and staff support functions are performed. Multipurpose conference room is useful for clinical audits, seminars, change of shift reports, and case discussions. A Clean Utility room is necessary for storage of clean materials and a Soiled Utility room is used for decontamination of soiled materials. Staff lounge with full kitchen appliance decreases staff absences from the ICU during service hours. On-call rooms with beds, television, internet, and table facilitate staff to have adequate rest when it is possible. ICU director and shift head need an office space. Toilet and shower services must also be available on the unit.

Family Support Zone

The Family Support Zone should consist of spaces which would be outside of the patient rooms to serve both family and visitors. This will also permit consultations, rest, visitor nourishment, and prayer activities in an isolated walled-off section. Chairs should recline sufficiently for the family and/or visitors to rest and nap.

ICU Classification

The ICU may be classified based on the following alternate basis: (1) Level (Level 1, Level 2, Level 3); (2) Purpose—(a) Standard (ideal or standard), (b) General (used for all purposes), (c) Specialized (medical, neurological, or surgical), (d). Age group (adult ICU, pediatrics, neonates); (3) Specific organ system (cardiovascular, neuro, renal, respiratory); (4) Clinical syndrome (burn, trauma, stroke, poisoning); and (5) based on Client (neonatal, pediatric, obstetric) [1, 5].

Level I ICU is also referred to as high dependency unit. This can be located in primary district hospitals, where close monitoring, resuscitation, and short-term ventilation for less than 24 h have to be performed. Trained general practitioners and nurses work in this unit. Specialist physicians might be in charge of the critical patients based on their expertise and availability. Teleconsultation with critical care physicians elsewhere is available at all times.

Level II ICU can be located in a general regional hospital. Here trained professionals including residents, doctors, nurses, and specialists supervise patient care and are able to undertake more prolonged patient ventilation and maintenance. Laboratory, radiology, and pathology accesses are modest but are available and are mandatory.

Level III ICU is a highly specialized unit located in a major tertiary hospital. It provides dialysis, cardiac catheterization laboratory, clinical pharmacy, physiotherapy, and rehabilitation services. This unit is overseen by intensivists, emergency, and critical care physicians and anesthesiologists. Further availability of nephrologists, gastroenterologists, neurologists, and other sub-specialists is almost always available on call.

General Intensive Care Unit
This represents a multi-disciplinary care unit. In consideration of critical complications of all disease entities, this type of unit offers specialized care to acute stabilization of the presenting life-threatening condition. A closely interacting team of Emergency and Critical Care specialists, Anesthesiologists, and Intensivists provides joint diagnostic and therapeutic interventions as they are needed. Consultations with other specialty areas, including surgeons, are made based on the individual patient's needs. This is a cost-effective strategy for LMICs since it permits a centralized system of resource management.

Medical Intensive Care Unit
The medical intensive care unit is dedicated to the care of adult patients with life-threatening medical conditions requiring frequent observation, specialized monitoring, and medical treatment. These include illnesses such as diabetic ketoacidosis, gastrointestinal bleeding, drug overdose, respiratory failure, sepsis, stroke, and metastatic cancer.

Surgical Intensive Care Unit
The surgical intensive care unit is dedicated primarily to the management of postoperative patients, including patients who have undergone major abdominal surgeries, craniotomies, thoracotomies, unstable multiple traumas, and any preoperative or acutely ill patient with a presumed surgical disease who requires continuous monitoring or organ support, regardless of cause.

Pediatric Intensive Care Unit
All critically ill children are managed in the pediatric intensive care units. Children who have recently undergone surgery and are at risk of deterioration are also managed in the pediatric intensive care unit.

Neonatal Intensive Care Unit
The neonatal intensive care unit (NICU) is dedicated to the management of premature, high-risk, and critically ill neonates. NewbornsInfants undergoing urgent operations following delivery (e.g., Diaphragmatic hernia, TE fistula) are cared for in NICU. Neonates with congenital disorders and birth complications are also managed in the NICU.

ICU Organizational Models

Intensive care services are an important and costly resource, which once established must be consistent, safe, and efficient [10].

Open Model
This organizational model allows many members from various specialties in the hospital to manage their patients in the ICU. This leads to inconsistencies in management, confuses and misleads the staff, and is unreliable and inefficient. It introduces many errors in judgment and in patient mismanagement [13].

Closed Model
In this model a limited number of ICU-certified physicians are responsible for the overall activities in the ICU. Based on the need judged by the full-time staff other specialists can be consulted. In most cases, patient's own physician or surgeon can assist in the care of their patients through suggestions and advice to the responsible ICU staff. This model leads to favorable outcomes and improved patient survival [13].

Hybrid Model
This model combines aspects of open and closed models in a systematic manner, usually combining responsibilities in patient management by joint rounds at which decisions are made. Availing many specialists at a time is not cost effective for LMICs.

ICU Standards

The number of ICU beds typically comprise 1 to 10% of a hospital's total bed capacity. Multidisciplinary ICUs require more beds than does a single specialty ICU. ICUs with fewer than four beds are not financially viable, and those with more than 20 beds may be difficult to manage. An ICU should be situated close to one or more important locations, such as the operating room, radiology department, acute wards, and emergency room. There should be a sufficient number of elevators available to transport seriously ill patients to various locations quickly and without delay. An ICU should have only a single entrance and exit point. Any traffic of medical personnel or supplies through an ICU should be prohibited.

ICU must feature places and/or rooms for support services, patient management talks, and public reception. A central station should be equipped with one or more telephones, two refrigerators, one for medications, the other for samples, and a central monitor for EKG and vital signs connected to each patient's bed. Patient records, if not electronic, or supplemental should also be maintained in this area. Each patient requires a floor area of 18.5 m^2 (200 sq.), with single rooms needing a greater area of 26–30 m^2 to comfortably fit patients, personnel, and equipment. All space restrictions listed above and in the comments are arbitrary and determined by the rules of the relevant health authorities. The distance between the bed centers should be at least 3 to 3.67 meters. Single rooms are essential for isolation purposes and for privacy. Three oxygen, two air, four suction, and 16 power outlets including a bedside lamp are optimal for level III ICU beds depending on size and function of the ICU.

The overall management should be led by a director who is a full-time physician and responsible to the chief executive director or medical director. Institution-based protocols on admission-discharge, IPC, sedation, enteral–parenteral feeding, lung protective ventilation, weaning, venous thrombo-embolism prophylaxis, and drug administration hospital should be clearly strictly adhered to.

A multidisciplinary committee should be established with main role of conducting clinical oversight and audits and an Ethics Committee should be available to help resolve ethical dilemmas.

ICU Staffing

The ICU structure depends on institutional human resource capacity.

Medical Staff

Large hospitals require larger teams. Intensivists are the most effective senior medical staff appointed to the leadership roles in ICUs. They can share their supervisory functions with other intensivists or specialists in various fields depending on the medical focus of the ICU. Other Emergency and Critical Care physicians and Pulmonologists or Anesthesiologists can also fulfill the supervisory ICU role. In very limited resource areas critical care trained physicians like surgeons, internists and pediatricians can also assume leadership ICU function (Fig. 11.1).

Nursing Staff

The head nurse should be an Emergency and/or Critical Care trained and experienced nurse. Alternatives include BSc critical care nurses. He/she should be experienced in the use of health information systems, in guiding quality improvement projects, and be familiar with enforcing IPC standards. The head nurse's duty extends to creating conducive environment among the nurses, physicians, and various working units in the ICU like pharmacy, laboratory, and physiotherapy.

The major hospital's teaching tertiary care ICUs require trained and critical care certified nurses. Nurse-to-patient ratio in tertiary units should aim for a ratio of, 1:1 in all mechanically ventilated patients, and not accept anything lower than 1:2 ratio. A ratio of 1:2 is acceptable for those patients who need only close observation and are not supported by a mechanical ventilator.

Allied Service Staff

Physiotherapy, social workers, dieticians, radiology services, and respiratory therapists are an important and essential workforce responsible for the overall effective and safe patient management. Biomedical department services are also required on a regular basis to service, repair, and install old and new equipment.

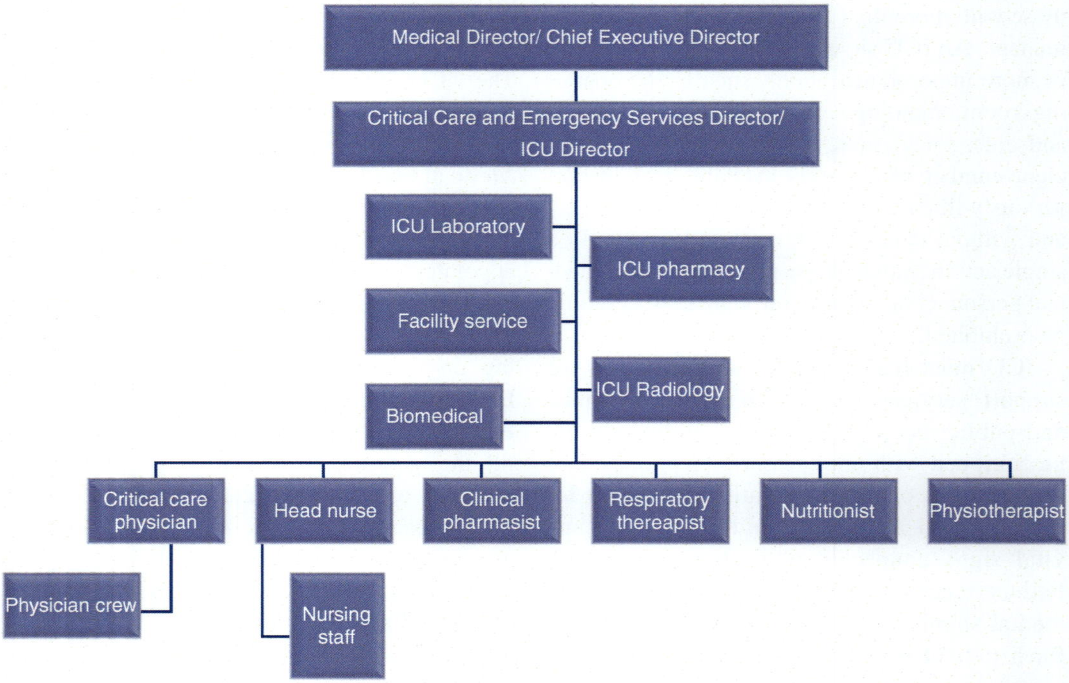

Fig. 11.1 ICU structure

ICU Equipment

Common equipment in an ICU includes mechanical ventilators to assist breathing through an endotracheal tube or a tracheostomy tube; cardiac monitors for monitoring blood pressure, cardiac rate and rhythms; equipment for the constant monitoring of respiratory rate and pulmonary functions in patients on ventilators; a web of intravenous lines, feeding tubes, nasogastric tubes, suction pumps, drains, and catheters, along with the various collection receptacles; syringe pumps; and a wide array of intravenous drugs to treat the primary condition(s) for which the patient was hospitalized. Medically induced comas, maximal analgesia to the point of anesthesia, and induced sedation are commonly needed ICU tools which require specialized monitoring equipment and close nursing attention to detailed observation. For further reading refer Annex I.

Monitoring in ICU

Intensive care units rely heavily on continuous monitoring and maintenance of patient's vital functions to improve survival and recovery of critically ill patients. Continuous monitoring of vital signs permits identification of critical changes in the patient's progress and helps to guide therapeutic interventions. Early recognition of patient deterioration and timely intervention are critical in saving patients' lives and are the main reason to be cared for in an ICU. Particular emphasis is placed on the following:

Noninvasive Monitoring

- Vital signs—preferable continuous SPO_2, BP, Respiratory rate, Temperature and O_2 flow rate.
- Neurological function—GCS—format.
- Renal function—hourly/daily, input–output balance.

- Respiratory functions—adequacy of coughing, respiratory patterns, bilateral air entry (check list on mechanical ventilator).
- Others including pain and response to pain management—Analgesia protocol, positioning, IPC protocols, nutritional status documentation, relevant lab results.

Invasive Monitoring of Patients
- CVP.
- Arterial lines.
- ICP.

Monitoring of Equipment's Function and Sterility/Hygiene
- Amount of various drainages—NGT and chest tubes, flow rate, and correct placement.
- Endotracheal tubes—position, fixation, and patency; dressing changes.
- Oxygen supply equipment (tanks)—empty, full, flow meter, and backup BMV.
- Perfusers' functionality, availability, and electric connectivity.
- Infusions—type of fluid, infusion rate, label (type, time, rate of flow) and hand covering format.
- Folly catheters—urine output amount every 12 h; day of insertion and functionality.
- Suction devices—amount of drainage from suction tubes; suction machine sterility and functionality and dressing change.
- Emergency drugs—daily inventory—availability and crush cart resupply.
- Mechanical Ventilator—monitor for the following parameters: VT, RR, MV, FIO_2, PEEP, Mode, I: E, PSV, patient synchrony; check daily for Alarms, humidifiers, Tubing, Filters, Power, Cleanness, and Safety.

Specific Medical Conditions

Shock: Patients with shock are initially admitted to the emergency department (either Adult or Pediatric). Institution-based protocols considering the availability of resources should be followed for individual patients. Overall fluid resuscitation starts based on the etiology of the problem. Nonresponders will be started on inotropes after a major effort at determining the diagnosis but not delaying treatment to achieve a favorable outcome. Mostly the available drugs are Adrenaline and Dopamine. For septic shock patients, broad-spectrum antibiotics are usually initiated before a sample for blood culture is obtained, since the microbiology lab is limited for selected critical patients. Oxygen is provided intra-nasally or via face mask, either from concentrator machines or oxygen cylinders based on availability. Serial follow-up is made by nurses, medical interns, and residents with consultants as needed, especially surgeons who are also responsible for newly coming emergency patients. Since monitors are not readily available in emergency and intensive care rooms in LMICs pulse oximetry and manual blood pressure cuffs are used routinely. This makes the follow-up laborious and inadequate. Baseline Laboratory investigations are done when a laboratory is available, while ECG and ultrasound evaluations are also desirable when available in station hospitals in LMICs. Culture for blood and body fluids can also be obtained more readily at initial meeting prior to antibiotics and transfer to an ICU. Patients continue to obtain adequate cardio-respiratory support and serial follow-up while being investigated for a precise diagnosis, either surgical or medical in a better-focused manner, with appropriate consultations as necessary. Manual defibrillator is usually available in an emergency room, but not routinely used, frequently because it needs repair and/or lack of training in its use. Another possible reason is late detection of cardiac arrests due to poor minute-to-minute follow-up in an understaffed busy setting.

Scarcity of equipment, trained personnel, shortage of supplies, and lack of biochemical and microbiologic profile measurements are some of the limitations in ICUs in LMICs, especially in remote station and even in regional hospitals, but rarely in tertiary centers.

Sepsis: Patients with sepsis are initially directed to emergency departments, just like patients with shock. Medical interns and emergency room residents provide the first evaluation, collaborating with specialists as necessary. Based on locally adapted Surviving Sepsis Campaign guideline, patients are resuscitated and empirical antibiotics are administered, usually before a sample for culture is taken (forgetting to do this is a major error which must be avoided). Basic laboratory testing, targeted radiologic examinations, and focused ultrasound tests are used to investigate these patients. Because of limited access, lengthy lineups, and local emergency service constraints, most patients with sepsis in LMICs progress to septic shock. Admission to ICU is usually prioritized for other critically ill patients due to the inadequate number of ICU beds unless these patients deteriorate to septic shock at which point, they may get the privilege of critical care unit management or get to the operating room if surgically indicated.

Arrhythmia: Dysrhythmia is often fatal due to failure to detect it or because of lack of appropriate anti-arrhythmic drugs that can be used in a timely fashion. Detailed knowledge of ECG interpretation as well as understanding of classification of type of arrhythmias is the first and critical step in leading the intervention. Unfortunately, this is frequently not recognized by staff in station or regional emergency areas in LMICs where adequate cardiac monitoring is rare. The commonest types of arrhythmias are atrial fibrillation, supraventricular tachycardia, and ventricular tachycardias. The widely available anti-arhythmic agents include digoxin, adenosine, amiodarone, and metoprolol, which are frequently not readily available in emergency rooms but must be available in the ICUs.

Challenges and Future Directions for ICUs

Operating critical care services in LMICs presents significant problems, in contrast to ICUs in HICs. These include financial constraints, scarcity of trained personnel, both doctors and nurses, restricted infrastructure for transportation, technology, communication, and administrative leadership. Even if the sufficient support was available, access to essential medications and supplies remains generally limited. The government's procurement approach usually does not facilitate acquisition of necessary resources. The exorbitant cost of treatment, which is frequently unaffordable for the majority, prevents admissions to ICUs and results in even greater cost in lives and loss of the workforce. This is partially due to an inadequate health insurance system and/or minimal universal health care. The staff generally has low motivation, lack of satisfaction because of lack of enthusiasm for ICUs by health authorities. This in turn leads to a vicious cycle of decreased specialized knowledge, and experience. Determination of priority of admissions to the limited number of ICU beds raise significant ethical issues. Delayed referral systems and late initiation of care significantly affect the outcome of the critically ill. Lack of preventive and corrective maintenance of equipment due to the absence of supplies and biomedical staff shortage hinders the delivery of optimal care.

The lack of accurate patient data from defined regions and countries and the shortfall in human resource management will be addressed by the growth of technologic tracking and by the specialized training of highly competent young professionals. The interest of the international health community in assisting in improvement of critical care in this environment should help to advance ongoing efforts. Introducing ICU professional skills and novel technologies to the existing system will further improve the care of the sickest patients. Vigorous advocacy, policy change, and a paradigm shift are required to address the critical care challenges in LMICs.

Conclusion

The intent of this chapter is to provide a brief road map on how to approach the establishment of an ICU in various areas of an LMIC, depending on the sites and types of hospitals, ranging from rural station hospital to regional hospital in a larger city, to tertiary centers in capitals and large urban areas, the emphasis is on training and employment of expert intensivists and/or providers of critical care by other specialists.

Emphasis is also placed on training and expertise of nursing and other ancillary staff, on nurse/patient ratios, on availability of supplies and equipment, and on staff interaction and collaboration with consultants and other caregivers. Appropriate staffing is adjusted to the size and type of ICU which may be multidisciplinary or specialty focused and will vary as to size and staffing according to the type of hospital it subserves; this includes the tertiary type as most advanced and the largest, regional which is smaller, and the station hospitals which are smallest and least advanced, usually found in rural areas. Laboratory, radiology, anesthesia, and specialist support for the different ICUs also vary in availability from most advanced hospitals to the smallest station hospitals. To achieve significant progress in this area, public and government enthusiasm is required to provide financial, technical, professional, and health care community collaboration and support.

Annexes

Annex I

List of equipment

- 24-hours monitoring and the provision of oxygen
- Adequate lighting for bedside procedures.
- Anesthesia machine.
- Arterial line monitoring.
- Bag valve mask.
- Beds with removable headboard and adjustable position.
- Blood Analyzer.
- Central venous catheters, arterial catheters.
- Central venous pressure monitoring devices.
- Chest tube, pigtail catheter, chest drainage system.
- Continuous end-tidal CO_2 monitoring.
- Continuous pulse oximetry.
- Defibrillators.
- Dialysis unit.
- Difficult airway management equipment.
- Echocardiography and ECG.
- Emergency resuscitative equipment.
- Fluid and bed warmers.
- Foley catheters.
- Hypo/hyperthermia blanket.
- Infusion pumps.
- Insert tons of airway equipment here such as direct laryngoscopes, Glide Scopes, bougies, etc.
- Insert tons of wound care supplies.
- Intra cranial monitoring devices.
- Nasal cannula (including high flow), non-rebreather masks.
- Nebulizer.
- Non-invasive monitors.
- Non-invasive positive pressure ventilation (e.g. BiPAP, CPAP) machines.
- Oxygen concentrators, oxygen cylinder, concentrator with flow meter.
- Paracentesis kit.
- pericardiocentesis set,
- Portable Clinical Lab. Devices.
- Portable light.
- Portable X-ray machine.
- Sterile gowns and sterile drapes.
- Suction machines including Yankauer tips.
- Telemedicine capability.
- Telemetry.
- Thoracentesis kit.
- Tracheostomy set.
- Transvenous pacemaker kits and external pacemaker device.
- Ultrasound machines.
- Ventilators and monitors.
- Weight scale.

Annex II

ICU quality indicators

1. Compliance with hand hygiene protocols
2. Providing information to families of patients in the ICU
3. Appropriate sedation
4. Appropriate pain management
5. Appropriate sepsis management
6. Early enteral nutrition
7. Prophylaxis for GI bleed in those undergoing invasive mechanical ventilation
8. Inappropriate transfusion of blood products

9. Semi recumbent position for patients on invasive mechanical ventilation
10. Ventilator associated pneumonia
11. Prevention of catheter related bloodstream infections (CRBSI), and catheter associated urinary tract infections (CAUTI)
12. Early administration of acetyl salicylic acid in acute coronary syndrome
13. Early reperfusion therapy in STEMI
14. Monitoring ICP in severe traumatic brain injury with CT findings
15. Surgical intervention within 3 h in traumatic brain injury with subdural and/or epidural hematoma
16. Perceived Quality Survey at discharge from ICU
17. Presence of ICU trained medical professionals in the ICU
18. Maintaining adverse events register
19. Length of stay
20. Tracheotomy rate
21. Mortality rate
22. Pressure ulcer
23. Rational use of antibiotics (development of drug resistance)
24. Readmission rate
25. Re-intubation rate
26. Fall rate
27. Presence of CC trained pharmacist/clinical pharmacists
28. Presence of key ICU drugs and supplies.

References

1. Marshall JC, Bosco L, Adhikari NK, Connolly B, Diaz JV, Dorman T, et al. What is an intensive care unit? A report of the task force of the World Federation of Societies of Intensive and Critical Care Medicine. J Crit Care. 2017;37:270–6.
2. Towey RM, Ojara S. Intensive care in the developing world. Anaesthesia [Internet]. 2007;62(s1):32–7. https://doi.org/10.1111/j.1365-2044.2007.05295.x.
3. Lagarde E. Road traffic injury is an escalating burden in Africa and deserves proportionate research efforts. PLOS Med [Internet]. 2007;4(6):170. https://doi.org/10.1371/journal.pmed.0040170.
4. Netshisaulu KG, Malelelo-Ndou H, Ramathuba DU. Challenges experienced by health care professionals working in resource-poor intensive care settings in the Limpopo province of South Africa. Curationis [Internet]. 2019;42(1):1–8. https://doi.org/10.4102/curationis.v42i1.1921.
5. Okech UK, Chokwe T, Mung'ayi V. The operational setup of intensive care units in a low income country in East Africa. East Afr Med J [Internet]. 2015;92(2):72–80. https://www.ajol.info/index.php/eamj/article/view/118829
6. Craig J, Kalanxhi E, Hauck S. National estimates of critical care capacity in 54 African countries [Internet]. medRxiv; 2020 [cited 2022 Aug 22]. p. 2020.05.13.20100727. https://doi.org/10.1101/2020.05.13.20100727v2
7. Ayebale ET, Roche AM, Kassebaum NJ, Biccard BM. Africa's critical care capacity before COVID-19. South Afr J Anaesth Analg [Internet]. 2020;26(3): 162–4. https://doi.org/10.10520/EJC-1d759b8c72.
8. Atumanya P, Sendagire C, Wabule A, Mukisa J, Ssemogerere L, Kwizera A, et al. Assessment of the current capacity of intensive care units in Uganda; A descriptive study. J Crit Care [Internet]. 2020;55:95–9. https://www.sciencedirect.com/science/article/pii/S0883944119310597
9. Riviello ED, Letchford S, Achieng L, Newton MW. Critical care in resource-poor settings: lessons learned and future directions*. Crit Care Med [Internet]. 2011;39(4):860–7. https://journals.lww.com/ccmjournal/Abstract/2011/04000/Critical_care_in_resource_poor_settings__Lessons.34.aspx
10. Institute FG. Guidelines for design and construction of health care facilities. ASHE (American Society for Healthcare Engineering of the American Hospital ...; 2010.
11. Guidelines for intensive care unit design*: Critical Care Medicine [Internet]. [cited 2022 Aug 24]. Available from: https://journals.lww.com/ccmjournal/fulltext/2012/05000/Guidelines_for_intensive_care_unit_design_.26.aspx
12. Bazuin D, Cardon K. Creating healing intensive care unit environments: physical and psychological considerations in designing critical care areas. Crit Care Nurs Q [Internet]. 2011;34(4):259–67. https://journals.lww.com/ccnq/Abstract/2011/10000/Creating_Healing_Intensive_Care_Unit_Environments_.4.aspx
13. The-optimal-icu-organizational-structure.pdf [Internet]. [cited 2022 Aug 23]. https://criticalcareshock.org/files/2018/10/the-optimal-icu-organizational-structure.pdf

12 How to Create a Post Anesthesia Care Unit for Recovery After Surgery and Anesthesia in a Low- and Middle-Income Country

Tricia Brentjens and Rebecca Havlir Martinez

They may forget your name, but they will never forget how you made them feel.

– Maya Angelou

Abbreviations

BP	Blood pressure
ECG	Electrocardiogram
HICs	High-income countries
ICU	Intensive Care Unit
LMICs	Low- and middle-income countries
ORs	Operating rooms
PACU	Post Anesthesia Care Unit
POCUS	Point of care ultrasound
PONV	Postoperative nausea and vomiting
RNs	Registered nurses
RR	Recovery room
RR	Respiratory rate

T. Brentjens (✉)
Department of Anesthesiology, Columbia University Irving Medical Center, New York, NY, USA
e-mail: tb164@cumc.columbia.edu

R. H. Martinez
Department of Anesthesia and Critical Care Medicine, University of California, San Francisco, San Francisco, CA, USA
e-mail: rebecca.martinez2@ucsf.edu

Introduction

Once patients have completed their care in the operating room, healthcare centers usher patients to a formal area for their initial recovery from anesthesia and surgery. Often termed a Recovery Room (RR) or Post Anesthesia Care Unit (PACU) these areas serve primarily to monitor patients in the immediate postoperative period after surgery as they emerge from general or regional anesthesia or sedation, providing vital medical services to patients and enhancing the safety and efficiency of the hospital system. Common postop issues include respiratory depression, hemodynamic instability (hypo/hypertension), postoperative nausea and vomiting (PONV), pain control, altered mental status, shivering and monitoring for postop bleeding.

The first PACU was established in the 1940s in the post-World War II era as surgical interventions and repairs became more common and survivable. Initially, RRs were poorly funded and staffed. However, backed by an intensive governmental investment in improving the standard of health care, these areas of the hospital quickly flourished. Establishing RRs became a priority after abysmal rates of post-anesthesia complications were reported in 1947 in the Journal of the

M. A. Hardy, B. R. Hochman (eds.), *Global Surgery*, https://doi.org/10.1007/978-3-031-28127-3_12

American Medical Association. This 11-year retrospective study identified 47% of anesthesia-related postoperative deaths as preventable. The commission recommended clustering patients together in the immediate postoperative period for improved direct observation of patients, which was predicted to prevent 33% of all post-surgical deaths [1].

Thus, the PACU was born to serve as an observational unit where nurses provide specialized postoperative care with physician oversight. The combination of skilled nurses trained to recognize and intervene in common post-anesthetic and surgical complications as well as physical proximity to the operating rooms where physicians remain actively engaged in caring for other patients facilitates the rapid identification and response to respiratory and hemodynamic instability, greatly improving patient safety.

Indeed, the core mission of the PACU to facilitate safe care of the post-anesthesia and surgical patient has remained the same nearly a century later and applies equally in high-income countries (HICs) and in low- and middle-income countries (LMICs). PACUs have been shown to enhance recovery from anesthesia and are correlated with improved surgical outcomes [2]. This is in part because a PACU clusters patients who have a higher likelihood for acute events that require early intervention and occasionally immediate emergency response; it is therefore staffed by professionals trained in the recognition and response of postoperative complications. PACUs also have transitioned to areas of the hospital that are optimal for triage as occasionally it is unknown if during the post-surgical period a patient will progress toward a trajectory of stability or deteriorate requiring a higher level of care than can be offered on a traditional inpatient ward [3].

Beyond what was traditionally envisioned, PACUs also have been recognized to facilitate optimal healthcare resource utilization. As patients can be ushered out of operating rooms and recover from anesthesia in a separate space, RRs allow "hospitals to improve their caseloads, reduce turnover times in the operating room, and even help to manage a shortage of beds in the intensive care unit" [4]. The flexibility offered by PACUs as areas that can be transformed to provide critical care space in times of extreme hospital duress and capacity was demonstrated most recently during the 2020 Sars-CoV-2 pandemic which tested the capacity of healthcare delivery systems worldwide. During localized case surges, existing PACUs were supplemented with personnel and services, and then converted into full intensive care units (ICU) [5].

In this chapter, we will review the essential components to establish and run a functional PACU. There will be attention given to setting up the physical space, personnel and training requirements, a very brief review of some common emergency scenarios, and finally steps toward perpetual quality improvement.

Physical Space and Equipment

The PACU should be located in close physical proximity to the operating rooms (ORs) which both minimizes transport times between operating rooms and the recovery area and allows for rapid response by additional staff in the case of an emergency and for possible return to the OR. PACUs are primarily open units with ideally one or two enclosed private rooms designed for patients in need of strict contact or airborne isolation needs. This facilitates a "shared care" model where providers in or walking through the PACU can quickly evaluate a patient and recognize changes that require attention and intervention. PACUs should have delineated spaces for each patient, ideally with a bed or a reclining chair. As with all units, natural light as well as sufficient airflow is optimal for patient safety and satisfaction, though as patients often spend only limited periods of time in the RR, these qualities can be prioritized less when necessary.

The monitoring of vital signs is an important component of delivering safe care in the PACU. A variety of equipment should be available for use in both monitoring and to intervene in emergency situations. Ideally, the PACU should have the ability to continuously monitor electrocardiogram (ECG), oxygen saturation, and intermittently monitor blood pressure (BP), respiratory rate (RR), and temperature. The most critical monitor is perhaps the pulse oximeter which can provide both a heart rate and blood oxygen saturation. Interestingly, continuous pulse ox monitoring was not found to decrease mortality [6], suggesting that intermittent checks combined with routine physical exams for cyanosis may be sufficient. Rapid availability of either manual or automatic BP monitoring is also essential as hemodynamic changes can be a harbinger of pending distress. It is preferable to have continuous ECG monitoring for all patients, especially those at high risk for arrhythmias or ischemia. In an ideal situation, all monitors would send data to a central monitoring area where one person can observe changes and initiate prompt bedside response to deviations from expected values, although we realize that this is not likely in many global healthcare situations in LMICs.

Equipment necessary for respiratory and airway support should be kept in the PACU as well as the operating room areas if feasible. Nasal cannulas and facemasks are necessary to provide supplemental oxygen. Ideally, every patient spot in the PACU would have an oxygen supply but we realize that in LMICs this may not always be possible and recommend the availability of portable oxygen tanks (safely and secured stored and checked regularly). Necessary items for airway support include: a bag-mask-valve system, oral and nasal airways, laryngeal mask airways, endotracheal tubes, intubating blades, boogies, and an end-tidal carbon dioxide colorimeter. More specialized airway equipment such as a video laryngoscope may provide further safety for patients requiring reintubation. A variety of styles are available on the market including the CMAC, Glidescope, and McGrath, though each of these requires a system either to sterilize specialized blades and/or replaceable components that are single-use only. Fiberoptic bronchoscopes provide a level of additional safety but are incredibly resource intensive in terms of both physical maintenance and routine staff familiarity with their safe usage; these scopes, if available, may be better suited in a designated operative space and transported to the PACU in case of emergency. If wall suction is not available, ideally a source for portable suction should always be available.

One technology worth potentially investing in is ultrasound. This imaging modality has significant diagnostic and therapeutic utility. Evolving technology includes handheld ultrasounds which plug into smartphones and require minimal maintenance and are relatively inexpensive. Point of Care Ultrasound, POCUS, has become an increasingly popular tool to allow prompt diagnosis of many conditions. Lung POCUS can easily diagnose pulmonary congestion, pneumothorax, or pleural effusion. Cardiac POCUS can allow for a quick assessment of global function, wall motion abnormalities, and pericardial effusion. Abdominal POCUS can assess for volume status and free fluid. It has been shown that ultrasound availability in the PACU narrows the differential diagnosis as well as decreases the length of stay in the PACU [7]. While ensuring proper training of the person interpreting the images is paramount to safe use of the technology, multiple free resources are available online from sites such as YouTube.com and nysora.com among many others (see Chap. 18).

Personal protective equipment for staff such as gloves and masks should be stored in this area along with bed linens. Gloves and supplies should ideally be latex free as many patients and healthcare professionals have latex allergies. Separate clean and dirty utility areas should be maintained. Necessary supplies range from routine wound care supplies including gauze, dressing supplies, and tape to supplies for vascular access including tourniquets, alcohol wipes, angiocatheters, and needles in a variety of gauges. Fluids, such as normal saline and lactated ringers, as well as IV tubing should be available. Syringes are needed for both the administration of medications and drawing of blood. Laboratory tubes for available blood tests should be stored. Each item should have a designated space that is well labeled to facilitate both ease of access and prompt identification of low-supply count. Storage of supplies in a centralized well secured area that is conveniently located to minimize foot traffic by nurses out of the immediate care vicinity of the patients is ideal. This area should be well protected from illegal entries and theft which may be very tempting for the patients and for the staff. Other equipments to consider are oro- and nasogastric tubes, foley catheters, and chest tubes. Bakri balloons may be lifesaving and should be prioritized to provide care for the patient with post-partum hemorrhage. An example of a cart system to organize supplies is shown in Fig. 12.1.

The availability and storage of routine and emergent drugs used in perioperative care is extremely important. Commonly used medications for administration in the recovery room include opioids for pain control (fentanyl or morphine being preferable because of long shelf life and easy storage), non-opioid analgesics (including paracetamol and ibuprofen), anti-emetics such as ondansetron and metoclopramide, and antibiotics. As some of these drugs can be habit-forming if improperly administered, it is recommended that a system to minimize abuse be implemented and maintained for staff and patient safety. Additionally, medications to treat hypertension, hypotension, and bronchospasm should also be available. These include first-line drugs such as epinephrine and atropine; second-line drugs may include phenylephrine and ephedrine. Albuterol inhalers and or nebulizers for treatment of bronchospasm should be stocked.

Personnel, Roles, and Training

Successful operation of a PACU begins in the preoperative area and in the operating room. In these spaces, high-risk patients can be optimized, analgesia can be administered, and a plan for the recovery can be formulated. The person providing care for the patient in the operating room should accompany the patient to the recovery area and provide a sign-out to the primary PACU provider, usually a specialist nurse, including a brief medical history, allergies, surgery overview, anesthesia overview, complications intraoperatively, and a plan for anticipated postoperative course, including orders for any pain and nausea control regimens.

The PACU should be overseen by a trained physician, typically an anesthesiologist or anesthetist, or a pulmonologist. Depending on the training system where the hospital is located, the senior-most person may be a physician or a nurse. Providers with this training are best equipped to lead a team response to both common and major events of instability. Their primary role is to oversee the functioning of the unit and respond to emergencies. Many times, the supervising anesthesiologist may continue to provide routine care to other patients in the operating room, but a system should be in place to make this person immediately available to respond and provide

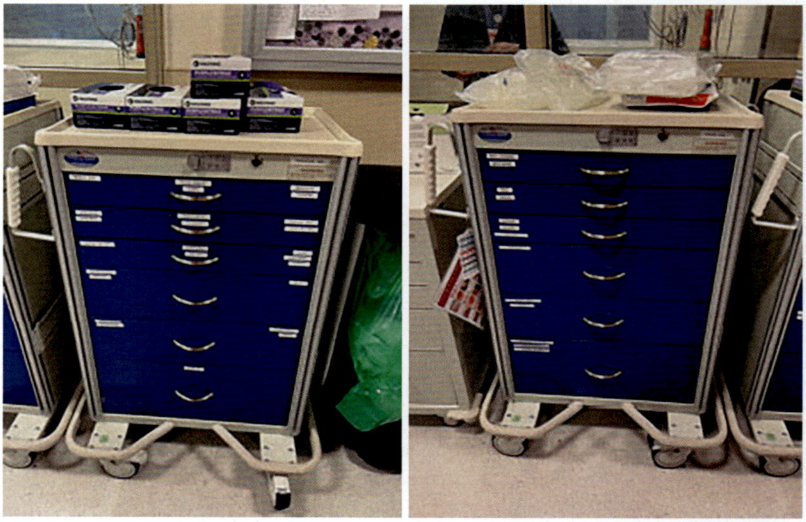

Fig. 12.1 An example of locked storage systems for organizing and containing basic supplies that may be helpful in the care of the PACU patient

care and treatment of patients in the recovery area.

The primary providers of care in the PACU are the nurses. Ideally, one nurse would be assigned to care for no more than four patients at a time, although this ratio will depend on the acuity of the patients and the amount of support available. If a patient is critically ill, they may even require 1:1 care. Nurses serve a variety of critical roles in caring for patients in the recovery room. Nurses assess the patient for hemodynamic stability, acquire regular vitals, perform physical exams to monitor for bleeding and other postoperative complications, evaluate patients for pain and nausea and provide medication as needed per postop orders, draw labs, assess for cognition and recovery from anesthesia and readiness to transition out of the PACU. Nurses are typically the first-line providers to initiate a call to action when recognizing a deteriorating patient. Indeed, communicating their critical findings to the supervising practitioner is among the important roles nurses serve in the PACU.

Nurses, given their direct bedside roles, also often serve beyond the role of care providers in the recovery room: they are often the frontline communicators with patients and their families. While surgeons typically discuss with patients and their families a summary of a patient's surgery, logistically, this task often falls on the nurses who are more readily available at the bedside to answer questions. Nurses should be comfortable answering questions that are standard practice in their clinical setting, but should also feel supported in reaching out to the lead physicians who may have more specific answers to any questions. Communication by the nurse is therefore not only between healthcare providers but also between the patient and the healthcare system.

In terms of more advanced procedures, the role of nurses in the recovery room and their scope of practice varies widely based on region. A review of multiple international hospitals found a wide range of supervision required for nursing care [8]. For example, while most nurses do not supervise patients on ventilators independently, at some institutions this is common. It is important that the scope of practice of the nurses in the PACU be established and clear in order to provide appropriate educational and logistical support to those undertaking more specialized responsibilities. As there is a high level of potential acuity in the PACU, it is recommended that PACU nurses not only have a solid foundation of nursing knowledge and experience, but also undergo additional orientation and continuing specialist education prior to caring for patients and during their stay in PACU. Training for a nurse should include a period of shadowing their colleagues to understand the logistics, set up and flow of the space, and an understanding of common emergency scenarios and responses. It is advisable that PACU RNs spend some time orienting in an ICU setting to gain more familiarity and expertise monitoring these types of patients. It is recommended that nurses in the PACU be competent and comfortable in participating in advanced cardiac life support. Many times PACU nurses are those who have already practiced care delivery in the ICU but are interested in a career shift.

Ancillary staff also provide critical elements of safety to the patients in the PACU. Trained pharmacists may be able to assist in medication prescription, reconstitution, and administration. People who are on the environmental service team can offload work from the usually busy nurses by ensuring the space remains clean and safe. Notably, families may also at times fill this role and provide simple food to facilitate recovery when appropriate.

Common PACU Issues and Emergencies

Common postoperative issues include respiratory depression, hemodynamic instability (hypo/hypertension), PONV, pain control, altered mental status, shivering and monitoring for postoperative bleeding. The first step in any emergency response is to ensure staff safety and communicate a need for assistance from a broader team. There are a multitude of emergency scenarios that may occur in the PACU. We recommend that

Table 12.1 Common PACU issues and emergencies

Issue	First priority	Other additional steps
Bleeding (post-surgical)	– Contact surgeons – Apply pressure (if possible) – Administer fluids – Blood transfusion if necessary	– Acquire baseline labs – Establish further IV access – Contact operating room to initiate possible re-exploration if appropriate per surgical recommendations
Bleeding (post-partum)	– Contact obstetrician – Fundal massage – Insert Bakri balloon – Administer fluids – Activate transfusion on standby	– Acquire baseline labs – Establish further IV access – Contact operating room to initiate possible re-exploration if appropriate per surgical recommendations
Hypotension	– Place patient in trendelenberg – Administer fluid bolus – Initiate vasopressors if needed	– Determine the source of shock (cardiogenic, hypovolemic, distributive, obstructive) – Bedside POCUS
Hypertension	– Evaluate and treat pain – Administer antihypertensives if needed	– Examine wounds or surgical site for bleeding – Restart home medications if needed
Altered mental status	– Evaluate cause – Maintain patient in safe recovery environment (for both patient and staff) – Reorient patient – Administer sedatives as needed for safety	– Consider cross-sectional imaging if AMS is sudden onset, accompanied by other neurological deficits, and/or fails to resolve in an appropriate time trajectory
Chest pain/ myocardial ischemia	– Administer oxygen – Obtain EKG – Consider administering ASA 325 mg chewed	– Establish steps for potentially activating transfer of further care
Hypoxia/ respiratory depression/arrest	– Administer oxygen – Sit patient upright – Consider administration of naloxone if appropriate	– Consider CXR/POCUS – Consider plan for airway support
PONV	– Administer antiemetics – Administer IV hydration – Maintain patient in the upright position	– Consider placement of NGT if refractory emesis and aspiration risk
Pain	– Administer multimodal analgesics as appropriate, including paracetamol, NSAIDS, opioids	– Discuss with surgeons and anesthesiologists possible iatrogenic pain causes if the pain is out of proportion to expected trajectory/physical exam
Sepsis	– Administer fluids. – Start broad-spectrum antibiotics – Initiate vasopressors if needed	– Acquire labs such as CBC and lactate – Consider imaging if the source of sepsis is unclear

each institution develops its own evidence-based rules and protocols for responding to common emergency scenarios, as well as reviews them regularly with on-site staff to remain prepared to act promptly, effectively, and safely to improve patient care when these instances arise. It is beyond the scope of this chapter to provide complete algorithms for all potential complications. Outlined in Table 12.1 is a list of some steps that can be initiated during the immediate response to common issues and emergency situations that arise in the PACU.

Quality Improvement

The PACU serves an additional important role of being a testing ground for innovation in the hospital. As a high-throughput center of patients whose efficiency and safety standards affect both out and inpatient services, the reach of the PACU's influence as a leader among the hospital wards cannot be underestimated. Quality improvement projects can be trialed, studied, and implemented with wide rippling effects. Throughput optimization, in particular, can help improve safety for patients in the PACU as well as the rest of the admitted patients in the hospital.

Conclusion

Overall, the PACU is a cornerstone of supporting functional and safe operating theatres and hospitals. When establishing or optimizing a PACU, particular attention should be given to space, personnel, supplies, and preparation of emergency responses while caring for this diverse patient population.

References

1. Cutugno C. Evolution of postanesthesia care units: a legacy of politics, funding, and patient safety concerns. Policy Polit Nurs Pract. 2013;14(3–4):142–50.
2. Simpson JC, Moonesinghe SR. Introduction to the postanaesthetic care unit. Perioper Med (Lond). 2013;2(1):5.
3. Prien T, Van Aken H. The perioperative phase as a part of anesthesia. Tasks of the recovery room. Anaesthesist. 1997;46(Suppl 2):S109–13.
4. Schad S, Booke H, Thal SC, Bentley AH, Booke M. The recovery room: transition from a sleepy postoperative unit to a vibrant and cost-effective multipurpose perioperative care unit. Clinicoecon Outcomes Res. 2021;13:893–6.
5. Mittel AM, Panzer O, Wang DS, Miller SE, Schaff JE, Hastie MJ, et al. Logistical considerations and clinical outcomes associated with converting operating rooms into an intensive care unit during the coronavirus disease 2019 pandemic in a New York City Hospital. Anesth Analg. 2021;132(5): 1182–90.
6. Pedersen T, Nicholson A, Hovhannisyan K, Moller AM, Smith AF, Lewis SR. Pulse oximetry for perioperative monitoring. Cochrane Database Syst Rev. 2014;2014(3):CD002013.
7. Ramsingh D, Singh S, Canales C, Guran E, Taylor Z, Antongiorgi Z, et al. The evaluation point-of-care ultrasound in the post-anesthesia unit-a multicenter prospective observational study. J Clin Med. 2021;10(11).
8. Dahlberg K, Brady JM, Jaensson M, Nilsson U, Odom-Forren J. Education, competence, and role of the nurse working in the PACU: an international survey. J Perianesth Nurs. 2021;36(3):224–31 e6.

13 How to Establish and Maintain a Functional Operating Room in a Low-Resource Environment

Robert Neighbour, Richard Raker, and Richard Smiley

To know just what has do be done, then to do it, comprises... philosophy of practical life.

– William Osler

Abbreviations

HICs	High-income countries
LMICs	Low- and middle-income countries
ORs	Operating rooms
PACU	Postoperative care unit

Introduction

The World Federation of Societies of Anesthesiologists recommends minimum standards for the safe practice of anesthesia [1]. Most low-resource settings are unable to achieve these. A survey of 590 facilities in low- and middle-income countries (LMICs) showed that 40% of hospitals had no anesthesia machines, 35% had no access to oxygen, and many had limited availability of essential medications, lack of support services such as laboratory and blood bank, and lack of technologies such as advanced airway devices and invasive monitors [2]. These standards were designed for permanent installations where local practitioners practice in LMICs. The general lack of national or regional infrastructure such as power, clean water and lighting in many low-resource areas of the world is well documented but this is particularly problematic in health care facilities This is often compounded by environmental factors such as temperature, humidity, dust, and insect infestation. Working within these constraints requires an understanding of the issues and their causes, much additional planning, and most importantly, always, flexibility.

When practitioners from high-income countries (HICs) plan to work in LMICs, they usually try to bring equipment, supplies, and make physical improvements in an attempt to at least approach the prescribed standards. To accomplish this a good sense of the existing status and framework is essential. Available equipment, often donated from HICs, despite good intentions, is frequently outdated, broken, or inappropriate for local needs. Even materials brought for specific missions often end up less than useful

R. Neighbour (✉)
Institution of Engineering and Technology, Diamedica (UK) Ltd, Barnstaple, UK
e-mail: r.neighbour@diamedica.co.uk

R. Raker · R. Smiley
Columbia University Vagelos College of Physicians and Surgeons, New York, NY, USA
e-mail: rkr1@cumc.columbia.edu; rms7@cumc.columbia.edu

M. A. Hardy, B. R. Hochman (eds.), *Global Surgery*, https://doi.org/10.1007/978-3-031-28127-3_13

due to electrical incompatibility and lack of spare parts or repair/maintenance expertise.

Overall Physical Structure and Layout

One of the first important tasks of the surgical/anesthesia visiting teams is to assess the physical structure of the actual operating room; size of the room, condition and flexibility of the operating table, lighting, storage, etc. Obviously, some inventory of the surgical instruments available should be made. The anesthesiologist will want to inspect the anesthesia machine and ventilator, oxygen and other gas sources as well as suction. In the case of a team that is traveling to a site for a brief temporary surgical mission, or a longer visit that requires the creation of a more permanent installation and project, some of this assessment and inventory can be done before arriving at a site, by phone or email communication and of course now, the easy availability of photographs and video.

An assessment should also be made of how patients arrive at the hospital and are transferred within the hospital to the operating room area. Many patients may not arrive at hospital by conventional means, internal transfer may be very slow and during this they may be exposed to the elements. They may be, unaccompanied by medical staff, and their medical information may be limited; the transferring patients may not have the use of oxygen or other equipment, monitoring, or drugs. Many of these limitations may not be modifiable, or may be only capable of being changed minimally, if at all. Any deficiencies must at least be understood and considered.

The postoperative areas should also be inspected or inquired about. Is there a dedicated postoperative care unit (PACU) or can one be created near the ORs? What will be the monitoring availability and standard of personnel, and are oxygen and airway management devices available, is there ventilation capability? Similarly, where will the patient be housed after recovery before being discharged? Is there a unit and team to support intensive care (e.g., mechanical ventilation, prolonged homodynamic monitoring, intravenous infusion pumps)? The resources available in the postoperative area will impact on the nature of surgery that is possible, and on the anesthesia management options.

Personnel

The needs and concerns regarding personnel will vary greatly depending on the specific nature of the surgical/anesthesia enterprise, but unless all personnel and expertise is being brought in to the low-resource environment some attention must be paid to what expertise or training the staff at the site possess. It is well known that there is a critical shortage of surgeons, anesthesiologists, and obstetricians in LMICs [3] and in fact, anesthesia care is often provided by non-physician or non-nurse personnel [4]. In general, “task sharing” occurs, where non-specialized physicians, nurses, or less qualified health care workers fill the provider gap. Will there be someone who can get equipment or supplies and medications for the anesthesia team in an emergency, help with patient positioning, or even perform more “medical” tasks such as preparing syringes with drugs, or providing cricoids pressure during an intubation? On the surgical side, are there staff who can perform the roles of scrub technician and circulator, or surgical assistant? The need for interpreters, perhaps capable of handling multiple languages, should not be underestimated.

Electricity

The presence and reliability of utilities needs to be determined, by report or by inspection. The reliability of electricity is problematic in many low-resource environments, and should be assessed by communication with local practitioners. There are two common “grid” electrical supply formats in the world, 220-volt 50 Hz and 110-volt 60 Hz. Ensuring that any equipment purchased or donated to a facility is the correct voltage and frequency is a necessary foundation for equipment survival. Voltage can be altered for either format by the use of a transformer, but this will not change the frequency, and incorrect frequency will often result in early equipment failure. Fluctuations and failure of grid supply are common and can cause damage to equipment and risk to the patient if the operator is unprepared.

What is plan B when the electrical power goes out? What equipment will fail without external power, and which devices are critical? Voltage stabilization, protection devices, and battery back-up systems are available and should be considered at the supply stage along with emergency lighting, but if these are not available, a plan for that (expected) emergency is required. Many facilities have an alternative power supply such as a generator but these are unlikely to start automatically following a grid failure. Generators require manual starting, assuming they have fuel, are ready, and an operator is available. It is always worth reviewing the process and availability prior to it becoming necessary. If they are available battery back-up systems, that will prevent interruption of electrical power for OR devices should be maintained in a fully charged state. An increasingly common device is the UPS (Uninterruptible Power Supply). These should be switched on before use to ensure the battery back-up is available, and batteries charged and switched off after use to ensure the batteries are available when needed.

Electrical safety in many low-resource locations can also be less than optimal. Circuit breakers and fuses may not be present or functioning properly. Attention should be paid to the potential of shock hazard caused by unshielded wires, overloaded sockets, and trailing leads, particularly in theaters where there is liberal application of water for cleaning.

Environmental Conditions and Considerations

Extremes of weather, temperature, and humidity can have a range of unexpected consequences beyond the obvious uncomfortable effects on the medical personnel and patient. Ambient temperatures approaching 50 °C (120 °F) are uncomfortable, but are also approaching the boiling point of volatile anesthetic agents and, where available monitoring does not include this parameter, caution should be shown. Even in locations such as Sub-Saharan Africa patients get cold, and in many situations the air-conditioning systems used by staff exacerbate this. Patient warming equipment and fluid warming equipment are not often available and unconventional patient warming may be common. For example, filling of gloves with warm water and wrapping in cotton or aluminum foil are common methods of warming babies and small children.

Oxygen Supply

Oxygen in low resource areas of the world can be expensive and is often unavailable; it may be a major element of a hospital's budget. Despite being classified by WHO as an essential medicine, it is often a scarce resource in these locations and should be considered as such. If oxygen is supplied in cylinders (as opposed to an oxygen concentrator) the anesthesiologist has obligations to ensure its availability before commencing with a procedure and to protect continuity of supply and avoid unnecessary or excessive use. Many cylinders are not in optimal condition. Regulators and tubing may be subject to leakage. The small back-up cylinders that are mandatory in HICs may be empty or unavailable.

In many areas the common alternative to pressurized oxygen supplied in cylinders or piped gas systems is the use of oxygen concentrators, which entrain ambient air and remove most of the nitrogen with the use of molecular sieves. These devices can provide dry oxygen at up to 95% purity at either 5 or 10 liters per minute. They are a very good source of oxygen, generated at the point of use, and avoid logistical problems associated with the movement of oxygen cylinders. However, oxygen concentrators do require a constant supply of stable electrical power, some regular maintenance, and have limited outlet pressures. The limited outlet pressures make the oxygen supply unsuitable to use with many conventional anesthetic machines, although there are anesthesia devices and ventilators specifically designed to run at these lower oxygen supply pressures such as draw-over circuits. Concentrators can be particularly useful in PACUs and ICU areas postoperatively where positive pressure ventilation may be less often needed [5].

In extreme situations the anesthetic technique may have to be altered based on the available oxygen, even to the point of accepting a lower FiO_2 than would normally be utilized in HICs, in appropriate patients. The routine use of supplemental oxygen during regional anesthesia or mild sedation, as is common in HICs, might have to be re-assessed, based on patients' needs and clinical condition. It should also be noted that postoperative areas may not have the availability of oxygen expected in better-resourced areas.

Anesthesia Machine

There are a number of common equipment constraints. The simple lack of available equipment, such as the situation where suction may be shared between the surgeon and the anesthetist, or the unavailability of the ideal airway equipment including endotracheal tubes, or supraglottic airways, can usually be overcome with some negotiation and flexibility in technique. However even if anesthetic techniques are going to be very restricted, some means of delivering a volatile anesthetic agent, maintaining an airway, and ventilating the patient are going to require a functioning anesthetic workstation.

The usual inputs to the modern anesthetic workstation in a well-resourced location would be three gases; oxygen, air, and nitrous oxide, as well as a constant, assured, and stable electrical supply. In the low-resource setting, it is more likely to be simply an oxygen source and a reasonable electrical supply, with, hopefully. a backup electrical supply. Since in most cases a surgical team will not bring completely functional anesthesia machines on a mission, understanding the available machine(s) and their constraints before use is vital. It may be an unfamiliar type, with complex gas circuit arrangements, and have non-functioning elements and limited monitoring. It is essential to carry out the normal recommended pre-use checks (hopefully, but not always, guided by an instruction manual) followed by an assessment and trial of the effect of loss of inputs such as electrical power failure or gas supply, and a plan for what the response to that situation would be. An alternative to the standard anesthetic system is the use of low-resistance systems suitable for draw-over circuits [6]. Although the agent use may be higher, the reduction in oxygen usage by using it to supplement room air entrainment offsets this cost implication particularly with a spontaneously breathing patient. It should be noted that the requirement for patient monitoring is also considerably reduced.

The most common inhalational agent in use in many locations is still halothane, with isoflurane as a secondary agent. Sevoflurane is starting to be introduced as a result of reduction in its cost and its utility for inhalational induction. The reduction in agent use (and cost) with semi-closed circle systems is useful, however only if a constant supply of active soda lime is available. The common response to a lack of soda lime is to increase gas flows to ensure removal of carbon dioxide; this can then result in excessive use of available oxygen. Vaporizers are infrequently calibrated and output inaccurate. Appropriate adjustments for vapor pressure and output will need to be considered in locations significantly above sea level.

The most common circuit configuration for patients under 10 kg in these locations is the Mapleson F, Ayres T piece, and familiarity with this circuit would be essential for any anesthesiologist working with children in a low-resource setting.

Anesthesia Supplies/Equipment, Monitoring, and Medications

The availability of a seemingly endless supply of consumables is restricted to very few, well resourced, areas of the world; the situation in the world of LMICs can be very different. Reprocessing or cleaning for reuse devices that are made to be disposable in HICs is a most common scenario. As such the anesthesiologist (and surgeon) should ensure an understanding of the cleaning processes available in a particular location. It is possible that some form of autoclave or chemical sterilization will be available, but this is not assured.

One of the most common causes of medical equipment failure in low-resource situations is the lack of any planned, routine maintenance. Most LMIC hospitals do not have readily available and competent technical support personnel. Equipment is likely to be donated from multiple sources, it may be "refurbished," may not have had maintenance manuals supplied, and spare parts are likely unavailable. It is common in well-resourced hospitals to have equipment redundancy; if an anesthesia machine or monitor fails to operate properly it is removed from the clinical arena and replaced while it is quite likely repaired. When a hospital does not have this redundancy, the equipment often continues in service with minor fault conditions, which can of course suddenly become more serious or total.

The need for specific amounts of anesthesia supplies and drugs depends on the nature and variety of surgical procedures planned or anticipated, but there are basic, essential needs that almost all operating rooms and surgical missions will require. Some missions, especially for orthopedic or gynecologic surgery, may involve procedures that will be performed under regional (spinal or peripheral nerve block) anesthesia, and thus sufficient equipment (needles, sterile kits, or the ability to properly sterilize equipment) and drugs (local anesthetics and perhaps adjuvants) will need to be secured, while sedatives and general anesthesia drugs and equipment, while necessary, will be needed in much less volume. If local supplies of medications are to be used, it must be realized that shortages and limited availability are common. Some sources of drugs in LMICs are not reliable as far as the actual concentrations and efficacy of the drugs supplied, and unfamiliar medications (or names) may be present in place of more familiar ones. Here again, flexibility, a good reference source, as well as attention to the possibility of failure to see the expected drug response on occasion, is warranted.

As noted above, it is impossible to define the proper amount of or specific medications that will be needed on any given surgical missions because of the significant differences that depend on the nature of the expected procedures. In fact, patients may be asked to supply medications for their surgical procedure The World Health Organization (WHO) has published and continuously updated a list of "Essential Medications" that should be available in health facilities worldwide [7]. While this list is still somewhat aspirational for many locales, it is a good starting point to assess how far any given facility or country is from achieving a reasonable inventory of medications. A listing of anesthetic and other perioperative medications, excerpted from the entire WHO list may be useful. We have not included antibiotics (again an availability issue) or other very specialized medications that might be needed for specific procedures or patient populations, but this list can serve as a checklist to assess whether the needed medications will be available for most intraoperative and perioperative situations.

Accustomed to monitoring the anesthetized patient with a full set of vital signs and ventilator/gas data, the practitioners will also experience the limited capacity to monitor LMIC patients. WHO and the World Federation of Societies of Anesthesiologists have recommended minimum guidelines for safe surgical practice but LMICs are unable to meet them, with the possible exception of monitoring O_2 saturation [8].

Blood Products

The source and availability of blood products may be dependent on location and often governed by strict national protocols. Visiting medical staff must make themselves aware of the national rules. In most LMICs, especially in the lower-resourced group of countries, blood products may be very difficult to obtain, and family members or friends are often required to donate blood in order for patients to receive blood (either directly from them or from banked stores, if such exist, with the concept being that the family donation will maintain the stores). Final cross-matching may have to be done at the bedside. Often the product available is whole blood, as there may be no blood bank to separate the blood into individual products. This is of course an advantage in many cases, as fresh whole-blood transfusion should usually eliminate the need for separate coagulation factors (plasma, cryoprecipitate) to be administered. As with almost all other aspects of perioperative care in LMICs, there will be a wide variety of scenarios, and the only consistent advice is to be aware of the conditions and constraints and to be prepared.

Summary

It is a daunting task to consider working in and setting up a safe OR for anesthesia and surgery in an LMIC or other resource-limited environment, because there are so many ways that resources can be limited compared to what practitioners are used to in the developed world. Any of these limitations or deficiencies may significantly affect the range of surgical procedures that can be undertaken, and/or the safety or even feasibility of any anesthetic or surgical techniques and choices. One might even paraphrase Tolstoy's famous line about happy and unhappy families and suggest that ("happy") ORs in the developed world are rather "all alike," while those that in under-resourced areas ("unhappy") are all lacking resources "in their own way."

References

1. Lee S, Onye A, Latif A. Emergency anesthesia in resource-limited areas. Anesthesiol Clin. 2020;38(1):213–30.
2. Vo D, Cherian MN, Bianchi S, Noël L, Lundeg G, Taqdeer A, et al. Anesthesia capacity in 22 low- and middle-income countries. J Anesth Clin Res. 2012; 3:207. https://doi.org/10.4172/2155-6148.1000207.
3. Meara JG, Leather AJ, Hagander L, Alkire BC, Alonso N, Ameh EA, et al. Global surgery 2030: evidence and solutions for achieving health, welfare, and economic development. Lancet. 2015;386(9993):569–624.
4. Kempthorne P, Morriss WW, Mellin-Olsen J, Gore-Booth J. The WFSA global anesthesia workforce survey. Anesth Analg. 2017;125(3):981–90.
5. Howie SR, Ebruke BE, Gil M, Bradley B, Nyassi E, Edmonds T, et al. The development and implementation of an oxygen treatment solution for health facilities in low and middle-income countries. J Glob Health. 2020;10(2):020425.
6. Vande Lune SA, Lantry JH, Mason PE, Skupski R, Toth A, Zimmer D, et al. Universal anesthesia machine: clinical application in an austere, resource-limited environment. Mil Med. 2020;185(5–6):e550–e6.
7. WHO model list of essential medicines - 22nd list, 2021. https://www.who.int/publications/i/item/WHO-MHP-HPS-EML-2021.02. Accessed 23 April 2022.
8. Gelb AW, Morriss WW, Johnson W, Merry AF, Abayadeera A, Belii N, et al. World Health Organization-World Federation of Societies of Anaesthesiologists (WHO-WFSA) international standards for a safe practice of anesthesia. Anesth Analg. 2018;126(6):2047–55.

14 How to Establish a Trauma and Disaster Response Service in Low- and Middle-Income Countries, Including Staff, Transportation, Testing, Triage, Resuscitation Training, and Facilities

Emnet Tesfaye Shimber

Few people plan to fail, they just fail to plan.

– Lee Whistler

Abbreviations

ATLS	Advanced Trauma Life Support
BEC	Basic Emergency Care
DMAT	Disaster medical assistance teams
EMS	Emergency medical service
EMT	Emergency Medical Team
ER	Emergency room
IMS	Incident Management System
LMICs	Low- and Middle-Income Countries
MCM	Mass Casualty Management
VAC	Vacuum-assisted closure
WHO	World Health Organization

How To Establish a Trauma Disaster Response Service

A disaster is an occurrence disrupting the normal conditions of existence and causing a level of suffering that exceeds the capacity of adjustment of the affected community. The normal functioning of the health system is inadequate to manage the urgent and massive demands posed by disaster. This requires, therefore, the use of a different operating plan and approach than the usual management of individual emergent health issues [1].

Disaster management can be anticipated and planned for based on previous trends and situational analysis or sometimes, unfortunately, cannot be anticipated. The sudden effect of a disaster will be magnified in underprivileged settings, especially in low- and middle-income countries (LMICs) [2]. There is no uniform planning procedure because the hazard profiles of each country vary greatly. However, the presence of fundamental concepts aids in problem detection and mitigation. Differences in geography, infrastructure, economy, political climate, and emergency response systems can be used to explain this variation [3].

Without appropriate planning for unexpected emergency situations, hospital health systems can easily become overwhelmed in their attempts to provide care to many groups of patients simultaneously during a critical event. Limited resources, a surge in demand for medical services, and the frequent disruption of communication and supply lines create a significant barrier to the provision of effective health care. To

E. T. Shimber (✉)
Hawassa University School of Medicine, Hawassa, Ethiopia

M. A. Hardy, B. R. Hochman (eds.), *Global Surgery*, https://doi.org/10.1007/978-3-031-28127-3_14

enhance the readiness of all health facilities and to cope with the challenges of a disaster, health facilities need to be prepared to initiate fundamental priority action at the first knowledge of a disaster [4]. Disasters go through four stages: mitigation, preparedness, response, and recovery. Each stage requires careful planning and quick execution. Finding potential risks, assessing vulnerabilities, and estimating the degree of damage are the fundamental steps [2].

LMICs serve large populations with limited number of trained staff and lack of resources. A large proportion of the patient health burden in LMICs consists of young persons who require urgent trauma and emergency services. The relative paucity of specialized neuro-trauma, ortho-trauma, and intensive care management services in LMICs necessitates a well-organized and practiced plan for emergency disaster conditions that may occur unexpectedly [2].

With the current resource and professional personnel constriction and with an overwhelmed health care system, maintenance of routine basic services has remained the main focus of care. During a disaster, an interruption of standard communications or shortage of critical equipment and supplies can disrupt operations of essential health facilities. There is also an unanticipated rise in the number of admissions which alone can overwhelm any hospital beyond its functional reserve. Preparedness and timely action facilitate containment and effective and safe management of the disasters as well as prevention of post-disaster consequences [5].

As part of disaster preparedness, disaster medical assistance teams (DMAT) or Emergency Medical Team (EMT) need to be established as part of most regional or national planning efforts. The composition of the team should range from various health professionals to support staff, and include nurses, technicians, firemen, policemen, and social workers. The team works best during preparation for anticipated critical incidents but can also be very effective in emergency, unexpected situations, once it has learned how to work together efficiently. Training coverage ranges from Basic Emergency Care (BEC) course to Mass Casualty Management (MCM). The BEC course is geared toward preparing medical providers on the frontline to recognize, evaluate and treat life-threatening conditions and to be able to triage effectively when necessary.

Trauma System

Trauma often involves injuries that affect anywhere from a few to a large number of individuals at the same time. Mass casualty is an incident which frequently places the event beyond the existing capacity of the health system. An event which involves many casualties differs from mass casualty in that it is represented by a variety of cases which present at the same time but may not exceed the capacity of an existing health system. Trauma care is underrepresented and inadequate in most of LMICs because of scarcity of sufficiently trained professionals, lack of specialized equipment and supplies, and insufficient preplanned organization at various levels of care to be able to deliver the expected standard of care. Lack of infrastructure and human and non-human resources lead to significant mortality and morbidity during both natural and man-made disasters [5]. Trauma care must begin at the scene of injury in order to be most effective. A new concept in most African countries is that bystanders or community first-aid responders must be able to and be trained to immediately initiate trauma care on site [6]. This may be followed by pre-hospital care by Emergency Medical Team (EMT) which are frequently unavailable. As a result of initial care by "amateurs", victims of trauma arrive to hospital (if transportation or roads are available) without receiving competent medical care in the golden hour of resuscitation [7]. In hospitals in LMICs emergency rooms (ER) trauma activation systems are not yet sufficiently mature to allow any responsible physician to treat the trauma patients successfully [8].

The primary objective of a trauma system is to eliminate the risk of death or permanent disability following traumatic events. Unfortunately, in many developing countries, a trauma system is non-existent or, immature. It is therefore essential to advocate the need for an organized and effective trauma system to the national and regional governments, community, and other stakeholders to bring it to the level of that found in high-income countries (HICs). This is particularly important since the incidence of surgical trauma in LMICs, and especially in Africa, is higher than anywhere in the world and represents the majority of surgical interventions [9].

Infrastructure of Trauma System

Since injury may be a complex phenomenon, it needs the inclusion of distinctive methodologies. As a result, considering the following pillars is crucial [10].

Leadership

Leadership is a process that enables all members of a group to achieve a common goal. Overall trauma system leadership needs high-level national and regional involvement and the support of the countries' ministries of health, transportation, environment, security including police and fire departments, and insurance agencies. The multisectorial steering committee should support policy development, approve major decisions, and uphold system standards. A technical team should concentrate on developing national guidelines, gathering data, and monitoring the current system with a particular focus on quality and efficiency. The integration of community first responders, an EMS team (if one is present), the local health department, and hospital administrations entails system leadership in a particular city or even hamlet. Case management requires leadership of emergency professionals and surgeons selected from multitask teams necessary for specific types of trauma. A failed system is the result of fragmented leadership and poor coordination.

Technology

Essential assistive technology, such as wheelchairs, crutches, splints, and orthotics, is often in short supply in LMICs during the immediate response to disasters. After stabilization of acute trauma and termination of the disaster, long rehabilitation strategy requires early planning and is also largely dependent on these assistive devices which are frequently in low supply during disaster relief operations This lack of assistive technology affects not only those with new injuries, but also those who may have displaced or damaged assistive technology because of the disaster or conflict. The overall consequence of such inadequacies will be prolonged bed rest for the victims who may suffer all the known complications of limited early mobilization (e.g., pulmonary emboli) or whose discharge home may be delayed, which further impacts rehabilitation capacity. Long-term rehabilitation strategy involves early preparation and is heavily dependent on these supportive technologies after acute response of the disaster. Also consideration of non-functioning or damaged device replacement should be in place. The overall effect of these shortcomings will be prolonged bed rest for the victims, who may experience all the known risks of limited early mobilization (such as deep venous thrombosis and pulmonary emboli), or whose discharge home may be postponed, which further reduces their ability to recover. Other technology areas include video conferencing, tele-consultation, and virtual reality assist to advance trauma training and research. Few technological areas incorporate identification by the use of Global Positioning System (GPS), initiation of a call to dispatch centers by emergency access numbers, coordination of care by utilizing telemedicine, trauma education technologies, and arrangement of assistive devices. Technological advances in trauma management have already improved patient outcomes in the pre-hospital care, in the emergency room, in the operation theatre, in the intensive care unit, and during inpatient care, primarily because of improved monitoring, communication, ventilators, and even dressings (vacuum-assisted closure—VAC). Management of patients using newer technologies like laparoscopy, invasive monitoring, endovascular techniques, as well as modern computerized mechanical ventilator has contributed significantly to improvement of trauma care and recovery, but their adoption in LMICs is very slow and selective to tertiary centers because of the high cost of the equipment and the need for trained technical support to repair and maintain it.

Personnel

In addition to proper health care training, individuals who work in trauma centers must have specialized trauma-focused training and experience. A multidisciplinary team of physicians, nurses, paramedics, and administrators must be involved in directing and training of trauma teams. The number and type of professionals included in each team depends on the size and designated level of the facility. Level III centers may require fewer trauma-trained professionals to provide initial acute stabilization care and to arrange transfers to better-equipped facilities. Level II centers are intermediate units that provide general care and inpatient services and may choose to care for patients who don't need highly specialized orthopedic, thoracic, vascular, neurosurgical, or other care. The most advanced center is Level I with full complement of various ICUs' intensivists and other highly specialized professionals in most areas of medicine and surgery, in addition to having dedicated rehabilitation, physiotherapy, psychiatry, and social services.

Transfer protocols must be consistent and transparent, written in collaboration with all stakeholders from various hospitals, departments, trauma leaders, and health care authorities who must be ready to fund the effort. Such protocols must be the main guidelines for triage and deciding which patients are transferred to which appropriate facility and when and how this should take place. Trauma specialists with extensive experience of major trauma, and other clinical specialists for complicated conditions that may be part of a traumatic injury are in short supply in LMICs. This raises many problems which can be partially resolved by appropriate triaging and division of labor among the various stakeholders. Continuity of care in most serious cases depends heavily on the level of experience of rehabilitation professionals.

Education and Training

Trauma education programs include short-term training which facilitates acquisition of basic medical knowledge and clinical skills, in addition to many specialized programs focused on both very narrow medical and surgical areas and/or on broad areas of organization, supervision, recruitment, fundraising, and on education itself via practical supervised practice exercises. Trauma evaluation and management course is an introductory course for medical students in many African countries, which can be easily extended and expanded to instruct professionals working in low-level centers (Levels II, and II). More advanced training courses, including Advanced Trauma Life Support (ATLS), are not widely available although they are required and essential in low-resource settings. The cumulative effect of inadequate medical education among non-medical professional staff puts Trauma programs in LMICs at a major disadvantage which can only be corrected by an increase in organized advocacy aimed at the public, the doctors, and at the policymakers, especially those in health ministries of LMICs.

Information Management

Numbers speak more than words. While there are major digital advances in information management in HICs, health information management system is generally poor in LMICs. The accurate statistics on trauma in the system are not available but are estimated to be high. It has become clear recently that more accurate data may influence national and professional changes favorably and most importantly, influence significantly the budgetary allocations to improvement of national trauma care which is badly needed in most LMICs. Due to disproportionate growth of population in existing living conditions most of the societies in LMICs are vulnerable to injury. All advocacies, public education, and planning are being made based on available information. The WHO trauma registry system is being utilized only in a few settings. Trauma database should be one of the priority areas in all health facilities.

Finances

Injuries often occur in emergency conditions in areas where victims may not be financially ready for health care. Few governments give free service while others request large compensation. To alleviate this discrepancy all stakeholders should work to optimize health insurance coverage. Trauma care is very costly and requires significant resources. The cost of imaging, operation, and rehabilitation care is high compared to standard medical care. Training and research are the other financial need areas.

Disaster Preparedness and Response.

Disaster preparedness plan is a process which includes development of emergency plans and early warning systems to respond rapidly and cope effectively during disaster situation.

The disaster-planning phase is a continuum of activities starting from (1) baseline assessment, (2) event management, and (3) rehabilitation process. All stakeholders must agree on their role in the communal effort so that they can all rely and have confidence on this jointly created infrastructure. The implementation of the specific plan is the response phase. Disaster response may involve EMTs, fire brigades, police departments, and industries. All should respond in a coordinated manner.

The response phase focuses primarily on emergency relief, i.e., saving lives, providing first aid, minimizing and restoring damaged systems, such as communications and transportation, and providing care and basic life requirements to victims (food, water, and shelter). Response activities need to be continually evaluated and adjusted to the changing situation.

The preparedness, planning, and periodic drills enhance the ability of a hospital's team to respond to most of the challenges encountered in trauma and to continue to function in disasters. Constant growth and improvement must remain the goal of the team, even during times when it is not needed so as to remain well prepared when eventually faced with a medical and social disaster.

Transportation

Proper transfer protocol is necessary to ensure availability and proper selection of types of transport. Basic and advanced ambulances can be deployed based on the need. Air ambulances can be arranged by using military helicopters in resource-limited settings. In places where the disaster happens near a water source boats can be refurbished to serve as ambulances. Availability of the various modes of transfer must be planned, foreseen, and practiced. The plans will differ according to the site and the extent of the disaster.

Triage

Jump START triage (Simple Triage and Rapid Treatment) is a simple triage system that can be performed by lightly trained lay and emergency personnel. It was developed at Hoag Hospital in Newport Beach, California for use by emergency services. It is based on the principle of walking and non-walking victims.

Triage separates the injured into four groups:

- The injured who are beyond help.
- The injured who can be helped by immediate transportation.
- The injured whose transport can be delayed.
- Those with minor injuries who need help less urgently.

It also sets priorities for evacuation and transport as follows:

(a) Deceased are left where they fell. These include those who aren't breathing and where efforts to reposition their airway were unsuccessful.
(b) Immediate or Priority 1 (red) evacuation by an ambulance (or by other means like a helicopter) is reserved for those who are in critical condition and need immediate (or within

1 h) advanced medical care in order to survive.

(c) Delayed or Priority 2 (yellow) victims can have their medical evacuation delayed until all Priority 1 patients have been evacuated. These individuals are in stable condition but require careful medical or surgical management.

(d) Minor or Priority 3 (green) victims are evacuated after all Priority 1 and 2 victims have been evacuated. These will not need advanced medical care for at least several hours. Continue to re-triage in case their condition worsens in which case they will jump to a higher Priority. These Individuals are able to walk and may only need bandages and antiseptic.

Essential Components of Disaster Preparedness

The following components serve to summarize the technical processes and operational mechanisms required to ensure the effective, and safe function of a preparedness plan:

Disaster Management Committee

Establishing a disaster/emergency/committee is the first step for making a disaster plan for the nation as well as health care facilities. If one already exists, it needs to conform to the universal established requirements for the country or the region as appropriate.

Compositions:

- The Chief Executive Director of the institution.
- Member/members from hospital management board.
- The chiefs/heads of various clinical departments supporting the emergency services.
- The chiefs/heads of various ancillary departments.
  - Including radio-diagnosis, laboratory/pathology, blood bank, and forensic medicine.
  - Infection control.
  - Pharmacy and pharmaceutical supplies.
- The chief nursing service director/matron.
- Heads of Administrative Departments including; finance, procurement, and asset management.

Note that:

- There should be a backup member for each category, in case the assigned member(s) in charge of a section is unavailable to perform tasks during the event of an emergency/disaster.
- The copy of the preparedness plan should be communicated and available for each department of the hospital.

Incident Command System

Incident command system (ICS) is necessary to ensure effective control and avoid duplication of action. There needs to be a unified command system which should be based on the individual hospital hierarchical chain of command.

All emergency operations must be managed by an ICS. It is a method for dealing with disasters when the situation requires coordination of all hospital activities through a single loop of command post communication system.

ICS is managed by six main command post leaders:

Commander—Chief Executive Director.

Operation leader—Chief of Disaster Management Team.

Logistics—Chief of Pharmacy and Purchasing unit.

Finance/administration—Chief of Finance.

Information—dissemination of news and progress.

Public health—Chief of Public health.

Each other hospital unit, area, or department continues to maintain the same leaders or directors as they have per their regular routines, regardless of their additional function on the ICS.

Chain of Command

Whenever the hospital units, areas, or departments need to communicate with ICS, they should do so via the Command Post leader assigned to that particular function.

How to Activate Disaster Response

Disaster Alert should be provided to the hospital staff and/or patients when activation of Emergency Operations is probable or anticipated in the near future. The information should include the type of causalities, place of disaster (distance from the center), and estimated number of victims. The plan is activated after the first patients arrive at the hospital and/or when the team moves to the scene of disaster or of emergency.

Only the Incident Commander has the authority to activate the hospital disaster response. He/she must announce the following notice to the hospital staff with a loudspeaker and available social media platforms: "Attention! Attention! Attention! All staff and visitors, Disaster Activation is now in effect for the emergency that has happened in the city, please implement the Hospital Disaster Plan". This should be announced in the official language of the country and the local language of the area.

Initial Assignment of Responsibilities

As soon as there is a disaster alert declared, the communication loop between the disaster team and stakeholders should be put into operation. All off-duty staff should be prepared for possible recall to the hospital by the hospital director.

Disaster store should be replenished with emergency drugs and resuscitation equipment. The key or the combination to the store should be placed with the director of ER and be available for 24 h each day of the ongoing disaster activities.

Surge Capacity

Newly arriving patients require admission for definitive treatment. It is therefore necessary to put into effect plans to increase the bed capacity of the hospital. This can be achieved by opening areas with nursing supervision that are not employed for other reasons, to accommodate hospital beds and necessary equipment for the new patients. This can be achieved by the following actions:

- Discharge elective cases.
- Discharge stable recovering patients.
- Stop admitting non-emergency patients.
- Convert waiting/non-patient care areas into makeshift wards.
- Transfer patients to lower level health facilities.

Planning for Disaster Beds

Critical areas including ERs, ICUs, and ORs should be cleared of many of their current routine functions and of their impending functions (e.g., postpone elective surgeries; discharge non-emergent, etc.). Open space on surgical wards and even in the corridors may serve as temporary areas for admission of patients who are in the ER irrespective of their clinical diagnosis. Mechanical ventilators, suction machines, monitors, and other ICU equipment should be used according to their availability anywhere they are needed at the time of disaster. There might be sharing of resources in all service areas of the hospital as per the Operation Leader.

Patients can be admitted to ER utilizing all possible spaces including stretchers, boards, or beds. Patients should be marked with their paper triaging category based on the severity of injury when initially found. This facilitates identification of the patients and the severity of their injuries. This also guides the selection of the management approach for each individual patient. All Public hospitals should be part of the disaster response team.

As mentioned previously the injuries are triaged and therefore marked by the following Categories: RED, YELLOW, GREEN, AND BLACK.

Other Services

All ancillary services must be notified of the alert. Representatives of the services must make themselves available to provide their expert services when called on by the responsible physicians caring for the victims.

Imaging service will be provided by members of the radiology department staff including CT-scan, X-ray, and Ultrasound services when requested by the physicians providing care.

Laboratory service: Both emergency and central laboratory service should resume full capacity especially if the disaster is at night. Personnel should be recalled from home to increase the skeleton night roster. Extra blood for transfusion should be prepared and provided by the blood bank as soon as possible. Obtaining any available blood from other hospitals may be necessary and recruitment of new donors should be initiated to replenish the available blood stores both for victims of the disaster and for daily needs of regular patients.

Pharmacy service: All disaster trauma patients may partially rely on the disaster mini-stock. This should provide all the necessary equipment and medications. More drugs should be obtained from the ER or other pharmacies without any restriction.

Security service: Apart from guards on each shift, there should be reassignment of two guards to the ER gate to prevent unauthorized entry to any visitors, reporters, and anyone who is not either a patient or member of the team or of the staff. City police assistance might be needed in case of an uncontrolled crowd or disorderly and insistent visitors.

Chart and recording room: If electronic medical records are not available, paper-based charts should be employed in the ER for all victims to maintain accurate records at frequent intervals. Charting new medications, vital signs, intake & output, unusual events during treatment or evolution of the original injury must be recorded in a timely manner right after its occurrence. A designated person must record basic components of the history and of the procedures.

ER staff arrangement: Patients should be admitted to ER without any delay. Triaging can be done simultaneously with the patient admission evaluation. All available ER staff on the shift should be reassigned to the RED ZONE while the disaster team takes care of all the other trauma categories.

The disaster team, most of whom visit the ER frequently, includes General surgeons, Neurosurgeons, Orthopedic surgeons, ER physicians, Surgery residents, midwives, lab techs, ER nurses, ICU nurses, Pediatric ER nurses, OR nurses, Ortho nurses, pharmacists, anesthetists, anesthesiologists, and support staff dedicate most of their efforts in the areas where they are usually assigned. Further arrangement of human resource will be done based on necessity and is directed by the Operation Leader.

Initial management meeting after first phase response: Following the initial rush of patients to the ER following a disaster and disposition of the first wave of victims, a brief pause must be taken to conduct an initial management meeting following the first phase response. During that time discussion must be directed to improve the flow of patients, if possible, and make minor adjustments in distribution of staff, formation of new patient areas, and establishment of priorities, especially in ICUs and ORs. This is briefly summarized below.

1. Discuss the overall situation with Command Post Staff.
2. Establish action priorities based on the first response.
3. Detail resources that are now available or in shortage.
4. Report the current state to stakeholders.

Visitor's Policy

Accompanying persons are not permitted. All visitors should be directed to the waiting area so as not to interfere with the busy traffic of patients and their providers in the ER. Others should leave the compound as soon as possible. This could be challenging in highly dense areas so that different strategies can be considered to control the crows.

Trauma Resuscitation Training

Trauma resuscitation is a multidisciplinary and multiprofessional process practiced daily in trauma management. The team should have a pre-defined role with one leader. Skill and knowledge have been shown to increase with regular simulation and practice drills.

The training encompasses and intends to evaluate first aid practice in staged emergency-scene events. This practice includes evaluation of competence in communication among EMS team and their ability to appropriately transfer victims to the nearby health facility.. Part of such training includes initial evaluation of expertise in hospital triage, need for subsequent intervention, and eventual decision regarding placement. The training also includes learning about external communication and liaison system which must be practiced effectively in any disasters that cause significant damage. After completing the training, each participant must receive performance-based feedback and instructed on how to improve their efforts.

There is also a need for training of non-medical personnel such as policemen, firemen, and especially EMT personnel, in how to treat the patient and how to transfer the patient to an appropriate health facility. Before arrival at the hospital, pre-hospital providers (generally non-physicians) should transmit information about the mechanism of injury, the status of the patient, and initial treatments given in the field. This information can result in furthering the management plan. All the necessary equipment and resources may be prepared on the basis of this initial report. After the patient arrives at the health facility a written handover should be done to inform the local staff of all the necessary details needed for continuity of care. Essential elements that should be obtained in this report include details about the injury event, vital signs obtained at the scene and during transport, pertinent physical findings, and the initial treatments administered along with the response to these treatments. In the receiving hospital activated trauma team should then assume responsibility for the patient based on standard protocol.

Disaster Drill

A drill is a practical exercise which teaches the application of skills and techniques that would be needed in real situations to manage hypothetical emergency situations which simulate real damage and injuries that may be encountered in a disaster or an emergency. Such drills require the actual mobilization of personnel and the use of material resources, communication, collaboration, triage, disposition, and treatment in the field. During the drill an experienced and knowledgeable supervisor evaluates on a scoring sheet the procedures, tools, skills, individual and institutional capacity, and everything else pertinent to management of an emergency/disaster in relation to the institutional plans for disaster preparedness and response. The overall aim of the drill is to identify specific weaknesses that can be targeted for improvement and to promote continuing efforts to strengthen hospital disaster preparedness.

How To Coordinate a Response in the Setting of Public Health Emergency

COVID-19 Lessons from Different Environments

A pandemic at large and epidemics in a regional context have had a significant negative impact on social, psychological, and economic sectors so far. The COVID-19 pandemic overwhelms the health care system not only in LMICs but also in resource intense countries. Collaboration and integration among different stakeholders may reduce the effect of public health emergencies. Health care systems in LMICs are known to be weak. In the face of a highly transmissible pandemic, they become more fragile since they have a little reserve. Accessibility and efficiency of health care systems prevent, detect, and treat disease effectively through primary health care. Shifting of resources for COVID-19 care is expected to compromise the effectiveness and use of other services. Health systems worldwide were challenged by the increasing number of patients with COVID-19. This overwhelmed health care systems everywhere to a greater or lesser degree and therefore compromised the delivery of other health care to non-COVID patients due to various factors. These included marked and rapid decrease in available supplies and even equipment, like ventilators, and partially because of decrease in personnel due to illness or fear of exposure to the virus, stigma, misinformation, and limitations on contacts. When health systems are disrupted and people fail to access needed care, both direct mortality from an outbreak and indirect mortality from preventable and treatable conditions increase dramatically The optimization of infection prevention and control via vaccinations and mask and distance precautions is the core part of maintaining non-COVID-19 health care system.

The challenges to weak health care systems are magnified in these situations because of the need for shifting of professionals (already inadequate in number) for COVID-19 care and isolation of staff and needed personnel who may be infected. This causes additional disruption of delivery of non-COVID care. The supply of drugs and equipment is also disrupted due to factories shifting to COVID-19-related protective equipment production, which may lead to a mismatch of demand and supply.

Pandemic response strategy should consider engagement of non-health sector organizations, international partners, local community members, and media to promulgate energetically all possible preventive measures, including masking, isolation, frequent washing, and especially vaccination when available.

Conclusion

This chapter on the management of disasters and emergencies focuses on organization of a standard approach to consistent and responsible leadership, frequent re-evaluations and re-adjustments of personnel, resources, hospital capacity, and transport systems to accommodate a changing number of victims with variable injuries. Emphasis is placed on a careful triage system which also may need to be adjusted periodically. The focus of this chapter is how to combine fixed and relatively rigid approaches to the management of victims of disasters and at the same time maintain flexibility to accommodate moment-to-moment changes within the relatively fixed infrastructure needed to maintain discipline and cooperation among the providers and non-professional staff.

References

1. World Health Organization. WHO guidance on preparing for national response to health emergencies and disasters. 2021.
2. Henderson LJ. Emergency and disaster: pervasive risk and public bureaucracy in developing nations. Public Organ Rev. 2004;4(2):103–19.
3. Mohamed Shaluf I. An overview on disasters. Disaster Prev Manag Int J [Internet]. 2007;16(5):687–703. https://doi.org/10.1108/09653560710837000
4. Asghar S, Alahakoon D, Churilov L. A comprehensive conceptual model for disaster management. J Humanit Assist. 2006;1360(0222):1–15.
5. Callese TE, Richards CT, Shaw P, Schuetz SJ, Paladino L, Issa N, et al. Trauma system development in low-and middle-income countries: a review. J Surg Res. 2015;193(1):300–7.
6. Eisner ZJ, Delaney PG, Thullah AH, Yu AJ, Timbo SB, Koroma S, et al. Evaluation of a lay first responder program in Sierra Leone as a scalable model for prehospital trauma care. Injury [Internet]. 2020;51(11):2565–73. https://www.sciencedirect.com/science/article/pii/S0020138320307087
7. Anderson PD. Health organization world, prehospital trauma care systems, World Health Organization (2005), 2005 62 p. ISBN: 92-4-159294X. 2006.

8. Wesson HKH, Bachani AM, Wekesa JM, Mburu J, Hyder AA, Stevens KA. Assessing trauma care at the district and provincial hospital levels: a case study of hospitals in Kenya. Glob Road Saf Updat Ten Low-Middle-Income Ctries [Internet]. 2013;44:S75–80. https://www.sciencedirect.com/science/article/pii/S0020138313702171
9. Callese TE, Richards CT, Shaw P, Schuetz SJ, Paladino L, Issa N, et al. Trauma system development in low- and middle-income countries: a review. J Surg Res [Internet]. 2015;193(1):300–7. https://www.sciencedirect.com/science/article/pii/S0022480414008956
10. Borgohain B, Khonglah T. Developing and organizing a trauma system and mass casualty management: some useful observations from the Israeli trauma model. Ann Med Health Sci Res. 2013;3(1):85–9.

How To Select a Database Software for Surgical Data in Low- and Middle-Income Countries

15

Henry M. Spotnitz and Matthew E. Spotnitz

A man only becomes wise when he begins to calculate the approximate depth of his ignorance.

– Gian Carlo Menotti

Abbreviations

DOD	Day of Discharge
DOS	Date of Surgery
Dx	Diagnosis
RDBS	Relational database structures
SQL	Structured query language

Introduction

Some databases are optimized for multiple users and provide flexibility in data content, whereas others are better suited for homogeneous data content and fewer users. Database options include flat file and relational structures (RDBS). Flat files contain information and a program that accesses it. A common example of RDBS is a Microsoft Excel spreadsheet. The structure is simple and programming is not demanding. Data entry and retrieval is straightforward. However, applications are limited. RDBS consists of information that is distributed over multiple tables. The data are entered and retrieved by the structured query language (SQL) [1, 2].

How To Choose a Program

There are advantages and disadvantages to each kind of database. For small populations, flat file databases have benefits of being inexpensive and easy to implement. Because of the widespread use of flat files, many surgeons are likely to be proficient with them. Alternatively, there is an abundance of resources to help people who are not familiar with their use. Flat files may be efficient for tracking a small number of variables that are relevant to a surgical service, such as basic patient information, the type of operation, and the length of stay in an ambulatory care service. However, for larger and more complicated data sets, RDBS offers unique advantages. The distribution of data over multiple tables allows for different data formats to be stored, as well as the relationships among them. For large data sets, SQL queries are more efficient than searching a flat file and those queries are also efficient at filtering duplicate entries. Furthermore, the RDBMS structure allows for access to multiple users. Disadvantages of RDBMSs are that they

H. M. Spotnitz (✉) · M. E. Spotnitz
Columbia University Vagelos College of Physicians and Surgeons, New York, NY, USA
e-mail: hms2@cumc.columbia.edu; mes2165@cumc.columbia.edu

M. A. Hardy, B. R. Hochman (eds.), *Global Surgery*, https://doi.org/10.1007/978-3-031-28127-3_15

require more hardware and expertise for implementation, maintenance, programming, and use [1, 2]. RDBMSs are well suited for synthesis of the surgical data across domains of the electronic health record. RDBMS designs allow tracking surgical patients across different services in a healthcare system. This allows investigators to study non-operative management, resource utilization, and long-term outcomes. Furthermore, RDBMSs are better suited for high-volume access, which allows for clinicians from different specialties to access data concurrently. In summary, the decision for whether to implement a flat file or RDBMS depends on the size and complexity of the data as well as the number of users. For simple data that are used by a small number of users in resource-constrained settings, flat files are likely best. Alternatively, RDBMSs are best for large, complicated data sets that are used by a large number of users.

Data Entry

Creation of a database requires a computer and a programmer who can enter data and modify the database as needs develop. The simplest way to start a surgical database is to purchase an inexpensive computer and software. These purchases should be directed by the programmer who will operate the system. These steps will be directed by an overall strategic plan.

The primary purpose of a new database is to maintain records of surgical procedures. These records are necessary to provide follow-up care for patients who return to the primary care center at infrequent intervals.

The following are critical patient data

MRN This is a numerical index that is unique to each patient and is used to track critical data.

Names (demographics) are critical for patient identification and should not be duplicated

First Name
Last Name
Date of Birth
Sex

Once demographics are entered, they should remain unique to the patient and should not be changed.

In contrast, data specific to a surgical procedure are highly variable and specific:

Date of Surgery (DOS)
Date of Admission for Surgery (DOA)
Date of Discharge (DODC)
Name of Operations performed: Op1,2,3…..
Surgical Complications: Comp1,2,3…
Surgical Diagnosis:Dx1,Dx2, Dx3
Surgical Team:
Surgeon
Assistants
Anesthesiologists

Surgical procedures can be uniquely identified by a CONCATENATED INDEX consisting of the MRN and DOS strung together as in "MRN*DOS."

Getting Started

A relatively simple approach to surgical data uses a flat file with the following entry form:

First Name
Last Name
SEX
DOA
DODC

These data would be entered into the computer system at the time of admission and would be updated daily.

Indexes and Multiuser Configurations

Multi-user databases provide the ultimate flexibility and are based on multiple independent tables of data linked by indexes. HELIX and SQL are marketed examples.

Summary

Database structures are essential for surgical follow-up and quality improvement. In the simplest form, these consist of punch cards, but current developments are based heavily on multiuser databases and indexing. For a new surgical unit, flat files offer effective, simple data management and effective patient follow-up.

References

1. Scheider MAE, Siebels J, Schmitt C. Data base management in interventional electrophysiology—the relational advantage. J Intervent Cardiac Electrophysiol. 1998;2:333–41.
2. Stein L. Creating databases for biological information: an introduction. Curr Protoc Bioinform. 2013;42:9.1.1–9.1.10.

Websites

https://www.techwalla.com/articles/difference-flat-file-relational-database, https://otiskopp.com/flat-files-vs-relational-databases/, http://carltonmatthews.com/flat-file-vs-rdbms/

Part II

Education and Training

How to Establish Surgical Teaching, Guidance, and Simulation Practices in Low- and Middle-Income Countries

16

Shamir O. Cawich, Paul Shridath Ramphal, Marlon Mencia, Chris Dodgion, and Alazar Berhe Aregawi

A mentor must expect their mentees to supersede their own performance in order to consider themselves successful.

– V. Naraynsingh

Abbreviations

AHPBA	Americas Hepato-Pancreato-Biliary Association
ARRIVE	Animal Research Reporting In Vivo Experiment
CaSES	Caribbean Society of Endoscopic Surgeons
CCOS	Caribbean College of Surgeons
GPD	Gross domestic product
HICs	High-income countries
ICU	Intensive care unit
LMICs	Low- and middle-income countries
MDT	Multidisciplinary team
MIS	Minimally invasive surgery
MISTELS	McGill Inanimate System for Training and Evaluation of Laparoscopy
NASKHO	Netherlands-Caribbean Foundation for Clinical Higher Education
SAGES	Society of American Gastrointestinal and Endoscopic Surgeons

Background

There are many low- and middle-income countries (LMICs) scattered across the globe, each with different healthcare systems and their individual challenges. This may range from landlocked nations on the African continent with large land masses and scattered populations that may be difficult to access to the small island nations of the Caribbean geographically separated by the Caribbean Sea. Most are independent nations with their own languages, customs, governments, healthcare systems, infrastructure, and medical customs. Some of these nations are small states, with populations as low as 5000 persons [1]. These characteristics present several

The original version of the chapter has been revised. A correction to this chapter can be found at https://doi.org/10.1007/978-3-031-28127-3_46

S. O. Cawich (✉) · M. Mencia
University of the West Indies, St Augustine Campus, Trinidad and Tobago

P. S. Ramphal
University of the West Indies, Princess Margaret Hospital, Nassau, Bahamas

C. Dodgion
Surgery Medical College of Wisconsin, Milwaukee, WI, USA
e-mail: cdodgion@mcw.edu

A. B. Aregawi
College of Medicine and Health Sciences, Hawassa University, Hawassa, Ethiopia

M. A. Hardy, B. R. Hochman (eds.), *Global Surgery*, https://doi.org/10.1007/978-3-031-28127-3_16

challenges to both surgical practice and to surgical education, which make them quite different from that in developed, high-income countries (HICs).

Specific Challenges

The practice of surgery and therefore its teaching in LMICs may be affected in the areas discussed below.

1. Lack of Subspecialty Services
Nations with small populations cannot attract subspecialty trained surgeons as the workload is often too small. In these circumstances, most operations that would normally be performed by subspecialty surgical teams are now performed by general surgeons at low volumes. Additionally, in many countries of the world, there are limited educational opportunities for surgical specialization, and therefore supply of subspecialty care is inadequate. This means that general surgery teams will perform a wide cadre of procedures, but each at low volumes.

An immediate concern arises: Several authors in the latter part of the twenty-first century demonstrated significantly reduced morbidity and mortality when complex operations were performed in high-volume hospitals and by high-volume surgeons [2]. However, this would not be possible in small nations, such as the Caribbean Islands. Even in the more populous islands of the Anglophone Caribbean, there were no hospitals that qualified as high-volume facilities in the year 2021 [3].

This creates the situation where patients who require complex operations have no choice but to consent to surgery in the LMICs or to travel to high-volume hospitals in developed nations. The high-volume centers are often located in HICs, and only a fraction of persons can afford healthcare in these centers. Even in 2014, Naraynsingh et al. [1] documented that only 4 of 19 Caribbean countries had the services of a urologist and in 2022 only 5 of 19 Caribbean countries had access to hepatobiliary surgeons. Even when a specialist center exists within the Anglophone Caribbean, transporting patients between the nearby islands proves impractical as there is no provision for cost-sharing between the countries. Many other cases such as replant surgery, vascularized free tissue transfer, myocutaneous flaps, and neonatal surgery are performed by the general surgeons.

2. Limited Opportunity for Multidisciplinary Cooperation
A multidisciplinary team (MDT) approach to therapeutics has become standard of care in modern healthcare delivery systems [4–6]. There are numerous advantages associated with the structured forum to exchange information and ideas, including improved working relationships, expedited investigations, adherence to evidence-based treatment, and ultimately improved clinical outcomes [7]. Unfortunately, the MDT approach to disease management is not routinely practiced in LMICs [4, 5]. Again, this may be partly due to the small population size and small cadre of specialists and subspecialists. In healthcare systems like these, it has become commonplace for a small cadre of doctors to assume responsibility for healthcare for the entire nation. Subspecialty support is often unavailable, and general surgeons must be versatile, often performing operations that range from gynecology, obstetrics, orthopedics, and neurosurgery, all in the same week. These doctors often have no choice because they may work in remote and isolated areas [5]. The phrase *sole practitioner culture* was coined to describe this situation where medical decisions are made autonomously by attending doctors in an autocratic manner, with very little collaborative input and without routine application of MDT principles [4, 5].

3. Limited Equipment (Hardware)
LMICs often have underfunded healthcare systems and provide only basic levels of healthcare to the population. Policy makers prioritize their spending, and often, only a small fraction of their gross domestic product (GDP) is directed for healthcare. Therefore, surgeons in these nations are challenged to provide innovative effective high-quality care in a setting where resources are limited. This may occasionally be

difficult without regular access to basic drugs (antibiotics, anesthetic agents, analgesics, etc.) or materials such as vascular grafts or laparoscopic equipment.

Specialized surgical equipment is often unavailable. A simple example is the practice of minimally invasive surgery (MIS) that has been well accepted across the globe. The advantages of early mobilization, minimal scarring, decreased pain, and early return to work are well documented for a variety of operations. In the English-speaking Caribbean, only few countries are able to offer regular MIS services because many do not have the requisite expertise and/or equipment. For example, Naraynsingh et al. [1] documented that as recently as 2014, laparoscopic stacks were only available in public hospitals in 25% of countries in the Caribbean. Therefore, surgeons are simply unable to offer laparoscopic operations, even if the expertise exists. In addition to hardware acquisition, the additional financial burden of equipment maintenance and the high cost of disposable instruments and consumables limit laparoscopic surgery seriously in LMICs [1].

4. Operative Consumables

As the move away from open surgery to laparoscopic and robotic surgery continues, more consumables are being utilized, such as stapling devices or ultrasonic dissectors. Frequently, the cost of these consumables is beyond the limited budgets of hospitals in LMICs, and consequently, surgeons would use sutures instead of staples or cautery dissection instead of ultrasonic dissectors. West Indian surgeons have navigated around this issue by sterilizing and re-purposing single-use instruments (Fig. 16.1).

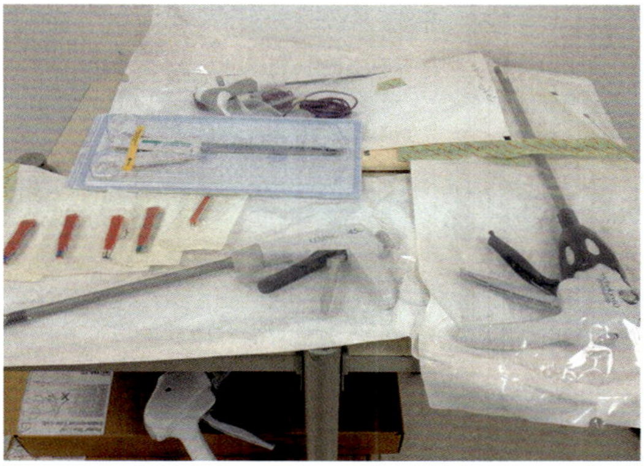

Fig. 16.1 Single-use laparoscopic consumables have been sterilized and re-packaged for continued use in low-income nations

5. Blood Products

The stark reality is that in low-resource settings, there is a relative lack of blood products. This limits the type of care that can be delivered. For example, complex procedures such as major liver resections or aneurysm repairs that may require large volumes of blood products often cannot be done. Surgeons in the LMICs of the Caribbean have partially compensated for this by increasing the use of tranexamic acid in surgery as it is relatively inexpensive and has reduced transfusion rates in our practice. In addition, many of LMICs also deal with the concomitant problem of interpersonal violence. The high burden of trauma patients often consume what little blood products are available.

It is not uncommon that surgeons have to proceed with complex operations, such as major liver resections, pancreatico-duodenectomy, or abdominal aortic aneurysm that usually would require standby products, with only one unit of packed cells available. Most surgeons will agree that such a situation is less than desirable and may be outright dangerous, unless a cell saver is available and is usable.

6. Intensive Care Unit Support

Intensive care is costly to deliver and to outfit. Therefore, many LMICs may not be able to afford the recommended number of intensive care unit (ICU) beds per capita population. Often, even when nations may have physical ICU bed space, the requisite consumables, staffing, and pharmacologic support are not readily available, effectively rendering the ICU unavailable. This again limits the support trauma patients can receive and limits the number of major cases that can be done safely.

7. Private Healthcare

The limitations outlined above in LMICs have increased patient demand for improved standards of care. Many private facilities have been created to fill this demand using the fee-for-service model of healthcare delivery. Although this offers some societal benefits as it increases the cadre of services available in the nation, it also creates disparity and inequity in healthcare.

Solutions to Specific Challenges

It is clear that there are many challenges to provision of surgical care and surgical teaching in LMICs. These are the realities, and it is obvious that many of these scenarios are imperfect. Many LMICs have devised innovative solutions discussed below to overcome these challenges.

(1) Surgical Education
Surgical education in LMICs differs significantly from that in HICs. While it is beneficial for surgeons practicing in resource-poor nations to be exposed to surgical care in high-volume hospitals located in developed countries, many of the practices cannot be readily transposed to their home countries. In the Caribbean, we recognized this difference and responded by forming professional bodies, which include 250 general surgeons practicing in the Caribbean nations. There are also subspecialty professional associations dedicated to the practice of liver and pancreatic surgery, The Caribbean Chapter of the Americas Hepatopancreatobiliary Association (AHPBA), a professional association dedicated to MIS, and the Caribbean Society of Endoscopic Surgeons (CaSES). The important aspect of these professional associations is their mandate to foster continued professional development specific to healthcare systems in LMICs. All societies host regular educational activities to develop regional surgical practice. A specific example relates to the practice of liver and pancreatic surgery in the Caribbean where in 2022, there were only seven subspecialty trained hepatopancreatobiliary surgeons. There are few opportunities for properly organized multidisciplinary care meetings as these surgeons are scattered across the region. However, through the Caribbean Chapter AHPBA, regional MDT meetings are held, and a trans-Caribbean support service using social media is maintained for real-time second opinions and technical support. The Caribbean Chapter AHPBA also hosts biannual educational events for tailored surgical education. These surgeons are all operating in similar conditions and are poised to give relevant support/advice to their colleagues.

(2) Multidisciplinary Cooperation
The benefits of a MDT approach to disease management have already been discussed. It is not routinely practiced in all LMICs because of the previously described *sole practitioner culture* [4]. With the well-documented benefits of this approach, inclusive of its educational value, it is important to introduce and establish MDT principles in LMICs with concern of the potential for opposition to change [4, 5].

We recommend that this should be done in a phased approach: Firstly, common interest clinician-led groups should be established. They can then provide a strong, unified voice to lobby for change. This would be more effective than the lobbying of only one or two isolated individuals.

As a second phase, all stakeholders should be approached and given a chance to participate in the process as to eliminate any individuals who may be overlooked and who had the potential to erect barriers [6]—this includes established clinicians. Institutional recognition is also important to facilitate technical support and dedicated staffing. In a facility at the Port of Spain General Hospital in Trinidad and Tobago, MDT principles were implemented as a self-driven venture, with interested individuals taking up roles for governance, documentation, audiovisual service, and meeting coordination. The established clinicians and institutional support followed, although they were not excluded in the early stages.

Many nations will have budgetary limitations, but these can be overcome by use of free software such as WhatsApp® (WhatsApp Inc., California, USA) and Google Mail® (Google Inc., Mountain View, CA 94043, USA) to disseminate information, Dropbox® (Dropbox Inc., San Francisco, California) to share clinical material/files, and OsiriX® DICOM imaging software (Pixmeo,

Geneva, Switzerland) to view radiologic images [7]. In the initial stages of our MDT, personal property was used such as personal computers, software, and audiovisual equipment [4]. The development of public–private partnerships is encouraged as there are many interested foundations and businesses as well as individuals who are willing to support healthcare development, by contributing financially and by providing their expertise [4].

Critical to success of MDT is for all core members to meet in advance and agree to protocols and to governance. For example, all participants agreed to document the information exchanged and to abide by any collective decisions made by the MDT. This reduced the potential for interpersonal conflicts during meetings [4]. It is important to maintain regular audits of outcomes of practices since this is the only way to demonstrate meaningful benefit of MDT to the healthcare system. Following introduction of MDT practice at a facility, there was a significant increase in participation and a major change in treatment plans in 48% of cases after a MDT discussion [4]. The other benefits included regular interactions between various disciplines, which led to a better understanding of the challenges each member faced in a system with limited resources [7] and allowed to effectively streamline patient pathways.

(3) Surgical Teaching Events

Healthcare systems in LMICs may not be able to care effectively for complex cases for a variety of reasons. Routine transfer of such patients to high-volume facilities is not only expensive and difficult to execute but also important in that the local surgeons are denied the opportunity to manage challenging cases, leaving them exposed only to minor cases. To overcome this, regular surgical teaching events have been held across the Caribbean region. Surgical workshops are planned, and regional experts are invited to the target country as speakers and as surgical proctors. The advantage of this exercise is that a large audience can be reached in target hospitals. The entire cadre of healthcare workers, including operating room nurses, surgical scrub technicians, surgeons, and support staff, are exposed to surgical teaching at the same time. This also improves the standard of care for the nation, which hosts the workshop [8]. Because regional experts are chosen as proctors/tutors, they are able to teach tailored surgical techniques, tips, and tricks that are relevant to LMIC healthcare systems since they also work in similar resource-poor environments [8].

The disadvantage is that this is a costly exercise. The limitation of high cost of this exercise can be overcome by developing public–private partnerships. As an example, there are two main suppliers of surgical consumables in the Caribbean, and under the public–private partnership arrangements, these suppliers fund the regional workshops. The benefit to these companies is that surgeons learn to use their consumables/equipment, and they are more likely to generate additional sales. We have found that the suppliers in the Caribbean have been supportive of this initiative [9, 10]. Surgeons, however, must be cognizant that close relationships with industry may create conflicts of interest.

(4) Simulation Practices

Although surgery was traditionally taught using the apprenticeship model, there has been a shift toward surgical education by simulation. Here, surgical trainees are interactively immersed into environments that replicate real-world scenarios [11]. Although surgical education via simulation is still emerging, this concept has been well accepted in other industries such as the aviation industry [12]. Simulated surgical education brings several advantages:

1. Patients are not exposed to the potential harm when residents learn procedures in the operating room.
2. Trainee surgeons acquire technical skills in a simulated environment so that they have amassed significant experience by the time they are called upon to operate on patients [10].
3. Simulators are always available for use and so provide extended practice opportunities that

are significantly more flexible than the operating room/clinical patient exposure [11].
4. There are reductions in operating time and associated costs when resident teaching is removed from the operating room.

Simulation can also be used to teach non-technical skills, such as communication, crisis management, teamwork, and professionalism, but this chapter focuses predominantly on teaching technical skills. Surgical skill sets can be taught through several simulation types, including benchtop models, cadaver models, live animal models, virtual reality simulators, laparoscopic simulators, and robotic simulators.

Benchtop Simulators for Open Surgery

Benchtop models use inanimate/synthetic material to teach and/or assess technical skills. These benchtop models may range from simple, crude models (Fig. 16.2) to interactive models (Fig. 16.3).

At the University of the West Indies, animal part models have been used, such as pig intestines to teach residents to perform bowel anastomoses (Fig. 16.4), pig aorta to teach creation of vascular anastomoses (Fig. 16.5), pig trotters to teach tendon repair (Fig. 16.6), and chicken breast to teach microwave ablation, use of energy devices, and staple firing (Fig. 16.7). There have also been reports of obstetric sphincter injury repair using pig tongue [13], endometrial resection, and ablation on pumpkin models [14]. Many other simple and inexpensive examples of benchtop models have been described.

Benchtop models are attractive for LMICs because they are inexpensive, safe, and made of locally available materials, require little maintenance, and provide unlimited opportunities for task repetition. They are probably the most likely modalities used in LMICs. Benchtop models allow residents to focus on other learning tasks when

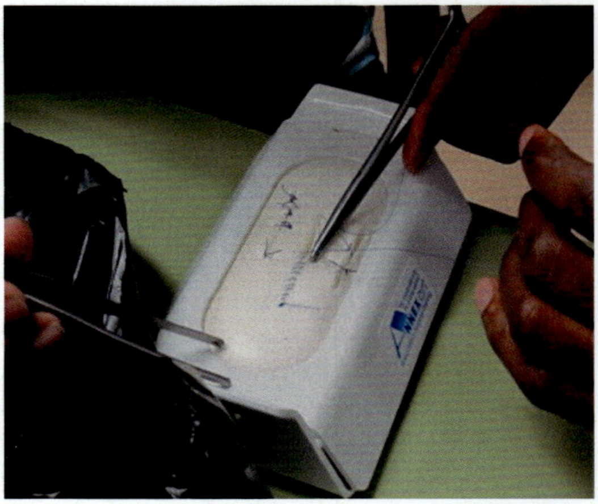

Fig. 16.2 Crude benchtop model used to teach suture closure of wounds

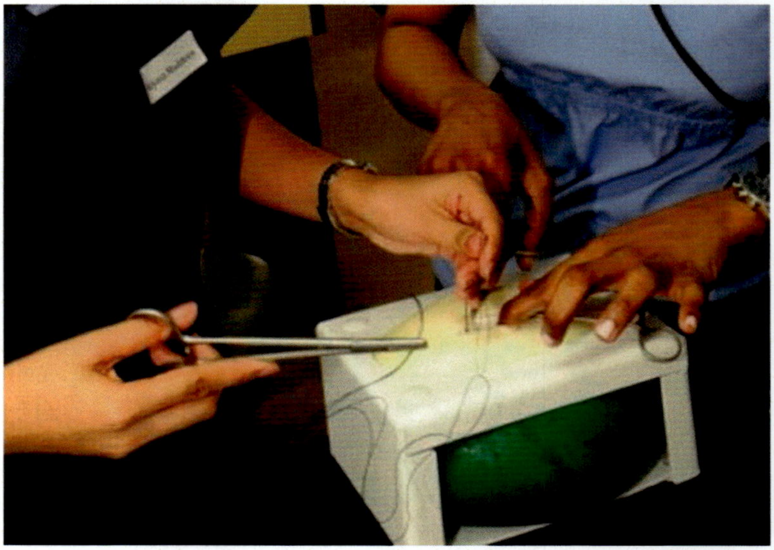

Fig. 16.3 A benchtop model to simulate fascial closure. A balloon is inflated within a box, and the trainee sutures overlying tissue to mimic the task of fascial closure without injuring underlying bowel

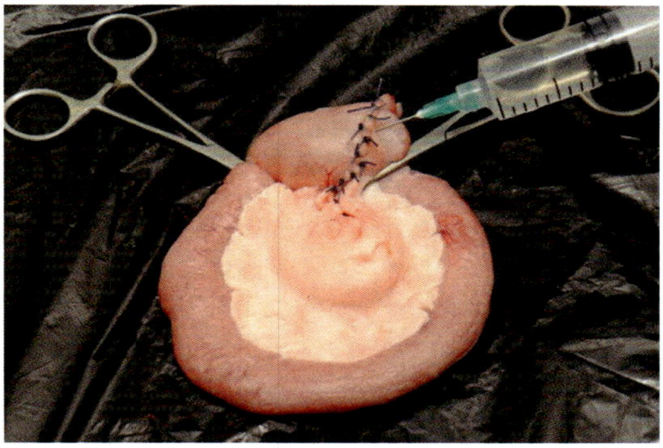

Fig. 16.4 Porcine intestine used to create a bowel anastomosis. The bowel was then injected with saline under pressure to assess for leakage/spillage

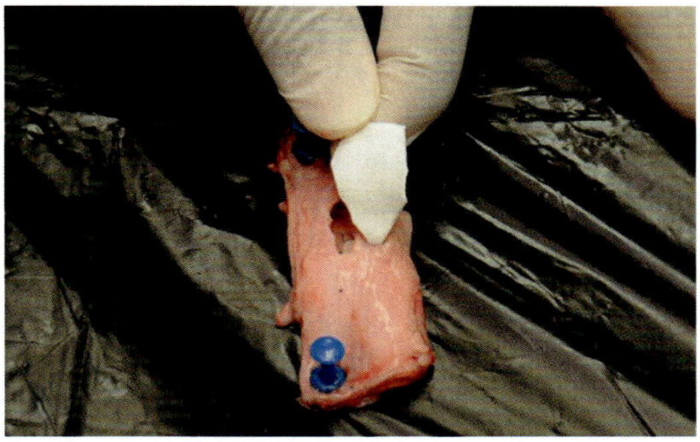

Fig. 16.5 A section of porcine aorta is used to teach principles of vascular anastomoses by creating a vein patch

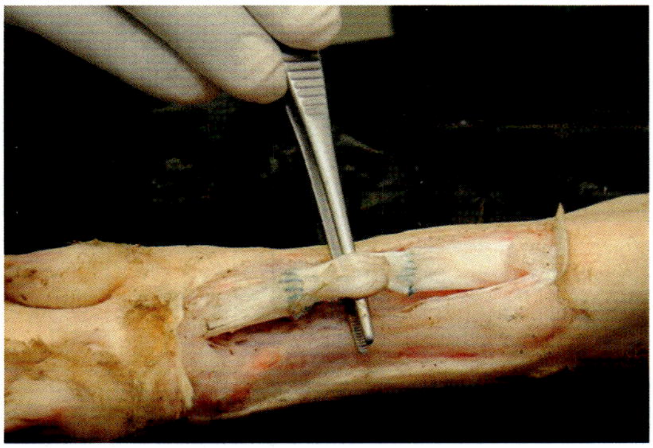

Fig. 16.6 Piglet trotters with tendon repair using a Kessler stitch

they go to the operating room [15] and result in demonstrable improvement in metrics for task performance [16, 17] and transfer of competency to the real operating room environment [16, 18].

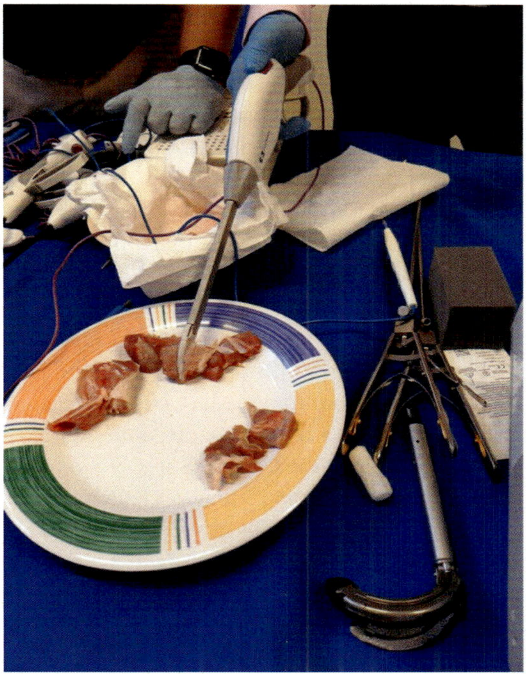

Fig. 16.7 Chicken breast used to practice operating energy devices and staple firing

There are also commercially developed inanimate models to teach skill sets such as cardiopulmonary resuscitation, endotracheal intubation, and/or thoracostomy placement on a mannequin. These are costly and are not always practical in LMICs. A potential advantage from partnerships for surgical education is that some equipment, such as mannequins or laparoscopic simulators, may be donated to the host institution. Unfortunately, they also come with the cost of maintenance and repair.

Full-task simulators are also available as benchtop models. For example, Lauscher et al. [15] designed the Berlin Operation Trainer where the surgeon stands in a simulated operating field in order to practice open GI anastomotic techniques. In Jamaica, animal tissue-based surgical simulation training models were being explored and utilized. The culmination of these efforts was the development of the world's first computer-controlled tissue-based simulator for teaching various aspects of cardiac surgery [19].

The cardiac surgical simulator was developed as a collaborative project between the University of the West Indies and the University of Technology in Jamaica, demonstrating that fruitful collaboration between academic institutions in LMICs was possible and could be very productive. The Cardiac Surgery Simulator was designed to provide a safe, anatomically accurate, and clinically challenging simulated operative environment to facilitate the teaching and acquisition of essential surgical skills. It facilitates trainees learning skills such as cannulation (Fig. 16.8) and cardiopulmonary bypass management and coronary and aortic anastomoses. As a full task simulator, the Cardiac Surgery Simulator also provides simulated clinical challenges and dilemmas that require the trainee to make decisions and take actions such as those that would be necessary in a real surgical procedure.

The entire functionality of the cardiac simulator with all its complexities is controlled by a laptop computer using proprietary software. The overall effect is to enable the trainer to take the trainee through parts of or a complete standard open-heart surgical operation, with the option of presenting the trainee with most of the possible adverse events that could arise during the conduct of such surgical procedures. The Cardiac Surgery Simulator has been described as a "flight simulator" for cardiac surgery, referring to the way pilots are trained to fly safely in optimal and adverse conditions and which has become standard training practice for airline pilots worldwide [20].

The Cardiac Surgery Simulator became one of the centerpieces of the Thoracic Surgical Director's Association Annual Boot Camp event spanning the period 2008 to 2022. It has been estimated that a minimum of one third of all US cardiothoracic surgical trainees were exposed to this simulator during the decade spanning from 2009 to 2019. A major point of note is that this demonstrated that innovations in surgical education can originate in LMICs, and these innovations can be equally applicable in HICs based on the intrinsic merits of the ideas as they are formulated and implemented.

Simulation for Laparoscopic Surgery

After laparoscopic cholecystectomy was demonstrated to be feasible and safe in the 1990s, there was rapid adoption of the minimally invasive approach. Laparoscopy almost became the standard of care for many abdominal operations. There was great emphasis on training and preventing complications [21]. Many surgeons pointed out that laparoscopy did not allow surgeons to have tactile feedback and depth perception and required new skill sets to operate instruments mounted on a long stick. Simulation seemed to be a natural fit to teach minimally invasive surgery. It allowed surgical residents to

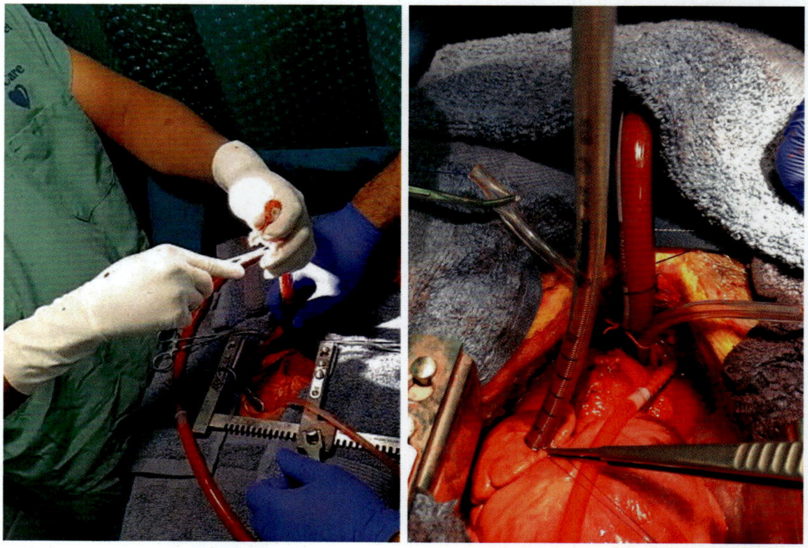

Fig. 16.8 Cannulation of the Cardiac Surgical Simulator for simulated cardiopulmonary bypass

become accustomed to these nuances and learn laparoscopic techniques in a safe environment outside of the operating room. Therefore, surgical residents would have already amassed significant skill by the time they are exposed to patients in the operating room [22].

Laparoscopic Trainers

Laparoscopic trainers may range from simple box trainers with feedback monitors to high-resolution virtual reality simulators. Virtual reality simulators provide realistic experiences that closely mimic the operative environment, but they are not affordable in many LMICs. Even when donated, they are difficult to maintain. For example, the Hawassa University in Ethiopia was gifted a virtual reality simulator but was no longer able to use it due to need for software upkeep. There are full-task or procedure-specific very expensive simulators that are dedicated to teaching entire operations. Virtual reality trainers use computer software to analyze tasks, and so they eliminate the need for a dedicated human proctor. They also have the advantage of comparing scores and/or allowing analyses of records. However, these advantages have not been shown to make virtual reality trainers superior to other simulators.

Most LMICs will have access to low-fidelity box trainers, which are portable and unlimited in availability. These are often partial task trainers that allow the resident to practice simple repetitive tasks such as object transfers, suturing, knot tying, clipping, and stapling. Other tasks, such as cutting a shape from a surgical glove or removing objects from the fingers of a glove, can also be taught as is done at the University of West Indies. These are basic skills that are used in every laparoscopic operation and are readily transferrable.

Laparoscopic Box Trainers

Laparoscopic box trainers are relatively inexpensive and consist of a closed box, camera, visual feedback monitor, and light source. A few authors have also described the use of homemade trainers from readily available and inexpensive materials [22, 23]. Several groups have invented programs to augment the use of trainers. Examples of these include the Royal College of Surgeons.

Laparoscopic Training course [24], the Fundamentals of Laparoscopy course from SAGES [25], and Curacao Laparoscopic Course [9], among others. The basic tenet is that residents are given standardized tasks to complete and are graded on accuracy and time to complete them. There has been sufficient evidence collected to show that structured programs are beneficial in training, resulting in improved performance metrics in the operating room [26].

Robotic Trainers

There has been significant progress in the adoption of robotics in surgery. The surgical robot has been widely adopted across the globe, especially the DaVinci robot (Intuitive Surgical Inc., Sunnyvale, California, USA), which has dominated the robotic landscape over the past two decades. While there is good evidence to validate these sophisticated, full-task robotic simulators, they are expensive and may be out of reach of many LMICs.

Live Non-survival Porcine Models

A common criticism of surgical simulators is that normal anatomic relationships are missing and tissue handling is unrealistic. For this reason, live animal tissue was thought to be more representative of the operating room experience because there is bleeding, movement with breathing, and more realistic tissue handling [27]. The two most common animals used are canine and porcine models, but many countries have existing laws against their use as surgical training models [27]. The non-survival porcine model is probably most common where the animals are anesthetized during the procedure and euthanized post-procedure; the porcine models have been shown to be effective for teaching a variety of operative procedures, but their use is limited by differences in legislation in each nation.

Cadaveric Models

Cadaver models are used commonly for surgical teaching because trainees can work with normal anatomic relationships and more realistic tissue characteristics [28, 29]. Many countries have existing legislation permitting cadaver use for surgical training [29]. Although cadavers are limited in supply, costly to procure, and difficult to store, they may be used by residents demonstrating to medical students in medical school anatomy laboratories.

Cadaveric models are reserved for complex procedures that require realistic tissue handling and anatomic integrity, such as surgical exposure in limbs for joint replacements, fiber-optic airway intubation, and endoscopic sinus surgery.

(5) Guidance in the OR

In LMICs, most general surgeons perform a wide repertoire of operations, each at low volumes. Although most surgeons are highly competent, they may not possess the necessary skill sets to complete advanced procedures. Surgical mentoring may be utilized as a method for development in this scenario. Formal mentorship is commonly used in fellowships following residency training, while in informal mentorship, one surgeon seeks out their own local or visiting mentors to increase their skillset for complex special operations, such as liver or pancreas resections. They also benefit from better networking while able to provide services that may not be normally available. This will reduce the need for outbound patient transfers, improve workplace satisfaction, retain healthcare staff, and increase access to essential surgical services within the healthcare system [30, 31].

The ideal mentor should be well trained, have significant operating experience, and must be a well-respected authority in their field. Good leadership qualities, interpersonal communication skills, patience, and professional integrity are other essential qualities. It is important for mentors to be emotionally mature so that they are not threatened by the potential success of their mentees.

Potential disadvantages from mentorship include gender, race or religious discrimination, trainee disenchantment, and abuse of authority [32, 33]. Unfortunately, it has been documented that many of these attitudes still exist and serve as barriers to development in LMICs, as well as in HICs.

A significant obstacle to mentorship in LMICs is that the mentor would have to travel for mentorship in the operating room. The cost to the mentor has been borne either by the mentee's institution or by public–private partnership with professional bodies or with industry [31]. To overcome such costs and inconvenience is to explore the concept of distance mentoring.

(6) Distance Mentoring

Distance mentoring differs from the traditional concept of physical mentoring by the fact that the mentor is not physically in the operating room, and this was triggered by the 2020 pandemic [34]. It involves a surgical mentor using videotelephony to guide a less experienced colleague to complete an operation. A carefully planned and effectively administered program of distance mentoring can be effective in stimulating progress in surgery in LMICs.

In the model originally published, readily available and inexpensive equipment was utilized [34]. A surgical resident was in command of the patient in the operating room and used two devices equipped with FaceTime (Apple Inc., Cupertino, California, USA) to live stream to the attending surgeon [34]. In the operating room, the first device was fixed onto the operating light or behind the surgeon to capture the surgeon's view, and another was placed on the ventilator stack facing backward to observe instrument handling in the operating field (Fig. 16.9). When necessary, the latter device was handled by circulating theatre staff to obtain closer views of the operating field while maintaining strict aseptic technique [34]. The attending surgeon was isolated in a separate room with two devices to observe both feeds and instruct residents during the live operation. The virtual mentor was available throughout the entire operation and instructed the mentee on steps to complete the operation.

This technique utilizes videotelephony to transmit audio-video signals in real time [35] and requires a high-resolution, uninterrupted power and Internet supply. Most modern personal computers and smartphones have built-in codec software to compress audio-video streams and transmit them as labeled digitalized packets on high-bandwidth connections using Internet Protocols [36]. The technology has become relatively cheap and transmits images with high resolution over the Internet at a low cost.

Apart from distance mentoring, videotelephony has found applications in distance education [36], virtual medical consultations [37], diagnostics [37], and transmission of medical images [34, 35]. The possibilities are endless,

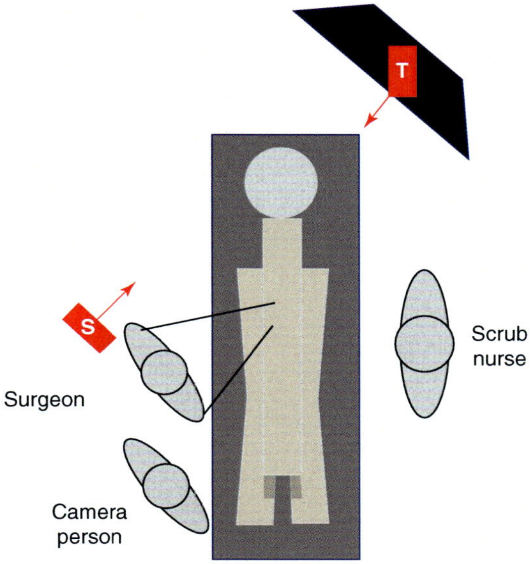

Fig. 16.9 Setup of operating room for distance mentoring. One smartphone (T) is positioned on the laparoscopic stack and records the operating field. The second smartphone (S) is positioned behind the surgeon's shoulder and captures images from the laparoscopic monitor. Both feeds are transmitted to the remote mentor who observes the instructions on two receiving devices. In this image, the operating room is set up to facilitate laparoscopic drainage of a giant left hepatic cyst

and the advantages are obvious, but there are also inherent drawbacks when using this technique, which can be grouped into three categories: (1) technology related, (2) procedure related, and (3) medicolegal.

Technology Related

These issues include signal latency, data transfer speed, system complexity, and compatibility. Signal latency refers to the time taken to transmit large digitalized data packages across the Internet. It becomes noticeable at >200 milliseconds and will appear as a lagged image on the receiving end of the transmission. It is affected by the data size, connection quality, and Internet bandwidth speed and can produce frustration and contribute to fatigue when using this technique. Most modern smartphones utilize MPEG4 codecs that can transmit high-definition audio-video signals at 2 megabytes per second, but they can still be limited by the quality and speed of the Internet connection. It is important to ensure system compatibility. In the Caribbean model, free proprietary software such as FaceTime (Apple Inc., Cupertino, CA, USA) was used to establish communication between supported devices.

Procedure Related

Eye contact is an important way to communicate nonverbal cues [35]. It is important to be aware of this; otherwise, there is the potential to transmit visual cues that may be confusing or misinterpreted [38]. It is important to appreciate the occurrence of appearance consciousness, the knowledge that one is on camera [35]; that adds a psychologic burden to the mentee to present an acceptable on-camera appearance, and this can potentially distract from concentrating on operative tasks.

Finally, for the mentor, there is the absence of stereopsis. Stereopsis is the act carried out by the brain exploiting parallax from differing views in each eye. It allows us to perceive depth and estimate distance. These are not possible in distance mentoring, as there is a single device camera recording the operating field and the surgeon, not allowing stereopsis. Therefore, the mentor is seeing the operative field in two dimensions, similar to the comparison between open and laparoscopic surgery.

Patient Safety/Medicolegal Issues

In any operative procedure, patient safety is paramount. There must be full disclosure to the patient, including the inherent drawbacks and incurred risks; this should also be documented as a part of the informed consent process. The most obvious concern is that the surgical mentor has no ability to physically intervene at the operation, whether it is to "take over the operation" or just to "demonstrate tips and tricks." It means that the mentor must be an experienced teacher with good communication skills. It is also important for the operating surgeon and mentor to build a bond of confidence in each other that will develop as the working relationship progresses. All contingency plans for potential complication during the operation must be discussed. Obviously, the operating surgeon should have sufficient skill to complete the operation and handle any complications that may arise. Predetermined thresholds that may trigger specific actions must be established prior to the operation, such as threshold for blood loss or for conversion to an open operation.

The mentor should know the operating surgeon sufficiently to determine whether they are within their capacity before embarking on telesurgery. This is clearly not something that will work with all surgeons and/or operations.

It is paramount that there is careful selection of straightforward cases following a planning meeting where all surgeons discuss detailed clinical information and plans for contingencies.

Telemedicine is a rapidly developing field, and so there are many potential medicolegal issues that will need to be addressed and are beyond the scope of this chapter.

Conclusions

Currently, there is rapid change occurring in healthcare delivery, with many new opportunities becoming available for surgical teaching. It is clear that simulation is becoming the new normal, but LMICs must adapt their teaching techniques to do so. There are also many other models used by LMICs that are valuable for other settings, including live animal models, cadaveric models, and innovative models such as distance mentoring techniques.

References

1. Naraynsingh V, Bahadursingh S, Maharaj R, Harnarayan P, Cawich SO. Surgery in the West Indies: a perspective from Trinidad. Current Med Res Prac. 2014;4:1126–9.
2. Schmidt CM, Turrini O, Parikh P, House MG, Zyromski NJ, Nakeeb A, Howard TJ, Pitt HA, Lillemoe KD. Effect of hospital volume, surgeon experience, and surgeon volume on patient outcomes after pancreaticoduodenectomy: a single-institution experience. Arch Surg. 2010;145:634–40. https://doi.org/10 1001/archsurg.2010.118.
3. Cawich SO, Kluger MD, Francis W, Deshpande RR, Mohammed F, Bonadie KO, Thomas DA, Pearce NW, Schrope BA. Review of minimally invasive pancreas surgery and opinion on its incorporation into low volume and resource poor centres. World J Gastrointest Surg. 2021;13(10):1122–35.
4. Cawich SO, Johnson PB, Shah S, Roberts P, Arthurs M, Murphy T, Bonadie KO, Crandon IW, Harding HE, Abu-Hilal M, Pearce NW. Overcoming obstacles to establish a multidisciplinary team approach to hepatobiliary diseases: a working model in a Caribbean setting. J Multidiscip Healthc. 2014;7:227–30.
5. Cawich SO, Pearce NW, Abu-Hilal MX. Surgical subspecialty training in HPB surgery for the Caribbean. West Ind Med J. 2012;61(S4):58.
6. Singletary SE. Mentoring surgeons for the 21st century. Ann Surg Oncol. 2005;12(11):848–60.
7. Cawich SO, Tennant IA, McGaw CD, Harding HE, Walters CA, Crandon IW. Infection control practice in the operating room: staff adherence to existing policies in a developing country. Perm J. 2013;17(3):114–8.
8. Cawich SO, Mahadeo C, Rambaran M, Amir S, Rajkumar S, Crandon IW, Naraynsingh V. Advancement of laparoscopic surgery in Guyana: a working model for developing countries. Adv Med Educ Pract. 2016;7:605–10.
9. Parker M, Ramdass MJ, Cawich SO, FaSiOen PR, Rosin D. A historical perspective on the introduction of laparoscopic basic surgical training in the Caribbean and factors that contribute to sustainability of such training. Int J Surg. 2019;72:6–12.
10. Wilson CB, Cawich SO, Simpson LK, Baker AJA. Starting a laparoscopic surgery service in a Rural Community Hospital in Jamaica: successes and challenges of the Percy Junor Hospital Experience. Caribbean Med J. 2014;76(1):8–11.
11. Montbrun SL, MacRae H. Simulation in surgical education. Clinic Colon Rectal Surg. 2012;25(3):156–65.
12. Reznick RK, MacRae H. Teaching surgical skills—changes in the wind. N Engl J Med. 2006;355(25):2664–9.
13. Oyama IA, Aaronoff MC, Burlingame JM. Obstetric anal sphincter injury repair workshop for residents. Hawaii Med J. 2009;68(6):133–5.
14. Kingston A, Abbott J, Lenart M, Vancaillie T. Hysteroscopic training: the butternut pumpkin model. J Am Assoc Gynecol Laparosc. 2004;11(2):256–61.
15. Lauscher JC, Ritz J-P, Stroux A, Buhr HJ, Gröne J. A new surgical trainer (BOPT) improves skill transfer for anastomotic techniques in gastrointestinal surgery into the operating room: a prospective randomized trial. World J Surg. 2010;34(9):2017–25.
16. Palter VN, Grantcharov T, Harvey A, Macrae HM. Ex vivo technical skills training transfers to the operating room and enhances cognitive learning: a randomized controlled trial. Ann Surg. 2011;253(5):886–9.
17. Grober ED, Hamstra SJ, Wanzel KR, et al. The educational impact of bench model fidelity on the acquisition of technical skill: the use of clinically relevant outcome measures. Ann Surg. 2004;240(2): 374–81.
18. Datta V, Bann S, Beard J, Mandalia M, Darzi A. Comparison of bench test evaluations of surgical

skill with live operating performance assessments. J Am Coll Surg. 2004;199(4):603–6.
19. Ramphal PS, Coore DN, Craven MP, Forbes NF, Newman SM, Coye AA, Little SG, Silvera BC. A high-fidelity tissue-based cardiac surgical simulator. Eur J Cardiothorac Surg. 2005;27(5):910–6.
20. Ramphal PS. High fidelity simulation as a cardiothoracic surgical training tool: early experience and future directions. Presented at the Royal Australasian College of surgeons, cardiac surgery training symposium and workshop, Melbourne, February 26, 2011.
21. Rosser JC, Rosser LE, Savalgi RS. Skill acquisition and assessment for laparoscopic surgery. Arch Surg. 1997;132(2):200–4.
22. Khine M, Leung E, Morran C, Muthukumarasamy G. Homemade laparoscopic simulators for surgical trainees. Clin Teach. 2011;8(2):118–21.
23. Kobayashi SA, Jamshidi R, O'Sullivan P, et al. Bringing the skills laboratory home: an affordable webcam-based personal trainer for developing laparoscopic skills. J Surg Educ. 2011;68(2):105–9.
24. Thomas WEG. Basic surgical skills courses: an educational success story. Ann R Coll Surg Engl. 1999;81(S):195–6.
25. Zheng B, Hur HC, Johnson S, Swanström LL. Validity of using fundamentals of laparoscopic surgery (FLS) program to assess laparoscopic competence for gynecologists. Surg Endosc. 2010;24(1):152–60.
26. Sutherland LM, Middleton PF, Anthony A, et al. Surgical simulation: a systematic review. Ann Surg. 2006;243(3):291–300.
27. Percie du Sert N, Ahluwalia A, Alam S, Avey MT, Baker M, Browne WJ, et al. Reporting animal research: explanation and elaboration for the ARRIVE guidelines 2.0. PLoS Biol. 2020;18(7):e3000411. https://doi.org/10.1371/journal.pbio.3000411.
28. Dunnington GL. A model for teaching sentinel lymph node mapping and excision and axillary lymph node dissection. J Am Coll Surg. 2003;197:119–21.
29. Supe A, Dalvi A, Prabhu R, et al. Cadaver as a model for laparoscopic training. Indian J Gastroenterol. 2005;24:111–3.
30. Gilbody J, Prasthofer AW, Ho K, Costa ML. The use and effectiveness of cadaveric workshops in higher surgical training: a systematic review. Ann R Coll Surg Engl. 2011;93(5):347–52.
31. Entezami P, Franxblau LE, Chung KC. Mentorship in surgical training: a systematic review. Hand. 2012;7:30–6.
32. Shiwani HM. Mentoring for surgical skills: a tool to share the workload. J Can Chir. 2007;50(6):432–3.
33. Cawich SO, Mahadeo C, Rambaran M, Amir S, Rajkumar S, Crandon IW, Naraynsingh V. Advancement of laparoscopic surgery in Guyana: a working model for developing countries. Adv Med Ed Prac. 2016;7:605–10.
34. Cawich SO, Mencia M, Thomas D, Spence R, Milne D, Naraynsingh V, Barrow S. Trauma surgery via distance mentoring: a model inspired by the 2020 pandemic. Trop Doctor. 2022;52(1):101–3.
35. Cawich SO, Griffith SP, Wilson C, FaSiOen PR, Burgess P, Thomas DA, Mencia M, Pearce NW, Kluger MD, Naraynsingh V. Distance mentoring in advanced minimally invasive surgery in the Caribbean: a model for low-resource environments. Curr Med Res Prac. 2021;11(3):125–32.
36. Gantenbein RE, Robinson BJ. Decoding CODECs. J Telemed Telecare. 2008;14(2):59–61.
37. Rosser JC, Fleming JP, Legare TB, Choi KM, Nakagiri J, Griffith E. Design and development of a novel distance learning telementoring system using off-the-shelf materials and software. Surg Technol Int. 2017;31:41–9.
38. Muhlbach L, Bocker M, Prussog A. Telepresence in videocommunications: a study on stereoscopy and individual eye contact. Hum Factors. 1995;37(2):290–305.

How to Teach Technical and Judgment Skills Effectively from Outside the Operating Room (Including Virtually)

17

Elijah W. Riddle and Carl E. Haisch

The supreme surgeon uses his supreme judgment to avoid situations that would test his supreme abilities.

– Unattributed aphorism (published in collection by Dr. Moshe Shein)

Abbreviations

ABS	American Board of Surgery
ACGME	Accreditation Council for Graduate Medical Education
BID	Briefing-Intraoperative Teaching-Debriefing
CME	Continuing medical education
COSECSA	College of Surgeons of East, Central and Southern Africa
FLS	Fundamentals of Laparoscopic Surgery
LMICs	Low- and middle-income countries
OPRS	Operative Performance Rating System
SCORE	Surgical Council on Resident Education
SiS	Step into Surgery

E. W. Riddle (✉)
College of Health Sciences, VinUniversity, Hanoi, Vietnam

Department of Surgery, Rutgers New Jersey Medical School, Newark, NJ, USA

C. E. Haisch
Division of Surgical Immunology and Transplantation, Faculty Development, Greenville, NC, USA
e-mail: haischc@ecu.edu

Introduction

The central goal of surgical training is progressive development of a trainee's surgical skill and judgment, culminating in the graduation of a safe, independent surgeon. Certainly, other competencies of an effective physician must be developed during training, including medical knowledge applicable to perioperative and multidisciplinary care, professionalism, interpersonal skills and communication, navigation of the healthcare system, personal and practice quality improvement, and lifelong learning. Yet the key ability differentiating a surgeon from other physicians is the ability to complete an operation safely and effectively.

Traditionally, trainees acquired surgical skills and judgment through an apprenticeship model with high volume of operative experience and pro-

M. A. Hardy, B. R. Hochman (eds.), *Global Surgery*, https://doi.org/10.1007/978-3-031-28127-3_17

gressive autonomy in the operating room. However, in the United States and Europe, various changes—including resident duty hour restrictions, increasing demands for operative throughput, and accreditation and legal restrictions on resident supervision—have cut into residents' volume and autonomy of experience during training. In response, many successful approaches to teaching technical skills and judgment outside the operating room have been developed. Visiting surgeons may find it challenging to teach in the operating room for many reasons in low- and middle-income countries (LMICs), including licensing limitations, legal restrictions, language barriers, and the imperative to avoid interrupting the practice of local surgeons or educational experience of local trainees. Beyond the individual surgeon, international partnering institutions may seek to maintain ongoing educational activities even when visiting surgeons are not physically present at the partner site. Thus, optimization of opportunities to teach technical skills and judgment outside of the operating room will be high yield for any training program.

In this chapter, we describe several practical approaches to teaching technical skills and judgment, with a focus on modalities that can be effectively employed outside the operating room. We will outline frameworks for the development of a surgeon that provide context for the teaching modalities and that may be useful for faculty development and intraoperative guidance. We will describe opportunities for integrating teaching of technical skills and judgment into existing structures and outline development of new teaching forums that may be in-person, virtual, or via independent study by trainees.

Needs Assessment and Faculty Development

A training needs assessment may be a valuable early step in determining the gaps and capabilities for teaching technical skills and judgment at a partner site. Chapter 6 describes a surgical needs assessment, which may overlap in many areas with a training needs assessment. In addition to understanding the local burden of surgical disease, the potential educator will want to investigate the local training program objectives, funding, teaching capacity, conference structure, and educational facilities. Published approaches to educational needs assessment in international settings include structured interviews [1], surveys of faculty and residents [2], and focus groups [3]. Close collaboration with a faculty partner from the host institution is critical to ensure proposed new educational activities or changes to existing activities will be appropriately received in the local cultural, regulatory, and training environment.

Ideally, teaching activities from visiting or remote partner surgeons would incorporate an element of "training the trainer," with a goal of developing local capacity to sustain the training long term. To that end, it can be helpful to deliver faculty development materials alongside the rollout of any new training activities. Local faculty or potential faculty surgeons should be invited to any training activities by a visiting surgeon and encouraged to participate or lead sessions once they have observed a few sessions. Visiting surgeons should encourage local surgeons to suggest changes or additions that may better adapt the activities to the local context. Trainees should also be empowered to take ownership of their educational activities. Explicitly outlining the objectives and format of any new training activity may improve local acceptance and provide critical background at sites without a long history of surgical training where the goals and objectives are not implicit. The ultimate faculty development strategy is to continuously train future surgical faculty from the current trainees by using teaching methods that the trainees buy into and want to carry forward for future generations. The bidirectional nature of communication between visiting or remote faculty and local faculty has been addressed in Chap. 4. This communication is crucial if training is to be successful.

Technical Skill

Most surgeons are familiar with the progressive acquisition of technical skills through consistent practice over time, both inside and outside of the

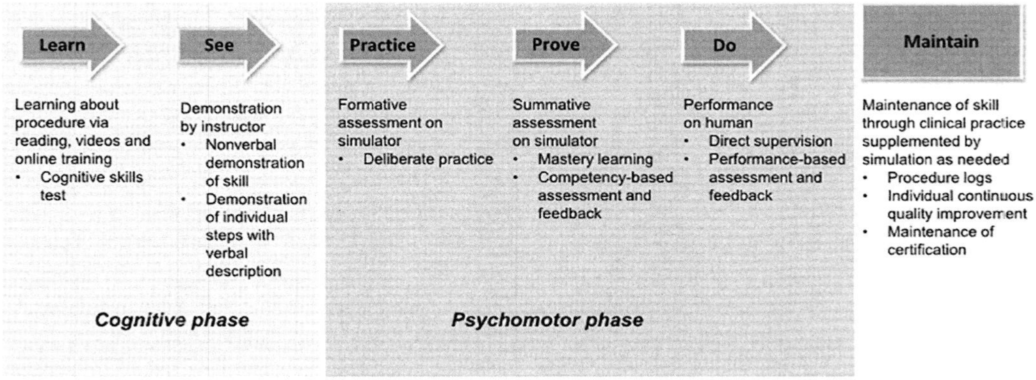

Fig. 17.1 A six-step process for skill development (from Sawyer, T, et al.—2015 Academic Medicine, 90(8))

operating room. Various groups have outlined this process using frameworks that may be helpful for directing educational efforts. Sawyer et al. described a six-step process for skill development, starting with a cognitive phase and then moving to a psychomotor phase before the final maintenance phase [4]. The six steps of their pedagogical framework include Learn, See, Practice, Prove, Do, and Maintain, as illustrated in the diagram below (Fig. 17.1). For simple skills and procedures, this entire six-step process may be accomplished in series. However, most surgical procedures are an accumulation of multiple technical skills that are acquired over time via repetitive cycling through the cognitive and psychomotor phases. The cognitive phase involves learning about the procedure through reading, didactic teaching, and multimedia modules, followed by seeing the procedure and hearing the steps described by an instructor. The psychomotor phase involves acquisition of manual skills through practice, ideally in a simulated setting first, and then performing the procedure in the clinical setting with supervision and feedback. It is important to note that many surgical procedures do not have high-fidelity simulation models, though core components such as knot tying, suturing, and laparoscopic maneuvering may be developed even with low-fidelity practice as described in Chap. 15. Overall, this framework shows clear opportunities for educational return outside the operating room in the cognitive phase, through curated reading or listening, lectures, surgical planning conferences, and video review, and in the psychomotor phase through simulation and feedback.

Surgical Judgment

Surgical judgment is considered an essential capability of a safe surgeon. However, surgical judgment cuts across many cognitive and perceptual domains, resulting in a wide range of definitions and a major challenge to develop and assess the attainment of this capability in trainees. Moulton and colleagues have proposed a framework for evaluating and teaching surgical judgment centered around the concept of "slowing-down moments" in surgery [5]. These are the critical moments of each operation when a surgeon must consciously or unconsciously slow down and make decisions. Slowing-down moments may be pre-planned, for patient-specific or procedure-related reasons, or situationally responsive when unexpected challenges arise. Within this framework, the authors note that three cognitive domains facilitate good judgment and distinguish levels of expertise—attention capacity, situational awareness, and automaticity. Targeting improvement in these domains outside the operating room can improve a trainee's judgment and facilitate improved opportunities for learning and exercising judgment in the operating room. For example, improving technical skills in simulation allows the trainee to devote less attention to these maneuvers in the operating room and provides more attention capacity for surveying the surgical field for cues to planned or unplanned slowing-down moments. Video review can augment actual operative experience in helping a resident discern operative anatomy, procedural steps, and cues for impending misadventures, improving their situational awareness and automaticity. Even more explicitly, faculty surgeons may push trainees to commit to planned slowing-down moments in preoperative surgical planning conferences or briefing discussions. They may assess and develop appropriate judgment in unplanned slowing-down moments by taking the trainees through boards-style scenarios or curated video review. This framework highlights the potential educational impact of a wide range of teaching activities.

Implementing Progressive Autonomy

Progressive autonomy, culminating in independence, is the foundation of surgical training. Introducing the concept of progressive autonomy may be challenging at sites without a history of surgical training, but shared mental frameworks and consistent language may help inculcate this critical idea. The "Zwisch Scale" has been proposed as a simple framework for categorizing trainee autonomy in a procedure or portion of a procedure [6]. Originally developed by Dr. Zwischenberger over years of use in his thoracic surgery fellowship, the scale includes four levels of faculty involvement that reflect progressive degrees of trainee autonomy—Show and Tell, Active Help, Passive Help, and Supervision Only (Table 17.1). The Zwisch scale provides a shared language and vision for development of trainee autonomy and can promote more granular goal setting and specific formative feedback for trainees.

Achieving progressive autonomy requires a concerted effort by faculty and trainees. Much of this effort occurs in the operating room, but key opportunities exist outside the operating room to set the stage for progressive autonomy, develop clear goals for development of technical skills and judgment, and coalesce the intraoperative teaching from each case to prepare the trainee to improve in the future. Roberts and colleagues have proposed the Briefing-Intraoperative Teaching-Debriefing (BID) model, which advocates optimizing three critical time points in the perioperative period [7].

During the preoperative briefing, the faculty surgeon should assess the experience and needs of the trainee and establish shared learning objectives for the case. The authors note that this interaction may occur even in the 2–3 minutes that are shared at the scrub sink or during the timeout prior to the start of the procedure. The learning objectives may include an explicit discussion of expected autonomy levels for all or part of the operation. The intraoperative teaching includes all guidance and instruction that the faculty surgeon provides the trainee during the case but ideally will be focused on the shared learning objectives developed in the preoperative briefing. If the circumstances of the case require the surgeon to take more control than anticipated, they may use the Zwisch scale to signal the transition to the trainee and to restore autonomy to the trainee when it is safe to do so. Finally, the post-operative debriefing includes a discussion of the learning objectives and signposted feedback regarding the key take-home points from the case. The debriefing may be accomplished during closing at the end of the case, if this portion is relatively automatic for surgeon and trainee, or may be reserved for a private setting after the case, particularly when more severe or potentially embarrassing feedback is necessary. This model emphasizes the critical educational importance of preoperative preparation and postoperative feedback, two time points where a visiting or remote partner surgeon may engage to teach technical skills and judgment.

Table 17.1 Zwisch proposed model for Teaching and Assessment in the operating room (level designated based on supervision provided for the majority of the key portions of the case)

Zwisch Stage of Supervision	Attending Behaviors	Resident Behaviors Commensurate with This Level of Supervision
Show and Tell	Does majority of key portions as the surgeon Narrates the case (i.e., thinks out loud) Demonstrates key concepts, anatomy, and skills	Opens and closes First assists and observes
Cues to advancement		When first assisting, begins to actively assist (i.e., anticipates surgeons' needs)
Smart Help	Shifts between surgeon and first assist roles When first assisting, leads the resident in surgeon role (active assist) Optimizes the field/exposure Demonstrates the plane or structure Coaches for specific technical skills Coaches regarding the next steps Continues to identify anatomical landmarks for the resident	The above, plus: Shifts between surgeon and first assist roles Knows all the component technical skills Demonstrates an increasing ability to perform different key parts of the operation with attending assistance
Cues to advancement		Can execute the majority steps of procedure with active assistance
Dumb Help	Assists and follows the lead of the resident (passive assist) Coaching regarding polishing and refinement of skills Follows the resident's lead throughout the operation	The above, plus: Can "set up" and accomplish the next step for the entire case with increasing efficiency Recognizes critical transition point issues
Cues to advancement		Can transition between all steps with passive assist from faculty
No Help	Largely provides no unsolicited advice Assisted by a junior resident or an attending acting like a junior resident Monitors progress and patient safety*	The above plus: Can work with inexperienced first assistant Can safely complete a case without faculty Can recover most errors Recognizes when to seek help/advice

*Implicit in all of these stages is the responsibility that the attending has to ensure optimal patient safety and outcomes. To that end, they may at any time correct behaviors that may lead to errors or, if an error has already occurred, to "take over" and correct the error.

Developmental Trajectories

Trainees should be progressively developing technical skill and judgment simultaneously over the course of their training. Faculty development and resident education using organized developmental frameworks can build a common vision among all shareholders in a training program. These frameworks guide assessment, feedback, and goals for deliberate practice. Huang et al. described five stages of development with associated narrative descriptions to enhance feedback and tracking of progress for trainees [8]. For a given procedure or as part of a global assessment, a resident may be designated as Technician, Anatomist, Anticipator, Strategist, or Executive (Table 17.2).

Similarly, the ACGME Surgery Milestones may be a useful tool for developing a shared understanding of an anticipated developmental trajectory and providing descriptive formative feedback (Fig. 17.2a, b, and c). The milestones for "Performance of Procedures," "Technical Skills," and "Anatomy" each include overlapping elements of technical skill and judgment. For the ACGME milestones, it is important to note that Level 4 is designated as the residency graduation target [9]. Programs hoping to assess resident progress in a more granular fashion may utilize the Operative Performance Rating System (OPRS) forms, initially developed at Southern Illinois University [10]. These forms include procedure-specific and global operative performance items. Completed forms can be utilized to provide specific formative feedback to trainees, and aggregate form data may provide useful information for understanding training gaps on a program level. The forms are currently a mandatory component of qualification by residents for American Board of Surgery (ABS) certification, and free links to the forms and a user's manual are available on the ABS website at the following link: https://www.absurgery.org/default.jsp?certgsqe_resassess.

Table 17.2 Descriptive assessment tool for intraoperative performance

Stage of development	Characteristics
Technician	Highly focused on individual technical skills; follows with some understanding of what is happening in a case.
Anatomist	Developing a "working knowledge" of anatomy and planes of dissection; focusing on translating conceptual knowledge of anatomy into purposeful action while operating
Anticipator	Actively participates and engages in the stepwise progression of a case; is able to anticipate next steps; focusing on learning operative principles including exposure and setup
Strategist	Begins to visualize cases as a richly textured "big picture"; applies planning and strategy to the case in a deliberate, goal-oriented fashion; exercises autonomy and agency; feels a strong sense of responsibility for the patient
Executive	Is confident and efficient; aligns cognitive and material resources for contingencies; can fluidly coordinate all aspects of an operation; anticipates potential complications

Patient Care 2: Intra-Operative Patient Care – Performance of Procedures				
Level 1	Level 2	Level 3	Level 4	Level 5
Demonstrates basic skills (e.g., knot tying, suturing)	Performs bedside procedures (e.g., central line, chest tube)	Performs common operations (e.g., hernia, cholecystectomy, appendectomy)	Performs complex operations (e.g., low anterior resection, paraesophegeal hernia, abdominal wall reconstruction)	Performs uncommon complex operations (e.g., Whipple, esophagectomy)
	Teaches basic skills to medical students and junior residents	Teaches bedside operations to junior residents	Teaches common operations to junior residents	Teaches complex operations to junior residents
Comments:				Not Yet Completed Level 1 Not Yet Rotated

Patient Care 3: Intra-Operative Patient Care – Technical Skills				
Level 1	Level 2	Level 3	Level 4	Level 5
Demonstrates limited tissue-handling skills	Inconsistently demonstrates careful tissue handling	Consistently demonstrates careful tissue handling	Adapts tissue handling based on tissue quality	Identifies innovative operative techniques, instrumentation, operative approaches, or significant improvement in established techniques
Requires prompting to identify appropriate tissue plane	Identifies appropriate plane but requires redirection to maintain dissection in the optimal tissue plane	Visualizes tissue plane, identifies and dissects relevant normal anatomy	Visualizes tissue plane, identifies and dissects relevant abnormal anatomy	
Moves forward in the operation only with active direction	Moves forward in the operation but requires prompting to complete the operation	Moves fluidly through the course of the operation and anticipates next steps	Adapts to unexpected findings and events during the course of the operation	
Comments:				Not Yet Completed Level 1 Not Yet Rotated

Medical Knowledge 2: Anatomy				
Level 1	Level 2	Level 3	Level 4	Level 5
Identifies normal anatomy (e.g., inguinal canal) during common operations	Identifies variations in anatomy (e.g., bile duct anatomic variations) during common operations	Identifies normal anatomy (e.g., gastric blood supply) during complex operations	Identifies variations in anatomy (e.g., replaced right hepatic artery) during complex operations	Develops simulation models for teaching anatomy and operations
Articulates the steps of common operations	Articulates the implications of varying anatomy on the steps of common operations	Articulates the steps of complex operations	Articulates the implications of varying anatomy on the steps of complex operations	Leads anatomy instruction for students and co-residents
Comments:				Not Yet Completed Level 1 Not Yet Rotated

Fig. 17.2 (**a**) ACGME surgery milestones - Performance of Procedures. (**b**) ACGME surgery milestones - Technical Skills. (**c**) ACGME surgery milestones - Anatomy

Conferences

Formal conferences are an important forum for teaching technical skills and judgment. Conference content will most commonly align with the cognitive phase of skill development, though it may be combined with psychomotor practice when paired with hands-on simulation activities. The necessity of teaching conferences as a component of surgical education is reflected in explicit requirements for training programs accredited by the ACGME. The ACGME requires "a course or a structured series of lectures that ensures education in the basic and clinical sciences fundamental to surgery…regular organized clinical teaching, such as grand rounds, ward rounds, and clinical conferences" and "a weekly morbidity and mortality or quality improvement conference." [11] Visiting or partnering surgeons may provide a significant boost to a training program by increasing the educational value of existing conferences and implementing new, education-focused conference formats.

At sites that have little or no prior experience with formal educational conferences, a first step may be identifying existing clinical conferences or routine meetings and adding a dedicated educational element. Many clinical facilities hold a daily sign-out meeting, morbidity and mortality or other quality conference, and surgical planning meetings. Below, we highlight ways that these conferences may add increased educational value as well as suggesting other conference formats that may be implemented toward the goal of teaching technical skills and judgment outside the operating room.

Morning Report

Many institutions hold a daily morning meeting to sign out overnight admissions and organize the clinical service for the day. Depending on the size of the institution and organization of the surgery department(s), this meeting may include all surgeons at the institution or only those divisions or surgeons who consistently receive acute overnight admissions. This type of conference has been shown to have a major educational potential [12], which can be optimized in several ways:

- Provide a consistent structure to the conference, and template the presentations.
- Select a dedicated "teaching case" at each meeting.
- Protect the educational time for trainees, and strongly recommend or require trainee and faculty attendance.
- Encourage and model Socratic questioning.
- Ensure resources are available to review and focus teaching around clinical data (i.e., ability to review radiology, clinical photos, laboratory values, etc.).
- When possible, review relevant literature, and provide follow-up on cases presented at prior conferences.

Morbidity and Mortality

Morbidity and mortality (M&M) conference is an essential forum for peer review, individual and institutional accountability, quality improvement, professional identity development, and education. M&M conferences vary in their specific structure across institutions. However, most M&M conferences include presentations by trainees with an emphasis on trainee education and surgical quality improvement. Generally, a key focus of the conference is discussion of changes in technique, judgment, or systems-based factors that could have averted an adverse outcome or that could prevent future adverse outcomes. The M&M conference is particularly well-suited for discussions of surgical judgment, especially when the conference is well attended by faculty who engage in frank discussions of the presented complications and deaths. Factors that have been proposed to improve the educational value of morbidity and mortality conferences include [13–15]:

- Consistent attendance by trainees and faculty surgeons.
- Designated conference moderator.
- Predetermined teaching point(s) for each case.
- Templated presentation format.

– Listing of complications using a defined system like Clavien-Dindo or National Surgical Quality Improvement Project (NSQIP).

Case Conference/Public Mock Oral Examination

Case conferences provide an opportunity to discuss surgical technique and judgment in cases that do not come under review at M&M. Programs may choose to emphasize "bread and butter" cases, rare diseases, interesting techniques, or a combination of these and more. Many programs that hold this type of conference will review one or two cases in a 1-hour conference. Frequently, residents prepare and present the cases, though faculty may also present. Ideally, most cases are pulled from clinical practice at the local site. A visiting surgeon may choose to present a case from their home institution to highlight surgical pathology or treatments that are rare or rarely implemented at the local site. The educational value of these conferences depends on the participation of experienced surgical faculty members to moderate the discussion and ensure teaching points are accurate. In many settings, the case will be worked through in an extended "boards style" questioning, often starting with the most junior learners for the basics of the history and physical exam and working up to senior trainees to discuss the intraoperative decision-making. The questioning may be formalized as a public mock oral examination. Harbor-UCLA Medical Center reported implementation of a series of six public mock oral board examinations each year, administered by the program director to senior residents in front of an audience of faculty, junior residents, and students. Examinees and the audience reported high satisfaction with the conference format, and the program reported improved pass rates on the oral board exams [16].

Surgical Planning Conference

Surgical indications and planning conferences provide a valuable opportunity to assess and develop trainees' judgment. Depending on the local context and surgical volume, these conferences may be held as often as daily, typically in the evening to review the next day's cases, or as infrequently as weekly or biweekly to review particularly complex cases. This conference format serves an administrative purpose as well, providing an opportunity to organize personnel and resources for scheduled cases. Typically, trainees prepare the case presentations, often using a template to maintain efficiency and ensure all critical information is reviewed. As noted in the paper by St. Martin, Moulton, and colleagues [5], a surgical planning conference is an ideal setting for faculty to probe the trainees' understanding of anticipated slowing-down moments. The preoperative discussion then scaffolds an intraoperative focus on key points in surgical judgment for that procedure.

Grand Rounds/Didactic Conference

Grand rounds and didactic conferences constitute the core of formal education for most surgical residency programs. These conferences may include discussions of technique and judgment among other important topics relating to the basic sciences and clinical practice of surgery. Often these conferences are conducted in a formal lecture format. While the lecture may be informative, it is unlikely to facilitate assessment or in-depth discussion of trainees' judgment. However, these conferences do provide an opportunity for trainees to encounter expert-level judgment and descriptions of expert technique. This is critical for the cognitive phase of procedural training and, especially for more senior trainees, may prompt development of more advanced learning objectives for technique and judgment in the operating room. Practically, grand rounds and didactic lectures are among the easiest formats to share virtually between remote partner sites and may be low-hanging fruit for educational collaboration.

Each conference format can clearly emphasize judgment and thought processes, which are crucial to surgical care. Traditionally, these conferences have been held in person. However, the travel and in-person gathering restrictions imposed by the COVID-19 pandemic forced most groups, from individual surgical training programs to international societies, into virtual formats. After an adjustment period, the virtual conferences proved efficacious in maintaining their clinical and educational functions. In many cases, groups saw increased attendance and reached attendees at more sites using the virtual format than the previous in-person format. The virtual format provided the added benefit of the option of recording the sessions for asynchronous viewing. As the world reaches a new normal, many programs are transitioning to hybrid in-person and virtual conferences to capture the benefits of each. The technology and experience of virtual conferencing that arose from the pandemic can be applied moving forward to facilitate educational opportunities between remote partners and for sites that previously had no access to these valuable conferences.

Simulation

Simulation presents a valuable opportunity for teaching technical skills and, in some cases, judgment, outside the operating room. Chapter 15 describes establishing simulation events. Ongoing opportunities to practice in a simulated setting are important for surgical trainees. Ideally, this is *deliberate practice*, a concept defined by Ericsson and colleagues that requires motivated learners, clear objectives, focused and repetitive practice, objective training goals, and specific feedback [17]. A visiting or remote partner surgeon may help guide the development of local simulation opportunities and actively teach trainees in person or virtually.

Specific simulation needs and opportunities may vary significantly between groups of trainees and clinical sites. Technical skills simulation ranges from basic knot tying and suturing to virtual reality endovascular and robotic procedures. The educational needs assessment should inform efforts in simulation. A valuable resource to guide the development of simulation capacity and augment simulation teaching with multimedia is the American College of Surgeons/Association for Program Directors in Surgery (ACS/APDS) Surgery Resident Skills Curriculum. This curriculum is available online (https://www.facs.org/for-medical-professionals/education/programs/acs-apds-surgery-resident-skills-curriculum/) at no cost to faculty and residents, though it is necessary to register for the program. The curriculum is divided into three phases. Phase 1 includes 16 modules focused on basic surgical skills. Phase 2 includes 15 modules focused on more advanced surgical skills. Phase 3 includes ten modules focused on teamwork and communication. Each module includes a faculty guide to setting up the simulation activity, and many modules include multimedia photo and video guides that trainees can reference to guide their ongoing practice.

Virtual engagement in simulation activities has been shown to be successful. Remote videoconference instruction has been shown to effectively augment trainees' practicing of basic knot-tying skills [18]. A collaboration between institutions in Canada and Botswana described "telesimulation" for intraosseus line insertion and laparoscopic skills [19, 20]. The telesimulation setup involved preparing a room at each location with the simulation model and two cameras attached to a laptop. One camera at each site was trained on the simulation model, while the other camera showed the person using the model. The two video feeds were transmitted to two screens in each location along with an audio feed via Skype, allowing the trainee and instructor to see and hear each other and view the movements on the simulation model in real time. In the laparoscopic skills telesimulation trial, 16 participants in Botswana were provided with a Fundamentals of Laparoscopic Surgery (FLS) DVD and access to a standard FLS simulator. All participants were instructed to practice the FLS skills for 2 hours per week. In addition, half the participants received 15 minutes per week of telesimulation mentoring from an instructor in Canada. At the conclusion of the 8-week trial, two surgeons from Canada traveled to Botswana to administer official FLS certification skills exams to participants. The participants in the telesimulation group had higher scores in every FLS task compared to the self-practice group, and eight of eight surgeons in the telesimulation group earned overall passing FLS skills scores, compared to only three of eight in the self-practice group. This setup may be adapted for simulation across a wide range of technical skills.

Notably, equipment for simulation, especially commercially available items, may be quite expensive. Basic technical skills, such as knot tying and suturing, can be taught with relatively little equipment. Expired suture or other consumables that can no longer be used for patients should be reserved for simulation. Expensive synthetic skin substitutes are not necessary to practice suturing—pig skin, chicken skin, or banana peels will suffice, and at least one of these is available in most locales. Even for laparoscopy, a wide range of low-cost simulators have been described for practicing basic skills [21]. For sites with a challenge to allocate even a few basic instruments for technical skills simulation, exploring opportunities at national or regional simulation centers may be productive. Finally, partner sites with well-developed simulation centers and curriculum may develop a focused simulation experience as part of any trainee exchange trips with partner programs.

Video-Based Teaching

Video-based teaching has been successfully implemented in surgical training across a wide range of specialties and settings [22]. Advances in video technology and proliferation of endoscopic procedures have made video-based teaching increasingly available and valuable in surgical training. Cameras may be comfortably head-mounted, incorporated in the surgical lights, or mounted in the operating room. Videos from cameras or endoscopes may be recorded for future viewing or live-streamed. These video resources provide an excellent opportunity for teaching skills and judgment outside the operating room.

Live-streaming of video allows a surgeon to replicate a "show and tell" approach to intraoperative teaching with a remote audience. When technical capabilities and time zones allow, this may be a very effective method of teaching intraoperative judgment and demonstrating technical skills. Live-streaming may especially be useful to teach cases that are rare at a partner site or when local teaching faculty is limited. Another promising technology is telementoring, where a remote surgeon views a live-streamed operation and provides commentary and direction in real time. Initially, this approach was primarily utilized in laparoscopic surgery with various platforms that allowed the remote surgeon to provide guidance and even make marks on the screen at the operative site [23]. More recently, telementoring systems have been developed that enable remote guidance and annotation on the surgical field in open operations via a tablet suspended over the operation [24] or through an augmented-reality headset that captures the operating surgeon's view and projects markings onto smart glasses [25]. The technical requirements and costs of these systems are variable, and programs would need to make an independent determination of their utility at a given site. Additionally, telementoring may introduce complicated questions about legal and ethical responsibility depending on the relative capabilities of the local and remote surgeons. However, the technology is promising as part of a training system and in settings where local surgeons may have no feasible options to transfer a patient.

Increasingly, video-based resources are being used as routine tools for education and preoperative preparation by trainees and surgeons in practice. A 2017 study found that 98.6% of respondents from a group of surgical faculty and trainees had used video to prepare for surgery [26]. A significantly higher percentage of trainees reported using videos as their preferred method of case preparation and used videos significantly more often compared to surgeons in practice. Trainees were more likely to use YouTube, SCORE, and WebSurg videos, while surgeons in practice were more likely to use videos from society webpages or commercially available videos. Finally, younger surgeons most valued didactic illustrations and narration in a video, while older surgeons most valued technical skill. Though this was a single-site study, it does raise important considerations for video-based teaching. Trainees are likely to use videos for case preparation and likely to seek videos from open access sites. Programs interested in optimizing video-based teaching may consider curating recommended videos or producing their own videos for resident review to ensure content is consistent with local technique, equipment, and standard of care.

In the postoperative setting, video-based coaching has proven beneficial for surgical trainees and for surgeons in practice [27]. This approach can improve technical skills and judgment as a complimentary tool for surgical training, surgical performance, and quality improvement. Surgical coaching has specifically been highlighted as a potentially valuable tool for continuous performance improvement and collaboration with surgeons in LMICs, helping to build surgical capacity and quality [28]. Hu and colleagues described a video-based coaching intervention for surgical trainees [29]. In their study, senior residents (post-graduate year 4 or 5) were video-recorded performing an open operation with their faculty supervisor. The video captured the operative field and operating room. The resident and faculty coach had a subsequent coaching session utilizing the video between 0 and 43 days after the procedure. The coaches received an instructional pamphlet on "Coaching Residents," but no other specific guidance was provided for the coaching session. The coaching sessions were audio-recorded, and researchers compared teaching in the operating room to teaching in the coaching session. Faculty surgeons made more teaching points per time in the coaching session than in the operating room. Teaching in the coaching sessions was also found to be more resident-centered, more focused on reflection and critical thinking by the resident, and more in-depth. Finally, the content of the coaching session complemented the intraoperative teaching, with significantly more focus on intraoperative decision-making and failure to progress in the coaching session and significantly more focus on progress through the case and anatomy in the operating room.

The Wisconsin Surgical Coaching Program was developed as a statewide initiative for surgeons in practice [30]. This program paired participating surgeons with peer-nominated surgeons who received special training in coaching techniques. Coaches were trained in a 4-hour in-person session supplemented with a coaching manual and instructional videos. Coaching sessions were 1 hour in length and included review of a video-recorded operation by the coachee. The activities of the session included goal setting, collaborative video analysis, feedback, and action planning, with a focus on technical, cognitive, interpersonal, and stress management skills. Coaches and coachees were satisfied with their participation, though no long-term outcome data has been collected to date.

Video is a valuable resource with many possible applications in surgical training. The specific uses of video at a given site will depend on local needs, technological capacity, and ethical or legal limitations on use of intraoperative video. Where feasible, video-based teaching can overcome barriers of time and distance to facilitate effective teaching in technical skills and operative judgment.

Independent Study

Independent study is a necessary component of surgical training. The effectiveness of most training opportunities, whether in the operating room, simulation, or conferences, relies on adequate preparation by the trainee. Local, visiting, and remote faculty may facilitate effective independent study by thoughtfully recommending resources to trainees and mentoring trainees as they develop lifelong learning skills. The lifelong learning strategies are critically important, as they will enable program graduates to efficiently and effectively assimilate new knowledge and techniques that will arise throughout their careers. In fact, one of the 18 ACGME Surgery Milestones, "Reflective Practice and Commitment to Personal

Growth," focuses on the developing surgeon's ability to design and implement an individual learning plan.

Ideally, recommended independent study materials will reference current evidence and technology but should also be relevant in the local context. The surgical and educational needs assessment should inform the provision and development of educational resources. In any setting, a library of at least a few current editions of surgical textbooks provides an excellent resource for trainees to develop foundational knowledge of surgical science, management, and technique. At sites with reliable Internet access and sufficient technology (computers, tablets, smartphones), a wide range of subscription and open-access educational materials are available.

The Surgical Council on Resident Education (SCORE) online portal, available at surgicalcore.org, includes hundreds of modules with learning objectives, detailed content, linked textbook and video references, and self-assessment via discussion questions and multiple-choice quizzes. The content covers a wide range of topics related to general surgery and fellowship-level content for some subspecialties, including pediatric surgery, surgical critical care, surgical oncology, and vascular surgery. Notably, SCORE merged with the American Board of Surgery in 2019, and the SCORE curriculum is now aligned with the content of the American Board of Surgery Qualifying Exam. Access to the SCORE program is available through a yearly subscription. Programs pay a $500 (USD) annual license fee and $175 for each trainee as of 2022. The annual program license fee includes accounts for the program director, program coordinator, and five faculty or administrative personnel. The program account includes the ability to create and manage assignments for trainees to tailor the curriculum to local program needs. The SCORE curriculum outlines and proposed weekly topic schedule for "This Week in Score" are available at https://surgicalcore.org/public/curriculum. The curriculum outlines and weekly topic schedule may be a valuable reference for faculty and trainees even at programs that cannot or choose not to subscribe to the full content.

Another commercial program is Decker Surgery, which offers continuously updated online curricular materials for surgery residents through the Surgery Weekly Curriculum™, in-training and board exam preparation materials, continuing medical education (CME) and maintenance of certification (MOC) opportunities, and a teaching slide library. Decker also offers a program designed for medical students called *Step into Surgery* (SiS). Decker's programs are available through individual, program, or institutional subscriptions at varying costs. More information is available at https://www.deckerip.com/products/surgery/.

The College of Surgeons of East, Central and Southern Africa (COSECSA) has developed an online learning platform for its members. School for Surgeons (www.schoolforsurgeons.net) is available to all COSECSA trainees, members, and fellows. Available content includes mandatory case studies and Surgery in Africa Journal Club modules for candidates. Through a collaboration with the Royal College of Surgeons in Ireland, the website links to several surgical and medical journals and textbooks. The website also has a focused section for surgical trainers with faculty development resources. Finally, the website hosts the Surgical Foundations in Basic Science curriculum, which was successfully introduced in January 2020 [31]. The curriculum is designed for independent study by trainees as preparation for flipped-classroom tutorial sessions with surgical faculty.

Increasingly, surgical societies are providing free online educational materials. Trainees can be directed to these materials for self-study if they have sufficient technological resources. Most North American societies publish their online materials in English, and visiting faculty must consider the relevance of materials that are not in the primary language of local trainees and faculty. Examples of free, online surgical society resources include:

- The Society of American Gastrointestinal and Endoscopic Surgeons (SAGES) has published the didactic content for their Fundamentals of Laparoscopic Surgery™ (FLS), Fundamentals of Endoscopic Surgery™ (FES), Fundamental Use of Surgical Energy™ (FUSE), and Safe Cholecystectomy programs online at fesdidactic.org. These programs are available to anyone who registers with a valid email address and are published in English, French, Spanish, and Chinese.

– The American Society of Colon and Rectal Surgeons (ASCRS) has several resources available through its website. For trainees, they have developed the ASCRS Trainee Boot Camp video series (https://fascrs.org/healthcare-providers/for-residents/colorectal-surgery-boot-camp) covering basic topics in colorectal surgical practice. Their Core Subject Update covers 24 core subjects in a rotating 4-year cycle. The recorded presentations by selected experts are available for viewing at https://fascrs.org/healthcare-providers/education/core-subjects.

Podcasts

Podcasts are an increasingly popular medium of entertainment and education [32]. Podcasts are audio-only recordings, typically available for free, and often listened to on mobile devices, though they are available on laptop and desktop computers as well. Access requires a compatible device and at least intermittent Internet access—most podcast episodes are available for download and thus do not require continuous Internet access.

The first surgery-focused podcast to gain popularity was *Behind the Knife* (behindtheknife.org), created in 2015 by a group of residents at Madigan Army Medical Center. *Behind the Knife* now has almost 500 episodes with a wide range of topics and formats including focused review of surgical diseases, interviews with leaders in their field, journal clubs and literature updates, and preparation for in-training and board exams. In 2018, an independent, bimonthly podcast focused on vascular surgery was developed. That podcast, *Audible Bleeding*, remains active and is supported by the Society for Vascular Surgery. More recently, many surgical societies have developed and published their own podcasts including the Society for Surgery of the Alimentary Tract (*SSAT Soundbites*), Society of American Gastrointestinal and Endoscopic Surgeons (*SAGES Stories*), Society of Surgical Oncology (*SurgOnc Today* & *Speaking of SurgOnc*), Society of Thoracic Surgeons (*Surgical Hot Topics*), and the Americas Hepato-Pancreato-Biliary Association (*The AHPBA Podcast* and *The AHPBA Podcast—Latin America*).

Podcasts can be a valuable tool for independent study by individual trainees or assigned to a group of residents for asynchronous education. Ideally, podcast recommendations are curated by a surgical faculty to optimize impact. The recommender should review the materials and consult the results of the local educational needs assessment or work collaboratively with local faculty and trainees to ensure the podcasts are contextually relevant and level appropriate for the assigned audience. Podcasts may be especially useful for education in surgical judgment, as many available episodes include experts discussing their approach to common and challenging surgical problems.

Conclusion

Teaching technical skill and judgment is the core of surgical training. Certainly, skill and judgment are primarily attained through experience in the operating room. Yet valuable opportunities exist to teach skills and judgment outside the operating room, augmenting and accelerating the trainee's progress toward independence. Visiting surgeons and remote partners may have limited opportunities to teach trainees in the operating room for a variety of reasons. However, these surgeons may still contribute significantly to the training of surgeons at partner sites. Conferences, simulation, video-based teaching, and coaching all provide rich opportunities for surgeons to supercharge the cognitive phase of procedural training and provide feedback that is necessary for effective deliberate practice in the psychomotor phase.

Advances in video technology, increasing use of videoconferencing, and improving Internet access make all these approaches feasible even from a vast distance. Additionally, trainees may be directed to reliable and ever-expanding sources of information for independent study, many of which are free and available to anyone with Internet access. Today's global surgeon should consider education and local capacity building as an essential part of their mission. Thankfully, resources and training methods are available to adapt training to a wide range of contexts, allowing global surgeons to train the next generation of safe, independent surgeons.

References

1. Peluso M, et al. Building health system capacity through medical education: a targeted needs assessment to guide development of a structured internal medicine curriculum for interns in Botswana. Ann Glob Health. 2018;84(1):151–9.
2. Cook M, et al. A consortium approach to surgical education in a developing country: educational needs assessment. JAMA Surg. 2015;150(100):1074–8.
3. Mocumbi AO, et al. Innovative strategies for transforming internal medicine residency training in resource-limited settings: the Mozambique experience. Acad Med. 2014;89(8 Suppl):S78–82.
4. Sawyer T, et al. Learn, see, practice, prove, do, maintain: an evidence-based pedagogical framework for procedural skill training in medicine. Acad Med. 2015;90(8):1025–33.
5. St-Martin L, et al. Teaching the slowing-down moments of operative judgment. Surg Clin N Am. 2012;92:125–35.
6. DaRosa DA, et al. A theory-based model for teaching and assessing residents in the operating room. J Surg Educ. 2013;70(1):24–30.
7. Roberts NK, et al. The briefing, intraoperative teaching, debriefing model for teaching in the operating room. J Am Coll Surg. 2009;208(2):299–303.
8. Huang E, et al. From novice to master surgeon: improving feedback with a descriptive approach to intraoperative assessment. Am J Surg. 2016;212(1):180–7.
9. Brasel K, et al. Surgical milestones work group; 2019. Surgery milestones, version 2. ©2019 accreditation Council for Graduate Medical Education (ACGME). Available online: https://www.acgme.org/globalassets/pdfs/milestones/surgerymilestones.pdf. Accessed 12 June 2022.
10. A User's Manual for the Operative Performance Rating System (OPRS). May 2012. Available online: https://www.absurgery.org/xfer/assessment/oprs_user_manual.pdf. Accessed 12 June 2022.
11. ACGME Program Requirements for Graduate Medical Education in General Surgery, effective July 1, 2020. Available online: https://www.acgme.org/globalassets/pfassets/programrequirements/440_generalsurgery_2021.pdf
12. Sanfey H, et al. Morning report: combining education with patient handover. Surgeon. 2008;6(2):94–100.
13. Abdelsattar JM, et al. Enhancing the educational value and faculty attendance of a morbidity and mortality conference. J Surg Educ. 2020;77(4):905–10.
14. Endicott KM, et al. Use of structured presentation formatting and NSQIP guidelines improves quality of surgical morbidity and mortality conference. J Surg Res. 2019;233:118–23.
15. De Vos MS, et al. Toward best practices for surgical morbidity and mortality conferences: a mixed methods study. J Surg Educ. 2018;75(1):33–42.
16. Aboulian A, et al. The public mock oral: a useful tool for examinees and the audience in preparation for the American Board of Surgery Certifying Examination. J Surg Educ. 2010;67(1):33–6.
17. Ericsson KA. Acquisition and maintenance of medical expertise: a perspective from the expert-performance approach with deliberate practice. Acad Med. 2015;90(11):1471–86.
18. Autry AM, et al. Teaching surgical skills using video internet communication in a resource-limited setting. Obst Gyn. 2013;122(1):127–31.
19. Mikrogianakis A, et al. Telesimulation: an innovative and effective tool for teaching novel intraosseous insertion techniques in developing countries. Acad Emerg Med. 2011;18(4):420–7.
20. Okrainec A, Henao O, Azzie G. Telesimulation: an effective method for teaching the fundamentals of laparoscopic surgery in resource-restricted countries. Surg Endosc. 2010;24:417–22.
21. Li MM, George J. A systematic review of low-cost laparoscopic simulators. Surg Endosc. 2017;31:38–48.
22. Ahmet A, et al. Is video-based education an effective method in surgical education? A systematic review. J Surg Edu. 2018;75(5):1150–8.
23. Antoniou SA, et al. A comprehensive review of telementoring applications in laparoscopic general surgery. Surg Endosc. 2012;26:2111–6.
24. Andersen D, et al. An augmented reality-based approach for surgical telementoring in austere environments. Mil Med. 2017;182(S1):310–5.
25. Rojas-Munoz E, et al. Surgical telementoring without encumbrance: a comparative study of see-through augmented reality-based approaches. Ann Surg. 2019;270(2):384–9.
26. Mota P, et al. Video-based surgical learning: improving trainee education and preparation for surgery. J Surg Educ. 2017;75(3):828–35.
27. Keller DS, et al. Video-based coaching: current status and role in surgical practice (part 1) from the Society for Surgery of the Alimentary Tract, Health Care

Quality and Outcomes Committee. J Gastroint Surg. 2021;25:2439.
28. El-Gabri D, et al. Surgical coaching for advancement of global surgical skills and capacity: a systematic review. J Surg Res. 2020;246:499–505.
29. Hu YY, et al. Complementing operating room teaching with video-based coaching. JAMA Surg. 2017;152(4):318–25.
30. Greenberg CC, et al. A statewide surgical coaching program provides opportunity for continuous professional development. Ann Surg. 2018;267(5):868–73.
31. Parker AS, et al. An online, modular curriculum enhances surgical education and improves learning outcomes in East, Central, and Southern Africa: a mixed-methods study. Ann Surg Open. 2022;3(1):e140.
32. Carpenter EL, et al. Surgical society podcasts: a novel way to engage and educate the community. J Surg Educ. 2022;79(3):565–7.

How to Teach Teamwork and Leadership Skills Effectively from Outside the Operating Room (Including Virtually)

18

Emad H. Asham, Korin E. Leffler, and Carl E. Haisch

When restraint and courtesy are added to strength, the latter becomes irresistible.

– Mahatma Gandhi

Abbreviations

LMICs	Low- and middle-income countries
M&M	Morbidity and mortality
PAACS	Pan-African Academy of Christian Surgeons

Introduction

First, we must define what a leader is. A leader is a person who has specific well-defined goals and a plan to lead others toward such goals. The leader is simultaneously committed to identifying, managing, and allocating resources to achieve the objective.

According to Bass's theory of leadership, there are three basic mechanisms that turn a person into a leader:

1. *The great event or great man theory*, when leaders are born under the pressure of a critical situation and rise to the occasion to lead.
2. *Trait theory*, for people who have natural abilities that qualify them to lead.
3. *Transformational or process leadership theory*, when an individual chooses to become a leader through learning skills.

The latter theory is the most accepted theory today [1]. In the past, many leaders used a transactional management style, which rewarded and punished certain behaviors. In contrast, transformational leadership theory emphasizes vision, empowerment, and support to inspire followers toward action and growth.

Real leaders have a clear vision of objectives and the ability to inspire and enable others to attain them. Leadership is essential in life—whenever two or three persons get together, one person will become the leader, within a family,

E. H. Asham (✉)
Department of Surgery, Methodist Hospital at Texas Medical Center, Houston, TX, USA
e-mail: ehasham@houstonmethodist.org

K. E. Leffler
Department of Pharmacology and Toxicology, Brody School of Medicine, Department of Advanced Nursing Practice and Education, College of Nursing, Pharmacology Liaison, School of Dental Medicine, East Carolina University, Greenville, NC, USA
e-mail: Lefflerk19@ecu.edu

C. E. Haisch
Division of Surgical Immunology and Transplantation, Faculty Development, Brody School of Medicine, East Carolina University, Greenville, NC, USA
e-mail: haischc@ecu.edu

M. A. Hardy, B. R. Hochman (eds.), *Global Surgery*, https://doi.org/10.1007/978-3-031-28127-3_18

small community, department of surgery, or an organization.

Surgeons assume leadership in three principle domains: first, as clinicians taking care of patients in the clinical arena; second, leading a surgical team in the operating room; and third, as managers in the administrative duties of day-to-day surgical practice. These administrative responsibilities can be as varied as heading a research laboratory, a residency program director, or a chief of a division within the department. With more interest in global surgery, leaders must be able to successfully intersect with surgeons from other areas of the globe and within varying environments and cultures. This interaction may occur at a national meeting with international guests, a visiting professorship, or an invited lecturer. The leader may also be asked to help develop new programs and infrastructure, to operate, and to train and send trainees to an international site for collaborative growth and experience in low- and middle-income countries (LMICs).

Surgical Leaders Are Visionaries

A surgical leader must have a clear vision of the goals of his department, must prioritize these goals, and have a plan to achieve them. Without a clear vision, the team will go astray. Good leaders know where they stand and where they are heading. They have the ability to inspire their staff to a common goal.

The young German surgeon Kurt Semm at the University of Kiel was an enthusiast about laparoscopy. When he performed the first laparoscopic appendectomy in September 1980 in the department of gynecology, he faced fierce opposition. This did not deter him from his vision for laparoscopic surgery, and he took the first steps toward his goal and changed the course of traditional surgery. Now laparoscopy is a well-established approach in any surgical practice [2].

If surgical leaders are to develop a vision and goals for their department, they must be scholars who keep abreast of new disease interventions and rapidly developing new technologies.

A good leader discerns the difference between knowledge and wisdom. As Isaac Asimov wrote: "The saddest aspect of life right now is that science gathers knowledge faster than society gathers wisdom" [3]. Knowledge is gathered by reading books and journals, listening to lectures, and attending conferences and symposia. Wisdom, on the other hand, is gleaned from years of experience; lifetime learning, not only about science but also about people; and most importantly, common sense. Wisdom entails a deep understanding of the zeitgeist and emotional intelligence. For example, the use of artificial intelligence in medicine needs to be understood; however, the leader must learn not only to know how to use this technology but to learn its strength, hazards, and weaknesses. The technology itself cannot provide the wisdom and intuition to make the critical decisions for its use in taking care of patients.

Leader Surgeons Are Humble

To aspire to leadership is an honorable ambition. The root of ambition is from the Latin word *ambitio*, which means to go around, to campaign for promotion. Leadership offers social visibility, peer recognition, popularity, and exercise of authority over others. Nevertheless, ambition must be tempered by humility; otherwise, it can lead to arrogance on the part of the leader and destruction of the team for which the leader is responsible. As Lord Acton said, "power tends to corrupt and absolute power corrupts absolutely."

Humility and leadership may appear to be an oxymoron. The traditional surgical hierarchical autocratic leadership model has been slowly phasing out recently. Humility of the chief executive officers (CEO) has been shown to contribute to the success of the enterprise and to improve outcomes. In an article in Forbes, Nicole Heimann highlighted how future CEOs are shifting from the heroic model to being humble [4]. Leadership should be viewed as an opportunity to serve rather than to seize power. This is clearly manifested in the traditional calling of surgical subdivisions a "service."

Surgeons should be humbled on regular basis by diseases that they cannot conquer, cancers that spread beyond the scalpel's reach, and terminal illnesses that cannot be cured. Indeed, human mortality is before the eyes of every surgeon's day and thus needs to keep their views of themselves in perspective. True leaders set their egos and emotions aside to be as objective as possible in all the important decisions they are obliged to make daily. The late British scholar and author C.S. Lewis wrote: "Humility is not thinking less of yourself but thinking of yourself less" [5]. To translate this to the daily life of a surgical leader, he/she must be approachable, courteous, and respectful to his staff. On a practical note, while on a short-term trip to an LMIC, one of the authors found that the local surgeons had scrubs that were of much lesser quality and ill-fitting compared to the pressed, clean, breathable cotton ones he takes and uses on every trip. He chose to wear the local ill-fitting scrubs to identify with the local staff. On the last day, he donated the scrubs he brought to allow the staff to explore if the scrubs could be produced locally.

Surgeon Leaders Are Good Managers

Not all managers are leaders, but all leaders are managers. Leader surgeons must manage their human resources including students, residents, new faculty, as well as existing faculty. They must also manage material resources such as office space, strategic planning, budgets, expansion, and adoption of new technologies. Surgical leaders have pecuniary responsibilities that need to intersect well with hospital administration concerning operations, finance, reimbursement, quality assessment, and assurance and conflict resolution. A good manager is a responsible steward with the resources entrusted in his/her hands. He/she should allocate these resources, whether human or materialistic, to achieve set goals. Efficient time management is an essential quality of good leadership. Good leaders are focused, have mechanisms to filter distractions, and know how to delegate responsibilities. They also remain happy in their life as well as in their work.

Micromanagement is the adversary of efficient leadership. It can cripple command, demoralize junior staff, and block progress. In the military realm, delegation to competent and confident staff down the chain of command has been shown to be very effective [6]. Autonomy must be entrusted and delegated to team members who are well trained and have a full grasp of the mission and goals of the team.

Leaders should use metrics to measure their progress and success. In the surgical world, there are several metrics to monitor the progress of the mission or of the department. For example, in the domain of surgical education, residency program directors can measure their success by how frequently they recruit high-quality residents and how reliably and well they perform and if they have good in-service examination scores and show good pass rates on the final board examinations. A surgeon leader uses the appropriate metrics to measure and evaluate the team performance, including the individual staff members' peer and mentees' evaluations, their surgical outcomes, and their patients' satisfaction. This must also include their overall behavior, empathy, and contributions to the team's effort. In LMIC settings, the influence of culture and environment plays a major role in development of such patterns of behavior. The structure of surgical services still mostly remains traditionally autocratic. In order to make rapid progress, it will need to evolve to more modern approaches appreciated by the new generation of surgeons.

Surgeon Leaders Walk the Talk

During the Second World War, in a French battlefield, an American battalion was given the order to advance inland through a large minefield. The commander decided to cross at the crack of dawn and so ordered his troops to camp for the night. Overnight, there was a heavy snowfall, and the minefield turned white. The captain of the battalion developed a plan. A soldier would step out and walk carefully through the field; if a mine exploded, the next soldier would walk to that point and take another path toward the goal of crossing the mine field. This would continue until the battalion crossed the field. There was dead silence among his men. While the soldiers were looking at each other, the leader of the battalion took the first step into the minefield, leading the way.

True leaders spend ample time with their troops. They do not reside in their ivory towers or behind glorified rhetoric and big desks. A leader surgeon does not shy away from taking night call. He/she is often seen in scrubs in the operating room, transferring his/her acumen of skill and knowledge to his/her residents and colleagues. He/she may even help transfer the patient to and from the operating table. A surgeon leader in white coat makes rounds with his team. It is essential for the leader of a surgical service to get to know his staff both on a professional and on a personal level, to recognize their strengths and their weaknesses, and to spot areas that need improvement or reward.

An additional quality of a good leader who leads by example is to care for those he/she leads, to listen to their professional and personal problems, to be trusted by them, and to take their concerns seriously. Recently, online evaluations have made the evaluation process mechanistic and far less human than when done face to face. The human interaction during evaluations or at a day retreat, at team sport event, or at a cookout outing can break barriers and strengthen both professional and personal relationships between the leader and his team members.

Care and attention for team members' welfare also needs to be part of hospital and organizational structure and commitment. An example of this quality is the Pan-African Academy of Christian Surgeons (PAACS). PAACS is a charitable organization that trains national surgeons in Africa according to the highest American standards. Part of the requirement to start a surgical residency program is to ensure the hosting hospital provides adequate living accommodations for the residents and their families. Moreover, the residents are compensated with a stipend that matches the cost of living in that country. PAACS also sponsors an annual retreat to support the residents' and their spouses spiritual and emotional well-being [7]. This type of bidirectional interaction between the hospital/institution and the individual team member is necessary not only to create a cadre of highly qualified surgeon-leaders but to retain them in the region or the country to prevent the existing "brain drain" in LMICs, mostly because of inadequate funding.

Surgeon Leaders Are Effective Communicators

Surgeons in leadership roles must master the art of communication on an individual and group level. On an individual level, a good leader surgeon sits down with his residents before a surgical procedure, discusses the patient's history and physical, and reviews the imaging studies. Just like in the war room studying battle fields maps, the surgeon leader clearly communicates the goal of the operation, the steps to achieve the goal, and the plan to avoid potential complications and defines the role of each team member.

Leaders are knowledgeable and articulate and know how to convey ideas, goals, and orders in a very clear and respectful manner. Morning rounds is a great opportunity to sharpen the skill of communication. A surgeon leader should serve as a model for the art of listening empathetically and patiently to the patient complaints. He/she needs to assess his/her team's ability to analyze the data, formulate differential diagnosis, and initiate a care plan.

Morbidity and mortality (M&M) conferences are a good occasion to practice the art of communication skills for the entire surgical department. Students and residents present the case, and surgeons pose questions and share their perspective. M&M conferences should never be a place for indictment of individual surgeons based on the case being presented. On the contrary, the conference should be a place for sharpening critical thinking, honest intellectual curiosity, and candid discussion to learn from mistakes. A good leader surgeon turns the M&M conference to be the soul of a surgical department.

Good leaders are not compulsive talkers. "He would not listen, he gives an answer before I had a chance to state the problem," once complained a junior faculty about the chair of his department. Sympathetic listening requires not only hearing the words but also understanding the meaning, the ethos, and the context of what the other person is saying.

Surgeon Leaders Handle Criticism

A surgeon leader makes numerous decisions on daily basis. Some will meet the approval of his/her team and the administration, and some will be criticized. Good leaders do not dismiss or ignore criticism. They listen and analyze carefully, seek counsel on the issue, and, if necessary, reconsider their decision.

In the business world, Fred Smith, founder of FedEx, was given a C grade by a Yale University management professor when he wrote a paper proposing a reliable overnight delivery service because the idea was deemed not feasible. Fred Smith followed his dream, and now FedEx is a gigantic global corporation.

In the surgical world, Thomas Starzl, the pioneer of liver transplantation, had to leave the University of Colorado. At that time, the University deemed that liver transplantation could not be performed safely in humans. Despite severe criticism, he never gave up his vision or goal and pursued liver transplants successfully at the University of Pittsburgh. Thomas Starzl worked tirelessly to transform liver transplantation from a dream to reality. Surgeons around the globe flocked to Pittsburgh to train under his tutelage and have made liver transplantation a therapy that has saved thousands of lives [8].

Surgeon leaders learn from their mistakes. In their book *Extreme Ownership*, two retired navy seals Jocko Willink and Leif Babin dedicated the first chapter to an important trait in good leaders—namely, total ownership of the operation or project they lead, including mistakes [9]. They were quoted as saying, "The best leaders checked their egos, accepted blame, sought out constructive criticism and took detailed notes for improvement. They exhibited extreme ownership." Admitting mistakes rather than shifting the blame down the chain of command and an honest analysis of why and how an error happened helps the whole team avoid future errors. Total ownership and taking the responsibility does not undermine the authority of the leader. On the contrary, it reinforces trust in leaders.

Leader Surgeons Are Good Mentors

Subordinates look up to leaders not only to learn the skill of the trade but also for inspiration, encouragement, and conflict resolution. True leaders create the space and allocate the time for mentorship of those on their team who exhibit leadership qualities. Even in the age of Zoom calls, a healthy mentor–mentee relationship can be developed and be rewarding to both. Good leaders recognize talents and know how to nurture and develop mentees. They do not miss the opportunity to learn from their mentees, appreciating that learning can be bidirectional. Residents, younger faculty, and colleagues may bring new ideas from unique backgrounds and education that can help achieve the goals of the leader and of the team.

Global Leaders Have Cross-Cultural Sensitivity

The Internet has connected people like never before and turned the world into a global village. Cross-culture communication is the new norm. Cultural sensitivity is important, and leadership across different cultures requires a particular skill set. Cultural differences should be regarded with respect, not on a superior-inferior scale. A good leader listens attentively, observes carefully, and gathers information to learn about the culture with which he/she wants to interact. The best way to learn about another culture is via immersion experiences. Visiting hospitals in LMICs, sharing the daily life of surgical colleagues, and realizing the differences in resources across the globe are an eye-opener and of high educational value.

Genuine leaders do not apply their methodologies, no matter how successful they may be, across different cultures without thoughtful adaptation to the local culture and resources. For example, not all that can be done laparoscopically in the USA can be done laparoscopically in Africa. Open surgery is still the cornerstone of African surgery. Laparoscopic equipment and instruments are not widely available. On the other hand, African surgeons are proficient in open surgery more than many newly trained western surgeons who trained in the minimally invasive era and rarely do open surgery. Listening, planning, and cooperating with the local leaders are of paramount importance. Learning can always be reciprocal.

Courtesy is the most important pillar of cross-culture leadership. Paying attention to differences such as time zones, holidays, or even working days (some countries expect a 6-day work week) is particularly important when organizing online meetings and events or visiting in person. Despite various cultural differences, e.g., ways to greet, address, or express thanks to others, there are also similarities that leaders can capitalize on. Mutual respect and integrity are highly prized within most cultures across the globe.

Leader Surgeon And the Digital (Virtual) World

There are currently many platforms that allow leaders to exercise their duties from a distance in the digital world including desktop or laptop computers and mobile phones. The COVID-19 pandemic and the lockdown brought these digital platforms to the forefront of daily life for the public, physicians, and the hospitals. Grand rounds, tumor boards, and M&M conferences can be conducted and attended online using digital platforms such as Zoom and Microsoft Teams. The use of virtual platforms was explored during the pandemic for use in simulation labs. Internet connection and digital media have increased possible learning platforms for learners worldwide and now provide additional learning opportunities. Surgical videos are great tools not only for surgical learning but also for evaluation of competency of surgical trainees by their leaders before certification [10].

Virtual surgical forums are increasing at a quick pace and are being utilized at an increasing rate. The American College of Surgeons sponsors many forums, as does the Academy of Master Surgeon Educators. One which has been very useful is the International Hernia Collaboration page on Facebook. This allows the exchange of expertise and sharing of innovations without traveling [11]. This type of sharing applies to many other specialties whose societies have initiated many webinars on sharing of information and innovation.

Intraoperative surgical consultation can be obtained live on FaceTime from any operating room in the world, provided there is a reliable Internet connection. One of the authors has been providing such pro bono consultation on regular basis to a network of surgical colleagues with whom he became acquainted during a series of short-term mission trips to an LMIC.

A word of caution: medicine cannot be 100% digitalized. Surgeon-patient relationship is the core of practicing surgery. The core of training and exhibiting leadership has traditionally required person-to-person contact and cannot be totally replaced using the digital medium. Eye contact and a gentle touch or tap on the shoulder can be soothing to the patient and learner. Hospitals remained open for emergencies and treating COVID-19 patient during the pandemic lockdown. Leader surgeons innovated how to do safe tracheostomies with extra protection from infection transmission via aerosolization [12]. Physicians, surgeons, nurses, physiotherapist, respiratory therapist, and all supportive staff took care of patients “in person.” However, digital platforms are very useful and can be employed to reinforce the human surgeon-patient relationship and inter-collegiality among leader surgeons and their staff.

Conclusion

This section of the chapter has briefly outlined characteristics of leaders, which are critical as people develop leadership skills. Being a follower is also part of being a leader at a different level and sometimes to a different population—each physician is a leader for a patient who seeks his/her care and advice. As has been previously mentioned, leadership is critical in the cross-cultural context. Special abilities are required, which demand adaptation to new cultural norms and humility as new challenges are met. As leadership and teamwork are taught, both the teachers and learners must be willing to learn from each other to make the relationship and the work successful.

Virtual Teaching in Leadership and Teamwork

The following section focuses on "how to" give the reader tools that can be used in person or virtually. The format is designed as a framework to teach virtually but can be adapted for in-person use. The reader is encouraged to change this as needed but to keep in mind the principles which are outlined (CEH).

Teaching soft skills like leadership and teamwork continues to be important. Doing this virtually requires careful rethinking on how these skills are to be transferred successfully to the mentees. The earlier part of this chapter enumerated the essential skills needed by surgeon leaders. Often, these important skills in surgery are not formally taught but rather are "caught" while on rounds and in the operating room. Since soft skills like leadership are "taught" in the same physical space with the teacher, there are many subtle cues which are not available in a virtual setting. These skills can be taught on a virtual platform, but this requires conscious changes in the approach by the teacher.

Developing online training in the essential skills of being a leader is more difficult and often must deliberately focus specifically on the goal of teaching leadership. Instead of relying on the learner observing these skills in the context of physical space, the teacher must model this on a virtual platform while emphasizing and demonstrating the same leadership skills during personal contacts, in the operating rooms, and in other clinical settings. The teacher must also remember this may need to be done in a cross-cultural context with authority and honesty, while interpersonal relationships and the community play an important a role in the learning environment [13]. Developing leadership skills in isolation and alone is very different than developing them while interacting during in-person group training. Instructors must intentionally consider the participant's isolation and technological disadvantage by purposely targeting a feeling of community and engagement within the virtual learning. It is still essential to maintain a small number of learners within the group to adequately promote leadership in the participants. Community interaction over a Webex link with more than six learners is very difficult, so it is recommended to try to keep groups at six learners or fewer. As one begins virtual training, it is imperative that the trainer knows the names of the individuals with whom he/she will interact and be familiar with each learner's basic key information.

Learning leadership skills virtually requires the lessons to be broken down into small segments. Multiple shorter segments ensure that each point is well understood and assimilated before proceeding to the next one. Group discussions are necessary to help understand the concepts, and this should be later combined with "homework" to reinforce the taught principles. The homework may consist of either direct information or be a case analysis, which will allow the learner to better understand the concept and to retain and retrieve the learned skills. Interaction among the mentees within the virtual environment helps one another to teach leadership and teamwork skills while at the same time solving clinical and/or surgical problems. The information used for teaching in case studies and complications must relate to real-world issues for them to be valuable for learning purposes. This offers an opportunity to have real-world interactions foster teamwork and leadership among the members of the small group of virtual learners. Discussion of solutions and problems should include and define the roles of the individual interprofessional healthcare team, composed of nurses, family members, and other medical specialists, to assure that the case example applies to real-life situations. Analysis of such real-life situations allow surgical learners to understand and embrace leadership roles and to reinforce their leadership skills. Interprofessional communication and collaboration skills are critical for the development of optimal healthcare outcomes and the establishment of innovative programs.

A solid review of leadership learning outcomes can also be done virtually. Clear and concise outlines of the key teaching points need to be emphasized when the learners interact with the trainer. At times, one-on-one coaching will be helpful to ascertain that the learner understands and is applying the leadership lessons appropriately. This is particularly true in a virtual situation where the learner is unable to individually ask content questions because of the virtual platform. Individual sessions, even if infrequent, encourage an authentic relationship between the trainer and the learner and allow for questions and deeper interaction. A mentor can then individually recommend areas for leadership growth and emphasize the positive leadership skills that the trainee already possesses. As is true in all learning, review and repetition at different time points are important for the lessons taught virtually to be retained and mastered. For this purpose, the teacher should build in regularly scheduled time for summary and review with the learners. This should be easily managed since the relationship between teacher and learners in a long-term surgical training situation allows time for skill building and advancement.

Example of an Approach to Teach Leadership Virtually

(The framework below illustrates how to teach leadership skills across a virtual platform.)

First Session: Assignment—Learners are asked to think about who they define as a good leader from their professional acquaintances and who they would consider as not a good leader and why. Have them write the key characteristics of each person and whether they are positive or negative. They then should create their own definition of a leader's characteristics and determine themselves if they fit into that definition. They should also define what character traits they want to see in a leader.

Second Session: Assignment—Learners should conduct a personality survey to learn about themselves and then initiate a survey to learn their perceived leadership style. The learner is then asked to incorporate the discussed skills defined in the first session prior to evaluating their own leadership strengths and where their weaknesses need to be addressed.

Third Session: Assignment—This session's selected assignment is to evaluate different types of leadership. It is to reflect on the question which one of the leadership types applies to which individuals in the group. A discussion among the learners should clarify if they individually view the information in similar or different ways. At this point, the mentor can also recommend additional (optional) outside reading material (notable books on leadership) if mentees would like to take their development a step further.

Fourth Session: Assignment—Follow-up on third session. Give a problem regarding activities on a surgical ward (possible examples: vital signs not being taken appropriately, medications given at the wrong time, wounds not being evaluated and reported on incorrectly, etc.). Have individuals solve the outlined problem with his/her leadership style and discuss the results. What are the strengths and weaknesses of each approach? Ensure a positive and non-judgmental learning space for the learners, and emphasize that this is an informal discussion and not subject to evaluation or criticism.

Fifth Session: Assignment—Distribute a reading assignment on teamwork, and discuss it virtually within the small group setting. Discussion should focus on how leadership styles impact teamwork and collect your learners' thoughts and conclusions on this topic. Ask learners to write a short reflection after the session on their thoughts regarding the intersection and appropriate balance between being a leader and working as part of a team.

Sixth Session: Assignment—Discuss how and why teamwork is important and how to lead a team to solve a problem. Then assign discussion of a surgical complication, and ask the group to focus on how to use teamwork to solve a real-world problem. Ask learners how they would approach the task of getting an unwilling team member to buy into helping to solve the assigned problem, even though he/she may not be willing to do that. How would they handle this dynamic?

Seventh Session: Assignment—Consider this as a summary session. Have each learner prepare and submit a summary of the main points learned from the previous set of six virtual exercises. Individuals should then each in turn present the highlights that resonated with each one and the reasons that it did. Facilitate a robust discussion regarding these concepts and welcome learner engagement. Summarize the key points you, as the teacher, would like to reinforce as conclusion and as a review.

Conclusion

In this section of the chapter, the authors have attempted to outline concrete steps, which can be taken to teach leadership and teamwork building virtually. This is clearly a work in progress. The seven sessions are a beginning that has proved constructive but leaves much more that can be done, especially within other cultural environments. There are already advanced degree programs on leadership that may be modified to the surgeons purposes and utilized following the initial steps to start training leadership in a cross-cultural context described in this second part of our chapter.

References

1. Bass B, Bass R. The Bass handbook of leadership: theory, research, and managerial applications. New York: Simon & Schuster; 2008.
2. Spaner SJ, Warkona GL. Brief history of endoscopy, laparoscopy, and laparoscopic surgery. J Laparoendosc Adv Surg Tech A. 1997;7:369–73.
3. Asimov I, Shulman JA, editors. Isaac Asimov's book of science and nature quotations. New York: Grove Press; 1990.
4. https://www.forbes.com/sites/forbescoachescouncil/2021/12/09/tomorrows-ceos-are-shifting-from-heroic-to-humble/?sh=355279da2d31. Accessed on 5.15.2022.
5. https://www.cslewisinstitute.org/resources/pride-and-humility/?gclid=EAIaIQobChMI9NqZzoqj-AIVghXUAR2wJQCYEAAYAiAAEgLQqPD_BwE. Accessed on 6.17.2022.
6. Steadman A. The military leader. Bloomington, IN: Westbow Press; 2018.
7. www.paacs.org
8. Starzl TE. The puzzle people. Pittsburgh: University of Pittsburgh Press; 2003.
9. Willink J, Babin L. Extreme ownership: how U.S. navy seals lead and win. New York: St. Martin's Press; 2017.
10. Laeeq K. Video-based assessment of operative competency in endoscopic sinus surgery. Am J Rhin Aller. 2010;24:234–7.
11. https://www.facebook.com/groups/herniacollab/about/
12. Prabhakaran K. Open tracheostomy for COVID-19-positive patients: a method to minimize aerosolization and reduce risk of exposure. J Trauma. 2020;89:265–71.
13. Dhaliwal G. Teaching medicine to non-English speaking background learners in a foreign country. J Gen Intern Med. 2009;24:771–3.

How to Organize and Provide ICU Care in Low- and Middle-Income Countries

19

Ananya Abate Shiferaw, Deborah A. Haisch, Dawit Kebede Huluka, and David H. Chong

Some people want it to happen, some wish it would happen, others make it happen.

– Michael Jordan

Abbreviations

ER	Emergency room
HICs	High-income countries
ICU	Intensive care unit
LMICs	Low- and middle-income countries
SSA	Sub-Saharan Africa
WHO	World Health Organization

A. A. Shiferaw
Department of Anesthesiology, Addis Ababa University College of health Sciences, Addis Ababa, Ethiopia

D. A. Haisch
Pulmonary and Critical Care Division, Weill Cornell Medical College, New York, NY, USA
e-mail: dah2020@med.cornell.edu

D. K. Huluka
Division of Pulmonary and Critical Care Medicine, Department of Internal Medicine, School of Medicine, College of Health Sciences, Addis Ababa University, Tikur Anbessa Specialized Hospital, Addis Ababa, Ethiopia

D. H. Chong (✉)
Division of Pulmonary and Critical Care and Sleep Medicine, CUNY School of Medicine, St. Barnabas Health System/CUNY School of Medicine, Bronx, NJ, USA
e-mail: dchong@sbhny.org

Introduction

Studies done in Africa show that the majority of admissions to intensive care unit (ICU) are associated with surgical conditions such as sepsis from a perforated viscous, multiple trauma, C-sections, orthopedics, and neurosurgical procedures [1–3]. The World Health Organization (WHO) mandates that ICU capacity be available in hospitals providing surgical services [4]. Postoperative patients, who made up the majority of critical care admissions in five sub-Saharan countries in a 2007 study, were found to have the greatest survival benefit from an ICU admission, highlighting the importance of critical care for postoperative patients in low- and middle-income countries (LMICs) [1].

Improving the availability and quality of critical care is essential for reducing the burden of preventable deaths in LMICs [5]. Currently, the overall high costs restrict access to ICU care in LMICs. There exists an urgent need to develop an affordable critical care model [5]. The substantial proportion of critical care costs in LMICs are due to staffing and fixed equipment costs as opposed to medication and laboratory testing costs [6]. The conventional high-income country model, based on resource-intensive units with expensive monitoring and life support equipment and large

M. A. Hardy, B. R. Hochman (eds.), *Global Surgery*, https://doi.org/10.1007/978-3-031-28127-3_19

numbers of highly trained staff, is unlikely to be an effective and sustainable model in LMICs settings [5].

Establishing Critical Care: The Ethiopian Experience

Back in early 1990s, foreign anesthesiologists established the idea of creating a surgical ICU when the first anesthesiology residency program was started in Ethiopia at Addis Ababa University. These anesthesiologists engaged with hospital administration and other key stakeholders and reached a consensus on a plan to start and grow a critical care program. Using a collaborative approach, a ward was created to accommodate six patients located in close proximity to the operating room that eventually was transformed into an ICU. The evolution to an ICU included constructing a nursing station, mounting monitors, and installing an infrastructure to connect oxygen tanks in a small room next to the ICU. Donations were solicited for the major essential ICU equipment; such purchases included four mechanical ventilators, six patient monitors, and six suction machines. Other equipment including a defibrillator, and intravenous pumps were procured. The foreign anesthesiologists trained the anesthesiology residents and nurses, thus completing the ICU care model. As the ICU progressed, the nurses and the resident physicians gradually developed, through supervision and training, the skills to independently manage critically ill surgical patients. The surgical ICU (SICU) program helped advance the capabilities of a medical ICU, which has been established earlier but were not able to provide mechanical ventilation support. Postgraduate residency training in critical care was expanded to other departments such as internal medicine, surgery, pediatrics, and gynecology as trainees came to the anesthesia managed SICU for a one- to three-month rotations. The SICU also provided rotations of other postgraduate students from all over the country and provided an opportunity to participate in a critical care training. Over time, the Ethiopian anesthesiology graduates grew to supervise and lead the teaching service and to they continue to expand critical care education.

The program continued to expand and to strengthen, thereby improved the quality of critical care. This led to the development and creation of a need-based adult critical care medicine curriculum. Invited foreign anesthesia faculty continued to visit for three-month rotations to deliver hands-on skill training and up-to-date teaching, in addition to virtual didactic lectures throughout the year. Partner institutions provided resources for faculty recruitment and helped cover travel-related costs. The SICU continues to be a hub for quality care and education for the SICU and other departments as well as outside teaching institutions locally, nationally, and internationally to advance critical care in all of Ethiopia and beyond (especially in sub-Saharan Africa (SSA)). Due to the high cost of ICU equipment and supplies, critical care in Ethiopia and many other LMICs continue to rely on foreign donations.

Pivoting to Address COVID in Ethiopia

The Ethiopian COVID response included having dedicated healthcare facilities and hospitals for COVID care, repurposing non-health facilities for COVID care, and devoting some health facilities to non-COVID essential services. The latter required an isolation center for COVID cases to stay until referral to a COVID treatment center or until recovery. Finally, COVID ICUs were established to help care for the most critically ill; ICU equipment like mechanical ventilators, monitors, and suction machines were procured or were obtained by donation specifically for the COVID response. Short-term ICU and COVID-specific training was established for all healthcare professionals involved in all the COVID centers. The COVID response increased the capacity of hospitals in terms of critical care service delivery as compared to pre-pandemic time. Importantly, COVID highlighted the need for more critical care capacity and training and has brought much needed attention to these requirements for adequate healthcare delivery to the local leaders and to the regional and national leaders and administrators.

What Does It Take to Set Up an ICU in LMICs?

The four major components that are vital to establish an ICU are (1) *infrastructure*, (2) *equipment and supplies*, (3) *education and training*, and (4) *establishing best practice models. Related discussion may be also found in Chaps. 12 and 14 which address the use of different types of iCU's.*

(1) and (2) Infrastructure, Equipment and Supplies

An ICU should have adequate *space* so that it can accommodate the essential equipment for providing mechanical ventilation, monitoring, suctioning, and resuscitation. Even though it is difficult to construct a new space in LMICs, it is possible to identify and reconstruct adequate available and appropriate space within a hospital setting. According to international standards, there needs to be a minimum, 12 m^2 per an ICU bed [7]. The ICU should also be located close to the operating theatres, or at least on the same floor, and relatively close to the radiology site, ER, and laboratory, if possible [7]. Easy means of patient transport such as a dedicated hallways and/or an elevator must be available whenever the ICU is located farther from these essential areas.

Uninterrupted supply of electricity is mandatory for safe delivery of critical care [8]. LMICs need to have a backup electricity system for ICUs (such as generators or a backup battery system) to protect patients for electricity interruption, which is not uncommon in many LMICs. Alternative sources of energy, like solar energy as needed, should be considered. A protocol on how to handle electricity interruptions must be put in place [7, 8]. Availability of water is also essential and challenging in most LMICs. Looking for alternative sources of water and a water conservation strategy must be implemented to safely deliver critical care. Hand hygiene infrastructure and assurance of environmental hygiene is absolutely essential for safe ICU care in LMICs [8].

Finally, an adequate and consistent oxygen supply is a crucial component of any ICU [8]. ICUs in LMICs need to choose the type of oxygen supply based on both availability and needs. A plan to procure a sustainable supply to ensure adequate oxygen delivery should be well developed and tested for efficiency, before setting up an ICU. A centralized distribution system for oxygen is recommended wherever mechanical ventilators are to be used [8].

Also ICU budgets and protocols should be developed and refined to maximize resources and focus on the purchase and maintenance (hospital staff and/or contract with the company) of essential ICU equipment. Whether that equipment is purchased or obtained by donation, maintenance is of utmost importance. Trained biomedical engineers should be on site to help with machine troubleshooting and fixing malfunctioning devices. The ICU team should also be trained on how to clean, utilize, and store equipment. Hospitals should dedicate a budget for maintenance, training of staff, and purchase of machine accessories such as ventilator circuits, monitor accessories, etc. The ICU leadership should work very closely with the hospital's administration, the ministry of health, and other stakeholders to assist with adequate resource allocation and planning.

A continuous education model for staff and providers for best proactive protocols must be provided. An education plan is essential for the successful implementation and sustainability of a successful ICU program.

(3) and (4) Education and Training, and Interdisciplinary Best Practice Models

Beyond the initial infrastructure and curriculum components of building an ICU, leveraging national and international resources can provide key support to ongoing education and initial research efforts in this context. These resources can provide additional specialist training, continuing medical education, mentorship, instruction in the conduct of research, methodology for data collection, and opportunities for development of collaborative interactions. An interdisciplinary team composed of physicians, surgeons, clinical pharmacists, gastroenterologists, internists, public health experts, nutritionists, nurses, and biomedical professionals should be established to facilitate development of protocols for (1) the management of common ailments, (2) utilization of equipment, (3) management of nutrition, (4) prevention and management of infection, etc.; it is critical to have regular planning and performance evaluation sessions to identify any gaps and to efficiently address any issues to establish a best practice model for delivery of ICU care.

Specialist Training Models

Multiple models for medical education have been used to train specialists in countries without a dedicated cadre of experienced staff on site. Most use a combination of foreign faculty with that of the local institution to develop an effective curriculum. Ideally, teaching should be on-site, but there are varying degrees of ongoing in-country training as well as in remote options.

One teaching model of an emergency medicine program was started with a initial needs assessment invited by the Ethiopian Ministry of Health's taskforce, which was performed in collaboration with a partner institution. These data included information about staffing, patient flow, and logistics concerning the emergency department where all training was to occur; the data also provided information on trainee education prior to residency and the availability and usefulness of the existing educational infrastructure including simulation, journal clubs, and bedside teaching. Finally, other factors were identified such as learner barriers and a needs assessment in the context of the existing framework for the learner environment. An assessment of disease burden and a survey of trainee ability to manage specific presentations was also considered. This granular data led to the formulation of program goals and of the resultant curriculum (including content and delivery plans). The plan was developed by the partner institution, with an outside visiting teaching attending physician invited for three months per year to implement this curriculum, which focused on fulfilling the previously formulated didactic and bedside teaching goals. In addition, an iterative feedback process allowed curriculum revisions after each month review, when the visiting attending was present. This feedback process eventually included "distance-bridging initiatives," including a formalized faculty-resident mentorship program and monthly videoconferences.

Similarly, a dedicated 2-year pulmonary and critical care fellowship training program (Eastern Africa Training Initiative) was developed in Ethiopia under the direction of one of the major medical schools in Addis Ababa. As with other programs, an initial needs assessment provided critical data to design the next steps. This program included an agreement by the school of medicine to recruit and pay fellow salaries, while a group of external invited volunteer faculty who would develop the curriculum and commit to be on-site for 80% of teaching and supervision during the initial years of the program. Currently, majority of the lectures are done remotely via Zoom, and internal attendings include previous graduates of the program. Additional training beyond the clinical scope includes training in research methodology (experimental design, data collection, statistical evaluations, etc.). The program culminated with a month-long observership in the United States at three major teaching hospitals to allow trainees to observe practices that might not be standard in their local setting (e.g., interdisciplinary intensive care unit rounds with respiratory therapy and nursing). This rotation also helped create networking opportunities for future collaborations. The program also helped the rotating fellows create research opportunities and the design an ICU database. Abstracts were submitted with joint authorships to major international conferences, and funds were solicited for fellows and attendings to attend and present their research. Fellows were also asked to successfully pass American Board-type annual examination to evaluate their and the program's effectiveness. To date, fifteen specialists have been trained in adult and pediatric pulmonary and critical care to serve throughout the region and country. Many of the graduates have been appointed to major hospitals throughout Ethiopia, consistent with their previous agreements with the Ministry of Health. Many are now leaders and department chairs in their home institutions. Two of those graduates are from other East African nations, Tanzania and Rwanda, and went back to their countries where they are actively serving their communities.

A similar training approach has been applied to other specialties and could also be applied in areas such as respiratory therapy, as well as in nursing. This type of approach to joint training could be employed to advance an education mechanism to implement high-quality intensive care delivery.

Impact of National and International Societies

Participation in regional and international professional societies and formation of relevant professional societies within countries may be important not only for accessing continuing education and research collaboration but may contribute significantly to the coordination of efforts and to setting public health agendas across regions and countries. The Society of Critical Care Medicine and the European Critical Care Society have created courses to help certify non-critical care practitioners to improve their care for these patients.

For example, during the COVID-19 pandemic, the Ethiopian professional societies which previously focused on pulmonary and critical care were the obvious source for much-needed guidance for Ethiopia's Ministry of Health in creation of management guidelines and ongoing education. The Ethiopian Thoracic Society and others helped guide the ministry with COVID management guidelines and assisted nationally with policy changes to (1) organizational structure; (2) record-keeping; (3) staffing and human resource capacity; (4) training and curriculum programs and practice guidelines (for physicians and nurses); and (5) existing relationships and collaborations, regionally and nationally.

Critical Care Improves Outcomes

In 2015, Dr. Paul Farmer's group conservatively estimated that 4.8 billion people in the world had no access to surgery. Ninety-five percent of the population in south Asia and central, eastern, and western sub-Saharan Africa did not have access to surgical care. In stark contrast, less than 5% of the population in Australasia, high-income North America, and western Europe lack access [9]. Approximately 16.9 million people die from conditions that require surgical care each year, the vast majority of them in low- and middle-income countries (LMICs) [10]. But even when patients can get surgery, the perioperative mortality after surgery is high, especially in Africa. The reasons are numerous; patients in LMICs often present late when the disease processes are more advanced. In one study, 57% of operations were for emergency indications, compared with around 25% emergency operations in cohorts from high-income countries (HICs) [11]. In the same study, the patients that were routinely admitted to a critical care unit immediately after surgery had a 2.4% mortality as compared to those who were admitted to a critical care unit to treat subsequent complications, which then led to a mortality which was in excess of four times at 9.7%. However, crucial resource challenges hamper the safe delivery of surgical and critical care in Africa. A quarter of hospitals do not have a reliable oxygen source, a third do not have reliable electricity, 70% do not have pulse oximeters, and 47% do not have a dedicated postoperative or critical care unit [12, 13]. In these studies in LMICs, the average provider-to-population density of specialist surgeons, anesthetists, and obstetricians was approximately thirty times lower than the recommended global minimum. The case for delay in expansion of surgical care and critical care in LMICs is primarily financial. It may also be delayed by insufficient total number of trained physicians, and especially specialists, complicated by significant "brain drain" because of poor physician income compared to that in HICs. Many essential surgical interventions such as C-sections, orthopedics, general surgery, and even hydrocephalus surgery are very cost-effective in resource-poor countries [14]. But the needs remain great. A 2020 review of critical care in the African continent reported an average of 0.3 ICU beds per 100,000 people [15]. A recent, on-the-ground study in Ethiopia confirmed only 0.3 public ICU beds per 100,000 populations [16]. Although higher than the rate of 0.1 reported for Uganda, this is far lower than the 8.9 previously reported in South Africa [17] and inadequate to meet the needs of Ethiopia. In contrast, the United States has 20–31.9 ICU beds per 100,000 people [18].

Summary

This chapter briefly summarizes the needs for ICU care in LMICs, especially for trauma and postoperative care to improve the overall survival outcomes. It addresses the staffing, the construction, the equipment, and the leadership required to establish well-functioning and effective ICUs in LMICs, using Ethiopia as an example. It also emphasizes the absolute need for multi-specialist collaboration and the need for specialist nurse training for the ICU to provide optimal care. Self-evaluation and periodic audits are needed to maintain and establish high standards of an ICU.

References

1. Towey RM, Ojara S. Intensive care in the developing world. Anaesthesia. 2007;62:32–7. https://doi.org/10.1111/j.1365-2044.2007.05295.x.
2. Okech UK, Chokwe T, Mung'ayi V. East Afr J Med. 2015;92(2).
3. Abebe K, Negasa T, Argaw F. Surgical admissions and treatment outcomes at a tertiary hospital intensive care unit in Ethiopia: a two-year review. Ethiop J Health Sci. 2020;30(5):725. https://doi.org/10.4314/ejhs.v30i5.11.
4. World Health Organization. WHO, surgical care at the district hospital; 2003. https://apps.who.int/iris/bitstream/handle/10665/42564/9241545755.pdf;jsessionid=6FC140F238332BF9FC34289BEBA60C23?sequence=1. Accessed 15 Aug 2020.
5. Turner HC, Van Hao N, Yacoub S, Hoang VMT, Clifton DA, Thwaites GE, Dondorp AM, Thwaites CL, Chau NVV. BMJ Global Health. 2019; https://doi.org/10.1136/bmjgh-2019-001675.
6. Agrawal A, Gandhe M, Gandhe S, et al. Study of length of stay and average cost of treatment in medicine intensive care unit at tertiary care center. J Health Res Rev. 2017;4:249. https://doi.org/10.4103/2394-2010.199329.
7. Rungta N, Govil D, Nainan S, Munjal M, Divatia J, Jani CK. ICU planning and designing in India – guidelines; 2010.
8. Papali A, Schultz MJ, Dünserr MW. Recommendations on infrastructure and organization of adult ICUs in resource-limited settings. Intensive Care Med. 2018;44:1133–7. https://doi.org/10.1007/s00134-017-4972-0.
9. Alkire BC, Raykar NP, Shrime MG, Weiser TG, Bickler SW, Rose JA, Nutt CT, Greenberg SL, Kotagal M, Riesel JN, Esquivel M, Uribe-Leitz T, Molina G, Roy N, Meara JG, Farmer PE. Global access to surgical care: a modelling study. Lancet Glob Health. 2015;3(6):e316–23. https://doi.org/10.1016/S2214-109X(15)70115-4.
10. Shrime MG, Bickler SW, Alkire BC, Mock C. Global burden of surgical disease: an estimation from the provider perspective. Lancet Glob Health. 2015;3(Suppl 2):S8–9.
11. International Surgical Outcomes Study group. Global patient outcomes after elective surgery: prospective cohort study in 27 low-, middle- and high-income countries. Br J Anaesth. 2016;117:601–9.
12. Meara JG, Leather AJ, Hagander L, et al. Global surgery 2030: evidence and solutions for achieving health, welfare, and economic development. Lancet. 2015;386:569–624.
13. LeBrun DG, Chackungal S, Chao TE, et al. Prioritizing essential surgery and safe anesthesia for the post-2015 development agenda: operative capacities of 78 district hospitals in 7 low- and middle-income countries. Surgery. 2014;155:365–73.
14. Chao TE, Sharma K, Mandigo M, Hagander L, Resch SC, Weiser TG, Meara JG. Cost-effectiveness of surgery and its policy implications for global health: a systematic review and analysis. Lancet Glob Health. 2014;2(6):e334–45. https://doi.org/10.1016/S2214-109X(14)70213-X.

15. Craig J, Kalanxhi E, Hauck S. National estimates of critical care capacity in 54 African-countries. medRxiv. Published online July 6, 2020. https://doi.org/10.1101/2020.05.13.20100727. Accessed 3 June 2021.
16. Kifle F, Boru Y, Tamiru HD, Sultan M, Walelign Y, Demelash A, Beane A, Haniffa R, Gebreyesus A, Moore J. Intensive care in sub-Saharan Africa: a national review of the service status in Ethiopia. Anesth Analg. 2022;134(5):930–7. https://doi.org/10.1213/ANE.0000000000005799.
17. Dünser MW, Baelani I, Ganbold L. A review and analysis of intensive care medicine in the least developed countries. Crit Care Med. 2006;34:1234–42.
18. Prin M, Wunsch H. International comparisons of intensive care: informing outcomes and improving standards. Curr Opin Crit Care. 2012;18(6):700–6. https://doi.org/10.1097/MCC.0b013e32835914d5.

20 How to Use Surgical Ultrasound in Resource-Limited Settings

Beth A. Schrope, Christopher Cassim, Shamir O. Cawich, Ayemoethu Ma, Catherine McManus, Robbie A. Rampersad, and Roshni Rao

The very first step towards success in any occupation is to become interested in it.

– William Osler

Abbreviations

ACR	American College of Radiology
AIUM	American Institute of Ultrasound in Medicine
ATA	American Thyroid Association
CME	Continuing medical education
dB	Decibels
FAST	Focused abdominal sonogram for trauma
FNA	Fine-needle aspiration
MHz	Megahertz
TGC	Time gain compensation
TI-RADS	Thyroid imaging reporting data system
USAID	United states agency for international development
USES	UltraSound essentials for surgeons
W	Watts

B. A. Schrope (✉) · C. McManus · R. Rao
Department of Surgery, Columbia University Vagelos College of Physicians and Surgeons, New York, NY, USA
e-mail: bs170@cumc.columbia.edu; cm3304@cumc.columbia.edu; rr3181@cumc.columbia.edu

C. Cassim · R. A. Rampersad
Department of Radiology, Eric Williams Medical Sciences Complex, Champ Fleur, Trinidad and Tobago

S. O. Cawich
Department of Surgery, University of the West Indies, St. Augustine Campus, Trinidad and Tobago

A. Ma
Department of Surgery, University of California, San Francisco - East Bay, Oakland, CA, USA

Background

Ultrasound Physics and Instrumentation

Critical to optimal utilization of ultrasound in clinical practice is a fundamental understanding of basic ultrasound physics. What follows is a concise review of the physical principles of ultrasound, correlated with practical applications to hands-on imaging techniques, modalities, and image interpretation. Finally, general recommendations for learning and practicing ultrasound are provided. Specialty-oriented training is also covered in the organ system sections.

An acoustic wave is a longitudinal, mechanical wave travelling through a medium, with alternating compression and rarefaction (expansion). Understanding the waves' behavior is facilitated

M. A. Hardy, B. R. Hochman (eds.), *Global Surgery*, https://doi.org/10.1007/978-3-031-28127-3_20

by a sinusoidal or transverse representation, with energy (both positive, compression, and negative, rarefaction) represented on the vertical axis and time on the horizontal axis (Fig. 20.1). Waves are described by their wavelength, frequency, propagation velocity, amplitude, and phase.

Wavelength is defined as the distance a wave travels per one complete cycle. Frequency is inversely proportional to wavelength and is defined as the number of cycles per second; 1 cycle/s is 1 Hz. Wavelength (λ, in meters) and frequency (*f*, in Hertz) are related by the speed of sound (*v*, meters per second) through a medium, which is a variable that is specific to the medium itself:

$$\lambda = \frac{v}{f}$$

The speed of sound through different biologic soft tissues varies slightly, but for the purposes of ultrasound imaging, an accepted speed used for calculations is 1540 m per second. For practical purposes, a smaller wavelength, and thus a higher frequency, results in better resolution or finer detail in the final image. Ultrasound is defined as acoustic energy with frequencies higher than that achievable with human hearing, about 20 kHz. Typical frequencies used in medical ultrasound imaging are in the range of 2.5 to 20 MHz. Note though that for reasons to be discussed forthwith, there are limitations on frequency selection that preclude just selecting the highest frequency possible for best resolution.

There are several descriptors of wave magnitude: amplitude, power, and intensity. The amplitude of the acoustic wave, measured in decibels (dB), corresponds to the amount of pressure in the medium as the wave propagates. Power is the amount of energy generated per unit time and is measured in Watts (W). Intensity is the power density within a given area and is expressed in W/m^2. In practical terms, these variables are manipulated by adjusting the power on the ultrasound equipment.

Phase describes the temporal location in the wave cycle and is measured in radians or degrees. It is difficult to appreciate absolute phase in the high frequencies of ultrasound, but the relationships between multiple waves can aid in interpretation of images. Two waves (incident and echo, perhaps) that are 180 degrees out of phase, for example, will cancel each other out.

With a basic understanding of the acoustic wave properties, we are now able to explore the behavior of the acoustic wave as it propagates through the medium, which is the essence of creating the image. Energy in any form is never lost but simply transformed. As ultrasound waves travel through a medium, they may be transmitted, refracted, reflected, scattered, or absorbed (Fig. 20.2). Initially, an acoustic wave is gener-

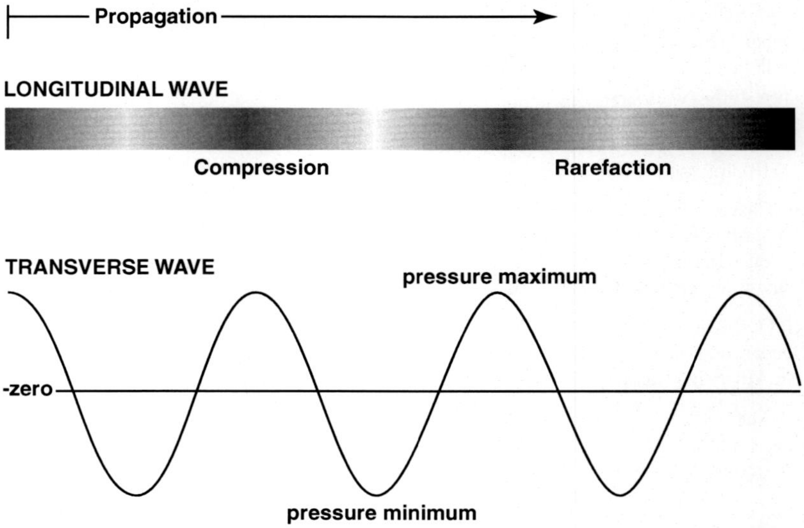

Fig. 20.1 An acoustic wave is a longitudinal wave travelling through a medium. It may be represented by a sinusoidal wave to more easily understand its properties

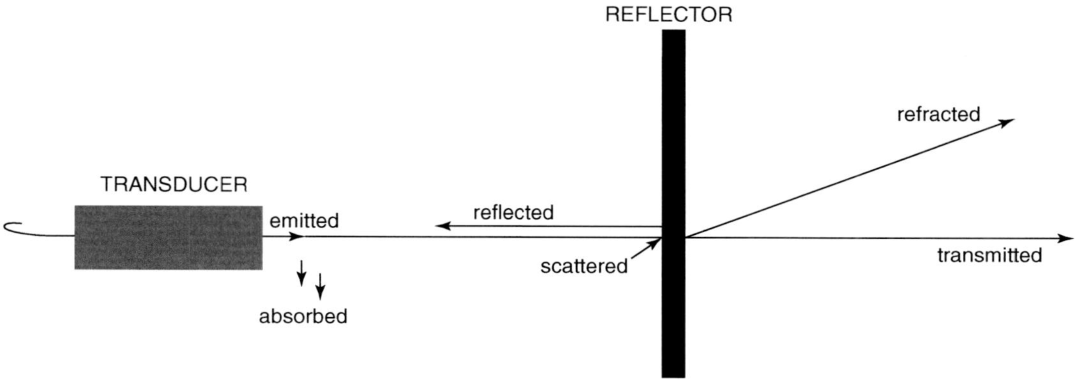

Fig. 20.2 Wave behavior in a medium

ated by a transducer that has the ability to transform electrical energy into mechanical energy (known as the piezoelectric effect). It is this acoustic energy that is transmitted through the medium. As the wave travels, it may encounter architecture in the medium that will change its direction. If the direction of change is at a forward angle, it is refracted; if the wave changes directed back toward the source (transducer), it is reflected. Scattering refers to a type of reflection and refraction due to very small details in the medium, on the order of the wavelength of the acoustic wave. The acoustic energy may also be "lost" in the medium through transformation to thermal energy (absorption), which relates to inherent properties of the medium. All of these behaviors are sensed back at the receiving aspect of the transducer, where the acoustic energy is transformed back to electrical energy, which is then used to compute the final image.

Each of these processes is influenced by the frequency of the incident wave. As a rule, the higher the incident frequency, the greater the energy "loss" or attenuation. The attenuation coefficient is a unique property of media, and for soft tissue, it may be approximated as 0.5 dB/cm/MHz. In the application of medical ultrasound, this influences your choice of transducer frequency; although a higher frequency of sound would result in clearer images (higher resolution), this is limited by the attenuation of the sound wave. In other words, you would use a lower-frequency transducer to reach deeper structures (at the sacrifice of image clarity), since the greater distance a wave must travel means it is attenuated more. Conversely, one would choose a higher-frequency transducer for more superficial structures (to optimize detail).

There are several different image options on commercial ultrasound equipment. Perhaps the most familiar is the B-mode or two-dimensional grayscale image. Depending on transducer construction, this may appear as a rectangular image or a wedge-shaped "sector" scan. Doppler ultrasound, which allows for flow velocity measurements based on the Doppler effect, may be superimposed on the B mode image for a duplex scan. In this mode, a cursor is directed to the point of interest (e.g., blood vessel) to assess for movement, which is displayed as color superimposed on the grayscale image. Arbitrarily, a red color may signify movement away from the transducer, and blue indicates flow toward the transducer. Most relevant here of course is direction of movement with different structures in the image relative to each other. Flow velocity may be quantified and displayed as well; triplex ultrasound is a term sometimes used to indicate B-mode image, color flow map, and velocity quantification on one image. Commonly used to assess heart valve motion in echocardiography, M-mode tracks velocity variation over time.

Scanning Techniques

Medical ultrasonography is a unique imaging modality in that the user's manipulation of the transducer or indeed the patient aids in image interpretation; thus, it is a dynamic and interactive skill. Practically, there are several key tips to successful ultrasound image interpretation. Starting with transducer selection, considerations include transducer footprint and frequency. Small anatomic regions such as the neck are best served with smaller-sized probes. Higher-frequency transducers deliver better image clarity, but attenuation of the acoustic energy limits frequency capability in imaging deep structures. Thus, thyroid or superficial vascular structures, for example, are well served by higher frequencies (7.5 to 10 MHz), but transabdominal imaging may require a 5 MHz probe. Many commercially available probes offer multifrequency probes, where a single probe can deliver a range of frequencies depending on user selection. Note that transducer orientation may be verified before every examination by touching one side of the probe and observing the corresponding area on the image where the signal is noted. Of course, coupling gel is mandatory with transcutaneous scanning; dedicated sonography gels can be used, but medical lubricants are also quite fine.

The image may be optimized with various front panel controls. In general, the desired anatomy should fill the image; thus, the user should adjust the *depth* to include the region of interest and nothing beyond. This of course magnifies the image but also mitigates any artifact from structures beyond the region of interest. In terms of "brightening" the image, two aspects of the signal may be manipulated. First, the *power* to the transmitted signal may be increased. This results in a stronger incident acoustic pulse, which may aid in targeting deeper structures. This can result in unacceptable "noise" or distortion of parts of the image, however. An alternative is to increase the amplification or *gain* of the received signal. Here one can select to amplify the signal from different depths of the image; this is typically referred to as Time Gain Compensation (TGC) and seeks to account for cumulative attenuation of the signal as it travels over a longer distance. Many commercial machines have a series of slide switches to change the gain at various depths in the image. Finally, *dynamic range* refers to the range of echo amplitudes processed and displayed by the system, from strongest to weakest, analogous to the concept of contrast in video applications. The strongest echoes received are those from the initial impulse and transducer-skin interface and will generally be similar from exam to exam. As the dynamic range is decreased, the echoes at the weaker end of the spectrum will be lost. For most imaging applications, the dynamic range should be kept at its maximum level to maximize the contrast of the image.

Image interpretation may be facilitated with the appreciation of a few simple principles, based on the physics lesson provided previously. Imaging artifacts are phenomena occurring as a result of ultrasound's interaction with the medium. Although artifacts can be considered "false" impressions, recognition and characterization of artifacts are vital to optimal image interpretation. It is also important to recognize the fact that ultrasound is a dynamic procedure, so artifacts can often be distinguished from genuine by scanning in different planes or by adjusting the system controls.

Acoustic properties of different soft tissues vary slightly, which aids in differentiation of structures (muscle, fat, solid organ, tumor, etc.). In addition, water is very different from soft tissue; thus, cystic structures are readily apparent and discernable from surrounding soft tissues. Specifically, the acoustic signal is minimally attenuated through water, so an artifact known as *posterior enhancement* can be diagnostic in evaluating cystic structures. Further, waves can "bounce" within the confines of a cyst creating artificial structures within the cyst on this image, which is known as reverberation artifact. Needles used for biopsy or aspiration display a particular type of *reverberation artifact* due to the large acoustic impedance mismatch between metal and water, known as a comet tail artifact.

Another type of reverberation artifact, referred to as *ring-down artifact*, occurs when there are small bubbles of air or partial liquids in the insonified field. A classic example is adenomyomatosis of the gallbladder, where acoustic energy reverberates between and within the bile-filled cystic spaces of the hyperplastic gallbladder epithelium.

Calcified structures such as bone or calcified stones, as well as air, also have different acoustic properties from soft tissues. For example, calcified gallstones will reflect acoustic energy much more strongly that surrounding soft tissues, leading to a *shadowing artifact* behind the stones. Air in the trachea will also strongly reflect acoustic energy, demonstrating an important landmark in neck imaging.

Training and Certification

Currently, many surgical residencies incorporate ultrasound training into their programs, thus enabling a graduating surgeon to incorporate ultrasound into their chosen practice fairly easily. And, as with any surgical skill, competence is gained through experience. Realistically, though, there are circumstances where a surgeon may not have had the opportunity to gain adequate training during residency, either due to deficit in the program or maturity in their careers. In this case, the acquisition of new skills should follow a standard rubric, namely, (1) didactic instruction by experts in the field; (2) hands-on training; (3) proctoring for an agreed amount of cases with eventual demonstration of satisfactory skill; and (4) continuing education, both practical (e.g., meeting a minimum number of cases per year) and quality assurance.

There are numerous excellent options for didactic online instruction in surgical ultrasound. The American College of Surgeons, for example, has published a comprehensive course, UltraSound Essentials for Surgeons (USES), available online for a nominal fee. The World Federation for Ultrasound in Medicine and Biology is another resource rich with online videos and courses, depending on an individual's particular interest. Indeed, hands-on training in ultrasound, as with any new skill, is best learned with a knowledgeable proctor. Fortunately, as ultrasound is a completely noninvasive entity with no known adverse bioeffects, a user can "practice" with known anatomy or pathology until they are comfortable with their skills, should a live proctor be unavailable. This may be the only option to gain competency in certain resource-limited areas of the world. In the case of surgeon-performed ultrasound, as with any surgical practice or skill, at minimum, periodic self-assessment of quality should be assured.

Neck Ultrasound

Ultrasound is an accessible and noninvasive diagnostic tool that often serves as the imaging of choice in the workup, diagnosis, and treatment of various thyroid, parathyroid, and lymphatic pathology. Advances in high-resolution imaging and the improved versatility of ultrasound have led to an exponential increase in point-of-care ultrasound exams [1]. For example, trained individuals can not only rapidly determine whether further workup is warranted, but they can also use the dynamic feedback to assist with procedures including biopsies of the thyroid or lymph nodes, cyst drainage, transcutaneous laryngeal ultrasonography of the vocal folds, and ultrasound-guided ethanol or radiofrequency ablation of thyroid nodules. Furthermore, surgeons often use ultrasound intraoperatively to evaluate for any progression of disease since consultation and to plan the ideal placement for the cervical incision. The focus of this section will be on the use of ultrasound to evaluate the thyroid, the parathyroid glands, and the cervical lymph nodes.

Thyroid

Sonographic evaluation is one of the initial steps in the workup of thyroid disease. A dedicated thyroid ultrasound consists of several components: a description of the thyroid parenchyma (heterogeneity, vascularity), the size of each thyroid lobe (length, width, and height), a description of any thyroid nodules, and an evaluation of the cervical lymph nodes (both central and lateral) [2]. A thorough evaluation of those features can aid in the diagnosis of thyroid nodules, thyroiditis, multinodular goiter, Graves' disease, and malignancy. When evaluating thyroid nodules, there are several important characteristics to note including location, size, echogenicity, composition (solid vs. cystic), vascularity, presence of calcifications, and borders [2, 3]. While certain ultrasound characteristics correlate with a higher risk of malignancy (microcalcifications, taller than wide shape, and irregular borders), the sensitivity of any individual characteristic is less than 70% [3–5]. Consequently, there are two validated ultrasound classification systems that are commonly used to assess and report sonographic features of thyroid nodules and to stratify the risk of malignancy of the nodule.

The American Thyroid Association (ATA) ultrasound classification stratifies thyroid nodules into five different groups: benign, very low suspicion, low suspicion, intermediate suspicion, and high suspicion (Fig. 20.3). Each category correlates to a different risk of malignancy that guides the clinician on whether a fine-needle aspiration (FNA) biopsy is warranted [6–8]. The American College of Radiology developed the Thyroid Imaging Reporting Data System (TI-RADS) in 2012 that utilizes a points-based system to assign nodules to five different categories: benign, minimally suspicious, moderately suspicious, or highly suspicious for malignancy (Fig. 20.4) [2, 9, 10]. While both the ATA and the TI-RADs classification systems have high sensitivity (92% and 74%, respectively), the ATA classification was found to demonstrate more consistent predictions for risk of malignancy among higher-risk nodules [11].

In general, the level of sonographic suspicion will guide the recommendation for a FNA biopsy. However, it is also important to take into account patient risk. For example, if a patient has known risk factors associated with thyroid cancer including exposure to radiation, a family history significant for thyroid cancer, new onset of symptoms (changes in voice), and a rapidly growing nodule,

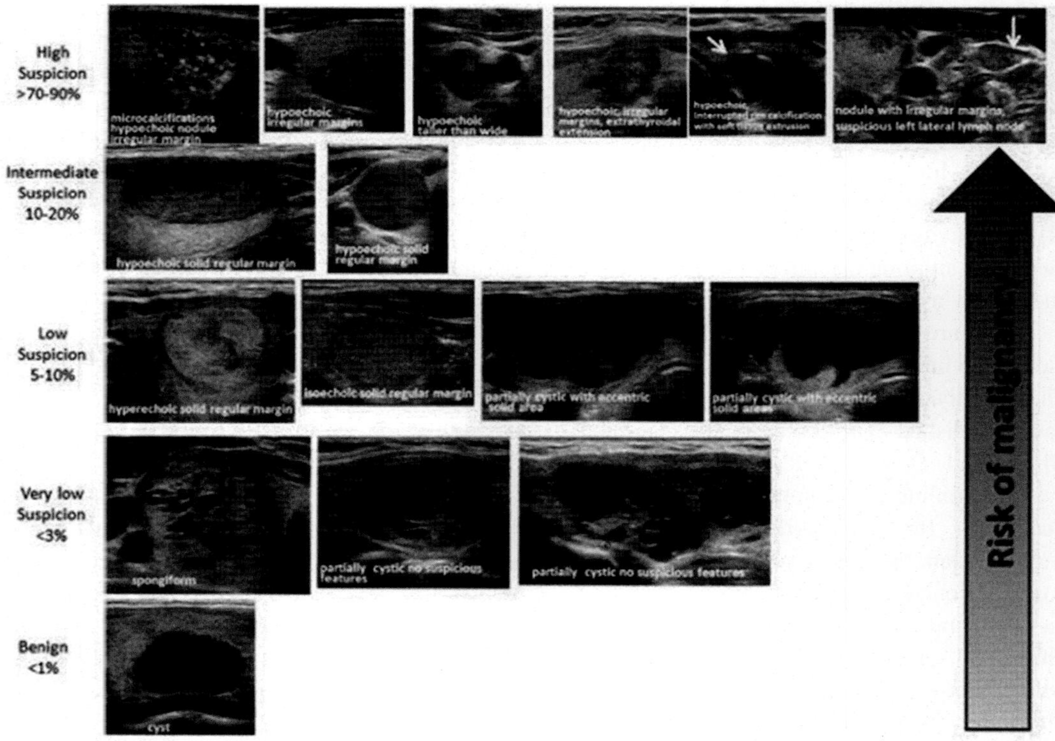

Fig. 20.3 American Thyroid Associate (ATA) ultrasound characteristics and risk of malignancy [2]

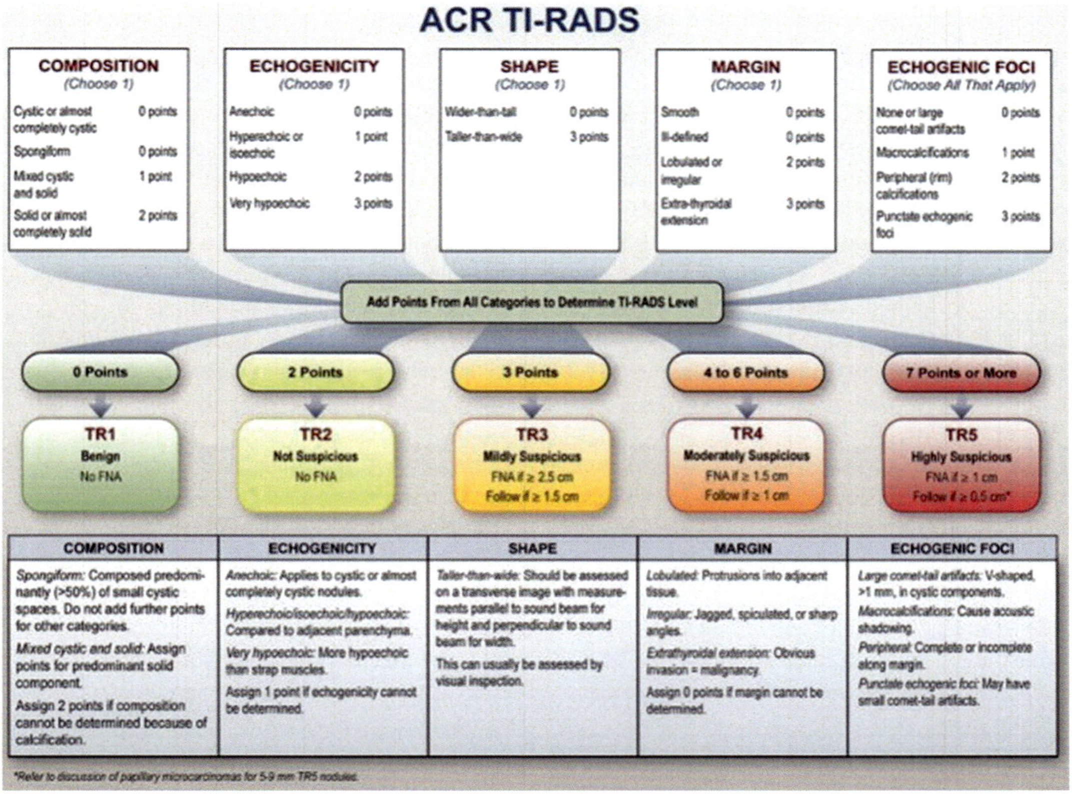

Fig. 20.4 American College of Radiology (ACR) Thyroid Imaging, Reporting and Data System (TI-RADS) [9]

an FNA should be considered at a lower size cutoff in all categories [12].

While the low cost and easy access of ultrasound are largely beneficial in the workup of thyroid nodules, especially in a resource-limited setting, these benefits of ultrasonography can result in an increase in incidental findings that contribute to the burden of overdiagnosis in our healthcare system [9, 13, 14]. Thus, it is imperative to use ultrasound in the neck selectively to help guide the workup and not simply as a routine extension of the physical exam.

Parathyroid

Ultrasound is often utilized for localization of enlarged parathyroid glands in the setting of hyperparathyroidism. Diseased parathyroid glands typically appear hypoechoic and homogeneous and have an extrathyroidal feeding vessel [15]. Although ultrasound is limited in the ability to provide functional information (as with a 99mTc-sestamibi scintigraphy) or anatomic detail for posterior and mediastinal glands (as with a 4DCT scan), one study found that it was the most cost-effective localization strategy [16]. Furthermore, another publication demonstrated that a surgeon performed preoperative ultrasound in a patient with primary hyperparathyroidism had a sensitivity of 76% and specificity of 97% to accurately localize a diseased parathyroid gland(s) [17].

Cervical Lymph Nodes

When evaluating a patient with neck pathology, it is important to perform a complete assessment of the cervical neck lymph nodes. Adults typically have hundreds of lymph nodes in the cervical neck, and fortunately, benign lymph nodes have several classic characteristics: small ovoid/flat shape, clear borders, homogeneous appearance, or echogenic hilum with vascularity (or a preserved "fatty hilum"). On the other hand, suspicious characteristics include a rounded appearance (or a long/short axis ratio < 2), loss of echogenic hilus (loss of fatty hilum), cystic change, ill-defined borders, peripheral vascularity, or calcifications [18]. One study indicated that the loss of a fatty hilum was the most sensitive finding for malignancy at 100%, but with a limited specificity of only 29% [19, 20]. The most specific characteristics for malignancy include cystic degeneration (100%), microcalcifications (100%), and hyperechogenicity (100%) [21]. However, as with thyroid nodules, no single characteristic is predictive of malignancy, and thus the absence of benign features and/or the presence of any suspicious characteristics warrants an FNA biopsy if the nodule measures greater than 8 mm [22].

Furthermore, the location of suspicious lymph nodes in the neck can be suggestive of different pathology. For example, thyroid cancer typically metastasizes to levels II–VI. However, lymphadenopathy in the posterior triangle increases the suspicion for nasopharyngeal carcinoma. If a lymph node is noted in the inferior portion of the deep cervical chain (known as "Virchow's node") with an absence of any lymphadenopathy caudal to that point, this is concerning for a metastasis [18].

Utilization and Training

The National Ultrasound Faculty of the American College of Surgeons offers several ultrasound courses at the annual Clinical Congress for students, residents, and faculty. Courses include an introductory ultrasound course for residents, a focused echocardiography/ICU ultrasound course, and a thyroid, parathyroid, and neck ultrasound course. Participants are required to complete an online course and subsequently gain hands-on experience during the practical session. Fortunately, more institutional-based programs are also being developed in response to the increasing need for clinicians to be proficient at performing diagnostic ultrasound [23, 24]. Still, the accessibility to a training course to learn ultrasound can be a barrier for clinicians in a resource-limited setting. Furthermore, according to the American Institute of Ultrasound in Medicine (AIUM), clinicians need to perform a minimum of 100 diagnostic thyroid, parathyroid, and neck ultrasound examinations to gain proficiency. Additionally, in order to obtain official credentialing, applicants need to document 15 CME credits dedicated to thyroid, parathyroid, and neck ultrasound [25].

Summary

Ultrasound is often the imaging modality of choice in the workup and diagnosis of thyroid, parathyroid, and cervical lymph node disease. The relative low cost and accessibility of ultrasound make it an ideal tool to use, especially in a resource-limited setting. With the ongoing development of ultrasound training programs, healthcare providers can reach proficiency and more effectively utilize this technology in low- to middle-income countries.

Breast Ultrasound

An ultrasound machine and skill set are versatile tools in diagnosing and managing breast symptoms in low-resource settings. It can eliminate an unnecessary visit to the operating room for excisional biopsies as well as guide further treatments and interventions. Having a correct linear probe with center frequency at 12 MHz and knowing how to adjust depth, gain, and focal zone are critical for the diagnosis and management of many breast problems.

Breast Screening

The incidence of breast cancer continues to increase worldwide [26], which is currently the leading cause of cancer-related deaths in females [27]. Screening for breast cancer allows for early detection and improved survival [28]. In Western countries, mammographic screening programs are widely utilized and readily available [27]. Mammography, however, requires specialized infrastructure that includes equipment, personnel, and trained radiologists. In low-resource settings, the infrastructure and expertise requirements may not be feasible on the large scale required to achieve oncologic benefit. Additionally, a trend toward younger age at diagnosis and subsequent denser breast tissue [29] may diminish the sensitivity of mammography [30] in many non-European populations. Ultrasound screening has been explored as an alternative to mammography. Advantages include its portability, lower cost, and potential to utilize trained community health workers for initial assessment rather than radiologists [27]. It can be a part of widespread asymptomatic screening [31] or utilized as part of specific programs that target high-risk or symptomatic populations [32]. A meta-analysis by Sood et al. [27] demonstrates an overall acceptable pooled sensitivity of 80.1% and a specificity of 88.4%.

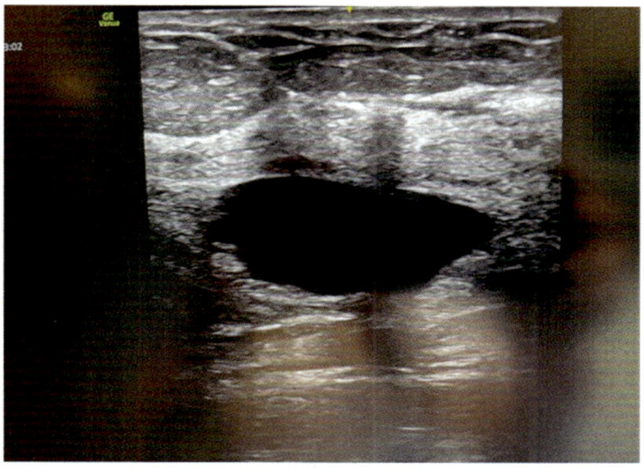

Fig. 20.5 Cyst with anechoic interior with regular borders, wider than tall appearance

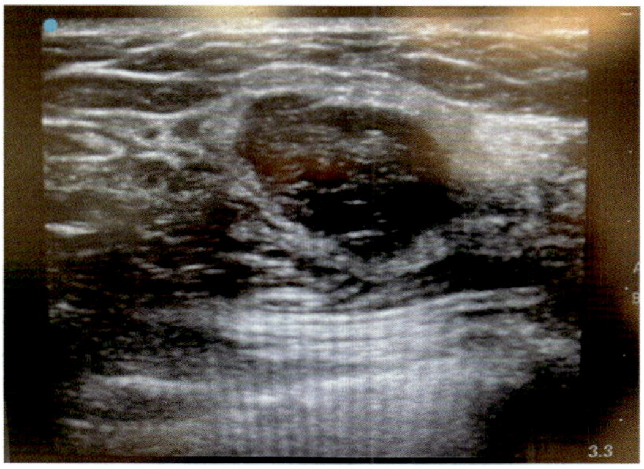

Fig. 20.6 Fibroadenoma with macrolobulations around the border and hypoechoic lesion of the breast

Palpable Mass

Focused ultrasound can be used for palpable breast masses to differentiate between cystic and solid lesions. Completely anechoic, collapsible, round lesions (Fig. 20.5) in an otherwise low-risk patient is a simple cyst that can be observed or, if symptomatic, can be aspirated by giving a small amount of 1% lidocaine and aspirating with a 22G needle until the cyst collapses. When clear, straw or green-colored fluid is obtained, it can be discarded as concordant and benign. The patient is usually counseled that there is a possibility of cyst recurrence in these situations. However, they are reassured by the benign nature of the palpable mass, and in symptomatic patients, immediate relief is usually observed. Bloody fluid aspirate should be sent to cytology for testing by preparing slides or rinsed in a container with CytoLyt® or formalin fluid. A clip or marker can be placed at the site of a bloody cyst to mark the area for future surgeries if needed. These cysts may need excisional biopsies to get a full diagnosis or at least observed with repeat ultrasound in 3 to 6 months.

For solid lesions seen as hypoechoic, other characteristics such as borders of the lesion and shadowing, together with patient risk assessment, help determine whether a lesion should be biopsied [33]. In an otherwise, young patient with a lack of family history of breast cancer, a wider than tall, hypoechoic lesion with regular borders is usually fibroadenomas (Fig. 20.6) and can be safely observed. For lesions with irregular borders, shadowing, or rapid growth or patients with a significant family history of breast cancer, ultrasound-assisted core biopsy can be performed. Once the pathology concordance is achieved, no further observation is needed for fibroadenomas. Discordant lesions should proceed with excisional biopsies or observed with repeat scans in 3 and 6 months.

Nipple Discharge

Another use of breast ultrasound is to evaluate patients with nipple discharge. In patients who present with pathologic nipple discharge, ultrasound of the retroareolar region may identify papillomas or a malignant lesion as the source of the discharge. Ultrasound-guided biopsies of these lesion can help diagnose a patient and prepare the patient for definitive surgery.

Inflammatory Disease

The most common use of ultrasound in breast care is to evaluate inflammatory diseases such as an abscess and cellulitis in the context of clinical presentations. Abscesses appear as a hypoechoic collection without vascularity with a thickened rim and increased echogenicity of breast parenchyma reflecting edema and inflammation [34]. Aspiration of the abscess with an 18G needle after local anesthesia under ultrasound is recommended for most deep abscesses [35]. In the situation where inflammatory breast cancer is considered, biopsy of the tissue or skin punch biopsy should be obtained.

Axillary Ultrasound

Particularly important in patients who are already diagnosed with malignancy is an axillary ultrasound during preoperative workup where up to 50% of positive metastatic node involvement can be detected [36]. For patients with a palpable axillary node, ultrasound can aid with biopsy to avoid injury to vascular structures. Findings of an irregular node with a thickened cortex should be biopsied to further stage the patient (Fig. 20.7). If the node has metastatic disease, patients may be a better candidate for neoadjuvant treatment rather than upfront surgery to downstage the disease in axilla. This can avoid challenging surgical situations in the operating room, perhaps avoid complete axillary dissection if there is no residual disease after neoadjuvant treatment, and decrease the risk of lymphedema for the patient. In addition to the axilla, ultrasound can also evaluate palpable cervical and supraclavicular nodes and biopsy as needed based on clinical exam.

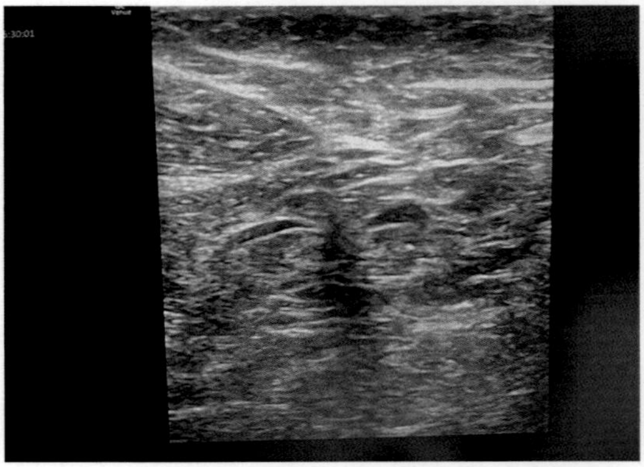

Fig. 20.7 Normal-appearing lymph node with intact hilum and thin cortex

Within a similar anatomic region, ultrasound can be utilized in breast care by providing regional blocks for surgeries such as pectoral I and II blocks in the perioperative setting for pain control [37].

Breast Ultrasound Certification

In the United States, the American Society of Breast Surgeons offers training courses and certification to surgeons, which are also accepted by the American College of Radiology. A minimum of 1-year experience with documented performance of at least 100 breast ultrasound exams among others is required before taking a written exam and submitting cases for the certification process.

Thoracic Ultrasound

An obvious application of ultrasound in the thoracic cavity is of course echocardiography, a complex and unique practice. With the exception of assessment for pericardial effusion, the heart is not commonly under the purview of the general surgeon. Yet this region of the body also houses organs that can fall under the practice of the general surgeon (and surgical intensivist). In particular, diagnosis and treatment of pneumothorax, hemothorax, pleural effusion, and even pulmonary contusions and rib fractures are all facilitated with ultrasound.

As the ribs are acoustic barriers, one must choose a small footprint transducer to image between the ribs to see into the thoracic cavity. Air also has a significant acoustic impedance mismatch from soft tissues, but this can be a diagnostic advantage.

Ultrasound can often be utilized quicker than conventional X-ray to detect a pneumothorax. Indeed, in experienced hands, ultrasound should be able to detect 90–100% of pneumothoraces [38]. Ideally, the patient should be sitting up about 30 degrees. The examiner starts with the lung apices, in the second rib interspace, because in the upright position this is most likely where air will accumulate. Start from the probe-skin interface, the first structure noted in the chest wall musculature. Distal to that is the pleura. The parietal and visceral pleura normally slide against each other, lubricated by a small amount of fluid. This sliding motion can be visualized with ultrasound and is often described as "ants marching" along the pleural interface (Fig. 20.8a). The dynamic advantage of ultrasound makes this even more apparent during the real-time ultrasound exam. If the image depth is too large, artefactual "A-lines" will be seen, which are reverberation echoes of the pleural line. In the case of a pneumothorax, air between the pleural surfaces prohibits this sliding motion, where the absence of motion can be detected with cine ultrasound. It is important to be aware that pleural sliding may also be absent in patients with lung damage from COPD or pleurisy, even if no pneumothorax is present. Finally, multiple interspaces must be evaluated to increase the accuracy of diagnosing NO pneumothorax.

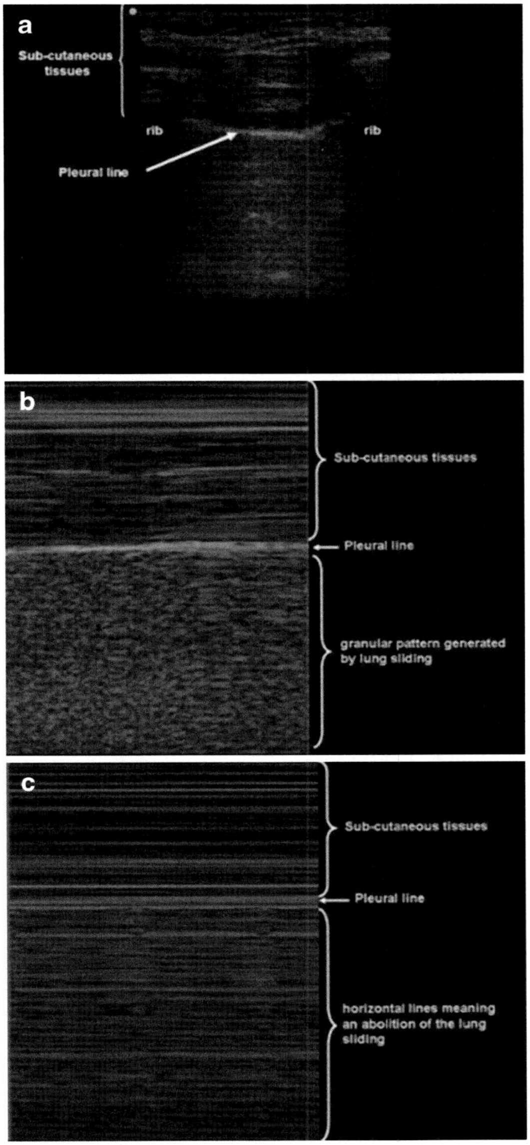

Fig. 20.8 (**a**) B-mode image of chest. The first layers seen are the musculocutaneous layers of the chest wall, followed by a hyperechoic pleural line. In the real-time view, the pleural sliding movement is more apparent and likened to "ants marching." (**b**) M-mode image of normal lung, where the chest wall (at the top of the M-mode) appears as waves, and the pleurae appear as grains of sand, due to the slight motion of normal pleural sliding. (**c**) M-mode image of a pneumothorax, where the grainy appearance of normal sliding pleurae is lost and replaced by a more defined appearance of lines or bars ("bar code sign") [39]

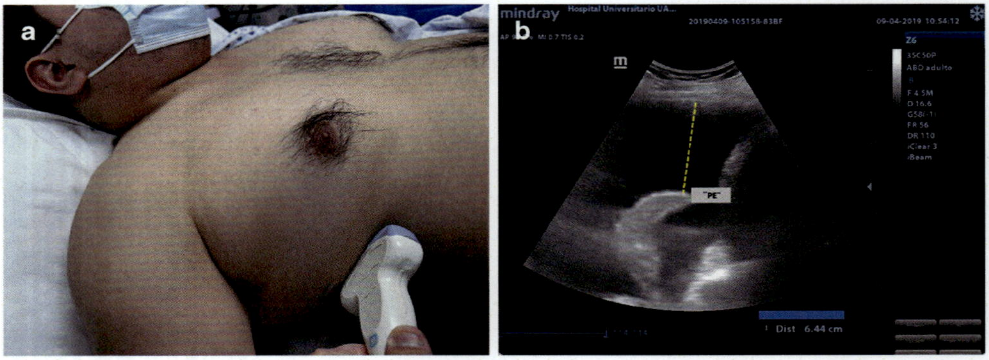

Fig. 20.9 (**a**) Probe position to obtain B-mode image at right. (**b**) Two-dimensional B-mode image of patient with pleural effusion. The hyperechoic structure is a partially collapsed lung. The yellow dotted line is spanning one axis of the fluid volume [40]

Further evaluation for pneumothorax can be quickly assessed by switching to M mode, which will characterize the motion of the lung with respect to the chest wall. In M mode, starting at the surface of the transducer, the pattern of the stationary chest wall looks like ocean waves. Deep to that, the motion of pleural sliding produces a grainy pattern similar to the appearance of sand on a beach (Fig. 20.8b). These findings are often described as the "seashore sign." In the case of a pneumothorax, the pleura is not moving, and the grains of sand are not present. Instead, a continued series of horizontal lines continues deep to the chest wall (the "stratosphere sign") (Fig. 20.8c). This is also referred to a "bar code pattern."

To assess for a pleural effusion, if at all possible (i.e., no spinal injury or mechanical ventilation), it is best to have the patient sit up to allow for fluid to accumulate at the lung bases. Alternatively, placement of the patient in the lateral decubitus position is preferable to a supine position. The ultrasound probe should be placed below the 11th rib in the midaxillary line for assessment of an effusion. The diaphragm should be apparent as a bright white line, and fluid if present can be seen as hypoechoic density above the diaphragm (Fig. 20.9). The lung may also be more hyperechoic than normal if it is collapsed. If fluid is visualized, a needle, wire, and/or catheter can all be placed under direct ultrasound visualization for drainage.

Ultrasound in the Emergent Setting

Its portability and ease of use make ultrasound an invaluable tool in the assessment for surgical emergencies. In this section, we will discuss more common scenarios including FAST exam, acute cholecystitis, acute appendicitis, and assessment for abdominal aortic aneurysm. In addition, tips for ultrasound-guided procedures such as percutaneous drainage of abscesses, ascites, or placement of cholecystostomy tube are reviewed.

Trauma

Blunt or penetrating trauma with potential for thoracoabdominal injury presents a scenario where speed of diagnosis and treatment is of the essence. Central to the sonographic evaluation for trauma is the FAST exam, or Focused Assessment with Sonography for Trauma. This is a simple-to-perform tool that will evaluate for free fluid in the anatomic spaces of the abdomen as well as the pericardial space. Unlike CT scan, this can be performed at the bedside or even in the field. Unlike diagnostic peritoneal lavage, ultrasound is noninvasive and of similar accuracy (and arguably a more thorough assessment as the pericardial space is also evaluated).

The FAST exam consists of four components or views (Fig. 20.10). These need not be com-

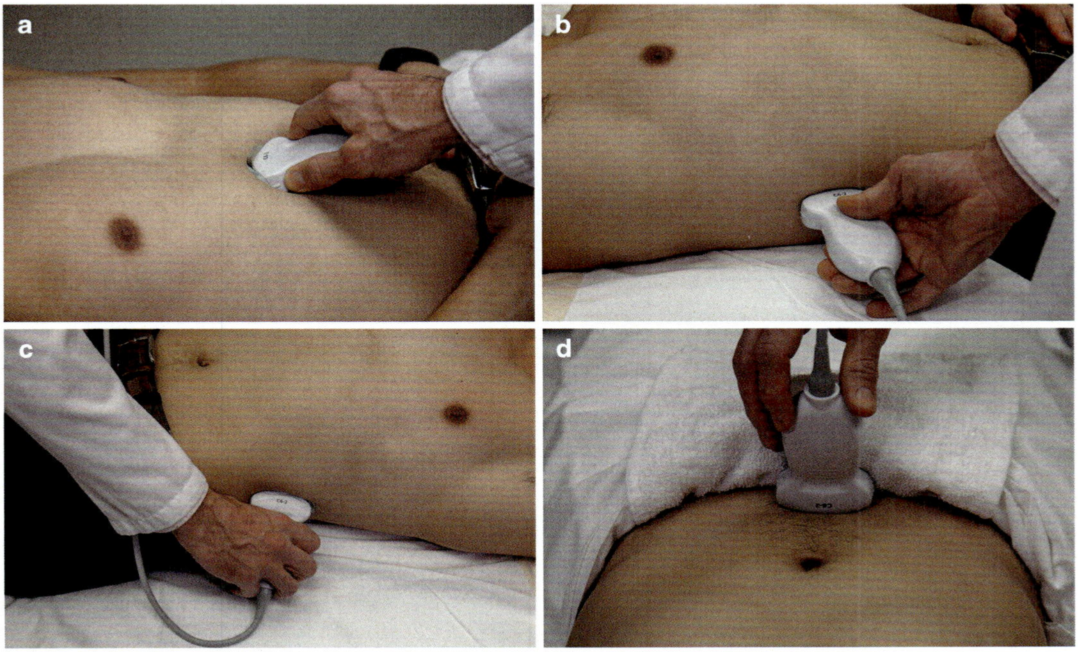

Fig. 20.10 Probe positions for FAST exam. (**a**) Subxiphoid cardiac view. (**b**) Right upper quadrant view. (**c**) Left upper quadrant view. (**d**) Suprapubic view [39]

pleted in any particular order. Approximately 200 cc of fluid is the minimum detectable volume. The "E-FAST" exam consists of additional views to assess the pleural spaces for free fluid.

First, starting in the right upper quadrant, we are looking for fluid in Morrison's pouch. In a non-fasting patient where bowel gas may interfere with transmission of acoustic energy more anteriorly, an excellent approach is to place the probe at the right anterior axillary line, between the 10th and 11th ribs. This allows the acoustic energy to transmit through the liver directly to the right kidney. If there is an intact interface between these two structures, as indicated by a white line, there is no free fluid (Fig. 20.11). In contrast, a hypoechoic area seen between the liver and the kidney is diagnostic of free fluid in Morrison's pouch (Fig. 20.12). The right inferior pleural can also be evaluated by directing the probe cephalad, looking for the hyperechoic right hemidiaphragm. A hypoechoic density signifying fluid present on the thoracic side of the diaphragm is a pleural effusion. Moving the probe slightly will allow one to discern the pitfall of the mirror image artifact, where reverberation echoes from

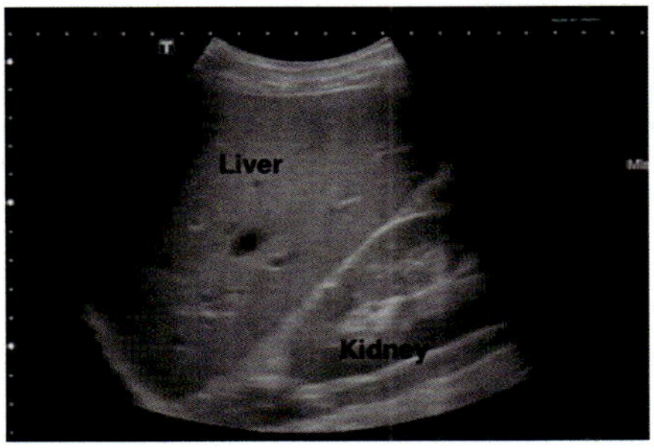

Fig. 20.11 B-mode image of a normal hepatorenal space

the liver may appear as if they are coming from the other (thoracic) side of the diaphragm.

The second view of the FAST exam is obtained in the left upper quadrant, to examine the splenorenal space. Similarly to the previously described view, the probe is placed on the left side at the mid-axillary line, between the tenth and 11th ribs (or even one interspace above). The goal is an image with the spleen-left kidney interface. Similar to Morrison's pouch, a thin hyperechoic interface between the kidney and spleen signifies a negative exam (Fig. 20.13), while a wider hypoechoic area between the kidney and spleen is diagnostic of free fluid (Fig. 20.14). The left

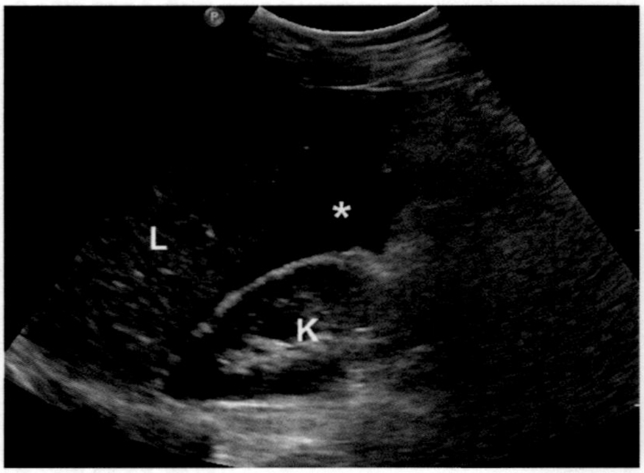

Fig. 20.12 B-mode image of positive FAST exam in the right upper quadrant. The hypoechoic signal between the liver and kidney (*) represents free intraabdominal fluid [41]

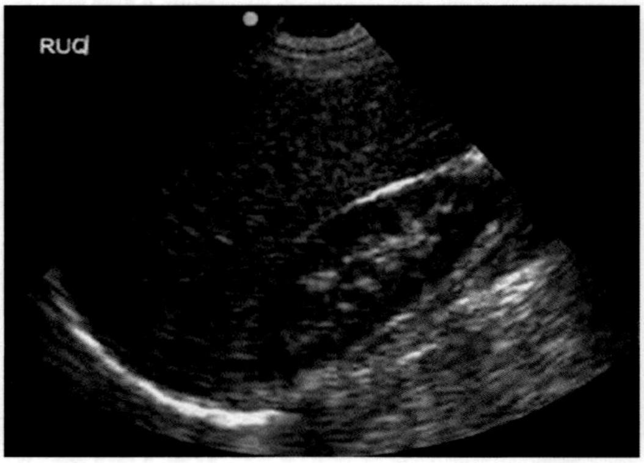

Fig. 20.13 B-mode image of normal left upper quadrant view of FAST exam

pleural space can also be evaluated by angling the

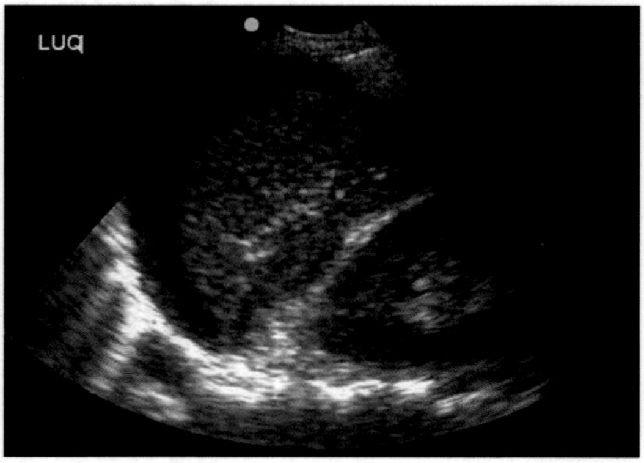

Fig. 20.14 B-mode image of left upper quadrant view showing free fluid in splenorenal space

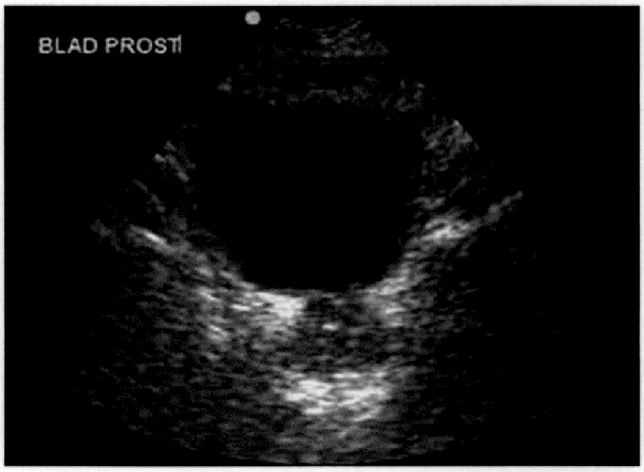

Fig. 20.15 Normal B-mode image of FAST exam, pelvic view

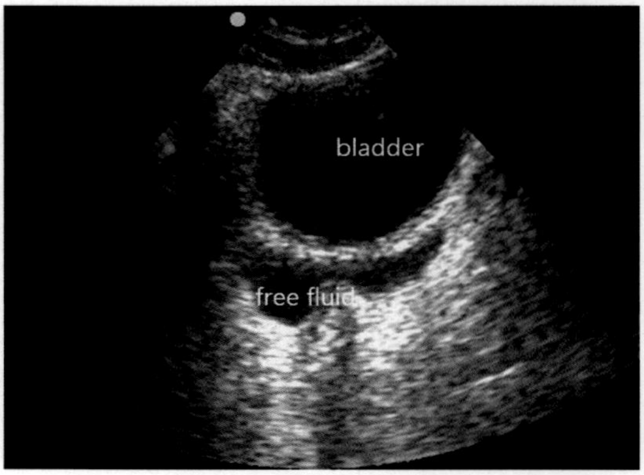

Fig. 20.16 Positive FAST exam, pelvic view

probe cephalad, directing the ultrasound through the spleen and left hemi-diaphragm.

Third is the evaluation of the pelvis. This is aided by a full bladder, so if a catheter is present, sterile saline may be instilled in the bladder (roughly 200 cc) and the catheter clamped for the duration of the exam. This avoids mirror image artifacts in the pelvis, resulting from strong echoes from the sacrum. The probe is placed in the suprapubic position and oriented posteriorly to inferiorly. With a relatively full bladder, that should be the only fluid-filled structure seen (Fig. 20.15). A positive FAST in the pelvis is the appearance of two fluid-filled structures in the pelvis, the bladder, and a pelvic fluid collection (Fig. 20.16).

Finally, the pericardial space is assessed. Placing the ultrasound probe in the subxiphoid position, orient it toward the left shoulder. A comprehensive cross-sectional view of the ventricles and atria is not required here; one simply needs to view a section of the ventricular myocardium. Normally, the myocardium is a soft tissue density surrounded by a subtle hyperechoic pericardium (Fig. 20.17). A pericardial effusion appears as a hypoechoic area between the myocardium and the pericardium (Fig. 20.18).

The Acute Abdomen

Central to evaluation for acute abdominal pain is of course physical examination, and holding an ultrasound probe in the hand can certainly be considered an extension of the physical exam. With some practice, numerous areas and pathologies can be evaluated with ultrasound. Imaging transhepatically to avoid interference from bowel gas, the gallbladder is easily evaluated for shadowing gallstones, pericholecystic fluid, and a thickened gallbladder wall, signs pathognomic for acute cholecystitis (Fig. 20.19). Moving to the right lower quadrant, placing the probe at McBurney's point, one can assess for a thickened appendix (Fig. 20.20), diagnostic of acute appendicitis. Accepted criteria for diagnosing acute appendicitis by ultrasound is the identification of an enlarged and noncompressible appendix, with its outer anteroposterior diameter under compression, measured in the transverse plane, of >6 mm.

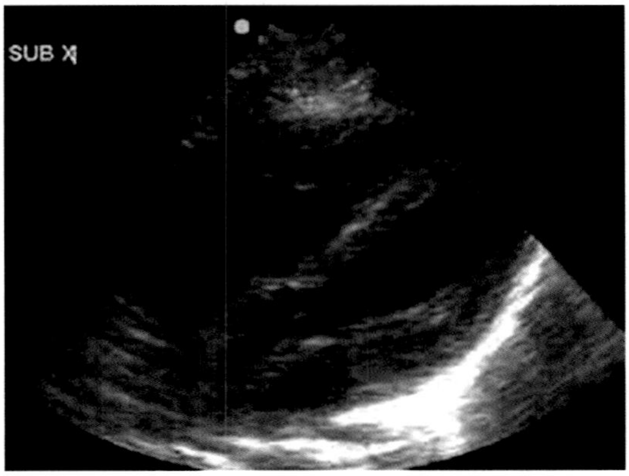

Fig. 20.17 Normal pericardial view of FAST exam

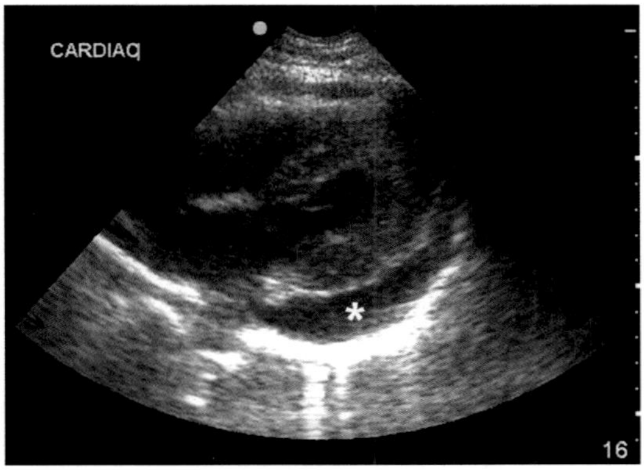

Fig. 20.18 Pericardial effusion detected with FAST exam. The asterisk (*) denotes fluid in the pericardial sac

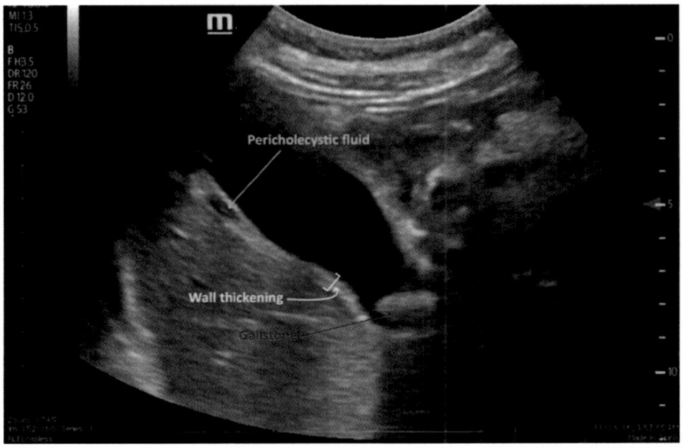

Fig. 20.19 B-mode image of acute cholecystitis. Note pericholecystic fluid and wall thickening indicative of edema and inflammation, as well as a gallstone impacted in the neck of the gallbladder [42]

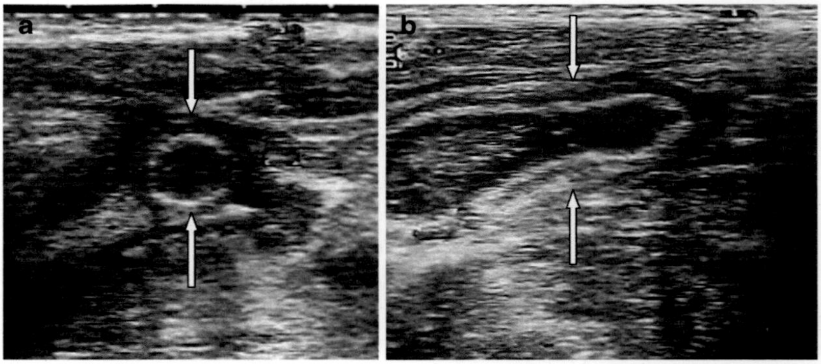

Fig. 20.20 B-mode image of acute appendicitis. Under compression with the probe, the maximal diameter of the appendix was measured to be 11 mm, meeting criteria for acute appendicitis. (**a**) transverse view; (**b**) longitudinal view [43]

Although the assessment of a normal aorta can be difficult in the non-fasting patient due to overlying bowel gas from an anterior approach, an abdominal aortic aneurysm can be quite apparent, particularly in a thin person. Lateral views are also worth attempting, as an enlarged aorta will push surrounding structures out of the way. The goal of the ultrasound exam is to identify the location of maximal aortic dilatation in the longitudinal plane and then to measure the diameter in the transverse plane. Diameters greater than 3 cm are considered aneurysmal (Fig. 20.21). Additionally, it is also useful to assess for evidence of leaking blood by the presence of free fluid around the aneurysm with the aid of the duplex setting.

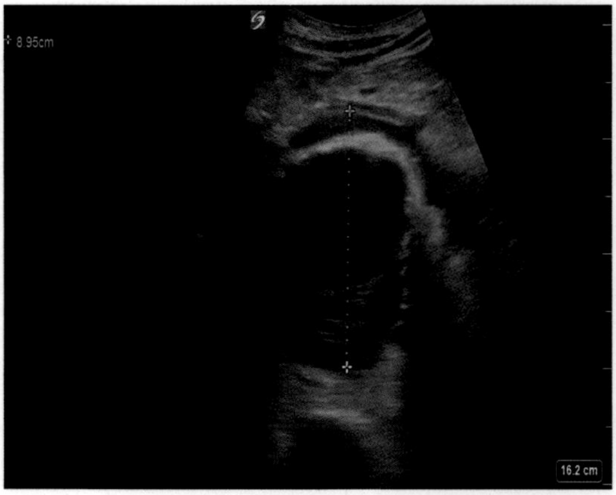

Fig. 20.21 Transverse view of abdominal aorta measuring 8.95 cm in anterior-posterior diameter at its largest point. The aneurysm had an anechoic center with echogenic material in the posterior lumen, representing cholesterol deposit. Free fluid was seen anterior to the aneurysm suggestive of rupture [44]

Ultrasound-Guided Procedures

Ultrasound can greatly facilitate many different types of procedures, including vascular access or drainage procedures. The target, whether it be a vein, an abscess, or an acutely inflamed and distended gallbladder, for example, can be visualized as the intervention is being performed. If at all possible, the instrument (needle, guidewire, catheter) can be imaged "in-plane," where the probe is held such that the needle, as it travels through the tissue, is visualized along its entire path (Fig. 20.22). If anatomy doesn't permit (structures such as ribs interfering), the target is imaged, and the needle is seen entering it only. To facilitate the early learner, needle guides for attachment to the probe are available, though as one gains experience, they tend to become more of a nuisance than helpful.

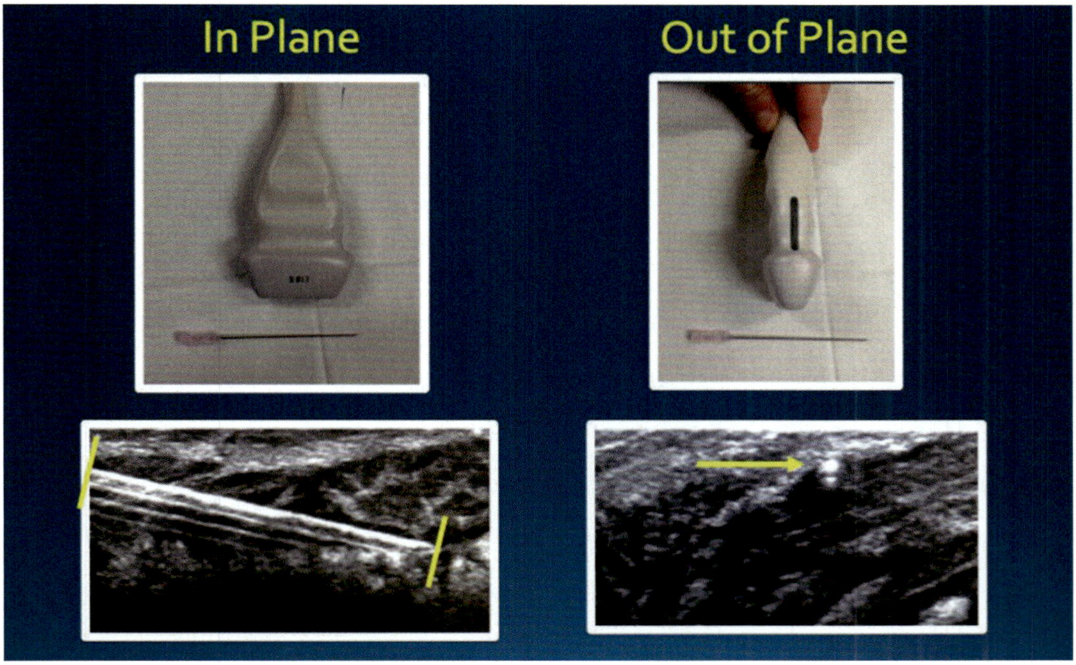

Fig. 20.22 In-plane versus out-of-plane imaging for ultrasound-guided procedures. Note the reverberation artifact of the entire needle in the in-plane approach, versus visualization of only a small cross-section of needle with the out of plane technique (This work is licensed under the Creative Commons Attribution 4.0 International License. To view a copy of this license, visit http://creativecommons.org/licenses/by/4.0/ or send a letter to Creative Commons, PO Box 1866, Mountain View, CA 94042, USA)

Abdominal Surgical Ultrasound

Ultrasound in the surgeon's hands can be invaluable for more precise and safe operations. Beyond diagnostic imaging, adding ultrasound to the surgeon's armamentarium guides interventions both in the operating room and at the bedside. This enables efficient and economical care, which is particularly imperative in resource-limited settings.

Liver Resection

Direct application of the transducer to the liver surface intraoperatively affords high-resolution images to be attained without signal attenuation from intervening tissue such as abdominal wall and/or air. When available, the surgeon may use intraoperative ultrasound to identify tumors deep in liver parenchyma that are not palpable. Typically, the surgeon will identify tumor margins and use this information to mark a parenchymal transection line, ensuring microscopic margin clearance (R0 resection). Often, sterile covers for the ultrasound probes are not available in low-resource centers. In these cases, we will still be able to utilize intraoperative ultrasound by placing the probes, along with acoustic gel, in a sterile surgical glove (Fig. 20.23).

Ablative Therapies

Ablation has become accepted as an alternative to resection for hepatic and renal tumors in appropriate cases. In the liver, ablative therapies have found application for hepatocellular carcinomas and colorectal liver metastases. The two most commonly utilized energy sources are microwave ablation and radiofrequency ablation. Although both techniques utilize differing energy

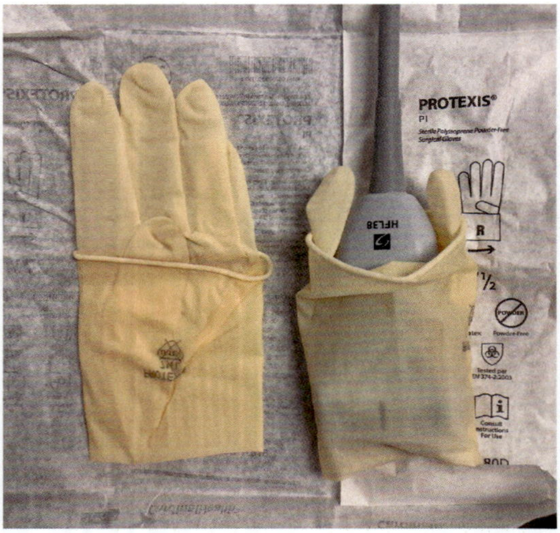

Fig. 20.23 Practice in resource-limited settings sometimes requires flexibility and ingenuity. In this case, a sterile surgical glove substitutes for a sterile probe cover for intraoperative ultrasound

sources, the ultimate aim is thermal destruction of all tissues in contact with the ablation antenna. Therefore, the antenna must be accurately placed within the center of the target lesion. This is often done by image guidance, either with CT guidance by our radiology colleagues or via intraoperative ultrasound (Fig. 20.24) in the operating room with a surgeon. Dedicated interventional suites may not be readily available in resource-limited regions, so the option for surgeon-performed procedures is an attractive one in these settings.

Targeted Biopsy

Ultrasound can be used to guide intraoperative biopsies for tumors that are difficult to target solely by palpation. As discussed in another part of this chapter, ultrasound-guided breast biopsy

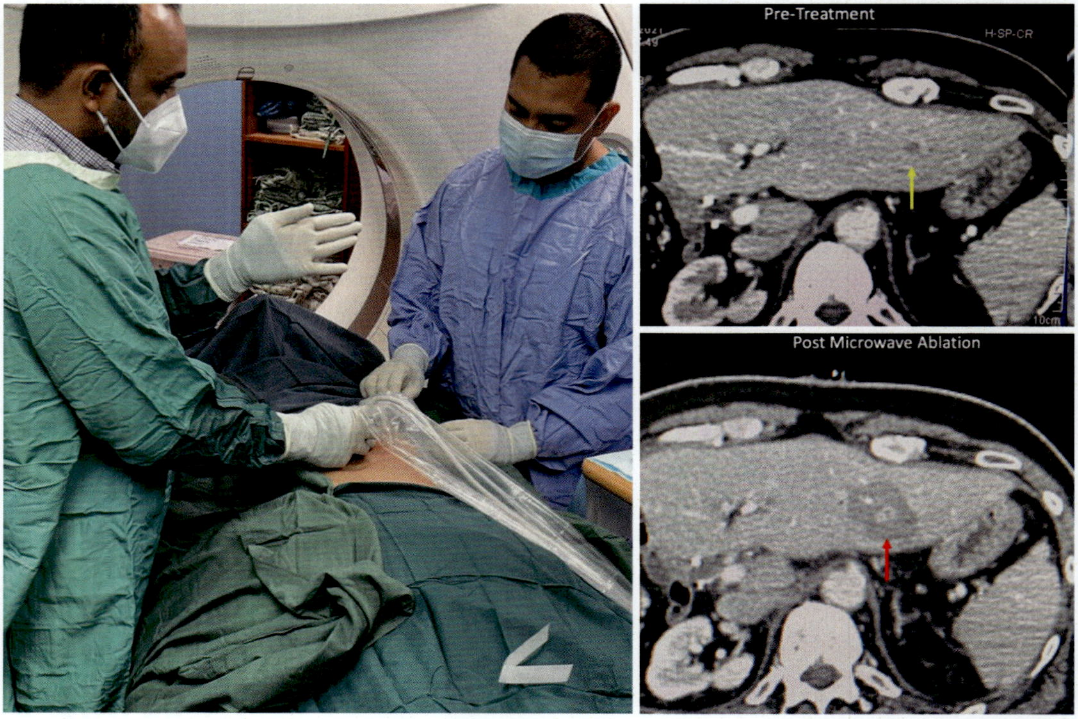

Fig. 20.24 Combined use of ultrasound and CT targeting during microwave ablation of colorectal liver metastases to the left hemi-liver. Inset: pre-ablation (yellow arrow) and post-ablation (red arrow) CT images are seen

has been shown to be superior to palpation-guided breast biopsy in terms of sensitivity, false negative rates, and repeat biopsy rates [45]. Targeted biopsies of the liver, kidneys, lymph nodes, prostate, and other miscellaneous lesions can be done under local anesthesia and with same day discharge.

Laparoscopic Ultrasound

Ultrasound can also be used at laparoscopic surgery with dedicated laparoscopic probes. These are usually specially configured linear array probes with ≤10 mm diameter that can pass through 12 mm laparoscopic ports, with a working shaft length of 35–40 cm to allow access to the viscera. The tip of the probe typically has multiple degrees of freedom to allow optimal scanning angles (Fig. 20.25). These modified laparoscopic probes usually operate at frequencies of 5–7.5 MHz with depth penetration from 4 to 10 cm [46]. In these cases, the ultrasound is usually operated by surgeons as radiologists may find it difficult to organize dedicated time in the operating room. Surgeons may have less exposure to the principles of ultrasound use during their surgical postgraduate training, and this exposure/training would normally be attained during fellowship training or post-training mentorship.

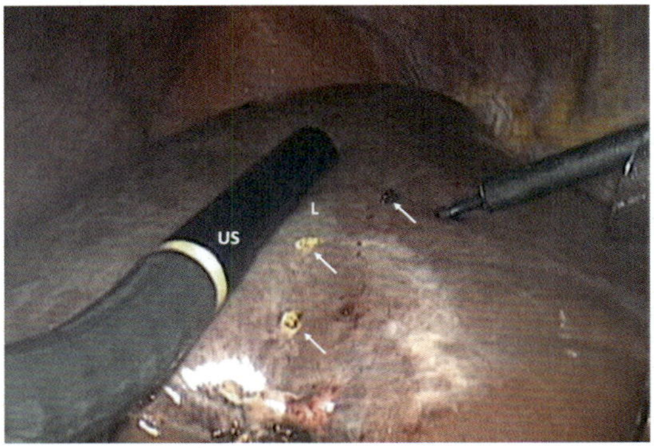

Fig. 20.25 Intraoperative use of a laparoscopic ultrasound probe (US) during liver resection. The instrument is flexed to maintain contact with the liver surface (L) and produce optimal scanning angles. Electrocautery is being used simultaneously to score the liver capsule (arrow), while intraoperative ultrasound ensures adequate resection margins

When available, laparoscopic ultrasound can be used as an adjunct to staging laparoscopy for a variety of malignancies, with only a few minutes of additional operating time and no increase in perioperative complications [47]. Diagnostic laparoscopy with laparoscopic ultrasound has been shown to upstage esophageal/gastric cancer patients in up to 40% of cases and prevent non-therapeutic laparotomy in 25% of cases [48, 49]. Laparoscopic ultrasound has been shown to increase the accuracy of staging in patients with hepatocellular carcinomas and colorectal liver metastases, with up to 20% of patients having additional lesions detected when compared to their preoperative CT scans [50, 51] and with management changes in up to 40% of cases [52]. Existing data suggests that laparoscopic ultrasound has 75–90% specificity and 80–100% sensitivity for staging in patients diagnosed with colorectal liver metastases and hepatocellular carcinomas [53, 54]. There is also value in patients with pancreatic adenocarcinomas, where vascular invasion and/or liver metastases may be detected, preventing non-therapeutic laparotomies in up to 30% of patients [55–58]. Laparoscopic ultrasound to evaluate periampullary carcinomas has been reported to have 85–100% diagnostic accuracy [56, 57, 59] and better sensitivity than CT scans to identify liver metastases, vascular encasement, and nodal involvement [59].

Laparoscopic ultrasound has also found application in patients without malignancies. It has been used as an adjunct to guide liver biopsies, resect giant hepatic cysts, identify bile duct anatomy, and detect common duct stones. The advantage is that it avoids the need for catheterization of the biliary system, prevents radiation exposure, reduces cost, and requires less time than intraoperative cholangiography [60, 61]. Current reports suggest that laparoscopic ultrasound has 90–96% sensitivity, 100% specificity, 98% positive predictive value, and 92% negative predictive value to detect choledocholithiasis [60–62]. A drawback is that the diagnostic yield is heavily user-dependent and has a steep learning curve.

While there is useful application in laparoscopic surgery, its use remains limited in the resource-poor nations for numerous possible reasons: (1) Dedicated laparoscopic probes (even entire ultrasound units reserved for the operating room) may not be universally available. (2) Operating room and biomedical engineering staff may be unfamiliar with the ultrasound machine for cleaning, sterilization, and maintenance. Surgeons would require additional training in imaging techniques, scanning parameters, and recognition of anatomic landmarks or subtle pathologic abnormalities.

Training and Certification

Often in severely resource-limited areas or low-income countries, training in new technologies is dependent on the movement of surgeons, either an experienced surgeon coming to mentor trainees or a local surgeon travelling for a mini-fellowship or training session elsewhere. Certainly, these expensive and time-consuming movements can be somewhat mitigated by online educational programs, which may be viewed prior to travel and hands-on training. Strategies for training and attainment of competency are addressed forthwith.

Skills and Equipment Acquisition in Resource-Limited Settings

It is readily apparent that ultrasound is a highly appropriate choice for surgeons and others in resource-limited settings. Lack of availability of even rudimentary equipment and training, as well as ongoing technical support, has made adoption difficult [53, 64]. There are success stories, however, to learn from [65–67]. Although most reported literature focusses on emergency ultrasound, surgeons may fall under a similar rubric and indeed are arguably more accustomed to adopting new skills than their medical counterparts.

Training

In 2016, Salmon et al. [65] suggested a framework for initiating and maintaining ultrasound curricula and practices on the African continent. Foremost is the integration of an ultrasound curriculum into residency programs. As with any new skill or technology, it is often the academic centers that pave the way forward for widespread adoption. "Champions," those who undertake dedicated training and integrate new skills into their practice, are the backbone of integrating new skills into residency programs. Once a program has been initiated, attention to continuing medical education and longitudinal training is paramount. Shared resources for training as well as durable equipment across a region is an important consideration, to ensure equitable access for all. Finally, regional standards for resource-limited locales can be based on accepted standards adopted from high-income countries.

For non-residency associated training, a review of the available literature [68] suggests that a short but intensive training period is sufficient for preparing clinical officers, nurses, and physicians alike to perform basic ultrasound exams. The more successful training program includes both lecture and practical experience and provides opportunity for continued upkeep of skills through review sessions and ongoing quality assurance after the training period ends.

Particularly for ongoing support, SonoWorld is a group of medical professionals launched in 1999 to provide free educational materials to ultrasound practitioners in developing countries around the world (https://www.sonoworld.com). With more than 170,000 registered members and over 150,000 monthly visits, SonoWorld reaches more ultrasound professionals worldwide than any other communication channel. The site has also become the world's largest single repository of ultrasound-related educational materials. With over 450 streaming video lectures by the most widely recognized authorities in the world, clinical cases, textbook chapters, and a wide range of other educational and informational materials, all free and readily accessible from anywhere in the world, SonoWorld is an excellent resource for basic and continuing education in ultrasound.

The explosion of telehealth options in the developed world is relevant to at least the issues of training and credentialing, as well as ongoing skills assessment. It has been suggested that images captured by non-physicians can theoretically be remotely transmitted to physicians anywhere in the world and successfully utilized to expand care [69] and assure quality control. Although randomized control studies are scarce for this scenario, one might argue that rapid adoption in parallel to data acquisition and analysis is reasonable given the extreme lack of resources in certain parts of the world.

Equipment Acquisition

In addition to access to operator training, equipment acquisition and maintenance can be a barrier to adoption of ultrasound in resource-challenged settings. This is due in part to financial constraints and in part to general lack of infrastructure and support. Fortunately, a growing movement among ultrasound equipment manufacturers is the development of lower-cost, "pared-down" equipment targeted to the developing world [70].

The Butterfly Network, a Connecticut-based company, launched its portable ultrasound prototype known as the Butterfly iQ in 2017 (https://www.butterflynetwork.com). The device costs approximately $2400 and is around the same size as a cell phone. The company's founder, Jonathan Rothberg, has donated scanners to multiple low-income countries as part of its Global Health Program, partnering with organizations such as Access Afya, Bridge to Health, MedGlobal, NYAGI, and others. The organization also has backing from external supporters such as USAID (United States Agency for International Development) and the Bill and Melinda Gates Foundation to help further its reach.

Installed in over 100 countries, GE Healthcare's Vscan also offers an affordable and portable solution for remote and resource-limited areas (https://handheldultrasound.gehealthcare.com). Starting at around $4500, the basic unit comprises of a wireless, two-sided probe coupled with a display the size of a smartphone.

California-based SonoQue offers a range of solutions in the form of iPhone/iPad-compatible transducers ranging from $1350 to $4400 (https://www.sonoque.com). Each wireless transducer relies on built-in WiFi, so no access to the Internet is necessary. Multiple probes are available to choose from, including a premium dual-head probe for maximum flexibility.

Clarius has developed a similar wireless probe technology compatible with both Apple and Android devices (https://www.clarius.com). This unit has been cleared for sale in many countries throughout the world, including developing nations. The units start at around $3000 and include a unique "endocavity" option. Purchase includes 60 min of 1:1 instruction; buying the membership option includes in-app video tutorials and availability of second opinion via telemedicine.

Similarly, Philips, a leader in hospital-based systems, offers its own portable ultrasound platform in Lumify (https://www.usa.philips.com/healthcare/sites/lumify/tele-ultrasound-solution). Here they partnered with (and recently acquired) Innovative Imaging Technologies Inc. (IIT), which developed a real-time collaborative tele-ultrasound solution (Reacts). The user of the Lumify system can interact with other Reacts users to share imaging data and seek advice as they are scanning the patient. Multiple different probes are available that connect to a range of compatible tablets including iPads and iPhones.

Summary

Although potentially daunting to the initiate, the adoption of ultrasound in various practices of surgery is an invaluable investment. In combination with online learning and through cooperation with clinical colleagues in other departments, regions, and countries, training, competency, and certification are possible. Equipment that is at a reasonable price point is readily available and often comes with online training and support. Surgeons of various specialties should strongly consider acquiring ultrasound skills and integrating it into their practice, no matter the setting they practice, for pre-, intra-, and postoperative care of their patients.

References

1. McQueen AS, Bhatia KS. Head and neck ultrasound: technical advances, novel applications and the role of elastography. Clin Radiol. 2018;73(1):81–93.
2. Haugen B, Alexander E, Bible K, et al. 2015 American Thyroid Association management guidelines for adult patients with thyroid nodules and differentiated thyroid cancer. Thyroid. 2016;26(1):1–133.
3. Papini E, Guglielmi R, Bianchini A, et al. 2002 Risk of malignancy in nonpalpable thyroid nodules: predictive value of ultrasound and color-Doppler features. J Clin Endocrinol Metab. 2002;87:1941–6.
4. Kwak JY, Han KH, Yoon JH, et al. Thyroid imaging reporting and data system for US features of nodules: a step in establishing better stratification of cancer risk. Radiology. 2011;260:892–9.
5. Moon WJ, Jung SL, Lee JH, et al. Benign and malignant thyroid nodules: US differentiation—multicenter retrospective study. Radiology. 2008;247:762–70.
6. Horvath E, Majlis S, Rossi R, Franco C, Niedmann JP, Castro A. An ultrasonogram reporting system for thyroid nodules stratifying cancer risk for clinical management. J Clin Endocrinol Metab. 2009;94:1748–51.
7. Tae HJ, Lim DJ, Baek KH, et al. Diagnostic value of ultrasonography to distinguish between benign and malignant lesions in the management of thyroid nodules. Thyroid. 2007;17:461–6.
8. Shimura H, Haraguchi K, Hiejima Y, et al. Distinct diagnostic criteria for ultrasonographic examination of papillary thyroid carcinoma: a multicenter study. Thyroid. 2005;15:251–8.
9. Tessler FN, Middleton WD, Grant EG, et al. ACR thyroid imaging, reporting and data system (TI-RADS): white paper of the ACR TI-RADS committee. J Am Coll Radiol. 2017;14:587–95.
10. Nam-Goong IS, Kim HY, Gong G, et al. Ultrasonography-guided fine- needle aspiration of thyroid incidentaloma: correlation with pathological findings. Clin Endocrinol. 2004;60:21–8.
11. Huang BL, Ebner SA, Makkar JS, Bentley-Hibbert S, McConnell RJ, Lee JA, Hecht EM, Kuo JH. A multidisciplinary head-to-head comparison of American College of Radiology Thyroid Imaging and Reporting Data System and American Thyroid Association ultrasound risk stratification systems. Oncologist. 2020;25:398–403.
12. Hamming JF, Goslings BM, van Steenis GJ, van Ravenswaay CH, Hermans J, Van de Velde CJ. The value of fine-needle aspiration biopsy in patients with nodular thyroid disease divided into groups of suspicion of malignant neoplasms on clinical grounds. Arch Intern Med. 1990;150:113–6.
13. Seim NB, Wood CB, Yancey KL, Mannion K, Netterville JL. Head and neck ultrasound in otolaryngology surgical missions. Ear Nose Throat J. 2019;98:535–6.
14. Brito JP, Gionfriddo MR, Al NA, et al. The accuracy of thyroid nodule ultrasound to predict thyroid cancer: systematic review and meta-analysis. J Clin Endocrinol Metab. 2014;99:1253–63.
15. Sung JY. Parathyroid ultrasonography: the evolving role of the radiologist. Ultrasonography. 2015;34:268–74.
16. Lubitz CC, Stephen AE, Hodin RA, Pandharipande P. Preoperative localization strategies for primary hyperparathyroidism: an economic analysis. Ann Surg Oncol. 2012;19:4202–9.
17. Solorzano CC, Carneiro-Pla DM, Irvin GL 3rd. Surgeon-performed ultrasonography as the initial and only localizing study in sporadic primary hyperparathyroidism. J Am Coll Surg. 2006;202:18–24.
18. Stack B, Moreno M. Neck dissection. 1st ed. 2018.
19. Frasoldati A, Valcavi R. Challenges in neck ultrasonography: lymphadenopathy and parathyroid glands. Endocr Pract. 2004;10:261–8.
20. Kuna SK, Bracic I, Tesic V, Kuna K, Herceg GH, Dodig D. Ultrasonographic differentiation of benign from malignant neck lymphadenopathy in thyroid cancer. J Ultrasound Med. 2006;25:1531–7.
21. Leboulleux S, Girard E, Rose M, et al. Ultrasound criteria of malignancy for cervical lymph nodes in patients followed up for differentiated thyroid cancer. J Clin Endocrinol Metab. 2007;92:3590–4.
22. Kuo JH, McManus C, Graves CE, Madani A, Khokhar MT, Huang B, Lee JA. Updates in the management of thyroid nodules. Curr Probl Surg. 2019;56:103–27.
23. Becker D, Tafoya C, Becker S, Kruger G, Tafoya M, Becker T. The use of portable ultrasound devices in low- and middle- income countries: a systematic review of the literature. Trop Med Int Health. 2016;21:294–311.
24. Beal E, Sigmond B, Sage-Silski L, Lahey S, Nguyen V, Bahner D. Point-of-care ultrasound in general surgery residency training. J Ultrasound Med. 2017;36:2577–84.
25. American Institute of Ultrasound in Medicine Training Guidelines for Physicians who evaluate and interpret diagnostic thyroid, parathyroid, and neck ultrasound examinations. Official Statement; 2019. www.aium.org
26. Broach RB, Geha R, Englander BS, DeLaCruz L, Thrash H, Brooks AD. A cost-effective handheld breast scanner for use in low-resource environments: a validation study. World J Surg Oncol. 2016; 14(1):277.
27. Sood R, Rositch AF, Shakoor D, et al. Ultrasound for breast cancer detection globally: a systematic review and meta-analysis. J Glob Oncol. 2019;5:1–17.

28. Corbex M, Burton R, Sancho-Garnier H. Breast cancer early detection methods for low and middle income countries, a review of the evidence. Breast. 2012;21(4):428–34.
29. Bae JM, Kim EH. Breast density and risk of breast cancer in Asian women: a meta-analysis of observational studies. J Prev Med Public Health. 2016;49(6):367–75.
30. McDonald JA, Rao R, Gibbons M, et al. Symposium report: breast cancer in India-trends, environmental exposures and clinical implications. Cancer Causes Control. 2021;32(6):567–75.
31. Shen S, Zhou Y, Xu Y, et al. A multi-centre randomised trial comparing ultrasound vs mammography for screening breast cancer in high-risk Chinese women. Br J Cancer. 2015;112(6):998–1004.
32. Sayed S, Moloo Z, Ngugi A, et al. Breast camps for awareness and early diagnosis of breast cancer in countries with limited resources: a multidisciplinary model from Kenya. Oncologist. 2016;21(9):1138–48.
33. Stavros AT, Thickman D, Rapp CL, Dennis MA, Parker SH, Sisney GA. Solid breast nodules: use of sonography to distinguish between benign and malignant lesions. Radiology. 1995;196(1):123–34.
34. Gunawardena RP, Gunawardena D, Metcalf C, Taylor D, Wylie L. Inflammatory breast disease: a pictorial essay with radiological-pathological correlation. J Med Imaging Radiat Oncol. 2017;61(1):70–6.
35. Rao R, Ludwig K, Bailey L, et al. Select choices in benign breast disease: an initiative of the American Society of Breast Surgeons for the American Board of Internal Medicine Choosing Wisely(®) campaign. Ann Surg Oncol. 2018;25(10):2795–800.
36. Diepstraten SC, Sever AR, Buckens CF, et al. Value of preoperative ultrasound-guided axillary lymph node biopsy for preventing completion axillary lymph node dissection in breast cancer: a systematic review and meta-analysis. Ann Surg Oncol. 2014;21(1):51–9.
37. Brenin DR, Dietz JR, Baima J, et al. Pain management in breast surgery: recommendations of a multidisciplinary expert panel-the American Society of Breast Surgeons. Ann Surg Oncol. 2020;27(12):4588–602.
38. Shah S, Price D, Bukhman G, Shah S, Wroe E. Manual of ultrasound for resource-limited settings, partners in health, 2011. ISBN: 978-0-9828968-0-8.
39. Galbois A, Ait-Oufella H, Baudel JL, Kofman T, Bottero J, Viennot S, Rabate C, Jabbouri S, Bouzeman A, Guidet B, Offenstadt G, Maury E. Pleural ultrasound compared with chest radiographic detection of pneumothorax resolution after drainage. Chest. 2010;138(3):648–55.
40. Rendón-Ramírez EJ, González-Villarreal M, Muñoz-Espinoza LE, Colunga-Pedraza PR, Moreno JF, Salinas-Chapa M, Mercado-Longoria R, Treviño-García KB, Cazares-Rendón E, Porcel JM. Pleural effusions identified by point-of-care ultrasound predict poor outcomes in decompensated cirrhosis. Ultrasound Med Biol. 2021;47(11):3283–90.
41. Wongwaisayawan S, Suwannanon R, Prachanukool T, Sricharoen P, Saksobhavivat N, Kaewlai R. Trauma ultrasound. Ultrasound Med Biol. 2015;41(10):2543–61.
42. Correa C, Spiegelman L. A case of acute cholecystitis. J Educ Teach Emerg Med. 3:1.
43. Topin F, Thierry AL, Catrevaux O, Barneux T, Menguy P, Bertani A, Massoure PL, Geffroy Y, Tourtier JP, Bougère J. Diagnostic accuracy of emergency physician-performed ultrasound for acute appendicitis in a remote location. J Emerg Med. 2016;50(6):859–67.
44. Briskey M, Elliott B, Cooper M. Diagnosis of abdominal aortic aneurysm with point of care ultrasound in the emergency department. Vis J Emerg Med. 2020;19:100727.
45. Hari S, Kumari S, Srivastava A, Thulkar S, Mathur S, Thotton V. Image-guided versus palpation guided core needle biopsy of palpable breast masses: a prospective study. Indian J Med Res. 2016;143(5):597–604.
46. Santambrogio R, Opocher E, Costa M, Cappellani A, Montorsi M. Survival and intra-hepatic recurrences after laparoscopic radiofrequency of hepatocellular carcinoma in patients with liver cirrhosis. J Surg Oncol. 2005;89(4):218–25.
47. Abdalla EK, Pisters PW. Staging and pre-operative evaluation of upper gastrointestinal malignancies. Semin Oncol. 2004;31(4):513–29.
48. Feussner H, Omote K, Fink U, Walker SJ, Siewert JR. Pretherapeutic laparoscopic staging in advanced gastric carcinoma. Endoscopy. 1999;31(5):342–7.
49. Stein HJ, Kraemer SJ, Feussner H, Fink U, Siewert JR. Clinical value of diagnostic laparoscopy with laparoscopic ultrasound in patients with cancer of the esophagus or cardia. J Gastrointest Surg. 1997;1(2):167–72.
50. Rau B, Hünerbein M, Schlag PM. Is there additional information from laparoscopic ultrasound in tumour staging? Dig Surg. 2002;19(6):479–83.
51. Santambrogio R, Opocher E, Costa M, Cappellani A, Montorsi M. Survival and intra-hepatic recurrences after laparoscopic radiofrequency of hepatocellular carcinoma in patient with liver cirrhosis. J Surg Oncol. 2005;89(4):218–25.
52. Thompson DM, Arregui ME. Role of laparoscopic ultrasound in cancer management. Semin Surg Oncol. 1998;15(3):166–75.
53. Barbot DJ, Marks JH, Feld RI, Liu JB, Rosato FE. Improved staging of liver tumours using laparoscopic intra-operative ultrasound. J Surg Oncol. 1997;64(1):63–7.
54. Foley EF, Kolecki RV, Schirmer BD. The accuracy of laparoscopic ultrasound in the detection of colorectal liver metastases. Am J Surg. 1998;176(3):262–4.
55. Tilleman EH, de Castro SM, Busch OR, Bemelman WA, van Gulik TM, Obertop H, et al. Diagnostic laparoscopy and laparoscopy for staging of patients with malignant proximal bile duct obstruction. J Gastrointest Surg. 2002;6(3):426–30.
56. Callery MP, Strasberg SM, Doherty GM, Soper NJ, Norton JA. Staging laparoscopy with laparoscopic ultrasonography: optimizing resectability in hepato-

biliary and pancreatic malignancy. J Am Coll Surg. 1997;185(1):33–9.
57. Pietrabissa A, Caramella D, Di Candio G, Carobbi A, Boggi U, Rossi G, et al. Laparoscopy and laparoscopic ultrasound for staging for pancreatic cancer: critical appraisal. World J Surg. 1999;23(10):998–1002.
58. Durup Scheel-Hincke J, Mortensen MB, Qvist N, Hovendal CP. TNM staging and assessment of resectability of pancreatic cancer by laparoscopic ultrasonography. Surg Endosc. 1999;13(10):967–71.
59. Catheline JM, Turner R, Rizk N, Barrat C, Champault G. The use of diagnostic laparoscopy supported by laparoscopic ultrasonography in the assessment of pancreatic cancer. Surg Endosc. 1999;13(3): 239–45.
60. Falcone RA Jr, Fegelman EJ, Nussbaum MS, Brown DL, Bebbe TM, Merhar GL, et al. A prospective comparison of laparoscopic ultrasound vs intraoperative cholangiogram during laparoscopic cholecystectomy. Surg Endosc. 1999;13(8):784–8.
61. Thompson DM, Arregui ME, Tetik C, Madden MT, Wegener M. A comparison of laparoscopic ultrasound with digital flourocholangiography for detecting choledocholithiasis during laparoscopic cholecystectomy. Surg Endosc. 1998;12(7):929–32.
62. Tranter SE, Thompson MH. A prospective single-blinded controlled study comparing laparoscopic ultrasound of the common bile duct with operative cholangiography. Surg Endosc. 2003;17(2):216–9.
63. Gopaul R, Bearman G, Stevens MP. Ultrasound use in re-source-limited settings: a systematic review. J Glob Radiol 2018;4(1):Article 4.
64. Shah S, Bellows BA, Adedipe AA, Totten JE, Backlund BH, Sajed D. Perceived barriers in the use of ultrasound in developing countries. Crit Ultrasound J. 2015;7(1):28.
65. Salmon M, Landes M, Hunchak C, Paluku J, Malemo Kalisya L, Salmon C, Muller MM, Wachira B, Mangan J, Chhaganlal K, Kalanzi J, Azazh A, Berman S, Zied ES, Lamprecht H. Getting it right the first time: defining regionally relevant training curricula and provider core competencies for point-of-care ultrasound education on the African continent. Ann Emerg Med. 2017;69(2):218–26.
66. Gbande P, Adam-bounou K, Sonhaye L, Agoda-Koussema LK, Adjenou K. Medical ultrasound practice in developing countries: example of Togo. Open J Radiol. 2018;8:217–22.
67. Spencer JK, Adler RS. Utility of portable ultrasound in a community in Ghana. J Ultrasound Med. 2008;27(12):1735–43.
68. Sippel S, Muruganandan K, Levine A, Shah S. Review article: use of ultrasound in the developing world. Int J Emerg Med. 2011;4:72.
69. Britton N, Miller MA, Safadi S, Siegel A, Levine AR, McCurdy MT. Tele-ultrasound in resource-limited settings: a systematic review. Front Public Health. 2019;7:244.
70. Harvey HB, Ahn R, Price DD, Burke TF. Innovating for the developing world: meeting the affordability challenge. AJR Am J Roentgenol. 2014;203(4):835–7.

21 How to Build an Academic Global Surgery Center: The UCSF CHESA Experience

Ava Yap, Patti Orozco, Zayna Tommalieh, David Bayne, Phyllis Kisa, Luggya Tonny Stone, Alex Emmanuel Elobu, Naomi Kebba, and Marissa A. Boeck

Building capacity dissolves differences. It irons out inequalities.
– A. P. J. Abdul Kalam

A. Yap
Department of Surgery, UCSF School of Medicine, San Francisco, CA, USA

P. Orozco · Z. Tommalieh
UCSF Center for Health Equity in Surgery and Anesthesia, UCSF Institute for Global Health Sciences, San Francisco, CA, USA

D. Bayne
UCSF Center for Health Equity in Surgery and Anesthesia, UCSF Institute for Global Health Sciences, San Francisco, CA, USA

Department of Urology, UCSF School of Medicine, San Francisco, CA, USA

P. Kisa
Makerere University College of Health Sciences, Kampala, Uganda

Paediatric Surgery and Paediatic Urology, Mulago National Referral Hospital, Kampala, Uganda

L. T. Stone
Department of Anesthesia and Emergency Medicine, Makerere University College of Health Sciences, Kampala, Uganda

Accident and Emergency, Mulago National Referral Hospital, Kampala, Uganda

A. E. Elobu
Gastrointestinal, General & Cancer Surgeon, Head of Colorectal Surgery, Mulago National Referral Hospital, Kampala, Uganda

N. Kebba
Cardiovascular and Thoracic Surgeon, Department of Adult Cardiac Surgery, Uganda Heart Institute, Kampala, Uganda

Faculty, Makerere University College of Health Sciences, Kampala, Uganda

M. A. Boeck (✉)
UCSF Center for Health Equity in Surgery and Anesthesia, UCSF Institute for Global Health Sciences, San Francisco, CA, USA

Trauma and Surgical Critical Care, UCSF School of Medicine & Zuckerberg San Francisco General Hospital, San Francisco, CA, USA
e-mail: marissa.boeck@ucsf.edu

M. A. Hardy, B. R. Hochman (eds.), *Global Surgery*, https://doi.org/10.1007/978-3-031-28127-3_21

Abbreviations

AAGS	Association for Academic Global Surgery
AAS	Association for Academic Surgery
ACGME	Accreditation Council for Graduate Medical Education
ADGHE	Anesthesia Division of Global Health Equity
CHESA	Center for Health Equity in Surgery and Anesthesia
COSECSA	College of Surgeons of East, Central and Southern Africa
CUGH	Consortium of Universities for Global Health
FIC	Fogarty International Center
GSSA	Global Surgery Student Alliance
HIC	High-income country
IGHS	Institute for Global Health Sciences
IGOT SMART	IGOT Surgical Management And Reconstructive Training
IGOT	Institute for Global Orthopaedics and Traumatology
LMIC	Low- and middle-income country
MOU	Memorandum of understanding
MU	Makerere University
NIH	National Institutes of Health
PIH	Partners in Health
UCSF HEAL	UCSF Health, Equity, Action, and Leadership
UCSF	University of California, San Francisco
UGHE	University of Global Health Equity
USAID	United States Agency for International Development
WIP	Work In Progress

Introduction/Background

Definitions of Key Concepts

Global Surgery

A field of healthcare which aims to "improve health outcomes & achieve health equity for all people who require surgical care, with a special emphasis on underserved populations & populations in crisis" [1].

Further, global surgery is "the enterprise of providing improved & equitable surgical care to the world's population, with its core tenets as the issues of need, access & quality…the patient requiring surgery as their focus" [2].

Academic Global Surgery

As a subset of global surgery, academic global surgery is dedicated to the training of surgical educators and the discovery of new knowledge to correct global disparities in access to surgical care [3].

Health Equity

Health being a fundamental human right, health equity is "the absence of unfair, avoidable, or remediable differences among groups of people. Health equity is achieved when everyone can attain their full potential for health and well-being" [4].

Public Health

Researchers, practitioners, and educators prevent disease and injury at the community and population level. Public health professionals identify the causes of diseases and disability and then implement large-scale solutions [5].

Resource-Constrained Settings

A locale where the capability to provide systems of care for its habitants does not meet population needs. In this context, this entails a local with limited capacity for vital healthcare access and safe services [6].

This chapter illustrates the Center for Health Equity in Surgery and Anesthesia (CHESA) experience in establishing an academic global surgery center. Readers should be mindful that the same steps and anecdotes will not be universally true for other prospective or established academic global surgery centers. CHESA is based in San Francisco, California, USA, and while health disparities are prevalent in this community and across the USA, this Center is located in a health-resource hub within a high-income country (HIC). Any dialogue around global engagement requires familiarity with the concept of decolonization (see Chap. 3). In the context of global health, decolonization is broadly defined as an effort to shift away from the historical dynamics of power and dominance to implement equitable systems to improve population health [7]. Recently, attention has been drawn to a dichotomy in global health, where global health organizations have historically lacked diversity and inclusivity, mirroring the society and values of Western high-income countries while maintaining a fixation on intervening in LMIC health systems [8]. The decolonization movement calls for the autonomy of previously underrepresented nations to build and sustain their own health systems and workforce, as well as increase inclusiveness of these nations in conversations within the global health community [9]. CHESA engages in all of its activities with these practices and priorities at the forefront.

Within global health, surgery and perioperative care have not received attention proportionate to their importance for overall health and well-being. The reasons behind surgery's stigma are varied, including but not limited to systematic barriers to accessing care, a misperception that surgical care is overly costly, and the variable definition of global surgery and all it encompasses [1]. In a field that heavily relies not only on equipment but also on trained surgeons, anesthesiologists, nurses, and others in the perioperative space, hospitals and clinics frequently have to navigate shortages and unequal distributions of resources while still aiming to provide quality care. The majority of people in the world do not have access to equitable, safe, and affordable surgical care, prompting academic and government institutions to build and foster creative models to address the problem [10]. As academic global surgery centers emerge, one aim has been to provide training and direct resources towards growing local perioperative workforce capacity, seeking to provide sustainable and prosperous solutions to varied barriers to safe surgical access around the world [11].

Academic global surgery centers have been established all over the world, and continue to increase in number, creating a network of centers in high-, middle-, and low-income countries focused on addressing both local and global healthcare challenges. In South Africa, an upper-middle income country, the Centre for Global Surgery was established in 2019 within Stellenbosch University. This center works toward promoting equitable surgical care in South Africa and sub-Saharan Africa through high-quality research, policy maker engagement, and education, with an overall mission to be a global surgery research center of excellence with collaborations within and outside South Africa [12]. Similarly, the University for Global Health Equity (UGHE) was created in 2019 in Rwanda, a low-income country. Initially envisioned by Partners in Health (PIH) in 2014 to build a university that would advance global health delivery, the university focuses on training future global health leaders and equipping them with the necessary skillsets to build effective, lasting, and equitable health systems. As of 2021, their programs included Bachelor of Medicine, Bachelor of Surgery, Master of Science in Global Health Delivery, Executive Education, and an Institute of Global Health Equity Research [13]. Specific to surgery, UGHE has a Center for Equity in Global Surgery, whose mission is to "create equitable access to quality, safe, and holistic surgical, obstetric, and anesthesia care for vulnerable populations provided through integrated, compassionate, and community-centric approach," with a focus on empowering local leaders and solutions [14]. The Harvard Program in Global Surgery and Social Change (PGSSC) is an example of an academic global surgery center in the USA, a HIC. PGSSC's mission advocates for "universal access to safe, affordable surgical, anesthesia, and OB/GYN care when needed." The Harvard Program exhibits its mission in surgical and health systems strengthening (i.e. fellowship) [15]. Additional academic global surgery programs in the USA include The Center for Global Surgery at the University of Utah [16] and the Global Surgical Track in the general surgery residency program at Baylor College of Medicine [17], among others in the USA, Canada, and across the globe.

University of California, San Francisco Center for Health Equity in Surgery and Anesthesia

The Center for Health Equity in Surgery and Anesthesia, abbreviated CHESA, is a center based at the University of California, San Francisco (UCSF) within the University's Institute for Global Health Sciences (IGHS). Led by the efforts of a surgeon and anesthesiologist at UCSF, as well as additional championing faculty, and the support of partners at Makerere University (MU) in Uganda, CHESA officially launched in March 2020 during the beginnings of the COVID-19 pandemic. The name of the Center is reflective of the global health equity focus of the group and the inclusion of the wide range of professionals working within surgery, anesthesia, and perioperative care. Inclusive of all related fields, current CHESA members represent anesthesiology, general surgery and surgical subspecialties, dermatology, nursing, pathology, public health, obstetrics and gynecology, and biostatistics, among others and with new additions continually welcomed.

CHESA's mission statement is "To advance equity in surgery, anesthesia, and perioperative care worldwide through ethical and innovative academic engagement." With this in mind, the Center has four guiding principles:

- Champion health equity for vulnerable populations.
- Elevate interventions prioritized by local and international partners.
- Harmonize approaches between local and international populations.
- Prioritize implementation and impact evaluation.

CHESA shows its commitment to these principles through its work, which has four focus areas: Fellowship Program, Education, Research, and Advocacy and Policy. CHESA's aims and structure are rooted in 20 years of partnerships and relationships established in the early 2000s by the Center's founding directors. The Center's formation has been an iterative process, with a focus on inclusivity to help unite and align many established and frequently parallel global health equity efforts at UCSF under the CHESA umbrella. Listed below are prior groups, individuals, and institutions which heavily contributed toward CHESA's creation [18].

Global Partners in Anesthesia and Surgery (GPAS): The formation of GPAS began with leads from UCSF and MU, with a focus on faculty and trainee exchange and mentorship while working toward addressing the surgical care crisis in Uganda. Over a decade, GPAS fostered collaborations that contributed to the foundation of CHESA.

Institute of Global Health Sciences (IGHS): Dr. Haile Debas is credited with creating IGHS in 1999, which was the first academic institution in the USA to use the term "global health" in its name. Today this institute is home to six centers: the Center for Global Health Diplomacy, Delivery, and Economics; Center for Pandemic Preparedness and Response; Center for Global Infectious and Parasitic Diseases; Center for Strategic Information & Public Health Practice; Center for Global Maternal, Newborn, and Child Health; and CHESA [19].

Anesthesia Division of Global Health Equity (ADGHE): Located within UCSF's Department of Anesthesia, ADGHE was a consortium of anesthesiologists based in the USA, Uganda, and Tanzania who collaborated on research pertinent to the use and training of safe anesthesia access and care. ADGHE eventually consolidated into CHESA, enriching the variety of members and advisors who work toward the goal of health equity in the perioperative space. Center for Global Surgical Studies (CGSS): Located within UCSF's Department of Surgery, CGSS launched in 2015 with the mission to tackle the global burden of surgical disease by improving access to quality surgical care in low-resource settings through education and research. The Center provided research mentorship to future leaders in academic global surgery, and established sustained partnerships with collaborators in LMICs. Elements of CGSS laid the groundwork for the subsequent founding of CHESA [20].

Institute for Global Orthopaedics and Traumatology (IGOT): Located within UCSF,

IGOT was founded in 2006 with the goal of addressing global disparities in orthopedic trauma care. IGOT's flagship innovation is the IGOT SMART (Surgical Management and Reconstructive Training) course. This course provides orthopedic surgeons in resource-limited settings with the skills to successfully perform surgeries to reduce the incidence of amputations. Through the IGOT Portal, educational material and the SMART course are available anywhere in the world with an online classroom format. IGOT and CHESA are active partners in distributing advanced educational tools and resources [21]. Health, Equity, Action, and Leadership Initiative (HEAL): Based in UCSF, HEAL's mission is to have health professionals train and practice in settings with vulnerable populations, both in the USA and internationally. The HEAL fellowship has two tracks, one track for "site fellows" who have roots in a HEAL partner site or community they currently serve and an alternative track for "rotating fellows" who rotate over two years. HEAL's initiatives aim to strengthen and bolster established yet underserved healthcare systems. In alignment with this mission, HEAL fellows are embraced as CHESA fellows, sharing the guiding principles of justice, solidarity, and equity throughout their work [22].

Components of a Center

In this section we will explore in more detail the components of a center, which include a fellowship program, education, research, and partnerships.

Fellowship Program

Academic scholarly training in the research, education, and advocacy of surgical practice in underserved settings is a keystone of a successful academic global surgical center. Historically, short-term international electives were the archetype for global surgical exposure and were highly sought after by American surgical residents [23]. However, these international rotations harbor the dubious reputation of "medical tourism" by solely accommodating the needs of the trainee traveling from a HIC [24, 25]. This unilateral approach is no longer sufficient nor accepted for equitable engagement in academic global surgery or to become an expert in this field. Similarly, technical skill-building courses for operative preparedness in LMICs are generally created for traveling HIC trainees but do not typically strengthen surgical capacity within the local setting [26]. Therefore, a concerted effort is needed to encourage crosstalk among HICs, LMICs, and underserved populations to promote equitable training opportunities which can be offered to the Global "South" and "North," as well as to resource-constrained communities within HICs.

While there is no broadly accepted set of competencies for academic global surgery, the Consortium of Universities for Global Health (CUGH) and the Accreditation Council for Graduate Medical Education (ACGME) have set forth guidelines on the essential components of comprehensive global health education (Table 21.1) [27, 28]. Nevertheless, HIC perspectives predominate existing global surgical curricula and perpetuate an imbalance in educational

Table 21.1 Published global health competencies

Consortium of Universities for Global Health	Accreditation Council for Graduate Medical Education
Global burden of disease	Medical knowledge
Globalization of health and healthcare	Patient care and procedural skills
Social and environmental determinants of health	Practice-based learning and improvement
Capacity strengthening	Interpersonal and communication skills
Collaboration, partnering and communication	Professionalism
Ethics	Systems-based practice
Professional practice	
Health equity and social justice	
Program management	
Sociocultural and political awareness	
Strategic analysis	

priorities [29]. Thus, a conscientious approach must be taken to build a training program that does not cater solely to HIC trainees and to adequately resourced population interests. The global surgical curriculum should be thoughtfully curated to meet the needs of scholars from diverse demographics and countries [30].

Instruction for these competencies can take various forms, from informal didactics to formal degrees. CHESA offers a plethora of training modalities, from multiyear funded research and clinical fellowships to summer internships. CHESA developed a health equity fellowship with a simultaneously flexible and structured curriculum modeled after the CUGH competency guidelines [31]. By following the CUGH framework, the aim was to make the scholarly objectives widely applicable to both low- and high-resource applicants, as the competencies can be universally employed to most surgical inequities. The curriculum embodies a full year of coursework spread over 11 domains. The content in each domain includes online modules, required and supplemental readings, lectures, and Socratic sessions, such as journal clubs and work-in-progress (WIP) meetings. Material is collaboratively decided on by multidisciplinary faculty and graduating fellows. Course content covers global and domestic health equity topics, research methodology, teaching, and mentorship. Fellows also have the flexibility to customize their own curriculum to fit their academic interests and goals, which allows support for fellows with different backgrounds, goals, and local resources.

Notably, LMIC trainees and clinicians are strongly encouraged to apply to CHESA's health equity fellowship. This recruitment strategy demonstrates the bidirectionality of the training program to optimize diversity and curriculum malleability. All fellows have access to institutional research resources, mentorship from a broad range of faculty, and funding tailored to their academic needs. Funding support is especially important for fellows from low-resource settings, providing the means to conduct research and other scholarly work that might otherwise not be financially feasible. These fellows from resource-constrained environments are uniquely positioned to understand the local disease burden and challenges, and will have insight into academic work that should take priority. Recruitment of fellows from LMICs guarantees that their critical perspectives are reflected in the health equity fellow curriculum and activities, ensuring the fellowship remains relevant to scholars from all backgrounds. Curriculum priorities are therefore not driven solely by HIC interests but rather established by contributors across resource settings that seek to broadly represent issues relevant to surgery and health equity globally.

In conjunction with the National Institutes of Health (NIH) Fogarty International Center (FIC), the University of California Global Health Institute (UCGHI) offers year-long funded GloCal fellowships for health professional students and postdoctoral fellows [32]. Fellows can be US citizens affiliated with the GloCal consortium or postdoctoral LMIC applicants from partner sites. To safeguard equitable project ownership, both mentors must be from both within the University of California system and the local partner site. Research aims are directed toward understanding and managing the disease burden in 21 designated LMIC sites in Southeast Asia, Sub-Saharan Africa, and South America, where longstanding collaborations have been established [33]. Previous surgically oriented GloCal projects have addressed hospital registry data deficits in Mozambique, trauma care in Tanzania, treatment of congenital anomalies in Uganda, and surgical oncology capacity building in Tanzania [34–37]. The FIC funds that support an LMIC fellow or principal investigator-initiated projects in international affiliated universities are excellent examples of the American government providing tangible support to academic global surgery initiatives [38]. The consistency of LMIC partnership is key to the sustainability of the program, as this exchange of international research fellows is built on the longstanding relationships with partnering sites.

The 1- or 2-year UCSF HEAL (Health, Equity, Action, and Leadership) fellowship is another global surgical opportunity linked with CHESA that is focused on clinical practice for board eligible or certified medical providers while maintaining core scholarly aspects [39]. The length of the fellowship is meant to allow for an immersive experience, where the fellow works as a full-time clinician at a partner hospital. Furthermore, the fellowship includes a fully funded Masters of Public Health or an equivalent degree for all fellows. The same theme of bidirectional exchange applies. HEAL fellows can either be "rotating" fellows, who are visiting US clinicians sponsored by UCSF, or "site" fellows, who are actively employed by HEAL partner sites and are rooted in their immediate communities. USA-based HEAL fellows have the option to work with domestic and international underrepresented populations. A fellow prerequisite is a full commitment to pursue a lifelong career of providing service to marginalized patients, with a recognition that they do not necessarily need to reside in the Global "South." Deployment sites for fellows range from the Navajo nation in New Mexico, USA, to Mbale, Uganda. The cross-sectional reach of the underserved transcends the division between HIC and LMIC, broadening the definition of the "global surgeon" to being one that strives to alleviate the surgical inequity irrespective of geographic location.

Junior investigators, such as undergraduate students, may choose to enroll in a shorter summer internship with CHESA. Students can work on health equity projects centered around the California Bay Area or tackle more far-reaching issues in international surgical health, with the guidance of an assigned mentor. Preference is again given to underrepresented minorities and first-generation trainees. For faculty members, CHESA also offers a Global MedEd Simulation Fellowship Program, which is a one-year non-ACGME program hosted at UCSF and co-sponsored by the World Federation of Societies of Anaesthesiologists (WFSA). This program is available for medical educators from LMICs. Fellows spend up to three months in San Francisco receiving intensive training on simulation methodology, then return to their home institutions to implement their projects, which are supported with stipends. The fellowship goals are to develop expertise in simulation as an educational strategy and to acquire a foundation to conduct scholarly work in simulation education.

Education and Expert Consultation

In addition to a formal fellowship pathway, an academic global surgery center can provide impactful education and access to expert consultants through association with other disciplines and professional societies. This access to multidisciplinary consultants and diverse skill sets is the hallmark of a holistic academic global surgery center.

At UCSF, an intensive 2-week global health pathway elective is provided by the Office of Graduate Medical Education and is free to students and trainees enrolled in the global health track. A series of 27 didactics led by local and international experts of all specialties from psychiatry to pharmacy exposes the learner to the fundamentals of global health from a wide range of perspectives. Global surgery comprises just one of the many sessions. The elective is designed to be a launchpad for students interested in the field who are seeking to become more involved in a specific area of global health.

Other academic surgical organizations have offered intensive training for leadership and research skills. For example, the College of Surgeons of East, Central and Southern Africa (COSECSA) and the Association of Academic Surgery (AAS) periodically hold a virtual Fundamentals of Research Course, which is open to all surgeon researchers for a nominal fee [40].

The course agenda ranges from abstract writing to effective presentation skills and includes breakout rooms for more in-depth discussion. Some of the skillsets touched upon are shown in Table 21.2. Virtual platforms lower the barriers to access and allows anyone with an Internet con-

Table 21.2 Essential and ancillary (nontechnical) skills relevant to academic global surgery, as showcased in the Fundamentals of Research Course [40]

Fundamental skills	Additional skills
Study design	Economic evaluation
Hypothesis generation	Implementation science
Abstract and manuscript writing	Policy making
Research presentation	Advocacy
Ethical considerations	Quantitative/statistical analysis
	Qualitative analysis

nection to participate in these educational opportunities. In fact, the COSECSA training curriculum for a general surgery resident requires completion of mandatory research and leadership courses [41].

Other essential skill sets to satisfy the global surgical competencies can be obtained within an equipped academic institution [40]. At UCSF, the Department of Epidemiology and Biostatistics provides robust, rigorous courses for learners to hone clinical research skills. Students can select from a myriad of topics. These can be enrolled as standalone classes, as fulfillment toward an Advanced Training in Clinical Research certificate, or as part of a Public Health Masters or Doctorate degree. An academic global surgery center can partner with these departments to create a pathway for trainees to take advantage of valuable educational experiences that may be distinct from the realm of surgery-specific knowledge.

For those who prefer to seek expert guidance, access to biostatistical consultation is highly beneficial for trainees and faculty members alike who are undertaking research projects involving quantitative data. Likewise, quality improvement committees may assist local teams in the development of hospital-level interventions to improve perioperative outcomes. Successful integration with other subjects requires a network of experts, which can be fostered within a university or a similar institution. Applied research methods such as analysis of cost-effectiveness, implementation science, qualitative analysis, and geospatial analysis can all be garnered through field expert consultants from these departments. Many are readily available to mentor or facilitate projects to ensure methodologic rigor of such approaches.

Research

Given the underlying goal to strengthen low-resource surgical systems, augmenting research capacity in LMIC and domestic resource-constrained settings is a main mission for an academic global surgery center. Research-related resources are not equitably distributed between high- and low-resource settings. Researchers from LMICs and domestic resource-denied communities face multiple roadblocks to performing quality investigations, ranging from minimal "protected time" to weak academic visibility to a general shortage of resources. The paucity of funding is a major limitation in the growth of research capacity in LMICs and domestic resource-constrained areas, as local institutions are often unable to support global surgical research, especially if it has not been made a local or national priority. In fact, the dearth of funding begets a dearth of accessible, reliable data to inform public health priorities, which in turn exacerbates the lack of research capacity in resource-denied settings [42].

Frequently, this resource deficit translates into inadequate access to practical tools such as specialized lab equipment, research personnel, statistical support, and data management infrastructure. Research reporting and publication are also unfairly stacked against investigators from LMICs and domestic under-resourced settings, as journal paywalls prevent published findings from reaching these investigators and open access fees are frequently prohibitive. Additionally, the language barrier is a major hurdle imposed on researchers who do not speak English, stifling communication to the broader academic community and hindering career advancement [43]. Thus, researchers from LMICs and domestic resource-constrained areas are forced to be reliant on HICs for both funding and resources to conduct research studies, which further perpetuates the power imbalance [44] extensively discussed previously in Chap. 3.

An equitable center can help lower these barriers by providing research funding and resources to investigators from international and domestic resource-denied communities who propose projects that are centered around local site interests [45]. The UCSF CHESA Fellow Fund allocates such unrestricted funding to support all fellowship endeavors, including career development skill courses to acquire the necessary research toolkit to succeed. Importantly, the funding criteria is not stipulated by HIC partners but directed by the LMICs and domestic resource-constrained research sites and partners, who are integral to the project conception and execution [46]. Ideally, the partnering LMIC and domestic resource-constrained sites could jointly contribute resources to increase the likelihood of long-term ownership [47]. Furthermore, academic global surgical centers are well positioned within an academic institution to provide the research support needed to disseminate the research findings. Technical assistance, such as grant writing workshops, scientific writing consultation, and library services, are made available to CHESA fellows under the purview of the university. This nurturing environment is the key to success for any aspiring researcher, regardless of his/her background.

Equity in global surgery research extends into project responsibility and recognition. Sensitivity to LMIC and local partner inclusivity in joint scholarly work is paramount. By providing a platform of affiliation, an equitable academic global surgery center is well poised to bolster ownership from LMIC and domestic community partners to ensure they steer the research agenda. CHESA seed funding has also helped to promote these research collaborative partnerships. An upfront memorandum of understanding (MOU) that a center can broker establishes the expectations for involved partners, such that there is minimal confusion over roles and recognition as the project progresses. This is especially important during the reporting of scholarly work. Domineering HIC authorship of LMIC and domestic vulnerable community projects has come under increasing scrutiny, as non-HIC authors get left in the middle of the author list or pushed into the acknowledgments section [48]. A designated academic global surgery center with preexisting connections with its partner sites can leverage its status to empower LMIC and domestic community partner authors to take on first and senior authorship roles.

Scholarship activity remains a major benchmark to evaluate the productivity of an academic center. Global surgery initiatives focus primarily on improving surgical care in low-resource systems, so that global surgical research typically has an activist agenda. Scholarly projects in global surgery are therefore not limited to the classic disciplines of basic science, translational, and clinical research. To adapt, academic global surgery centers can incorporate multifactorial research capabilities into its repertoire, including but not limited to economic evaluation, implementation science, qualitative analysis, and quality improvement. Other ways to disseminate global surgical initiatives can be in the form of opinion pieces and traditional media forums such as newspapers or magazine outlets, to engage a broader readership. Academic discoveries are most effective when creatively presented in a way that galvanizes or justifies some form of surgical capacity building.

Global surgery researchers can also risk working in silos as global surgery is diffuse and occasionally disjointed. Work may be duplicated, and the wheel is reinvented when multiple groups try to address the same issue without knowledge of the others' efforts, while synchronized efforts from several angles can more effectively and efficiently push the global surgical agenda forward. Furthermore, solutions for one site should be shared in a multidisciplinary forum, as they may be able to be adapted, repackaged, and reimplemented elsewhere. To streamline activity, global surgical organizations such as the Global Surgery Student Alliance (GSSA), the Association for Academic Global Surgery (AAGS), and CHESA have created centralized databases of ongoing academic projects [49, 50]. These repositories can connect like-minded investigators or groups to help synergize similar ideas and research methods, as well as to provide opportunities for involvement. A network of content experts can also be built within the Center, such that the discourse of global surgical research initiatives becomes routine. This communication can be facilitated by center-wide touchpoints or WIP meetings where representatives from different disciplines can present and discuss their work.

Partnerships

Partnership among LMIC, HIC, and domestic community stakeholders is at the Center's core. This can span many levels within the academic global surgery center, from faculty to trainee, and helps foster the intermingling of innovative ideas. The American Surgical Association Working Group for Global Surgery outlined successful characteristics of LMIC and HIC collaborations, which include a predetermined memorandum of understanding, needs assessment methodology, and identification of strategies to address priority needs [51]. However, many barriers prevent such partnerships from forming that stem from individual problems (e.g., insufficient income, family and clinical responsibilities, skepticism of global surgery efforts, ethical and safety concerns), difficulties with the community (e.g., lack of mentorship and colleagues), and immature systems (e.g., inadequate time, limited recognition, and poor administrative, political and financial support) [52].

Effective circumvention of these potential barriers requires a multilateral approach. Surgical subspecialties should be part of the core administrative team, such as orthopedics, urology, and gynecology, as international surgical delivery frequently does not differentiate subspecialties as the general surgeon (or even nonsurgical clinician) is tasked to treat every surgical problem. In order to improve surgical care in LMICs it is important to include surgical subspecialty training and subspecialty surgical care as a fundamental pillar of global surgery programs. Collaboration with other essential perioperative workforce members, including nursing and pharmacy, is also vital for a multilateral effort to enhance systematic surgical capacity, as is interface with nonclinician specialists such as epidemiologists, policy makers, and economists [53]. CHESA co-leads the UCSF World Health Organization Collaborating Center for Emergency, Critical and Operative Care, and is active in advancing the implementation of its emergency care program and providing technical input into the World Health Academy teaching modules. CHESA members work closely with their professional associations and non-government organizations to advance the global surgery and health equity agenda.

Prior to the establishment of CHESA in 2020, GPAS functioned with leads from UCSF and MU and focused on faculty and trainee exchange. During its tenure from 2010 to 2016, GPAS had 17 scholars. Two summarized experiences with the GPAS program are described by previous trainees below.

Dr. Naomi Kebba (2014 GPAS Scholar): Within the Department of Surgery at Mulago Hospital in Uganda, Naomi was able to pursue her passion in surgery and built her confidence as an academic leader. Enrolling in the GPAS program, she received extensive mentorship regarding her project: building an advanced trauma training curriculum designed for resource-constrained settings. Bolstered by a team composed of GPAS Scholars and UCSF faculty, this course was renamed the Kampala Advanced Trauma Course and still runs today.

Dr. Alex Elobu (2011 GPAS Scholar): Working within the Department of Surgery at Mulago Hospital, Alex joined GPAS with the aim of professional growth and mentorship. The uncertainty of job security after residency washed away once Alex was involved with GPAS, receiving further research training, publishing opportunities, collaboration with other hospitals, and having an opportunity to travel for an international conference. Using GPAS as a stepping stone toward a career in global and academic surgery, Alex continues to advocate for trainees who were in his same position years ago.

Advocacy, Allyship, and Policy

Center cohesion is evident in CHESA's response to recent civil and natural upheavals. Advocacy and allyship through the Center does not solely attend to domestic or international issues. Examples range from striking a united stance on stricter gun control after continued mass shootings in the USA to rapid mobilization of Center resources to address the immediate needs of victims from the COVID-19 pandemic, Haiti earthquake, and the war in Ukraine. In fact, the anesthesia arm of CHESA partnered with the US Agency for International Development (USAID) and the Public Health Institute Sustaining Technical and Analytic Resources Program during the height of the COVID-19 pandemic to assist with the COVID-19 response in LMICs. Together, they developed OpenCriticalCare, an open-source anesthesia educational platform with courses and other learning resources to help alleviate the critical care workforce shortage that occurred during the COVID-19 pandemic. During the 2021 Haiti earthquake, CHESA collaborated expediently with the charity MedShare, an international medical supply and personal protective equipment redistributor, to redirect critical medical equipment and supplies to the hardest hit areas. This was championed by Dr. Ernest Barthlemy, a CHESA fellow alum closely connected to the Haiti earthquake response. CHESA has been working on the early stages of development of a workforce strategy with the Ugandan Ministry of Health, to accompany a Surgery, Anesthesia, and Obstetrics National Plan. In addition, CHESA Advocacy and Policy lead Dr. Adrian Gelb has been advancing consensus metrics for global surgery post the Lancet Commission through the Utstein Consensus Group. Advocacy and allyship are critical and powerful components of a successful academic global surgery center. The ability to band together to coalesce diverse, like-minded groups allows for swift action especially in times of hardship.

Generalized "How To"

The effectiveness of an academic global surgery center's programming hinges on a well-defined operating model. Encompassing several domains including, but not limited to, leadership, finance, and governance, the purpose of the operating model is to translate strategy into results and provide a plan and structure for deploying people and resources to carry out the Center's mission. Each academic global surgery center's operating model is uniquely designed based on available resources and their strategic plan.

The purpose of this section is to share CHESA's experience in building its operating model to support its programming. It will offer generalized "how to" advice, describing what works for the Center at this point in its organizational history and noting some areas that need improvement to help the Center achieve better results over time. CHESA is a work in progress, and its operating model should and will evolve over time as it collaborates with a constellation of stakeholders including UCSF leadership, CHESA members, donors, and community-based partners in the USA and globally.

There are many existing resources that offer detailed technical guidance and recommendations for setting up a nonprofit organization or academic center's operating model. Few, however, focus on the intricacies of an academic global surgery center, let alone one like CHESA which focuses on advancing health equity in surgical, anesthesia, and perioperative care. Simultaneously, the generalized "how to's" presented in this section are not one-size-fits-all. CHESA does not have solutions to all the questions, nor does this section intend to give the impression that it does. However, CHESA's experience and lessons learned may prove useful to others in the process of conceptualizing or establishing their own academic global surgery centers or seeking to expand or bolster their existing programs.

How to Secure Funding

1. Secure endorsement from an institution that can financially support the center.
2. Develop a budget to inform funding goals.
3. Implement a resource mobilization strategy.

As with many mission-oriented organizations, securing funding to support the work while moving toward a sustainable financial model remains an ongoing challenge for CHESA. The Center is extremely fortunate to have the endorsement and backing of UCSF to provide startup funds for the first few years of operations. There is strong strategic alignment between CHESA and UCSF as a leading university dedicated exclusively to the health sciences and a pioneer in the field of academic global surgery. Before CHESA launched, various perioperative departments at UCSF had some support and interested faculty and trainees to advance global health and health equity priorities. Siloed, each department had too few resources to build a program, support trainees and carve out faculty roles for program directors. CHESA brought these departments together, bridging the divide among groups with shared goals. The Center enabled the pooling of resources in order to amplify the collective impact of these groups by sharing operational costs, leadership and fellowship support, mentorship resources and enabling joint projects. This is a distinguishing feature of CHESA's financial model.

The organization is partially funded by surplus from the surgery and anesthesia departments, as well as contributions from other departments like urology, orthopedics, and otolaryngology, who have agreed to dedicate faculty time and/or direct financial contributions to support CHESA activities, including the fellowship program, research, education, and advocacy and policy projects. This ensures that everyone has a vested interest in CHESA's success while further highlighting the critical, multidisciplinary nature of the Center.

To gain buy-in from internal UCSF decision-makers, CHESA's leadership leveraged existing university relationships and years of experience in global surgery, anesthesia, and perioperative care to highlight the imperative of the mission and to demonstrate the potential for greater impact by establishing the Center. To ask for this investment, CHESA needed clarity on what it sought to accomplish and how much these activities were expected to cost. With a history of previous global surgery partnerships and initiatives, the two main departments that came together to form CHESA – surgery and anesthesia – drew on previous project experience to develop a budget that included all components and activities that require funding (e.g., fellowships, event planning, staffing, etc.). A well-formulated operating budget facilitates the best use of limited financial resources by focusing on what is needed to achieve the primary goals and objectives of the Center. CHESA continues to monitor, oversee, and refine its budget, making course corrections as needs and priorities shift.

Securing an initial financial commitment enabled CHESA to hire a small team to establish and grow the Center. The UCSF departments and leadership backing CHESA seek a return on their seed investment, including the Center's ability to bring in more external funding from philanthropy, government, and other institutions. To accomplish this task, the Center is designing and delivering a resource mobilization strategy focused on harnessing and increasing existing university support, communicating impact, and pursuing external funding and strategic partnerships. As CHESA secures additional grants, it engages and offers the opportunity for other CHESA members to get involved and be supported.

Global surgery receives a much smaller proportion of funding from US government and non-governmental sources compared to other areas in global health, such as infectious diseases [54]. CHESA is cultivating relationships with other teams and organizations internal and external to UCSF to pursue business development opportunities that support shared outcomes. For example, a maternal and child health initiative that incorporates access to global surgery, anesthesia, and perioperative care as a key component to achieving the overall project outcome.

How to Recruit and Deploy Committed Faculty and Staff

1. Recruit faculty across all associated disciplines.
2. Bring in faculty and staff committed to center values.
3. Identify core staff who can adapt to diverse roles to support the center's management and growth.

In CHESA's experience, recruiting and retaining committed faculty and champions across multiple disciplines is critical to the Center's success. Under its current investment model, CHESA advocates to UCSF department chairs to protect varying levels of faculty time for center activities. This frees staff to do health equity work and to support the mission of CHESA while maintaining clinical commitments. CHESA invites representatives from across disciplines from UCSF and non-UCSF collaborating institutions in LMICs to be part of the Center's Leadership Committee (see next section). Furthermore, for some faculty recruits and prospective trainees at UCSF, a selling point for joining UCSF is the opportunity to participate in global surgery initiatives. CHESA facilitates opportunities for colleagues to get involved in this work, build networks, and collaborate with other faculty, staff, and partners. Access to faculty from various disciplines means CHESA can leverage diverse technical expertise when pursuing and collaborating on new projects and donor opportunities. Building these relationships expands CHESA's network of professionals involved in related health equity work, enhancing CHESA's visibility and potentially attracting new partners and donors.

CHESA engages faculty and staff aligned with its values of social justice, diversity, equity, and inclusion. These values are core to CHESA's programmatic approach and guide interactions and engagement with community stakeholders and partners from all settings, including domestic community partners and LMICs. CHESA prioritizes continuous learning and improvement in applying these values to the work as it pursues more equitable academic engagement in the global surgery, anesthesia, and the perioperative space.

Given the current size of the organization and limited resources, CHESA has hired full-time staff who can adapt and shift their support between multiple priorities related to finance, operations, business development, and project management, in collaboration with many stakeholders and partners internal and external to UCSF. Staff bring experience in global health and development and an interest in academia. As CHESA expands its programming and budget, the organization will plan to recruit professionals in dedicated roles such as communications and operations.

How to Set up the Governance

1. Test different organizational structures until you find what works.
2. Bring in diverse leadership to advise.
3. Clarify decision-making processes.

CHESA has gone through a few iterations in its organizational structure. For the first year, CHESA had multiple co-directors overseeing the Center's management and strategic direction. The Center opened participation to all members in technical working groups focused on education, research, and advocacy and policy. Setting up to promote inclusivity and collaboration, the structure unfortunately led to inefficient and unclear decision-making and accountability.

CHESA shifted its model so one director oversees the Center's overall strategic direction and management with multiple associate directors to facilitate the executive-level decisions and tasks for the Center. Administratively, there are currently two full-time staff (deputy director and program coordinator) and other faculty and staff of varying levels of effort up to 50% who help lead and implement center activities. CHESA's organizational structure is a work in progress being shaped by the Center's diverse leadership team who will periodically reflect on the effectiveness of the structure and make adjustments as necessary.

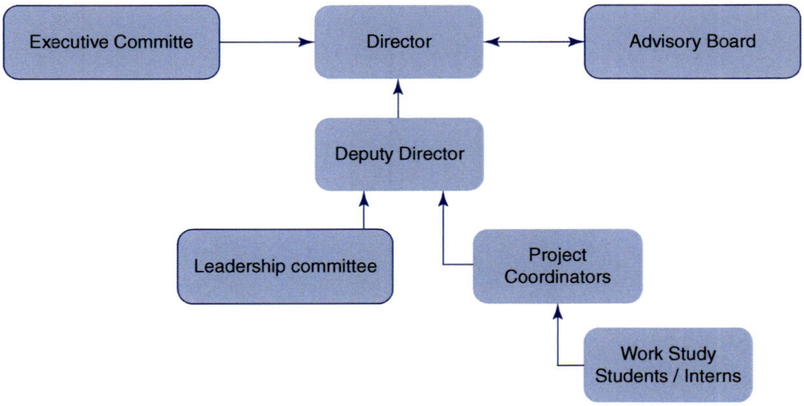

CHESA has set up three bodies to provide technical and strategic advice and help deliver center programming.

- **Executive committee:** Oversees the strategic direction of the Center. Chaired by the Director, the Executive Committee meets monthly for programmatic and operational updates and to engage in strategic decision-making at the organizational level.
- **Leadership committee:** Provides essential linkages between various perioperative specialties and departments at UCSF, CHESA, and our non-UCSF and international partners and works together to advance CHESA's mission. Included on the leadership committee are key leadership roles: directors and associate directors who oversee four focus areas for the center, namely, the fellowship program, education, research, and advocacy and policy. This is a shift away from the original working group approach, so specific leads are held accountable for direction and progress on Center priorities. The leadership committee invites participation from international collaborators from LMICs for their essential input and feedback on Center initiatives and provides a stipend for their participation. Each leadership committee member serves as a champion and liaison for CHESA with their home department or institution and provides technical input on CHESA's programming.
- **Advisory board:** Advises and counsels the CHESA director and executive committee on the strategic direction of the center. CHESA is grateful to have a diverse and highly accomplished board who guides the Center on its technical programing, as well as organizational strategies related to resource mobilization, partnerships, and communications. The advisory board members are connectors and thought partners to CHESA, providing vast experience in health care, philanthropy, and technology across the public, private, and nongovernmental organization sectors.

The CHESA structure sits within a large university system, which brings its own benefits and drawbacks. CHESA has access to office space and operational capabilities like communications, finance, supply chain, and legal departments. However, the university system is strictly administered by its own rules and regulations. It can be challenging for the Center to operate as nimbly as it would like when the umbrella administrative processes lack clarity or must move through multiple approval channels before a task is initiated or completed.

The organizational structure reflects CHESA's commitment to inclusivity, collaboration, and diverse perspectives. Clear decision-making processes are important for the Center to leverage the separate groups under its structure, as well as the many faculty, partners, and advisors who comprise these committees. This is an area that CHESA continues to improve as it balances the need to make timely decisions but in a way that encourages and leaves space for feedback and diverse input.

How to Promote Opportunities for Learning and Collaboration

1. Employ a social media strategy.
2. Act as a shared resource and bridge for collaboration at a local and global level.
3. Communicate the impact of your center's work.

CHESA employs a social media strategy through monthly newsletters, website updates, and social media channels (Twitter, Instagram, YouTube) to increase awareness of the challenges for achieving health equity in surgery and what the Center and its members and collaborators are doing to address this. CHESA shares regular opportunities for members to build bridges and connect with one another around shared interests and programs. This includes events like the WIP meetings for members to get immediate feedback and support from other experts and implementers to improve their health equity research projects. CHESA seeks to break down silos and enhance collaboration and learning across its community.

The WIP meetings are also used as a platform to share Center-wide updates.

CHESA has hosted open-access virtual Grand Rounds to discuss health equity topics related to surgery, anesthesia, and perioperative care, highlighting research and project experience in the USA and internationally. Health equity journal club is another avenue for members to connect and discuss literature and implications for members' ongoing projects or research and professional interests.

COVID-19 has made it challenging to organize in-person meetings and events to facilitate networking and learning across members. CHESA is exploring ways to strengthen the member community, including those who reside outside of the Bay Area and other countries.

Communicating impact is an area for improvement for CHESA, not only sharing data but improving CHESA's story-telling. Illustrating the organization's support and influence across system levels and geographies and its impact on a wide range of individuals from healthcare practitioners to patients is an important goal that has many important implications for the stakeholders. A strong communications strategy can help galvanize members and partners around the Center's mission and advance parallel efforts to build partnerships and cultivate new donor relationships.

Reflections

What Works

Although each academic global surgery center will be unique, we believe there are core principles for success that are universal.

Lead with Inclusion and Belonging From the beginning, CHESA set out to positively disrupt the global surgery space, with the first step being inclusion and a focus on the people as our most valuable asset. This led to the removal of "global" from the Center's name and inclusion of "anesthesia" to expand beyond surgery. These actions were aimed at promoting representation of all disciplines within the perioperative ecosystem, from nursing to dermatology, and ensuring those engaged in domestic health equity work felt included. We intentionally created minimal requirements for membership to encourage broad participation from our external collaborators across the globe, and we offered Center leadership roles with compensation to non-UCSF partners to ensure broad stakeholder representation. We also sought participation from people with diverse backgrounds to enrich the perspectives within CHESA.

Focus on Decolonization and Reduction of Implicit Bias We have placed decolonization and the reduction of implicit bias at the forefront of all our work, with an initial emphasis on awareness in order to identify and eliminate any bias. We acknowledge that an HIC academic center may historically represent a potential power imbalance to both local and global communities and partners. To address this potential conflict, we have sought to identify and address past injustices in order to rewrite the narrative and shift the center of gravity. It is not acceptable to proceed with work that is "about them, without them." It is essential to recognize partners as local experts and support them with our platform, resources, knowledge, experience, and advocacy, with a truly bidirectional exchange of ideas. We also sought to create a culture of listening and safety to encourage people who are vulnerable to be honest when raising possible issues or conflicts, as we consistently strive to optimize and equalize our work.

Engage from the Top-Down and Bottom-Up As many who are involved in health equity work can relate, diverse and creative approaches are frequently required for success. While support, recognition, and inclusion of our Center at the highest level was essential, including from the institution, relevant departments, divisions, and related centers, the importance of each individual Center member cannot be understated. These methods can be applied to all Center activities, including the fellowship, education, research, advocacy, allyship, and policy, partnerships, funding, and governance. Similarly, CHESA tackles projects from both levels – incremental at the point of education and research, and also at a higher level of policy and advocacy, as action via both approaches is needed to make progress.

Build on Long-Term Partnerships As highlighted previously, CHESA is founded on many longstanding relationships with local and international partners. Longitudinal engagement and investment show a commitment to and solidarity with the people, place, and work and build a level of trust that strengthens the relationship and enhances potential impacts. While exploring new sites and collaborations are also essential for the Center as we work to expand our work's footprint, this activity cannot come at the cost of existing, ongoing partnerships.

Stay Flexible and Adaptable It is critical to recognize the fragility of our work and the many factors that must align to allow for success, as well as how close many activities are to stagnancy or failure. Accepting this reality encourages us to remain flexible and open-minded and to routinely consider multiple avenues for an initiative's success, enabling us to pivot, adapt, and innovate when we need to take a different path. We have also realized timetables and priorities may not always align, and when this conflict arises, we must defer to our local partner's agenda and not force an issue for our own benefit. Occurrences will occasionally require a shift in the balance of effort and time in partnerships and will call upon everyone to remain malleable and to potentially let go of noncritical or unfeasible items while always keeping the end goal and purpose of our work in mind.

Conclusion and Challenges

Multiple obstacles have presented themselves during the development of our academic global surgery center. Many of our challenges are likely common across centers, and we continue to explore solutions.

How to Measure our Impact and Ensure the Center Has Value for its Members, Partners, Institution, Funders, and the Communities it Aims to Serve? We have consistently been confronted with how best to measure the value and impact of our Center and to constantly evaluate whether the work we are doing or considering engaging in aligns with our Center's mission and vision. Possible metrics for impact include sustained external funding and grants, membership roster, project tally, total research output (publications, presentations), courses taught, and fellows trained. Given our focus on people, our Center will gather stories from those who engage with CHESA to understand at a more granular level our Center's overall purpose and meaning for those who work and study with us and areas for improvement. There do not appear to be any agreed-upon metrics for an academic global surgery center based on review of existing center websites nor in the literature. This therefore remains an area in need of future exploration in an effort to hold all of us more accountable.

How to Sustain the Center? As discussed previously, at CHESA we developed a clear organizational structure which requires sustained engagement from multiple parties. We have struggled with staff retention, adequate protected time from clinical work for leaders to meaningfully participate, and with accountability. Many healthcare professionals engaged in global surgery work share this struggle due to competing clinical and academic responsibilities. To combat this, we have strived to confirm protected time from department chairs and/or provide compensation for time invested in the Center. We have also focused on hiring non-clinical staff and have involved work-study students to support the day-to-day functions of the Center and ensure continuity and sustained engagement. Furthermore, centers require longitudinal funding. While CHESA's initial support is largely from institutional funds, our goal is to transition to a larger proportion of grant and philanthropic support. Besides the inherent competitiveness of grants, an added challenge is the required academic institution indirect structure, which can range from 40 to 60% for indirect costs depending on the donor or funding agency, significantly decreasing the actual funds that can be used by the Center.

How to Achieve an Equitable Balance of Activities (e.g., Domestic Vs International, by Specialty)? While historically the field of global surgery was a synonym for international surgery, and frequently focused on surgery over other disciplines, at CHESA we have strived to dispel this misperception to include all health equity work in perioperative and anesthesia care, surgical diseases, and related disciplines under our Center's umbrella. Although many of our activities are focused in LMICs, we seek to increase participation and membership from individuals and groups doing both local and global perioperative health equity work, including domestic community organizations and members of vulnerable populations and underrepresented groups. CHESA's scope is intentionally broad, which we view as necessary to adequately represent the complex perioperative health equity landscape, and is in agreement with our inclusive mission, vision, and guiding principles. A broader alignment and use of access to care models and social determinant of health that are implemented in both domestic and international settings may catalyze cross-talk between these spaces and unify efforts.

How to Break Silos and Increase Awareness of the Center across Multiple Levels (Institutional, Local, Regional, National, and International)? Most individuals active in the global surgery space are unfortunately all-too-familiar with siloed activities. Without an ability to know what activities are occurring where and with whom, we are unable to avoid recreating the wheel and duplicating efforts, and therefore, opportunities for collaboration are stymied. We created and are maintaining a database of CHESA member perioperative health equity projects to catalog our Center's work and explore ways for members to collaborate to strengthen their activities. As part of our bigger global health community through UCSF's IGHS, we created a method of adding tags regarding one's relevant institutional center membership(s), research focus areas, and project locations that are listed on one's institutional profile webpage. This then links to an open-access database of IGHS professionals that can be searched by any of the above criteria [55].

Despite reaching out to meet with leaders and others engaged in a similar workspace, we continue to struggle at UCSF with limited institutional knowledge about our existence, purpose, and potential, not to mention global awareness. Albeit slower than desired, we have made progress and we realize this is not a unique problem for new organizations within much larger institutions. This has prompted us to continue and build on our activities in this space: direct outreach and meetings with stakeholders within UCSF, across University of California campuses, and externally; publicity and promotion of the Center's activities via a monthly newsletter to our members and CHESA social media channels (Twitter, Instagram, YouTube); brainstorming our branding; developing an informative, accessible website; open-access grand rounds programming; trainee-organized journal clubs; monthly member WIP meetings; and member representation of the Center via participation in various educational and academic activities locally, nationally, and globally. We also encourage members to list CHESA as an institutional affiliation on research conference abstracts, presentations, and publications.

How to Build and Sustain a Center during Massive Global Disruptions (e.g., COVID-19 Pandemic, Geopolitical Distress, War, Etc.) and Competing Interests? While "unprecedented" has been used to describe many world events since 2020, just as CHESA was coming into existence, our initial in-person retreat pivoted to virtual, our Center's community has come together to support each other in unparalleled ways. As highlighted previously, we raised our voices in support of various pivotal social justice movements and world events and sponsored fundraising activities for partners. While these unforeseen events may have temporarily diverted our attention from previous priorities, we relied on our Center's strengths, flexibility, and adaptability to respond to member, partner, and global societal needs. We did not face funding constraints during these times, which would be an added barrier some centers may face. This could severely limit a center's ability to continue even basic operations and activities due to inadequate staffing and resources. In addition, COVID related disruptions placed an additional emphasis on the need for close evaluation of surgical and anesthesia systems and perioperative infrastructure, and the oxygen ecosystem. CHESA was asked to work in these areas that will ideally translate to sustainable initiatives. Likewise, the social justice movement that has galvanized in the USA over the last several years put a focus on structural racism as a public health issue, and highlighted the need of our Centers to address this in concert with other partners.

Remote work impacted our ability to build our community in-person and contributed to difficulties with staff retention, yet it has also created opportunities to innovate and support broader digital engagement for CHESA members across the globe. We routinely reflect on what worked and what did not in order to change and grow. We recognize many within our Center's community are overburdened and underappreciated and inadequately supported, which were long standing challenges worsened by the COVID-19 pandemic and other local and global events. CHESA's goal is not to be an additional task or responsibility, but to be a supporter, facilitator, and advocate, with our member's wellness and prevention of burnout at our Center's core. There will always be competing priorities and inadequate time and resources to accomplish all our goals, but CHESA will continue to use our mission, vision, and member engagement to guide our activities. We aim for everyone within the CHESA community to thrive as we engage in this necessary and meaningful work together and move closer to achieving global perioperative health equity and justice.

Acknowledgments This chapter would not have been possible without the support of UCSF CHESA's leadership, including Director and Professor of Surgery Dr. Doruk Ozgediz. We are grateful to Dr. Kathryn Chu, Director of the Stellenbosch University Centre for Global Surgery and Professor of Global Surgery, for her critical insights and feedback on early chapter drafts.

References

1. Dare AJ, Grimes CE, Gillies R, Greenberg SLM, Hagander L, Meara JG, et al. Global surgery: defining an emerging global health field. Lancet. 2014;384(9961):2245–7.
2. Bath M, Bashford T, Fitzgerald JE. What is 'global surgery'? Defining the multidisciplinary interface between surgery, anaesthesia and public health. BMJ Glob Health. 2019;4(5):e001808.
3. Schecter WP. Academic global surgery: a moral imperative. JAMA Surg. 2015;150(7):605–6.
4. Health Equity [Internet]. World Health Organization. [cited 2022 Jul 21]. https://www.who.int/health-topics/health-equity
5. What Is Public Health? [Internet]. Johns Hopkins | Bloomberg School of Public Health. [cited 2022 Jul 21]. https://publichealth.jhu.edu/about/what-is-public-health
6. Geiling J, Burkle FM, Amundson D, Dominguez-Cherit G, Gomersall CD, Lim ML, et al. Resource-poor settings: infrastructure and capacity building. Chest. 2014;146(4 Suppl):e156S–67S.
7. Decolonising global health in 2021: a roadmap to move from rhetoric to reform | BMJ Global Health [Internet]. [cited 2022 Aug 22]. https://gh.bmj.com/content/6/3/e005604
8. Chawla B, Lindert J, Sharma D. Post-decolonisation: Global Health and Global Surgery's coming of age. Indian J Surg. 2022;84(2):259–61.
9. Alayande B, Forbes C, Degu S, Hey MT, Karekezi C, Khanyola J, et al. Shifting global surgery's center of gravity. Surgery. 2022;S0039606022003130
10. Shrime EB and MG. Surgery: the neglected stepchild of Global Health [Internet]. On the Ground. 1461165817 [cited 2022 Jul 21]. https://archive.nytimes.com/kristof.blogs.nytimes.com/2016/04/20/surgery-the-neglected-stepchild-of-global-health/
11. Bentounsi Z, Nazir A. Building global surgical workforce capacity through academic partnerships. J Public Health Emerg. 2020;4. J Public Health Emerg [Internet]. 2020 [cited 2020 Jan 1]; https://jphe.amegroups.com/article/view/6434
12. Centre for Global Surgery- About us [Internet]. Stellenbosch Univeristy. [cited 2022 Jul 21]. http://www.sun.ac.za/english/faculty/healthsciences/global-health/global-surgery/about-us
13. University of Global Health Equity [Internet]. UGHE [cited 2022 Jul 21]. https://ughe.org/

14. Center for Equity in Global Surgery [Internet]. University of Global Health Equity. [cited 2022 Aug 17]. https://ughe.org/center-for-equity-in-global-surgery
15. Harvard Medical School. Program in Global Surgery and Social Change, 2022. Aug 17 (2021).
16. University of Utah. Center for Global Surgery, 2023 April 23 (2023).
17. Baylor College of Medicine. Global Surgery Track, 2023 April 25 (2023).
18. CHESA Homepage [Internet]. CHESA. [cited 2022 Jul 21]. https://globalsurgery.org/about-us/
19. A history of the IGHS, 1999 to 2019 | Global Health Sciences [Internet]. [cited 2022 Aug 17]. https://globalhealthsciences.ucsf.edu/about-us/mission-and-vision/history-institute-global-health-sciences-1999-2019
20. Barg, Richard. "Department of Surgery to Create Center for Global Surgical Studies." UCSF Department of Surgery, January 6, 2015, https://surgery.ucsf.edu/news-events/ucsf-news/47422/Department-of-Surgery-to-Create-Center-for-Global-Surgical-Studies. 25 April 2023
21. Institute for Global Orthopaedics and Traumatology (IGOT) [Internet]. UCSF Department of Orthopaedic Surgery. [cited 2022 Jul 21]. https://orthosurgery.ucsf.edu/outreach/global/igot_program
22. University of California, San Francisco. HEAL Initiative, 2023 April 25 (2018).
23. Powell AC, Casey K, Liewehr DJ, Hayanga A, James TA, Cherr GS. Results of a national survey of surgical resident interest in international experience, electives, and volunteerism. J Am Coll Surg. 2009;208(2):304–12.
24. Melby MK, Loh LC, Evert J, Prater C, Lin H, Khan OA. Beyond medical "missions" to impact-driven short-term experiences in Global Health (STEGHs): ethical principles to optimize community benefit and learner experience. Acad Med. 2016;91(5):633–8.
25. Bozinoff N, Dorman KP, Kerr D, Roebbelen E, Rogers E, Hunter A, et al. Toward reciprocity: host supervisor perspectives on international medical electives. Med Educ. 2014;48(4):397–404.
26. Lin Y, Mukhopadhyay S, Meguid RA, Kuwayama DP. The Colorado Humanitarian Surgical Skills Workshop: a cadaver-based workshop to prepare residents for surgery in austere settings. J Surg Educ. 2018;75(2):383–91.
27. ACGME. Global Health Educational Curriculum [Internet]. American Council of Graduate Medical Education (ACGME); 2020. https://gme.cmhshealth.org/wp-content/uploads/2020/05/Global-Health-Curriculum-ACGME-2.24.20.pdf
28. Astle B, Guzman CA, Landry A, Romocki L, Evert J. Global Health Education Competencies Tool-kit [Internet]. 2nd ed. Consortium of Global Health; 2017. https://1cnvnq2oul8e2upwpp47ustn-wpengine.netdna-ssl.com/wp-content/uploads/sites/95/2020/05/CUGH-Global-Health-Toolkit-Web-Version.pdf
29. Jayaram A, Pawlak N, Kahanu A, Fallah P, Chung H, Valencia-Rojas N, et al. Academic global surgery curricula: current status and a call for a more equitable approach. J Surg Res. 2021;267:732–44.
30. Zivanov CN, Joseph JBA, MacLeod J, Kauffmann RM. Host perspectives on the expansion of unidirectional global surgery rotations in surgery residency programs. J Am Coll Surg. 2020;231(4):S125.
31. CHESA Fellowship [Internet]. UCSF Center of Health Equity in Surgery and Anesthesia. 2022 [cited 2022 Jul 20]. https://globalsurgery.org/chesa-fellowship/
32. GloCal Health Fellowship | UC Global Health Institute [Internet]. University of California Global Health Institute. 2022 [cited 2022 Jul 20]. https://ucghi.universityofcalifornia.edu/fellowships/glocal-health-fellowship
33. Research Sites | UC Global Health Institute [Internet]. University of California Global Health Institute. 2022 [cited 2022 Jul 20]. https://ucghi.universityofcalifornia.edu/fellowships/glocal-health-fellowship/research-sites
34. Cox R. GloCal fellow John Rose keeps surgery on global health agenda | UC Global Health Institute [Internet]. University of California Global Health Institute. 2017 [cited 2022 Jul 20]. https://ucghi.universityofcalifornia.edu/news/glocal-fellow-john-rose-keeps-surgery-global-health-agenda
35. Working Globally, Locally: GloCal Fellow Manages Tanzanian Project from California | UC Global Health Institute [Internet]. University of California Global Health Institute. 2021 [cited 2022 Jul 20]. https://ucghi.universityofcalifornia.edu/working-globally-locally-glocal-fellow-manages-tanzanian-project-california
36. GloCal Fellows 2021–2022 | UC Global Health Institute [Internet]. University of California Global Health Institute. 2021 [cited 2022 Jul 20]. https://ucghi.universityofcalifornia.edu/fellowships/glocal-health-fellowship/glocal-fellows-2021-2022
37. GloCal Fellows 2022–2023 | UC Global Health Institute [Internet]. University of California Global Health Institute. 2022 [cited 2022 Jul 20]. https://ucghi.universityofcalifornia.edu/fellowships/glocal-health-fellowship/glocal-fellows-2022-2023
38. Fogarty Funding Opportunities – Dates and Deadlines – Fogarty International Center @ NIH [Internet]. Fogarty International Center. [cited 2022 Jul 20]. https://www.fic.nih.gov:443/Funding/Pages/Fogarty-Funding-Opps.aspx
39. HEAL Fellowship Overview [Internet]. HEAL Initiative. [cited 2022 Jul 20]. https://healinitiative.org/fellowship-overview/
40. AAS/COSECSA Fundamentals of Surgical Research Course [Internet]. Association for Academic Surgery (AAS). [cited 2022 Jul 21]. https://www.aasurg.org/aas-cosecsa-fundamentals-of-surgical-research-course/
41. Training Curriculum: Fellowship in General Surgery – FCSgen(ECSA) [Internet]. College of Surgeons of East, Central & Southern Africa; 2017. https://

www.cosecsa.org/wp-content/uploads/2019/09/COSECSA-Overall-Curriculum.pdf
42. Holmer H, Bekele A, Hagander L, Harrison EM, Kamal P, Ng-Kamstra JS, et al. Evaluating the collection, comparability and findings of six global surgery indicators. Br J Surg. 2019;106(2):e138–50.
43. Busse C, August E. Addressing power imbalances in global health: pre-publication support services (PREPSS) for authors in low-income and middle-income countries. BMJ Glob Health. 2020;5(2):e002323.
44. Ollila E. Global health priorities—priorities of the wealthy? Glob Health. 2005;1(1):6.
45. Boum Y II, Burns BF, Siedner M, Mburu Y, Bukusi E, Haberer JE. Advancing equitable global health research partnerships in Africa. BMJ Glob Health. 2018;3(4):e000868.
46. Dieleman JL, Graves CM, Templin T, Johnson E, Baral R, Leach-Kemon K, et al. Global Health development assistance remained steady in 2013 but did not align with recipients' disease burden. Health Aff (Millwood). 2014;33(5):878–86.
47. Nordling L Nelson Torto: up for a challenge. Research Professional [Internet]. 2017 Aug; https://www.researchresearch.com/news/article/?articleId=1369817
48. Dimitris MC, Gittings M, King NB. How global is global health research? A large-scale analysis of trends in authorship. BMJ Glob Health. 2021;6(1):e003758.
49. Giles A, Ramirez A, Kim NE, Mehta A, Fallah P, Ovsak G. GSSA | Global Surgery Database [Internet]. Global Surgery Student Association. 2022 [cited 2022 Jul 20]. https://www.globalsurgerystudents.org/mentor-database
50. Global Surgery | Association for Academic Global Surgery [Internet]. globalsurgery. [cited 2022 Aug 10]. https://www.academicglobalsurgery.org
51. Debas H, Alatise OI, Balch CM, Brennan M, Cusack J, Donkor P, et al. Academic partnerships in global surgery: an overview American Surgical Association Working Group on Academic Global Surgery. Ann Surg. 2020;271(3):460–9.
52. Fallah PN, Bernstein M. Barriers to participation in global surgery academic collaborations, and possible solutions: a qualitative study. J Neurosurg. 2018;1–9
53. Peck G, Badillo J, Burbano M, Citron I, Domingues CDA, Lang R, et al. Nursing workforce in surgery and trauma care delivery: a global call to action. The Bulletin of the American College of Surgeons. 102nd ed. 2017 Nov 1;11–6.
54. Gutnik L, Yamey G, Riviello R, Meara JG, Dare AJ, Shrime MG. Financial contributions to global surgery: an analysis of 160 international charitable organizations. Springerplus. 2016;5(1):1558.
55. IGHS Affiliates Database [Internet]. UCSF Institute for Global Health Sciences. [cited 2022 Aug 1]. https://globalhealthsciences.ucsf.edu/resources/faculty-affiliate-program/ighs-affiliates-database

How to Build Research in Low- and Middle-Income Countries

22

Theresa Chin and Nia Zalamea

Research is formalized curiosity. It is poking and prying with a purpose.

– Zora Neale Hurston

Abbreviations

HICs	High-income countries
IRB	Institutional Review Board
LMICs	Low- and middle-income countries
QI	Quality improvement
WHO	World Health Organization

Background

Quality improvement (QI) and research are intertwined; they are similar in underlying concept of expanding knowledge, yet they differ in their specific goals (Table 22.1). Quality improvement focuses on the delivery of health care by implementing knowledge or evaluating a process or program, whereas research answers a question or hypothesis to create new knowledge that can be generalizable to a population [1, 2]. In QI, patients are subject to new initiatives as an inherent result of consenting to healthcare delivery, and protocols are adapted to a given healthcare system and adjusted therein to make improvements. On the contrary, in research, patients may be randomized to avert confounding data, or there may be a fixed protocol with a predefined population and methodology to avert bias when interpreting data. Research may be qualitative or quantitative and can include investigating processes or programs for generalizable knowledge for evidence-based medicine. QI initiatives can become research, and research methodologies can be used in quality improvement. When QI projects evolve and become research, ethical approval of the research is necessary to protect human subjects.

Creating a research program requires strategic planning and support, as it is an endeavor that cannot be done successfully alone. It will require time, effort, financial investment, and advocacy. This chapter is a framework from which to develop a research program (Table 22.2 and Fig. 22.1). It can be customized for building

T. Chin (✉)
University of California Irvine, Orange, CA, USA
e-mail: chintl1@hs.uci.edu

N. Zalamea
University of Tennessee Health Science Center, Global Surgery Institute, Memphis, TN, USA
e-mail: nzalamea@uthsc.edu

M. A. Hardy, B. R. Hochman (eds.), *Global Surgery*, https://doi.org/10.1007/978-3-031-28127-3_22

Table 22.1 Comparison of quality improvement and research

	Quality improvement	Research
Goal	• Implement knowledge • Evaluate a program or process • Improve healthcare delivery	• Produce to generalizable knowledge • Test a hypothesis • Answer a specific question
Risk	• No increased risk to patients, except possible breach of personal health information	• May have increased risk
Typical methodology	• Compares program, process, or system change to current or conventional standard	• Aimed to answer question or test hypothesis • Can be retrospective or prospective • Can be observational or interventional
Knowledge	• Implements existing knowledge to improve care	• Creates new knowledge or evidence

Table 22.2 Framework for building research capacity in LMICs

What is the current capacity for research?	• Knowledge of research methodology • Capability to do basic, translational, clinical, or outcomes research • Priority of research within the context of the healthcare system • Office or laboratory space, equipment, and supplies • Personnel resources (Translation services, biostatisticians) • Clinical and data services • Availability of an ethics committee or Institutional Review Board • Current data sources (medical record documentation, available registries)
Who are the stakeholders at your institution or community?	• Hospital leaders • Department or academic leaders • Nursing/Allied health representatives • Public health experts • Scientists • Government and nongovernment leaders
What collaborations or partnerships can be developed?	• Twinning models of institutional partnership • Regional or national collaborations • Nongovernmental organization partnerships • Medical society collaborations • Interdepartment collaborations • Industry or corporate partnerships
What to consider in a strategic plan?	• Support and completion of existing projects and other early successes to positively reinforce the potential of the program • Strategies to create tangible value early in the plan (grant funding, financial support from partner institutions, salary or time support from department leaders or partners, etc.) • Research ideas or methods that lead to subsequent projects • Win-win projects where all partners/collaborators benefit • Anticipation of potential failures and ways to avert them • Create a system of mentorship as it will encourage and train new researchers for sustainability and expansion • Develop a clear, simple action plan

Table 22.2 (continued)

What ethical issues should be considered throughout the program development?	• Autonomy, beneficence, nonmaleficence for all research subjects • Equitable authorship • Equity and transparency in partnerships and collaborations • Adequate financial compensation for research efforts • Management of the grant money and its disbursement in twinning partnerships • Local or cultural adjustments to the community • Systematic and unconscious biases
What to consider when implementing the action plan?	• Timeline and milestones • Scheduled reassessments • Realistic priorities
How to assess progress and modify for improvement or expansion?	• Available funding • Team feedback • External feedback

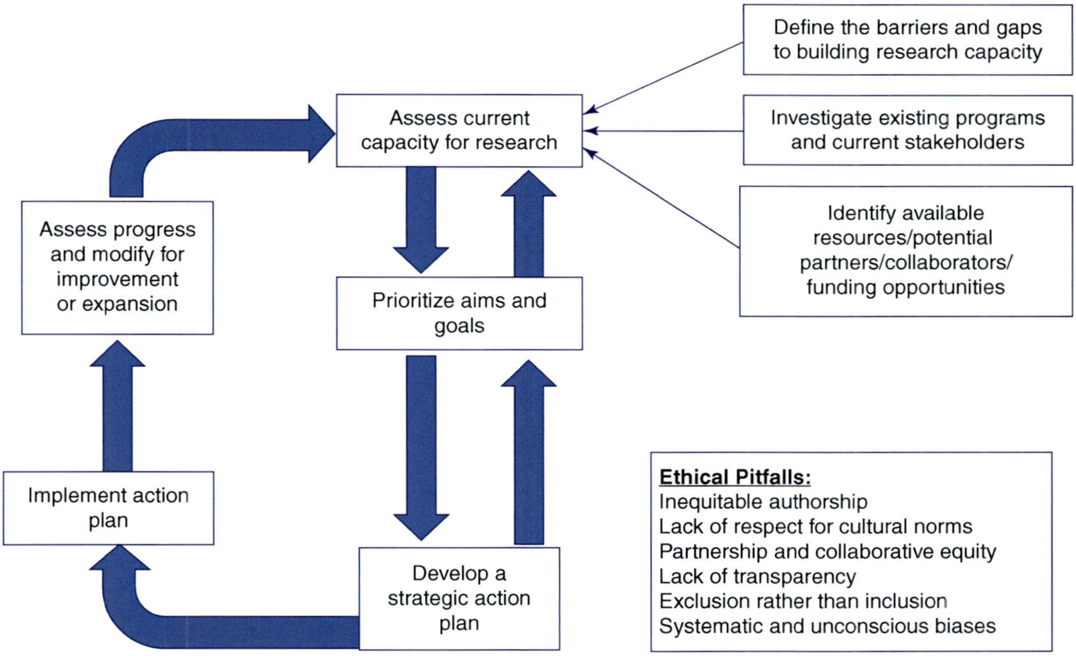

Fig. 22.1 Research program development

research capacity in LMICs and should be tailored to fit the local environment. The process of assessing need, defining aims and goals, and creating a strategic plan is dynamic and may change as new needs are identified, new ideas and goals are developed, and the strategic plan consequently changes. The leadership of any research program should be goal-oriented yet flexible.

A Framework for Developing Research in an LMIC

What Is the Current Capacity for Research?

A needs assessment gathers information to examine the current system and capacity for research in its current state. It is like doing an inventory in a store and allows the store owner to see which items are lacking. Someone who knows the local environment is vital to the needs assessment. Similarly, an inventory of a store is best done by workers in the store who know where every item is stored or displayed. Below are items to include in a broad assessment of research capacity of a given system and may not be completely comprehensive in all settings. Table 22.3 has a basic checklist of needs for a research program.

- *Knowledge of research methodology:* Are the researchers knowledgeable in study design and able to define a research question? Is it a research question that is applicable to the local population? Is it culturally and ethically feasible?
- *Capability to do basic, translational, clinical, or outcomes research*: clinical outcomes research as well as retrospective and prospective observational trials are frequently easier to start than basic science and translational research. Basic science and translational research may require testing or equipment not readily available in the clinical setting, such as polymerase chain reaction tests or other assays.
- *Priority of research within the context of the healthcare system*: Does the culture of the leadership and staff to prioritize research enough to contribute to the efforts? Research in a clinical setting requires additional time and effort beyond typical duties of clinician. Will the institution or department compensate the faculty to conduct research in either time or money? Will the local leadership advocate for research efforts to local government officials? Will the institutions be able to obtain access to research to improve the quality of care delivered? Is research required for faculty advancement? What are the metrics that are measured?
- *Office or laboratory space, equipment, and supplies:* Space can be shared or used for research and clinical obligations. Equipment and supplies include office equipment, computers, laboratory equipment, and consumable supplies/materials.
- *Personnel resources:* Research assistants, data manager or analyst, and clerical staff are frequently needed. People can fulfill multiple roles, but additional funding for personnel will improve the efficiency of the research as personnel specific for the research program can dedicate time to the project(s). If researchers are interested in publishing in journals that are in English, interpreter and translation services, though costly, may be necessary.
- *Clinical and data services:* Collaborating with the clinical lab can allow for more efficient work flow. Statistical assistance may be available in the school of public health. Data services may be available through the hospital system. The WHO has data registries available to LMICs such as burn or trauma. In countries looking to publish in a language that is not native, hiring of an interpreter and translator may be a previously unforeseen cost.
- *An ethics committee or Institutional Review Board*: to review research studies to ensure all research is conducted in an ethical manner.
- *Current data sources*: Does the medical record documentation have adequate detail and legibility (if paper) where a retrospective study could be performed? Does the healthcare system and cultural norms allow for patients to be followed prospectively?

Table 22.3 Basic checklist of needs for research programs

1. **Leader(s) of research efforts and/or principal investigator**
2. **Team member(s) knowledgeable in research methods and study design**
3. **Team members(s) to enroll and follow up patients and collect data**
4. **Team member(s) to manage the data, analyze, and interpret the data**
5. **Ethical board or institutional review board (IRB)**
6. **Equipment and supplies**
7. **Access to existing literature**

Who Are the Stakeholders at your Institution or Region?

Stakeholders are people who have a vested interest in the program and are important to the success of a research program. Local institutional leadership is essential to a *sustainable* research program because they are familiar with the culture, the local administration, and the feasibility within the local system. They may be leaders within the hospital, the department, or the academic institution. Support from the administration and local leaders helps to gain resources for the research program. These leaders can advocate and allocate resources for research. Administration and other leaders can work with editors of regional or international journals for equitable publishing and promotion.

Inclusion of other disciplines such as nursing or other allied health professions will improve the success of the research project and program and provide different perspectives for feasibility of select research studies. For example, public health faculty may be able to provide assistance for statistics or study design and, in exchange, authorship on research can benefit the faculty for academic promotion. Consider who may be affected by the research protocol. Think about nurses, pharmacist, other medical disciplines, and administration, information technology, equipment personnel, laboratory personnel. To be inclusive and culturally appropriate, representatives for all populations that are affected by research should be included in the research board. For example, if the study includes or affects indigenous populations, a representative of that population should be included in the study design and/or ethics board. It is helpful to include stakeholders early in the study design period or research program planning to maximize efficiency for study recruitment, enrollment, consent, data collection, and program development.

Investigate existing programs at the institution or local region. Learn from other programs that have thrived in similar environments. Sometimes, one may find that there are other people with similar interests at the same institution. In addition to available resources in the local area, there are many resources that are free or available at low cost on the Internet. Explore journals that have open access. Many institutions have free educational classes and webinars related to research. Many statistical programs that can be used for data analysis require a fee, but a few products are free and open access. Basic statistics can be calculated within a spreadsheet application, such as Microsoft Excel or Google Sheets. Advanced data analysis and interpretation often require additional training; however, collaboration with statisticians can bridge the gap and provide additional resources.

Develop a Strategic Plan for a Research Program

- A thoughtful strategic plan can be worth the investment over time. It can make the entire program more efficient, and creation of contingency plans can improve the potential for success. The basic checklist of needs in Table 22.3 will give you the necessary elements to get started.
- Identify early projects that can lead to other projects and continued research such as a dataset that can be used to answer more than one question. Projects that are "low-hanging fruit" and likely to be successful early on will be positive reinforcement for continued research efforts and support. These projects may be simpler in research methodology or already in progress. Publishing interesting case reports demonstrates an interest in the science of surgery and can lead to research topics or ideas. It will also introduce the complexities of submitting and revising a manuscript for publication.
- Many research questions arise from daily routine care for patients. There may be some clinical research projects in progress with basic data collection and tracking of patients. Consider investigating patterns of disease, a new or alternative intervention, a different population, patient outcomes, or efficacy of clinician behaviors. Conduct a literature review and see if your question is already answered. Is the existing literature generalizable to low- and middle-income health systems and populations? Are you identifying the problem or developing solutions to the prob-

lem? Is there another clinical question within a different population or subgroup?

- With new collaborations or partnerships, consider starting with projects where all involved benefit to be positive reinforcement to working together.
- Do others think the research idea is a good one that will have impact? What personnel is available to assist in your research? You may revisit this item throughout the research project. Seek help. Look for collaborations and mentorship. Find a local champion if you can't do it yourself.
- Are there personnel adequately trained in study design who can assist with creating studies? If not, consider expanding your search to identify potential collaborators or people who are willing to learn and train.
- Formulate a data management plan. This is to ensure that data, especially if it contains personal health information, is secure and protects patients and research subjects. Additionally, contingency plans to avert lost data either digitally or papers should be created. Electronic collection tools make it easier to analyze the data; however, paper collection tools may allow for ease of data collection, particularly if computers or tablets are not easily accessible or available. Paper collection tools can be more arduous since the data on the paper will need to be inputted to a computer program to be analyzed. This can lead to potential human errors in data entry. Aim to maintain the original data in the LMIC where the data is collected.
- Prioritize mentorship, because it is important to encourage new researchers to persevere early in their research career when successes are small or infrequent. Mentors can guide faculty on how to present and publish research or quality improvement projects. Mentors can be from the local LMIC institution and/or from partnering or HIC institutions. Telementorship can help with advancing research in LMICs, provided both parties are engaged and invested in the research project. Local mentorship is ideal as the mentor will understand the local infrastructure, system, and culture. Furthermore, engagement may be more sustainable with a local mentor.
- Create clear and simple action items as part of your strategic plan. This will help you monitor progress and allow the project to move forward.

Ethical Considerations

There are several ethical issues specific to LMICs. It is extremely important to maintain the highest ethical conscience to protect people and cultural communities and to preserve relationships and partnerships. Chapters 3 and 36 in this book focus on the ethical issues of both practice and of research in LMICs,

- The three principles of basic human subject research apply to all research regardless of geographic location or socioeconomic status:
  1. Autonomy: LMIC communities and patients should be able to make informed decisions about what is best for their communities and themselves.
  2. Beneficence: There should be benefit to the population of the LMIC either directly to the patients or to society.
  3. Non-maleficence: As possible, tactics to minimize risk to the community and individual patients should be employed.
- Credit and authorship for research efforts must be equitable and can be used to edify LMIC researchers. Some LMIC researchers are promoted based on publications, and their efforts should be considered. Strategies to ensure equitable authorship are described in the consensus statement by Morton et al. [3] and can include expectation of first or senior authorship from the initiation of the research project, structural reflexivity statements to describe how equity was maintained throughout the study, and adaptations to journal requirements that promote equity. Authorship can be discussed early in the project when the expectations of the LMIC and HIC partners are established.

- When researchers from high-income countries conduct research in a LMIC, early inclusion and heavy involvement of local LMIC personnel are vital to ensure that the research study confers maximum benefit with minimal risk, in addition to ensuring that the study is culturally appropriate. If available, ethical approval from both a local LMIC ethical board and the HIC institution should be obtained.
- Partnerships are a two-way relationship where both parties contribute resources and benefit. Collaborations occur when individuals or institutions work separately toward a unified goal. Both partnerships and collaborations should be equitable, and the communication should be bidirectional. In a partnership, decision-making should be shared, particularly in regard to shared resources. If a HIC institution or company is more authoritative and dictates the study plans, the lack of autonomy of the LMIC places those involved with the research at an increased risk of vulnerability.
- Access to the data should be equitable and ideally associated to where the bulk of the data is collected. Frequently, data is collected in LMICs but housed in HICs, limiting access to the data for LMICs for additional research and quality projects.
- When funding is available, LMIC partners should be adequately compensated. If the bulk of the labor is conducted at the LMIC, the bulk of the funding should be awarded to the LMIC.
- Addressing the impact of any research on the local community is essential to the trust of the community on biomedical research. Consider if the methodology is feasible with the resources available and if it inhibits the local community in other ways. For example, a laboratory test can be conducted for research, but it may delay or prevent other laboratory tests necessary for clinical care. Discuss with the local leaders if the research applicable to the LMIC setting is impactful for the patient population (i.e., will the research help the local people/society)?
- Take caution for people who may have alternative motivations. Some may be political or financial. Focus on what is best for the people and community and take heed to warnings from others with different perspectives.
- It can be hard to predict and foresee all systemic and unconscious biases that we all have. Regardless, once they come to light, they should be addressed with the highest ethical and equitable consideration and respect for others.

Implement Action Plan

- Successful action plans have timelines and milestones to keep the project on track. Be realistic in creating the timeline and milestones so that the program can be successful and sustainable.
- Schedule regular reassessments. In a new program, monthly or quarterly assessments may be needed to keep the program on track. As the program becomes more established, yearly review may be adequate to ensure the needs of all involved are being met.

Assess Progress and Modify for Improvement or Expansion

- Identify funding, if available. Funding is not required to start research; however, it is needed to sustain a program. Local institutional and governmental investment into the research program is one of the best strategies for sustainable funding. However, funding options through societies, academic institutions, nonprofit organizations, and even industry may provide an initial launching pad for research endeavors. Be mindful of conflicts of interest.
- Feedback from all members of the team and community will improve the efficiency of the team and can allow for growth of the program. It will also identify needs or gaps that may compromise the stability of the program and research team. There may be new resources or stakehold-

ers available and should be considered. As the program is successful, it will naturally expand as others become interested and want to partner or collaborate. However, take caution to expand too fast, as research requires time, money, and material resources that can easily be depleted.

- Feedback from outside sources can generate ideas for improving efficiency and introducing new resources. Outside sources may include other local leaders, society leaders, or other organizations that may have a vested interest in the population or community.

Conclusion

Research is a collaborative effort and requires persistence and multiple tries to be successful. Do not be discouraged! It can take multiple tries and relies on assembling the right team for success. Occasionally, merely starting a project and adapting to the needs of the project can lead to momentum and others joining and supporting the effort. It is practically impossible to be prepared for all aspects of research, so flexibility and adaptability are two qualities that can increase the success of a research program.

How can researchers in HICs edify LMIC researchers? Partnerships between institutions in HICs and LMICs can expand the available knowledge, experience, and resources to conduct research. However, the partnership may want to initially establish boundaries and formalize with a memorandum of understanding so that all institutions involved are treated fairly.

References

1. Baily MA, Bottrell M, Lynn J, Jennings B, Center H. The ethics of using QI methods to improve health care quality and safety. Hast Cent Rep. 2006;36(4):S1-40. https://doi.org/10.1353/hcr.2006.0054.
2. Finkelstein JA, Brickman AL, Capron A, Ford DE, Gombosev A, Greene SM, Iafrate RP, Kolaczkowski L, Pallin SC, Pletcher MJ, Staman KL, Vazquez MA, Sugarman J. Oversight on the borderline: quality improvement and pragmatic research. Clin Trials. 2015;12(5):457–66. https://doi.org/10.1177/1740774515597682. Epub 2015 Sep 15. PMID: 26374685; PMCID: PMC4699562
3. Morton B, Vercueil A, Masekela R, Heinz E, Reimer L, Saleh S, Kalinga C, Seekles M, Biccard B, Chakaya J, Abimbola S, Obasi A, Oriyo N. Consensus statement on measures to promote equitable authorship in the publication of research from international partnerships. Anaesthesia. 2022;77(3):264–76. https://doi.org/10.1111/anae.15597. Epub 2021 Oct 14

Part III

General Surgery: Organ-Focused Selected Interventions

How to Manage Urgent Neurosurgical Problems in Low- and Middle-Income Countries

23

Ernest J. Barthélemy, Tsegazaeb Laeke, and Kee B. Park

The essence of global health equity is the idea that something so precious as health might be viewed as a right.

– Paul Farmer

Abbreviations

ASDH	Acute subdural hemorrhage
BooTSTRAP	Beyond One Option for Treatment of Traumatic Brain Injury: A Stratified Protocol
BTF	Brain Trauma Foundation
CSDH	Chronic subdural hemorrhage
EDH	Epidural hemorrhage
LMIC(s)	Low- and middle-income countr(y/ies)
NCCTH	Noncontrast CT of the head and brain
SAH	Subarachnoid hemorrhage
SDH	Subdural hemorrhage
SSAH	Spontaneous subarachnoid hemorrhage
TBI	Traumatic brain injury
TICH	Traumatic intracerebral hemorrhage
TICN	Traumatic intracranial hypertension
TSAH	Traumatic subarachnoid hemorrhage

E. J. Barthélemy
Global Neurosurgery Laboratory, Division of Neurosurgery, SUNY Downstate Health Sciences University, Brooklyn, NY, USA

T. Laeke
Neurosurgery Division, College of Health Sciences, Addis Ababa University, Addis Ababa, Ethiopia

K. B. Park (✉)
Program in Global Surgery and Social Change, Harvard Medical School, Boston, MA, USA

Introduction

Neurosurgical disease is defined as any medicosurgical disorder or condition for which the diagnostic or therapeutic expertise of a neurosurgeon is required for its comprehensive management, treatment, and/or cure. In low- and middle-income countries (LMICs), the most common neurosurgical diseases include traumatic injuries of the head, brain, or spine (i.e., neurotrauma), spontaneous subarachnoid or intracerebral hemorrhages, and brain tumors. Treatment of these conditions in LMICs requires not only the extensive knowledge of nervous system anatomy, physiology, pathology, pathophysiology, and the medicosurgical management that comprises neurosurgical training, but also a thorough understanding of the socioeconomic and political

M. A. Hardy, B. R. Hochman (eds.), *Global Surgery*, https://doi.org/10.1007/978-3-031-28127-3_23

contexts within which patients suffer from neurosurgical disorders, and an ability to optimize resource utilization according to these contexts, especially when resources for effective neurosurgical care are limited or absent. This chapter introduces and describes some of the most common neurosurgical conditions encountered in LMICs and fundamental medical and surgical management strategies for optimizing the outcomes of patients afflicted with these conditions.

Neurosurgical Management of Brain Hemorrhage

Intracranial hemorrhage may occur within the tissue of the brain or in the various intervening spaces between the brain and the skull, as a result of primary or secondary brain insults. These hemorrhages, especially when they occur acutely, are usually neurosurgical emergencies that portend a poor prognosis if not rapidly diagnosed and treated. The most common causes of intracranial hemorrhage are nonpenetrating traumatic injuries of the head and brain. Various spontaneous vascular injuries of the brain may, however, also result in brain hemorrhage.

Traumatic Intracranial Hemorrhage

Trauma to the head that injures intracranial vessels results in traumatic intracranial hemorrhage. The mechanical force exerted upon the head, brain, and intracranial vessels varies according to the mechanism of trauma and dictates the type of intracranial vascular injury producing the resulting brain hemorrhage. For example, injury to veins and/or arteries at the periphery of the brain and its surrounding membranes (i.e., dura, arachnoid and pia mater) can result in extra-axial hemorrhages such as subdural or epidural hematomas, whereas injury to deep vessels within the brain can result in intra-axial brain hemorrhages such as contusions.

Acute Subdural Hematoma (ASDH)

Acute subdural hematoma (ASDH) refers to a rapid accumulation of blood forming extra-axial clots within the subdural space, i.e., between the outer dural membrane and the deeper brain parenchyma invested with pial and arachnoid meningeal layers [2]. ASDH is caused by a high-impact injury to the head that tears blood vessels within this space. It is commonly associated with injury to the underlying brain parenchyma, which may contribute to high associated morbidity and mortality, especially if not treated promptly [3]. Classically, the injured vessels are bridging veins between the dura mater and the brain surface, which tear as a result of acceleration-deceleration brain injury, resulting in hematoma formation in the subdural space.

Clinical Presentation

Patients presenting with large ASDH requiring neurosurgical management usually present with a loss of consciousness. Their Glasgow Coma Score (GCS) is generally less than or equal to 8/15, indicating a severe traumatic brain injury. Focal neurologic deficits such as motor weakness contralateral to the lesion (or less commonly, ipsilateral to large lesions with significant midline shift), generalized seizure, and/or anisocoria with pupillary dilation ipsilateral to the lesion are also clinical manifestations of a large ASDH requiring surgical evacuation.

The definitive diagnosis of ASDH requires a computed tomography scan of the head and brain without contrast enhancement (NCCTH), which therefore makes computed tomography imaging capability an indispensable resource for management of ASDH in all contexts. ASDH typically appears as a crescentic-shaped hyperdense lesion overlying the brain surface (Fig. 23.1). Associated NCCTH findings in patients with large ASDH include mass effect that effaces the sulcal and gyral anatomy of the brain surface compressed by the hematoma and a shift of midline structures away from the side of the lesion (Fig. 23.1).

Chronic Subdural Hematoma (CSDH)

Chronic subdural hematoma (CSDH) is a common neurosurgical condition characterized by a slow, progressive accumulation of hematoma and inflammatory products in the subdural space. It is

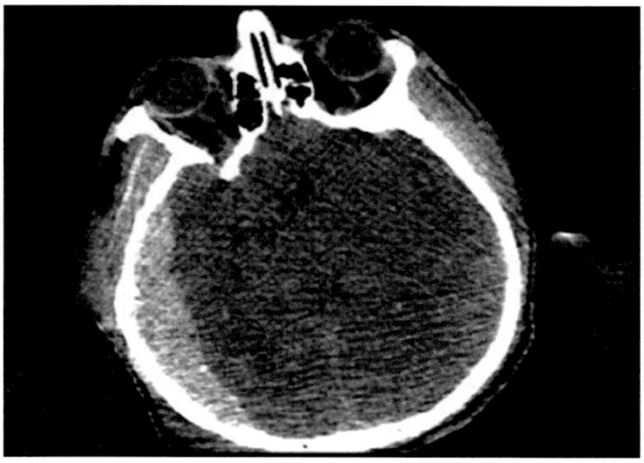

Fig. 23.1 Noncontrast CT scan of the head and brain showing a large, right-sided acute subdural hematoma compressing the temporoparietal convexity, with mass effect on the right temporal lobe, and midline shift from right to left

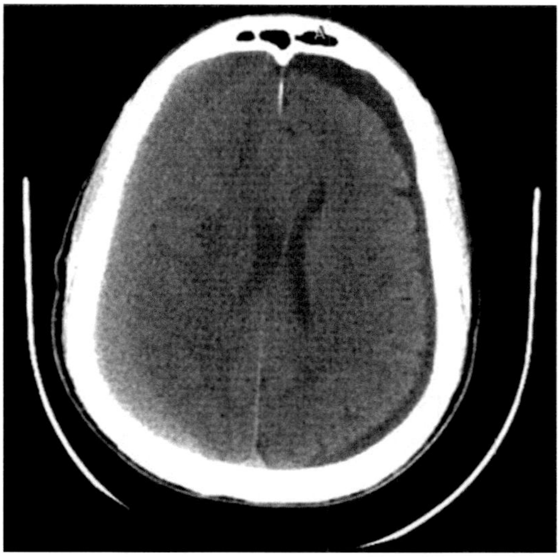

Fig. 23.2 Noncontrast CT scan of the head and brain showing bilateral chronic subdural hematomas. Note the more isodense appearance of the larger, right-sighted lesion as compared to the hypodense left-sided lesion. The asymmetry of lesions produces right-sided mass effect, with a leftward shift of midline structures. CT, computed tomography

classically thought to have a similar pathophysiology to that of ASDH, with chronification of a hematoma originally caused by tearing of bridging veins, along with an inflammatory process originally referred to as a, "pachymeningitis hemorrhagica interna." Recent studies continue to elucidate the role of multiple inflammatory and angiogenic factors in the pathophysiology of CSDH [4].

Clinical Presentation

Patients with CSDH are typically older patients having insidious onset of neurologic symptoms lasting for a few days to weeks before presentation. Patients can have different symptoms mimicking other neurologic conditions such as stroke and dementia. However, the most common symptoms found in patients with CSDH include gait disturbance, contralateral limb weakness, and alteration of mental status. Unlike ASDH, however, patients do not generally present with rapid loss of consciousness and are more likely to present with GCS scores higher than 8. As in ASDH, NCCTH is the gold standard for the rapid diagnosis of CSDH. It appears as a crescentic-shaped hypodense or isodense extra-axial lesion compressing the brain surface (Fig. 23.2). This lesion can also produce mass effect on the underlying brain parenchyma and a contralateral shift of midline structures.

Epidural Hematoma (EDH)

Epidural hematoma (EDH) is a collection of blood between the dura and the inner table of the skull. Mechanisms of head trauma resulting in EDH are similar to those that result in ASDH and commonly include road traffic accidents, falls, or assaults. ASDH and EDH may occur in isolation or concurrently. When occurring in isolation, EDH is commonly associated with a fracture of the temporal bone that classically injures the middle meningeal artery. Hence, EDH is frequently located in the temporoparietal region. It has been reported that EDH occurs in 14–35% of traumatic brain injuries and occurs less frequently than ASDH; however, lack of data from low- and middle-income countries (LMICs) on TBI renders the real incidence of EDH in LMICs underrecognized or unknown, and resource limitations in many of these contexts may contribute to higher incidence of EDH than that observed in high-income countries [5–7]. For instance, a prospective study from Ethiopia including over

1000 patients found EDH to be the most common extra-axial brain hemorrhage among patients with TBI, accounting for 39% of cases as compared to 7% of cases with subdural hematoma [8].

Clinical Presentation

EDH classically presents with a lucid interval, characterized by a brief loss of consciousness immediately after trauma, followed by the transient regaining of consciousness, and a subsequent definitive loss of consciousness without intervention. Nonetheless, patients with EDH can also lose consciousness immediately after the trauma or be fully conscious at hospital presentation. Headache, seizures, hemiparesis, and vomiting are also possible clinical findings. Some patients may also present with anisocoria when the EDH is large enough to result in mass effect that compromises the parasympathetic tone of the ipsilateral oculomotor nerve (cranial nerve III).

As in ASDH or CSDH, the definitive diagnosis of EDH is made by NCCTH. Imaging shows a lenticular-shaped hyperdense lesion pressing on the brain parenchyma and limited by the sutures of the skull (Fig. 23.3).

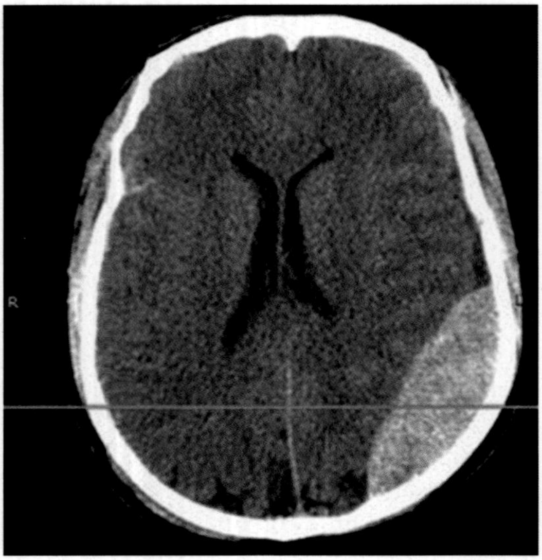

Fig. 23.3 Precontrast brain CT scan showing a left parieto-occipital acute epidural hematoma

Traumatic Subarachnoid Hemorrhage (tSAH)

Subarachnoid hemorrhage is bleeding in the space between the arachnoid membrane and the pia. The most common cause of subarachnoid hemorrhage is trauma. Traumatic subarachnoid hemorrhage (tSAH) often occurs along the convexity of the brain within its sulci, or within expansions of the subarachnoid space such as the cistern of the sylvian fissure or the basal cisterns of the skull surrounding the brain stem. Some components of tSAH are frequently found in moderate and severe traumatic brain injuries. TSAH can contribute to adverse outcomes by its pathophysiologic sequelae that include cerebral vasospasm, electrolyte imbalances, intracranial hypertension, and disruptions in cerebrospinal fluid dynamics producing hydrocephalus.

NCCTH in tSAH typically shows hyperdensity of cerebrospinal fluid (CSF) spaces that otherwise appear hypodense in normal computed tomography brain imaging, such as the sulci of the brain. The bright appearance of sulcal spaces or basal spaces such as the interpeduncular fossa, following traumatic brain injury, therefore suggests tSAH and sometimes can be associated with adjacent traumatic contusions of brain parenchyma.

Brain Contusions

Brain contusions occur when sudden deceleration force impacts the brain on the skull's bony prominences, commonly affecting the frontal poles, temporal poles, or lateral surfaces of the temporoparietal lobes. They may occur at the site of brain impact on the surface of injury (i.e., "coup" injury) or at a contralateral brain surface due to impact against the cranial vault resulting from the brain's ricochet or "contrecoup" movement away from the primary site of injury. Contusions consist of bleeding from cortical vessels that extends into the brain parenchyma, producing bruises of the brain tissue [9]. They occur immediately following injury, and/or they may expand several days following injury as evidenced on interval NCCTH images that may be obtained in the setting of neurological examination worsening. Contusions are typically not surgically evacuated unless they expand enough to contribute to life-threatening intracranial hypertension.

Management of Traumatic Intracranial Hemorrhage

Emergency Department Management (Spectrum of Resources)

Management of traumatic intracranial hemorrhage should follow standardized protocols designed by local authorities in trauma care to optimize patient survival and outcome following trauma, such as the Advanced Trauma Life Support (ATLS) Guidelines of the American College of Surgeons. Imminently life-threatening conditions such as airway obstruction, breathing difficulties, and threats to hemodynamic stability such as large-volume bleeding or circulation abnormalities should be prioritized before specialized management of brain injury.

The treatment options available for managing traumatic intracranial hemorrhage depend on the resources and context of a patient's local health system. Context-specific management options for TBI patients in LMICs were not broadly available until recently, with global neurosurgery publications that have started to address both policy-level recommendations for optimal neurotrauma care in LMICs and institutional and health system recommendations for resource-stratified protocolization of TBI care in LMICs [10, 11].

At the emergency department, patients with traumatic intracranial hemorrhage should have the head-of-bed elevated to 30 degrees. They should be provided with supplemental oxygen as needed to prevent hypoxia, with a pulse oximetry target range of 95–100%. Comatose patients with a GCS of less than 9 should be intubated for airway security and placed on a mechanical ventilator. Patients should also be kept euvolemic with a blood pressure target no lower than 90/60 mmHG. Analgesics are given to alleviate pain and to help prevent pathologic increases of intracranial pressure (ICP).

Patients with signs of intracranial hypertension such as dilated and fixed pupil, decerebrate or decorticate posturing, and rapid neurologic deterioration are administered a 1 gram per kilogram bolus of mannitol; however, mannitol is contraindicated in patients having hypotension or congestive heart failure. Prophylactic administration of mannitol is also contraindicated. Patients receiving mannitol infusion must undergo insertion of a urethral catheter into the urinary bladder in order to facilitate diuresis.

Surgical Treatment of Acute Epidural Hematoma

According to guidelines by the Brain Trauma Foundation, acute epidural hematoma with a volume of more than 30cm^3, a midline shift of more than 5 mm, and a hematoma thickness of at least 15 mm is considered significant and warrants surgical intervention [12].

The surgery involves performing a craniotomy and evacuation of the clot from the epidural space, as well as identification and cauterization of the injured blood vessel producing the hematoma. The scalp incision is made overlying the hematoma after localizing it from the NCCTH. The most commonly used scalp incision is a "trauma flap" which is also known as a "question mark" or "reverse question mark" flap. The flap is generally made around the frontotemporal area which is the most common site for epidural hemorrhage. After developing the scalp flap, the craniotomy is performed either by an electric-powered drill and craniotome if available or by manual drill and Gigli saws. The clot is then removed from the dura gently by using gentle saline irrigation, a spatula, and suction as needed. After removing the clot, tack-up stitches are applied which involve suturing the dura with the skull, or to peri-cranial tissue to close the potential epidural space. Applying tack-up stitches is important to prevent postoperative hematoma reaccumulation by obliterating the epidural space. The bone flap is then replaced once the hematoma is evacuated and the tack-up stitches are applied.

Surgical Treatment of Acute Subdural Hematoma

According to Brain Trauma Foundation guidelines, patients with an ASDH thickness of more than 10 mm or a midline shift of 5 mm should be surgically treated [12]. Patients having a GCS of less than 9 with ASDH thickness of less than 10 mm and midline shift of less than 5 mm should be treated surgically if their GCS drops by 2 between two neurological evaluations.

Craniotomy is the surgical procedure of choice for ASDH. The craniotomy can be converted to a decompressive craniectomy by leaving the bone flap off, which is more commonly performed in cases where there is heightened concern for significant postoperative brain swelling. A generous scalp flap should be done which accommodates a big bone flap. The decision to leave off the bone flap often depends on the extent of intraoperative brain swelling encountered. In the presence of significant brain swelling, replacement of the bone flap may both be challenging and poorly advised as the replaced bone may contribute to postoperative intracranial hypertension. In the case of decompressive craniectomy, the bone flap is either stored in a refrigerator with a temperature of around −80 degrees Celsius if available or is inserted into a subcutaneous tissue pocket developed in the lower abdomen (i.e., marsupialization) for future reconstruction of the skull once the brain swelling subsides. This is a much cheaper option especially in a resource-constrained setting. However, synthetic materials such as methyl methacrylate and titanium mesh could also be used for delayed, alloplastic cranial reconstruction.

Surgical Treatment of Traumatic Intracerebral Hemorrhage

Evacuation of traumatic intracerebral hemorrhage (tICH) is recommended if patients' neurological status deteriorates progressively and the deterioration is due to the tICH. Surgery to evacuate tICH is also indicated if the intracranial hypertension is medically refractory. However, any tICH with a volume of greater than 50 cm^3 should be evacuated regardless of the patients' condition. Patients with a GCS of 8 or less with a temporal or frontal tICH of greater than 20 cm^3 and midline shift of 5 mm or more should also undergo surgical treatment and evacuation of the hemorrhage.

Surgical Treatment of Chronic Subdural Hematoma

Patients with CSDH are usually elderly, with comorbidities. They may be on antiplatelet or anticoagulant treatment for cardiac or vascular conditions and thus have a propensity toward intracranial hemorrhage. Hence, if surgery is indicated, it is important to discontinue these drugs and reverse their effects before surgical treatment.

Symptomatic patients with CSDH should be surgically treated. The most common surgical technique is burr hole craniostomy. Intraoperative irrigation of the subdural space helps wash out the hematoma. Leaving drain in the subdural or subgaleal space postoperatively can help to significantly reduce the recurrence rate of CSDH. Moreover, following evacuation, lying patients supine with the head-of-bed flat in the first 24–48 h after surgery can facilitate re-expansion of the formerly compressed brain and reduce the risk of hematoma recurrence.

Spontaneous Bleeds

Spontaneous Subarachnoid Hemorrhage (sSAH)

Spontaneous subarachnoid hemorrhage (sSAH) frequently occurs in the fifth or sixth decades of life. It is more common in females. Risk factors for sSAH could be modifiable or nonmodifiable. Modifiable risk factors include hypertension, smoking, and heavy alcohol intake, while nonmodifiable risk factors include increasing age, female sex, family history, Japanese or Finnish ethnic origin, and history of subarachnoid hemorrhage [13, 14].

The most common cause of sSAH is aneurysmal rupture. It can be accompanied by intracerebral, intraventricular, or subdural hematoma. While 85% of all sSAHs are due to aneurysmal rupture, 15% are non-aneurysmal peri-mesencephalic. Aneurysmal sSAHs have worse prognosis than the non-aneurysmal peri-mesencephalic sSAH.

Clinical Features

The most common presentation of sSAH is "thunderclap" headache which is usually described by patients as the most severe headache they have ever experienced in their lifetime. The headache is commonly of sudden onset and reaches its maximum intensity within several seconds. In nearly half of such patients, the only presenting symptom is a headache. Hence, failure to recognize this differential diagnosis of sSAH can result in misdiagnosis of migraine and delay early treatment that may otherwise prevent death or severe disability. Other clinical features include nuchal rigidity or pain from meningeal irritation, alteration of mental status, or neurological deficits that may be referable to aneurysm location.

Similarly to traumatic brain hemorrhage, NCCTH is the frontline diagnostic modality of choice for sSAH. It is advised that all patients with sudden onset of headache and rapid worsening reaching maximum severity in an hour undergo an emergent NCCTH. The sensitivity of NCCTH depends on the time gap between the onset of symptoms and NCCTH acquisition: the shorter the time interval, the higher the sensitivity. An NCCTH taken within 72 hours has 97% sensitivity compared to an NCCTH taken after 5 days which has a sensitivity of 50%. NCCTH shows hyperdense blood products within the subarachnoid spaces which is suggestive of sSAH. Lumbar puncture is also another diagnostic test performed if the NCCTH scan result is inconclusive and the patient's clinical presentation is highly suggestive of sSAH. The stable presence of erythrocytes in each collection tube and/or xanthochromia in the CSF supports the diagnosis of sSAH (see below).

CT angiogram (CTA) is an important diagnostic adjunct to identify any ruptured aneurysms or other lesions that may be the source of hemorrhage. A digital subtraction catheter angiogram of the brain (DSA) is the gold standard diagnostic test for detecting the source of bleeding.

Table 23.1 Severity scores for subarachnoid hemorrhage: Hunt and Hess score, and corresponding WFNS score

Grade	Hunt and Hess	WFNS
I	Asymptomatic, or mild H/A and slight nuchal rigidity	GCS = 15
II	CN palsy, nuchal rigidity, moderate to severe headache,	GCS = 13–14 without major focal deficit
III	Mild focal deficit (other than CN deficit), confusion, or lethargy	GCS = 13–14 with major focal deficit
IV	Stupor, hemiparesis, early decerebrate rigidity	GCS 7–12 with or without major focal deficit
V	Deep coma, decerebrate posturing, moribund appearance	GCS = 3–6 with or without major focal deficit

Table 23.2 Modified Fischer Scale of SAH

Modified Fisher Score	Findings on noncontrast CT scan of the head and brain
0	No SAH
1	Focal or diffuse thin SAH without intraventricular hemorrhage
2	Focal or diffuse thin SAH with intraventricular hemorrhage
3	Focal or diffuse thick SAH without intraventricular hemorrhage
4	Focal or diffuse thick SAH with intraventricular hemorrhage

Moreover, it helps in planning treatment and, in settings with endovascular treatment capacity, may enable direct treatment and exclusion of the bleeding source from the brain's normal circulation. Cerebral catheter angiography is, however, an invasive and expensive procedure that is rarely available in resource-limited settings of LMICs. In most instances, CTA can replace DSA in diagnosing the cause of sSAH and planning treatment and requires only the ability to administer an intravascular contrast agent prior to computed tomography imaging.

sSAH is graded based on the clinical findings of the patient, the volume of hemorrhage, and whether there is extension of hemorrhage to the ventricles. These grading systems facilitate communication among the members of the treating team, assess the severity, and also predict the prognosis of patients (Tables 23.1 and 23.2) [14].

Management of sSAH

Patients with sSAH should be first treated for life-threatening emergency conditions. Their airway, breathing, and circulation should be secured and stabilized. Once the diagnosis of sSAH is made, the patients should ideally be admitted to the intensive care unit (ICU). If patients have acute hydrocephalus due to the sSAH, external ventriculostomy drain (EVD) insertion should be performed immediately for diversion of cerebrospinal fluid (CSF) into an external bag and collection system; this diversion can be converted to a ventriculoperitoneal shunt in delayed fashion. Of note, excessive diversion of CSF via EVD immediately following sSAH can potentiate re-rupture of a ruptured aneurysm (see below, "Eq. 23.1"). CSF diversion should therefore be limited to management of acute hydrocephalus and controlled to minimize the risk of re-rupture. Significant ASDH and intracerebral hemorrhages with pressure effect as a result of the sSAH occasionally occur and should also be evacuated.

The most common cause of death in sSAH is rebleeding from the ruptured aneurysm. Poor neurologic grade, hypertension at admission, and large aneurysm are risk factors for rebleeding. Clipping the ruptured aneurysm before it rebleeds is a life-saving procedure. It is suggested that clipping should be done immediately or within 72 h of the inaugural event [14]. The other alternative to clipping is endovascular coiling. The decision of using either of the two modalities depends on the clinical condition and age of the patients, location, size, shape of the ruptured aneurysms, and resources available for either mode of treatment.

Any patient presenting with SAH should be admitted and treated with the following initial orders.

Admission and inpatient orders

1. Patients should be admitted to the ICU.
2. Vital signs and neurologic status monitoring every hour.
3. Keep the head of the bed elevated to 30 degrees.
4. Keep the patient in a quiet place to minimize risk of bleeding: no loud noises, limited number of visitors, and limited level of external stimulation.
5. Keep NPO in case surgery is planned.
6. Maintain oxygen saturation above 90%; all those with GCS <9 should be intubated and put on mechanical ventilator.
7. Administer generous IV fluids to avoid cerebral salt wasting.
   - NS + 20 mEq KCl/L at ≈ 2 ml/kg/h. (typically 140–150 ml/h)
8. Normothermia should be maintained: acetaminophen is widely used.
9. Blood pressure: systolic blood pressure should be kept between 120 and 160 mmhg. It should not exceed more than 175mmhg as it has a high risk of aneurysmal rebleeding.
10. Medications to be considered:
    - **Prophylactic anticonvulsants**: widely used in many LMICs based on availability, dosing for phenytoin is typically 1 gm loading then 100 mg po tid; further dosing based on levels.
    - **Sedation**: IV propofol is often used for intubated patients.
    - **Analgesics**: fentanyl 25–100 mcg (0.5–2 ml) iv push, q 1–2 hrs as needed.
    - **Stool softener**: bisacodyl is frequently used; 5 mg po/day.
    - **Dexamethasone:** may help with H/A and neck pain due to meningeal inflammation by subarachnoid blood; often given before craniotomy.
    - **Anti-emetics**: ondansetron (4 mg IV over 2–5 min; can be repeated at 4 and 8 h and then every 8 h for 1–2 days) or metoclopramide (10 mg iv or po every 12 h).
    - **Calcium channel blocker:** nimodipine – 60 mg po or through nasogastric tube every 4 h started within 96 h of the onset of sSAH; titrate as needed to blood pressure parameters.
    - **Proton pump inhibitors:** omeprazole 20 mg po or iv every 12 h.

Spontaneous Intracerebral Hemorrhage (SICH)

Spontaneous intracerebral hemorrhage (SICH), also known as hemorrhagic stroke, refers to a sudden, acute rupture of blood vessels within the brain parenchyma. It is often precipitated or accompanied by malignant hypertension in the setting of some intrinsic neurovascular vulnerability attributable to risk factors that include longstanding uncontrolled hypertension, diabetes, connective tissue disorders, cerebral amyloid angiopathy, alcohol abuse, coagulation disorders, antiplatelet or anticoagulant therapy for preexisting cardiovascular conditions, or vascular anomalies such as arteriovenous malformations. Hemorrhagic conversion of ischemic stroke may also result in SICH. In high-income countries (HICs), hemorrhagic stroke is estimated to constitute about 10% of strokes, whereas in LMICs, hemorrhagic stroke accounts for 28–32% of acute strokes [15]. SICH typically presents with acute neurological deficits referable to the location of the mass lesion, such as right-sided hemiplegia accompanying SICH centered at the precentral gyrus of the left frontal lobe. Large volume SICH may produce severe intracranial hypertension and herniation syndromes if not rapidly treated. SICH may also extend into the ventricular system or be limited to the ventricular system, thereby resulting in acute alteration of mental status from obstructive hydrocephalus.

Initial Management of SICH

Initial management of SICH requires radiologic diagnosis with an NCCTH, followed by CTA to assess for an underlying lesion. As for any of the above-described hemorrhagic entities, the diagnosis can therefore not be confirmed without this minimum requirement of resources. Patients presenting to the emergency department with an acute neurologic deficit in the absence of trauma, and blood pressure elevation into malignant ranges of hypertension, e.g., >170 mm Hg systolic blood pressure, must be evaluated for a possible SICH in addition to other spontaneous neurovascular entities. Standard protocols of first-line care typically include assuring adequate airway security, breathing, and hemodynamic stability, with head-of-bed elevation to at least 30 degrees until NCCTH can be rapidly obtained to confirm the diagnosis.

Once SICH is confirmed, neurosurgical consultation is made, and typical admission orders are very similar to the initial management of subarachnoid hemorrhage (see above), with the exception of nimodipine administration. Orders should include admission to a neurointensive care unit with hourly neurological examination, maintenance of head-of-bed elevation to at least 30 degrees, strict control of blood pressure with a systolic blood pressure target of less than 160 mm Hg, and anticonvulsant therapy for seizure prophylaxis. Assessment and prognostication of SICH relies on a confluence of patient factors that include patient age, baseline function and preexisting patient comorbidities, neurological findings, and radiologic characteristics of the hemorrhage. These factors can be estimated by the intracerebral hemorrhage (ICH) score, a 0–6-point grading scale that integrates GCS score, ICH volume, presence or absence of intraventricular hemorrhage, presence or absence of an infratentorial origin of hemorrhage, and patient age into a composite estimate of 30-day mortality. ICH volume in this score is calculated using the ABC/2 method, in which the greatest diameter of the hematoma chosen from the slice in which it appears largest ("A") is multiplied by the diameter perpendicular to "A" (i.e., component "B"), multiplied by the estimated number of axial slices with hemorrhage multiplied by slice thickness ("C"). The product of these three components (A × B × C) is then divided by 2 [16]. The ICH score, as with other clinical scoring algorithms, should be validated in each context where it may be used since the original research informing the score was performed in a distinct population that may differ in important ways from other socioeconomic contexts. Such scores do, however, provide clinical tools that may prove useful in all contexts once they have been validated. The ICH scoring algorithm appears below (Table 23.3).

Surgical Management of SICH

SICH stemming from identifiable vascular lesions requires a management approach that may include endovascular embolization or treatment strategies, open microsurgical resection,

Table 23.3 ICH score. According to the original publication by Hemphill et al., scores from 0 to 6 are respectively associated with a 30-day mortality ranging from 0% for a score of 0 to 13% for grade 1, 26% for grade 2, 72% for grade 3, 87% for grade 4, and nearly 100% for grades 5 and 6 [16]. GCS score indicates the initial GCS on presentation or following resuscitation; volume of ICH is calculated using the ABC/2 method [16]

ICH score	
Component	Score
GCS score	
3–4	2
5–12	1
13–15	0
ICH volume, mL	
≥30	1
<30	0
Intraventricular hemorrhage	
Yes	1
No	0
Infratentorial origin of ICH	
Yes	1
No	0
Age	
≥80	1
<80	0
Total score	**0–6**

or a combination of techniques and approaches that are generally reserved for highly specialized referral centers. Surgical management of SICH without an underlying vascular malformation has otherwise been a controversial area, with earlier studies showing improvements in mortality for some patients, but without a definite improvement in function or in the neurological deficit produced by the original lesion. More recent surgical innovations in the realm of minimally invasive hematoma evacuation have shown some promise, with technologies such as endoport- and endoscope-assisted hematoma evacuation, or stereotactic aspiration and thrombolysis, increasingly replacing standard craniotomies and microsurgical techniques for optimizing surgical outcomes in SICH [17]. These technologies are, however, in an early phase of development and pose barriers to implementation in LMICs that include prohibitive costs and significant learning curves. A health equity-driven paradigm for neurosurgical capacity development in LMICs must, however, focus on disruptive innovation that makes these technologies available to patients in all settings who stand to benefit from these treatments. These innovations may include leveraging local engineering talent to develop minimally invasive technologies with more inexpensive yet equally durable and effective materials and strategic partnering with institutions in HICs to facilitate resource-sharing for transnational education, training, and research initiatives focused on decreasing the global burden of hemorrhagic stroke.

Management of Traumatic Intracranial Hypertension (TICN)

Intracranial hypertension refers to the pathological elevation of intracranial pressure. Normal intracranial pressure has globally been accepted to range between 0 and 20 mmHg for adults, with the exception of transient increases of intracranial pressure which occur during normal variations in human physiology during events such as coughing, sneezing, breath-holding maneuvers, or some forms of heavy lifting or physical exertion. Traumatic intracranial hypertension (TICN) refers to the sustained elevation of intracranial pressure beyond 20 mmHg as a consequence of traumatic injury to the head and brain. Following the paradigm of the Monro-Kellie hypothesis, which predicts that the closed system of the human skull can only accommodate a fixed volume of intracranial components, TICN may result from a post-traumatic increase in any of these components such as blood (e.g., from extra-axial or intraparenchymal hemorrhage), brain parenchyma (e.g., as a consequence of the various forms of brain edema), or cerebrospinal fluid (e.g., as a consequence of hydrocephalus from disruption of CSF dynamics or obstruction of CSF pathways [18].

Treatment of TICN

The treatment of ICN is paramount in the prevention of life-threatening posttraumatic events such as acute herniation syndromes, as well as in the optimization of cerebral physiology by maintaining adequate brain tissue perfusion, as predicted by the formula for cerebral perfusion pressure (CPP), which is calculated as the difference between mean arterial pressure (MAP) and intracranial pressure (ICP) [19]. See Eq. 23.1:

$$\text{CPP} = \text{MAP} - \text{ICP} \tag{23.1}$$

where CPP is cerebral perfusion pressure, MAP is mean arterial pressure, and ICP is intracranial pressure.

The management of ICN, especially in high-income country (HIC) contexts, is currently entering a realm of multimodality monitoring, which involves the placement of both external ventricular drains that allow intermittent or continuous CSF diversion as well as measurement of ICP when closed and intracranial monitors that detect several other parameters of cerebral physiology, such as brain temperature, oxygen tension of brain tissue, cerebral blood flow, and electroencephalography via depth electrodes. These monitoring modalities represent the current state of the art in neurocritical care monitoring and management for TICN, and new protocols integrating this data into the optimization of care are the subject of recent consensus efforts and intense research. The interested reader can reference several of these protocols, particularly as they relate to intracranial pressure and brain tissue oxygen monitoring for patients with severe TBI, on the resources page of the website of Global Neuro or in the articles produced by the Seattle International Severe Traumatic Brain Injury Consensus Conference (SIBICC) [20–22].

Nonetheless, the optimization of long-term outcomes for patients with TICN managed using these advanced modalities remains to be seen and comes with a cost of care that, taken together with the many other costs of a HIC intensive care unit, can exceed a daily expense of $20,000 per patient [23, 24]. The practitioner caring for victims of TBI with TICN in a low-resource setting therefore faces the challenge of managing TICN in a rapid and effective manner in the absence of many of the tools available in a HIC setting. Recently, a group based in Latin America developed a series of stratified protocols for optimizing TBI management in resource-constricted settings, representing the first such set of protocols that specifically consider common limitations encountered by neurosurgeons, neurointensivists, and emergency medicine physicians in low- and middle-income countries [11]. This "Beyond One Option for Treatment of Traumatic Brain Injury: A Stratified Protocol [BOOTStraP]" approach expands upon the prior "international" protocols from HIC environments, such as the recommendations of the Brain Trauma Foundation (BTF) and of SIBICC, by offering TICN management options that can readily be adapted to environments where BTF and SIBICC protocols cannot be enacted with integrity.

While a detailed recapitulation of the guidelines from BTF, SIBICC, or BOOTStraP is beyond the scope the scope of this chapter, the following principles of TICN management may be appreciated in all such protocols and can be used to guide the rapid relief of TICN in all contexts:

I. Rapid assessment and stabilization of the TBI patient at risk of TICN is key, including maintenance of a patent airway, adequate oxygenation, and perfusion. This includes safely securing the patient's airway with intubation if required, ventilating the patient as needed, and maintaining blood pressure levels that adequately perfuse the brain. Hypoxia and hypotension are well-described secondary brain insults that increase mortality in patients with severe TBI.

II. In the absence of monitoring modalities, acute TICN can be inferred from common changes to the clinical and neurological exam that result from impending herniation syndromes, such as worsening mental status, worsening Glasgow coma score, nausea and vomiting, changes in pupillary exam such as dilation and nonreactivity to light, and stereotyped posturing such as abnormal flexion or extension which may indicate brainstem compression.

III. When CT scanning is available, a rapid noncontrast head and brain imaging of a patient with TICN is key for identifying surgically treatable causes of TICN such as epidural or subdural hemorrhage, large intraparenchymal contusions, or diffuse posttraumatic brain swelling.

IV. Noninvasive gestures that can optimize ICP and treat acute TICN include head of bed elevation to at least 30 degrees to optimize jugular venous drainage, judicious use of transient hyperventilation to decrease intracranial volume through intracerebral vasoconstriction, use of sedation, analgesic and paralytic medications as available and indicated, and judicious bolus administration of hyperosmolar therapies such as mannitol or hypertonic saline. Note that sedating and/or paralyzing medications can compromise the neurological exam and result in lack of ability to reliably use the exam to manage patients with TBI.

V. Insertion of an external ventricular drain (EVD), when available, provides the most basic invasive maneuver enabling direct measurement of ICP, and a therapeutic maneuver that, through CSF diversion, can directly treat TICN. When CT scanning is available, CT imaging should be obtained prior to EVD insertion in order to account for possible posttraumatic alterations in brain anatomy that can render EVD placement difficult, or prohibitive. Otherwise, the standard technique, following patient positioning, hair removal, and skin sterilization, involves a stab-incision, or 1–2 cm parasagittal incision at a point corresponding to the intersection of the midpupillary line with a perpendicular line extending from the midpoint of an imaginary line connecting the external canthus to the tragus. A burr hole is then made at this site, followed by dural incision, and insertion of the EVD at a trajectory that targets the frontal horn and foramen of Monro in the ipsilateral lateral ventricle. The trajectory is classically found by insertion orthogonal to the skull, which can also be reliably obtained with the use of a tripod device such as a Ghajar guide [25] (see Fig. 23.4).

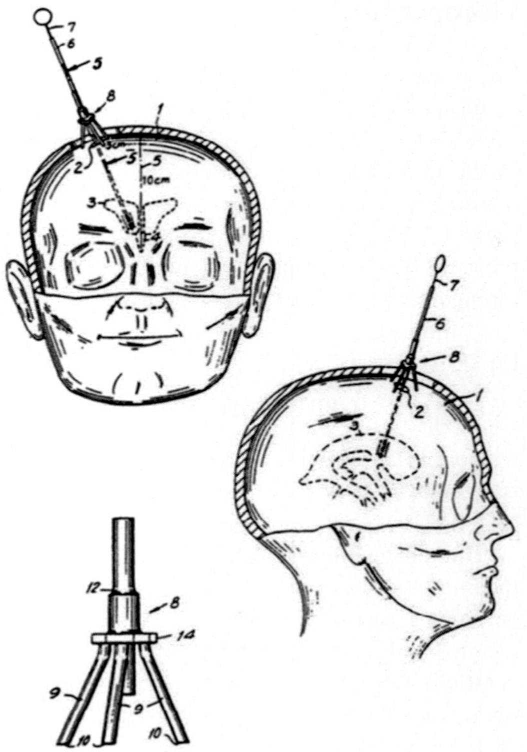

Fig. 23.4 EVD entry point with utilization of the Ghajar tripod guide. Reprinted with permission. Permission has been obtained

VI. While the role of decompressive craniectomy in treatment of severe TBI has remained a controversial issue, especially in the literature coming primarily from HIC environments, strong evidence supports the ability of decompressive craniectomy to definitively control TICN in severe TBI patients, with many other factors influencing whether this treatment ultimately improves mortality. In low-resource settings, findings and recommendations from HIC environments are recognized as lacking the external validity for generalized application, and there may be a role for early, primary decompressive craniectomy, particularly in settings where neurocritical care monitoring may be delayed or unavailable [26].

Diagnostic Lumbar Puncture

Overview

The lumbar puncture is a standard procedure in the medicosurgical care of patients with a range of neurological and neurosurgical diagnoses. The principal indication for a lumbar puncture is to exclude, or confirm, suspected central nervous system infection or spontaneous subarachnoid hemorrhage from rupture of an intracerebral aneurysm or other vascular malformation or anomaly of the brain. The principal contraindication for lumbar puncture is any lesion or anomaly that increases the risk of a cerebral herniation event, such as a space occupying mass, or other structural anomalies of the brain resulting in intracranial hypertension and/or obstructive hydrocephalus. Therefore, any suspicion of a space occupying brain mass or other structural lesions of the brain should be investigated with imaging where available, including CT scan of the brain. When CT imaging is not available to exclude such anomalies, the potential risk of causing a herniation event must be weighed against the potential benefit of performing cerebrospinal fluid analysis.

Procedure

The procedure for a lumbar puncture involves insertion of a lumbar puncture needle at a level of the lumbar spine caudal to the conus medullaris, in order to minimize the risk of injury to neural elements. Classically, needle insertion at the interlaminar space of the L4 and L5 vertebral body levels permits access of the lumbar cistern with minimal risk to neural injury. If the lumbar cistern cannot be readily accessed at this level, the L3–L4 level is also an appropriate target that is normally caudal to the conus medullaris.

The patient is classically positioned in a lateral decubitus position, facing away from the operator, with the chin of the patient tucked down toward the chest with the neck flexed, with the hips and knees of the patient flexed toward the abdomen in order to facilitate and maximize spinal flexion. This positioning optimizes access to the lumbar cistern by expanding the interlaminar space. In this position, the skin is prepared by cleaning and sterilizing the skin in standard sterile surgical fashion, using either iodine- or alcohol-based cleansers. Sterile drapes are then placed to isolate the area of lumbar puncture and to exclude any unsterile surfaces from the field. The operator then cleans her/his/their hands and dons a pair of sterile surgical gloves to perform the procedure. The L4–L5 level is identified by palpating the patient's iliac crest bilaterally and identifying the intercristal line at this level, where it intersects the spinous processes orthogonally.

The needle is inserted in between the L4 and L5 spinous processes, parallel to the floor, and with a slightly rostral inclination to mimic the angle produced by the flanking spinous processes. As the needle is inserted, it is gently advanced, feeling for haptic feedback from each of the connective tissue structures encountered before reaching the subarachnoid space. These are the skin and subcutaneous layers: the more dense supraspinous ligament, the thinner interspinous ligament, the ligamentum flavum, and the dural/arachnoid puncture which results in a sudden loss of resistance and egress of cerebrospinal fluid upon removal of the stylet from the spinal needle. If opening pressure is desired, it can be measured at this time by connection of a manometer to the spinal needle. Several milliliters of cerebrospinal fluid are collected for analysis and sent to a laboratory with biochemistry and microbiology capacity. Standard tests

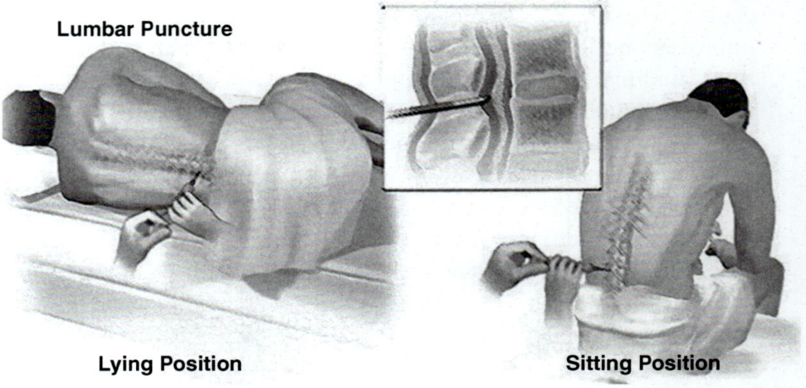

Fig. 23.5 Lumbar puncture technique

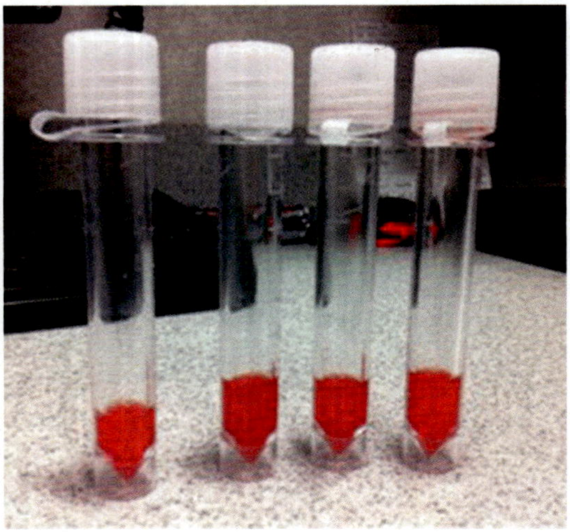

Fig. 23.6 Examples of red blood cell findings from lumbar puncture for subarachnoid hemorrhage

include protein, glucose, cell count, differential, and gram stain study, as well as culture to isolate organisms of interest. When performed to confirm a diagnosis of acute, or subacute subarachnoid hemorrhage, the studies of interest include cell count, and fluid appearance (see Fig. 23.5 for an illustration of the lumbar puncture technique).

Cerebrospinal fluid collection to diagnose acute subarachnoid hemorrhage requires four numbered tubes for CSF collection in order to reliably determine whether red blood cell count is due to traumatic lumbar puncture or due to spontaneous subarachnoid hemorrhage. In a traumatic puncture, the red blood cell count decreases each successive collection tube. In subarachnoid hemorrhage, the red blood cell count is consistently high in all four collection tubes (see Fig. 23.6 for an example of CSF appearance in subarachnoid hemorrhage).

Of note, analysis of cerebrospinal fluid for the purposes described in this chapter requires not only the materials found in a standard lumbar puncture kit prepared for this purpose but also the capacity for medical laboratory studies including assays for glucose, protein, cell count and differential, gram stain, and microbiology cultures. More sophisticated studies for viral assay or cancer workup require more sophisticated laboratory capacity; however, these analyses are beyond the scope of this chapter.

Neurosurgical indications for lumbar puncture beyond the above-described diagnoses included obtaining access for insertion lumbar subarachnoid drain, cerebrospinal fluid diversion to facilitate microsurgical resection of brain and skull base tumors, repair of cerebrospinal fluid fistulae, or reconstruction of posttraumatic cranial defects, or a diagnostic confirmation of communicating, normal pressure hydrocephalus. A comprehensive discussion of these lumbar puncture indications is, however, beyond the scope of this chapter.

Table 23.4 lists the common cellular and biochemical findings in the differential diagnosis for meningitis.

Table 23.4 Common findings of CSF studies. A guide for common findings in cellular and biochemical analysis of cerebrospinal fluid in the differential diagnosis of meningitis

Study	Normal findings	Bacterial infection	Viral infection	Fungal infection
Opening pressure	6–20 cm H2O	15–50 cm H2O	6–30 cm H2O	15–50 cm H2O
Leukocyte count	<5/uL	High elevation; usually >1000/uL	Mild elevation; usually <1000/uL	Mild elevation; usually <1000/uL
Differential	Lymphocyte predominance	Neutrophilic	Lymphocytic	Lymphocytic
Protein density	<60 mg/dL	High elevation; 80–500 mg/dL	Mild elevation; 80–500 mg/dL	High elevation; 80–500 mg/dL
Glucose density	>40% serum glucose, or > 40 mg/dL	Decreased	Normal[a]	Decreased

[a]Note that some viruses can produce a decrease of CSF glucose density. Source: adapted from the Internet Book of Critical Care [27]

Brain Tumors

Presentation

Brain tumors are among the most common disease entities in neurosurgery. The most common type of brain tumors in LMICs, especially in Africa, are meningiomas. Patients with brain tumors commonly present with headache which is usually worse in the morning. The headache is often accompanied by nausea and vomiting. Patients get temporary relief from the headache due to the hyperventilation associated with the vomiting. Moreover, patients with brain tumors present with progressive neurologic deficits such as weakness of the limbs, visual deterioration, cranial nerve deficit, or change in mentation. Seizure is also a common manifestation which could be focal onset or generalized. Patients with infratentorial brain tumors arising from either the cerebellum or the brain stem present with gait disturbance, ataxia, vertigo or diplopia.

Classification of Brain Tumors

Brain tumors are broadly classified as primary or secondary (metastatic). Primary brain tumors are those tumors arising from the brain tissue or surrounding structures. They can be of glial or nonglial origin.

The most common benign brain tumor in adults is meningioma, while glioblastoma is the most common malignant brain tumor. In children, the most common tumors are pilocytic astrocytoma and medulloblastoma.

The most widely used classification of brain tumors is the World Health Organization (WHO) classification of Central Nervous System tumors. It provides nomenclature and grading of CNS tumors which are important for treatment planning.

Diagnostics for Brain Tumors: Challenges and Approaches

Magnetic resonance imaging (MRI) is the diagnostic of choice for brain tumors followed by computed tomography (CT). Contrast-enhanced MRI and CT scan help characterize brain tumors. CT is an important imaging modality to assess the bone involvement by the tumors and to diagnose calcifications associated with the tumors.

Access to these imaging modalities is limited in LMICs and the cost is also expensive [28]. As a result, patients with brain tumors are diagnosed late, and it is common to see patients who had advanced diseases with big tumors. Available MRI machines also have low resolution and the CT scans are usually 16 to 32 slices [29]. Interpretation of imaging findings is also limited due to the shortage of radiologists. Neurosurgeons are usually expected to interpret imaging findings and plan treatment accordingly.

Spine Stabilization and Urgent Repair and/or Decompression

Overview

Traumatic injuries of the spine can pose multiple challenges to neurosurgeons and orthopedic spine surgeons in any context. The variability of resource availability in LMIC settings can aggravate these challenges at every stage of care. While the principles of prehospital care, including spinal immobilization in any patient with suspected spinal injury, can be generalized to several key principles and maneuvers, definitive diagnosis and management are more challenging and ideally undertaken by a team with specific spinal surgery expertise, which is generally the domain of neurosurgeons, or spine surgery-specialized orthopedists.

The generalities of spinal anatomy can be found in any standard medical textbook. The regions of greatest interest by frequency of injury in the existing spine trauma literature include the sub-axial cervical spine and the thoracolumbar spine. Other regions, including the cranio-cervical, cervicothoracic, sacrum, and sacropelvic regions, may also be injured and require tailored approaches to care; however, spinal anatomy and biomechanics render the cervical spine and the thoracolumbar region, most susceptible to injury in the most common mechanisms of spinal injury, including motor vehicle accidents, falls, occupational injuries, and athletic injuries. We will therefore focus on managing suspected injury to the cervical, or thoracolumbar, spine.

In the vast majority of cases, indications for surgery require radiological demonstration of the patho-anatomy of spinal injury, with clinical neurological and/or destabilizing musculoskeletal findings referable to radiological findings. In HIC contexts, the challenges of determining surgical indications for neurotrauma have resulted in the development of several predictive algorithms and frameworks that may be useful in resource-restricted settings, if and when such frameworks are validated. They include the classification schemes of AO Spine, the Subaxial Cervical Spine Injury Classification Scale (SLICS), and the Thoracolumbar Injury Classification and Severity Scale (TLICS) [30]. At the time of writing, an international collaboration led by a group based in Columbia, South America, is producing detailed algorithms to guide practitioners in low- and middle-income countries, as was recently done for traumatic brain injury with BOOSTRAP TBI [11].

Nonsurgical Stabilization

Options for nonsurgical stabilization of the injured spine are limited primarily to orthotic braces and more invasive cervical spine stabilization devices. Orthotic braces include the cervical collar, the cervicothoracic brace, the thoracolumbar sacral orthosis (TLSO), and the lumbosacral orthosis. More invasive options for cervical spine stabilization without surgery include a halo orthosis or, when available, Gardner-Wells cervical traction tongs. All of these devices are associated with a cost of production or acquisition that must be considered within the socioeconomic constraints of the context where they may be used.

Noninvasive orthoses range in rigidity from soft, more flexible braces that may remind patients to limit movement without providing significant support to the far more rigid and/or custom-made orthoses that more securely restrict harmful movement of injured spinal segments. The principal role of such braces, particularly in the cervical spine, is to transiently provide immobilization of injured spinal segments until definitive care can be provided. They may also have a role in conservative management of spinal injury and/or postoperative recovery from a spinal fusion to facilitate arthrodesis of the segments of interest.

Halo orthosis may be used as a conservative management approach in craniocervical spinal injury when surgical correction cannot be performed or when a nonsurgical treatment appears to be possible with more definitive immobilization than can be achieved with a cervical collar. Traction using Gardner-Wells tongs is reserved for patients with subluxation injuries of the cervical spine that can be treated with closed reduction using cervical traction.

Rapid Surgical Decompression/ Repair

The two principal modalities of surgical care for spinal injury include decompression and stabilization. Decompression refers to the surgical removal of traumatic lesions that compress either the spinal cord, or conus medullaris, or nerves. While some lesions, such as traumatic herniation of cervical discs, require an anterior approach, adequate spinal decompression for most traumatic indications can be accomplished from a posterior approach in the cervical, thoracic, or lumbar spine, with the patient position prone. As described above, indications for surgery should be confirmed with imaging. Spinal MRI without contrast is the most useful study for definitive assessment of neural elements of the spine with suspected injury; however, MRI may also be an absent or prohibitively expensive resource in many LMIC settings. In these cases, computed tomography imaging can provide invaluable information about osseous patho-anatomy and facilitate deductions about soft tissue injury. At minimum, X-ray studies should be available to guide surgical decision-making.

Ideally, neurophysiologic monitoring would provide a means of assessing neurological compromise and the patient with spinal injury both before and after positioning the patient for surgery. Blood loss should be anticipated before surgery, minimized using meticulous hemostasis, and factored into the plans for surgery so that availability of blood for transfusion is confirmed if significant blood loss is anticipated.

The general procedure for laminectomy begins with carefully flipping the intubated and sedated patient prone, avoiding any uncoordinated or sudden movements during this maneuver that might exacerbate an existing injury. If intraoperative X-ray is available, such as a C-arm, then the site of surgery is localized using intraoperative X-ray. If this imaging is not available, then localization must be done using preoperative imaging studies and anatomic landmarks; for fracture dislocations, a palpable step-off readily identifies the side of interest. Hair is removed, and a midline incision as planned. After a standard sterile surgical prepping and draping, an incision is made over the level(s) of interest, and a subperiosteal dissection is performed, exposing the spinous processes and laminae at the levels of interest. Care is taken to protect the facet joints and their overlying capsules. Using a combination of available rongeurs and osteotomes, the spinous processes, supraspinous and interspinous ligaments, and the laminae are removed, taking care to preserve the facet joints, and the pars interarticularis, bilaterally. Care is taken to prevent injury to any neurovascular elements, or violation of the thecal sac; however, in the setting of trauma, there may already be a traumatic cerebrospinal fluid fistula. This is primarily repaired as possible using appropriately sized suture and/or local autograft of fat and/or muscle. Synthetic adhesives, such as *DuraSeal Exact*, can be helpful if/when available to augment such dural repair.

Upon completion of decompression procedures, if no stabilization is required, then the wound is closed in layers, starting with approximation and primary closure of the fascia incision, followed by successive superficial levels of subcutaneous, and finally epidermal closure.

Surgical Stabilization

Stabilization refers to placement of spinal implants, such as screws and rods, to rigidly, internally immobilize destabilized levels for healing and, when indicated, to facilitate osseous fusion of injured levels. In the cervical spine, lateral mass screws are typically placed, using one of the screw insertion techniques that aim to achieve good bone purchase while minimizing the risk of injury to the vertebral arteries, or cervical spinal nerves. The An technique for screw insertion places the screw entry point in the lateral mass at approximately 1 mm medial to the center and uses a cephalo-lateral trajectory with cranial inclination of about 10–15 degrees and lateral trajectory of about 25–30 degrees [31].

Screws placed in the thoracic and lumbar spine generally target the particles. At these levels, intraoperative X-ray is a vital tool for assuring accuracy of screw placement. When not available, classic anatomical landmarks and some intraoperative techniques may be used to achieve the best approximation of pedicle trajectory. One example of intraoperative technique that can optimize pedicle screw placement in the absence of adequate intraoperative imaging is the concept of lamina-pedicle perpendicularity, described by Elfiky et al. [32, 33] This technique, utilizing the nearly orthogonal orientation of each thoracic or lumbar pedicle to the sagittal inclination given by the edge of the inferior lamina, has shown remarkable accuracy in its ability to estimate the location of thoracic and lumbar screws for safe screw placement.

Upon completion of screw placement at indicated levels, rods typically made from titanium or other biologically compatible metals are bent as needed to achieve the desired spinal curvature or correction and subsequently secured to the heads of the screws for completion of internal fixation. Following internal fixation of indicated spinal levels, arthrodesis may be initiated by facet capsule disruption and decortication of the joint surfaces at each pair of intervening intervertebral joints. Generally, bony fusion across spinal levels of desired arthrodesis requires 3 months or more of healing time. Stabilization of fusion levels with instrumentation facilitates early mobilization and rehabilitation in the postoperative period, which in turn enables patients to more quickly resume activities of daily living and, as possible, professional activities. In resource-limited contexts, the lack of spinal instrumentation can therefore pose a barrier to optimal clinical and socioeconomic outcomes following spine surgery. Surgeons treating patients with spinal pathology in LMICs must therefore carefully consider the risks and benefits of intervention when the tools required for optimal treatment may not be available. In these contexts, a health equity-driven agenda for advancing neurosurgical capacity may require a combination of charitable support from international medicosurgical device companies, strategic partnerships with institutions in HICs for global neurosurgical program development, and a long-term plan for local health system strengthening designed to fully address unmet needs for neurosurgical care [34].

Summary/Conclusion

The field of neurosurgery constitutes a vast array of pathology requiring human and material resources that are often inadequate, or completely absent from the healthcare systems of LMICs. Despite these challenges, a growing number of clinicians, researchers, educators, and health policy experts and advocates are recognizing the unmet need for neurosurgical care around the world and the impact of the indispensable requirement to respond to this need in order to advance global health equity, economic welfare, and social justice [1, 35]. This chapter introduces selected neurosurgical disorders, management strategies, and techniques that the authors have found to be especially relevant to the prevailing burden of neurosurgical diseases in LMICs.

References

1. Park KB, Johnson WD, Dempsey RJ. Global neurosurgery: the unmet need. World Neurosurg. 2016;88:32–5. https://doi.org/10.1016/j.wneu.2015.12.048.
2. Pascual JM, Prieto R. *Chapter 133—Surgical management of severe closed head injury in adults*. Elsevier; 2012. doi:https://doi.org/10.1016/B978-1-4160-6839-6.10133-9.
3. Seelig JM, Becker DP, Miller JD, Greenberg RP, Ward JD, Choi SC. Traumatic acute subdural hematoma: major mortality reduction in comatose patients treated within four hours. N Engl J Med. 1981;304(25):1511–8. https://doi.org/10.1056/NEJM198106183042503.
4. Weigel R, Schilling L, Krauss JK. The pathophysiology of chronic subdural hematoma revis-

ited: emphasis on aging processes as key factor. GeroScience. 2022:1–19. https://doi.org/10.1007/s11357-022-00570-y.

5. Gutowski P, Meier U, Rohde V, Lemcke J, von der Brelie C. Clinical outcome of epidural hematoma treated surgically in the era of modern resuscitation and trauma care. World Neurosurg. 2018;118:e166–74. https://doi.org/10.1016/j.wneu.2018.06.147.
6. Algahtany MA. Extra-axial hematomas due to road traffic accidents and their outcome: a ten-year study. Eur Rev Med Pharmacol Sci. 2022;26(1):120–9. https://doi.org/10.26355/eurrev_202201_27757.
7. Nevalainen N, Luoto TM, Iverson GL, Mattila VM, Huttunen TT. Craniotomies following acute traumatic brain injury in Finland—a national study between 1997 and 2018. Acta Neurochir. 2022;164(3):625–33. https://doi.org/10.1007/s00701-022-05140-x.
8. Laeke T, Tirsit A, Kassahun A, et al. Prospective study of surgery for traumatic brain injury in Addis Ababa, Ethiopia: trauma causes, injury types, and clinical presentation. World Neurosurg. 2021;149:e460–8. https://doi.org/10.1016/j.wneu.2021.02.003.
9. Hilton D. The neuropathology of traumatic brain injury. In: Whitfield PC, Welbourne J, Thomas E, Summers F, Whyte M, Hutchinson PJ, editors. Traumatic brain injury: a multidisciplinary approach. 2nd ed. Cambridge University Press; 2020. p. 12–23. https://doi.org/10.1017/9781108355247.
10. Corley J, Barthélemy EJ, Lepard J, et al. Comprehensive policy recommendations for head and spine injury care in low- and middle-income countries. World Neurosurg. 2019;132:434–6. https://doi.org/10.1016/j.wneu.2019.08.240.
11. Rubiano AM, Vera DS, Montenegro JH, et al. Recommendations of the Colombian consensus Committee for the Management of Traumatic Brain Injury in Prehospital, Emergency Department, Surgery, and Intensive Care (Beyond One Option for Treatment of Traumatic Brain Injury: A Stratified Protocol [BOOTStraP]). J Neurosci Rural Pract. 2020;11(1):7–22. https://doi.org/10.1055/s-0040-1701370.
12. Bullock MR, Chesnut R, Ghajar J, et al. Surgical management of TBI. Neurosurgery. 2006;58(3):S2-1-S2-3. https://doi.org/10.1227/01.NEU.0000210361.83548.D0.
13. Tawk RG, Hasan TF, D'Souza CE, Peel JB, Freeman WD. Diagnosis and treatment of unruptured intracranial aneurysms and aneurysmal subarachnoid Hemorrhage. Mayo Clin Proc. 2021;96(7):1970–2000. https://doi.org/10.1016/j.mayocp.2021.01.005.
14. Rouanet C, Silva GS. Aneurysmal subarachnoid hemorrhage: current concepts and updates. Arq Neuropsiquiatr. 2019;77(11):806–14. https://doi.org/10.1590/0004-282X20190112.
15. Langhorne P, O'Donnell MJ, Chin SL, et al. Practice patterns and outcomes after stroke across countries at different economic levels (INTERSTROKE): an international observational study. Lancet. 2018;391(10134):2019–27. https://doi.org/10.1016/S0140-6736(18)30802-X.
16. Hemphill JC, Bonovich DC, Besmertis L, Manley GT, Johnston SC. The ICH score: a simple, reliable grading scale for intracerebral hemorrhage. Stroke. 2001;32(4):891–6. https://doi.org/10.1161/01.str.32.4.891.
17. Vitt JR, Sun CH, Le Roux PD, Hemphill JC. Minimally invasive surgery for intracerebral hemorrhage. Curr Opin Crit Care. 2020;26(2):129–36. https://doi.org/10.1097/MCC.0000000000000695.
18. Mokri B. The Monro-Kellie hypothesis: applications in CSF volume depletion. Neurology. 2001;56(12):1746–8. https://doi.org/10.1212/wnl.56.12.1746.
19. Depreitere B, Meyfroidt G, Güiza F. What do we mean by cerebral perfusion pressure? Acta Neurochir Suppl. 2018;126:201–3. https://doi.org/10.1007/978-3-319-65798-1_41.
20. Hawryluk GWJ, Aguilera S, Buki A, et al. A management algorithm for patients with intracranial pressure monitoring: the Seattle International Severe Traumatic Brain Injury Consensus Conference (SIBICC). Intensive Care Med. 2019;45(12):1783–94. https://doi.org/10.1007/s00134-019-05805-9.
21. Chesnut R, Aguilera S, Buki A, et al. A management algorithm for adult patients with both brain oxygen and intracranial pressure monitoring: the Seattle International Severe Traumatic Brain Injury Consensus Conference (SIBICC). Intensive Care Med. 2020;46(5):919–29. https://doi.org/10.1007/s00134-019-05900-x.
22. Global Neuro. SIBICC severe TBI algorithms. https://globalneuro.org/EN/resources/sibicc-stbi-algorithm.html. Published 2020. Accessed May 8, 2022.
23. Raj R, Bendel S, Reinikainen M, et al. Costs, outcome and cost-effectiveness of neurocritical care: a multi-center observational study. doi:https://doi.org/10.1186/s13054-018-2151-5.
24. Dasta JF, McLaughlin TP, Mody SH, Piech CT. Daily cost of an intensive care unit day: the contribution of mechanical ventilation. Crit Care Med. 2005;33(6):1266–71. https://doi.org/10.1097/01.CCM.0000164543.14619.00.
25. Chau CYC, Craven CL, Rubiano AM, et al. The evolution of the role of external ventricular drainage in traumatic brain injury. J Clin Med. 2019;8:9. https://doi.org/10.3390/jcm8091422.
26. Clavijo A, Khan AA, Mendoza J, et al. The role of decompressive craniectomy in limited resource environments. Front Neurol. 2019;10(FEB):1–6. https://doi.org/10.3389/fneur.2019.00112.
27. Farkas J. Meningitis & encephalitis. The Internet Book of Critical Care.
28. Frija G, Blažić I, Frush DP, et al. How to improve access to medical imaging in low- and middle-income countries ? eClinicalMedicine. 2021;38:101034. https://doi.org/10.1016/j.eclinm.2021.101034.

29. Helal AE, Abouzahra H, Fayed AA, Rayan T, Abbassy M. Socioeconomic restraints and brain tumor surgery in low-income countries. Neurosurg Focus. 2018;45(4):E11. https://doi.org/10.3171/2018.7.FOCUS18258.
30. American College of Surgeons. *Best practices guidelines spine injury*; 2022. https://www.facs.org/media/k45gikqv/spine_injury_guidelines.pdf.
31. Komotar RJ, Mocco J, Kaiser MG. Surgical management of cervical myelopathy: indications and techniques for laminectomy and fusion. Spine J. 2006;6(6 Suppl):252S–67S. https://doi.org/10.1016/j.spinee.2006.04.029.
32. Elfiky TA, Patil ND, Luk KD, Faheem ME, Samartzis D. The concept of lamina–pedicle Perpendicularity: part 2: thoracic spine. Asian Spine J. 2021;15(2):252. https://doi.org/10.31616/ASJ.2019.0334.
33. Elfiky TA, Patil ND, Luk KDK, Faheem ME, Samartzis D. The concept of lamina–pedicle perpendicularity: part 1. Lumbar spine. Asian Spine J. 2021;15(1):81. https://doi.org/10.31616/ASJ.2019.0114.
34. Park KB, Iv V. Spinal implants in resource-limited settings: "keep it simple.". World Neurosurg. 2016;86:36–8. https://doi.org/10.1016/j.wneu.2015.09.101.
35. Corley JA, Haglund M. Letter: how neurosurgery fits into the global surgery 2030 agenda. Neurosurgery. 2016;79(4):E544–5. https://doi.org/10.1227/NEU.0000000000001351.

24 How to Manage Urgent Problems in the Neck: Foreign Bodies in the Trachea and in the Esophagus in Children and Adults and Other Surgical Problems in Low- and Middle-Income Countries

Philip Vareed Alexander

Be calm and strong and patient.

– William Osler

Abbreviations

A-P	Anteroposterior
CT	Computerized tomography
SCIWORA	Spinal cord injury without radiologic abnormality

Trachea

Foreign Bodies in Children

Clinical Vignette

A 6-month-old male infant was brought to the emergency room with sudden difficulty in breathing. He was seen holding a shelled peanut prior to presentation. On examination, the child was in severe respiratory distress with use of accessory muscles of respiration, indrawing of the intercostal muscles and subcostal recession. An X-ray showed compensatory emphysema of the left side and some hyperinflation of the left upper lobe. He was taken up for bronchoscopy when half a shelled peanut was extracted from his right bronchus.

P. V. Alexander (✉)
Lady Willingdon Hospital, Manali, India

Foreign body inhalation is life threatening especially in those under 2 years of age. The child may present acutely with observed aspiration and choking or they may present insidiously with undetected aspiration. Peanuts and food items are the usual culprits in children under 2, whereas non-food items are aspirated by older children [1]. Balloons, round objects, failure to disintegrate, and swelling up of irritant vegetable matter complicate extraction and increase morbidity [2]. Most foreign bodies lodge in the bronchus, unless they are large and cause tracheal obstruction [3]. There is no predilection in children for the right bronchus as there is in adults.

Coins are a commonly ingested or aspirated. An A-P X-ray will differentiate the site of obstruction, whether in the airway, where the coin will be seen edge-on (since it sits sagitally in the trachea) or in the esophagus, where its face will be visualized on the film (since it sits coronally in the esophagus) (Fig. 24.1).

Only 15% of aspirated foreign bodies are radio opaque and identifiable on a plain X-ray. Secondary signs need to be relied upon to diagnose radiolucent object aspiration. Cough, wheeze, and diminished breath sounds are the

M. A. Hardy, B. R. Hochman (eds.), *Global Surgery*, https://doi.org/10.1007/978-3-031-28127-3_24

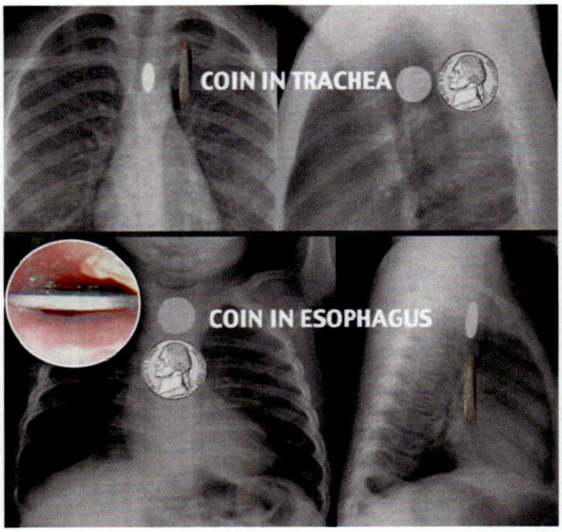

Fig. 24.1 Coin in the esophagus (Image courtesy Dr. Gerald Diaz)

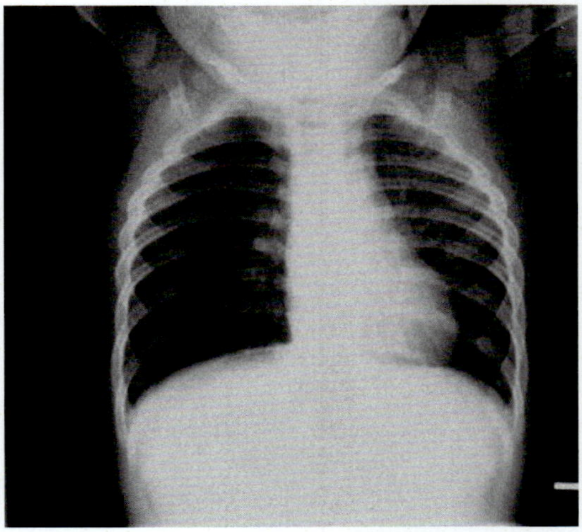

Fig. 24.2 Inspiratory chest radiograph in a 12-month-old boy with a 2-month history of wheezing demonstrates moderate hyperlucency and hyperexpansion of the right hemithorax. A mild deviation of the mediastinum toward the left chest is noted (Courtesy of Brit B. Gay, Jr., MD, Radiology Department, Egleston Children's Hospital, Atlanta, Ga)

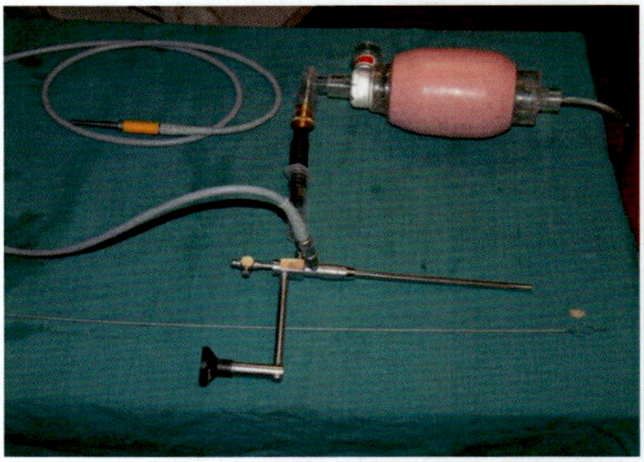

Fig. 24.3 Demonstrating use of a rigid nephroscope for bronchoscopic extraction of foreign bodies. Note the use of the irrigation port for ventilation using a syringe as a connector

classic triad, but additional subtle signs include flaring of ala nasi, stridor, intercostal recession on the affected side, and hyperinflation of the opposite lung (Fig. 24.2). Distal hyperinflation seen on the X-ray is indicative of partial bronchial obstruction, with progressive inflation but inadequate expiration. Complete obstruction can cause distal collapse with compensatory hyperinflation of the opposite lung. Mediastinal shift, obstructive emphysema, and atelectasis are other secondary signs (Fig. 24.2).

If time permits before intervention, a CT scan is usually conclusive in demonstrating the obstruction and the offending object. Delayed presentation or undetected foreign body may primarily present as a pneumonia.

Foreign body aspiration in children is a life-threatening emergency condition and mandates bronchoscopic removal [4]. Bronchoscopy has altered mortality dramatically. In remote areas, bronchoscopy can present quite a challenge. Many remote locations lack anesthetists. Close monitoring and ventilation are precariously balanced during the bronchoscopic extraction. Most centers lack the rigid or flexible bronchoscope needed for this procedure [5]. Referral to a higher center may take anywhere between 8 and 10 h so the attending is caught between a rock and a hard place and is hard pressed to make the right decision. We describe the use of a rigid nephroscope in the extraction of a peanut from the trachea of a 3-year-old child (Fig. 24.3), which is a demonstration of adaptation often necessary in remote and rural surgery. The side irrigation port was used for ventilation and a Dormia basket was used to extract the offending peanut (Fig. 24.3).

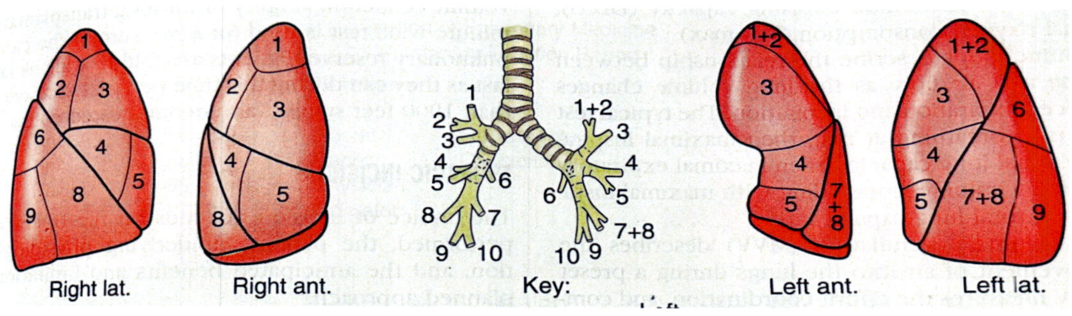

Fig. 24.4 Segments of pulmonary lobes in left and right lungs correlated with the anatomy of the bronchial tree (source: Sabiston Textbook of Surgery, 17th Ed. Putnam Jr., JB, Chapter 57, p. 1765, Elsevier Publisher)

Intravenous steroids and antibiotics are always indicated in management, and delayed presentation or stubborn foreign bodies could be re-approached bronchoscopically after a 5–7-day course of steroids.

Airway Foreign Bodies in Adults

Unless the foreign body is large, and there is acute aspiration as in "café coronary" or aspiration of nails or pins held in the teeth during work, foreign body aspiration in adults is usually more subtle and undetected and presents late as a chronic cough or a delayed pneumonia trending toward a lung abscess. It usually occurs in the elderly or debilitated who have trouble with their swallowing reflex. The radiologic signs of hyperinflation are not replicated in the adult lung, though a CT scan will either demonstrate a pneumonia or suggest the obstruction. The angulation of the right main bronchus permits objects to lodge in it (Fig. 24.4).

Complete obstruction is usually supraglottic or pre-carinal tracheal. Supraglottic obstruction can be relieved with direct laryngoscopic extraction with Magill forceps, while pre-carinal clearance may be obtained by endotracheal intubation obtaining tracheal clearance by pushing a tracheal foreign body into the bronchus, converting a complete obstruction into a partial one, amenable to later elective bronchoscopic extraction. Though rigid bronchoscopy is still the most successful, flexible bronchoscopy in skilled hands has been reported with equivalent success [6]. The rigid nephroscope system we have described (Fig. 24.3) can also be utilized in adult patients.

Esophagus

Foreign Bodies in Children

Clinical Vignette

A 1-year-old male child was brought to the emergency room with history of swallowing a coin. The child was comfortable and in no acute distress and able to swallow and keep down solids and liquids. An X-ray demonstrated a coin in his esophagus identified by its coronal presentation. The child was taken up for endoscopy under anesthesia and the coin extracted with the help of a Foley catheter whose balloon was inflated distal to the coin to withdraw it back into the oropharynx.

Foreign body aspiration is not uncommon in infancy from 6 months of age to 3 years. At this age the child is passing through the oral phase of development when everything goes into his or her mouth and can be easily inhaled or swallowed [7]. It is at this age that parents should be careful to keep small objects away from children. The ingestion may or may not be witnessed.

Esophageal ingestion is usually asymptomatic, and the offending object may transit through the gastrointestinal tract uneventfully if it has negotiated through the pylorus. Those with a developmental delay may be particularly prone to recurrent ingestion or inhalation. Death from

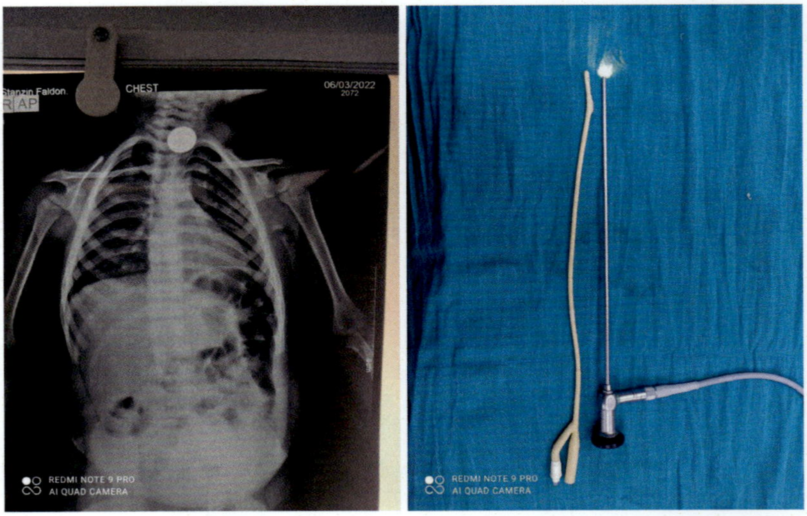

Fig. 24.5 Demonstrating the use of a cystoscope to extract a coin from the esophagus under vision with a Foley catheter passed alongside it

ingestion of a foreign body is rare except if the offending object is a coin battery which mandates extraction [8].

Children have a predilection to put all objects into their mouth. Coins are the most frequently ingested, but then there is a huge variety of other swallowed objects. Witnessed or reported ingestion usually brings the child to the doctor. The child is in no acute distress and is usually quite placid considering the amount of fuss that swirls around him or her post-ingestion. Large swallowed objects can cause distress and near-complete obstruction can cause drooling. Coins can be easily identified by an X-ray with its placement in the coronal plane. The recent utility of coin batteries in a plethora of gadgets make for a dangerous and critical situation since these can erode and perforate through the esophageal or intestinal lumen and mandate extraction. The definitive management has to be endoscopy under general anesthesia. Intubation secures the airway and a pediatric endoscope with an array of graspers, and snare is an essential armament to tackle the situation.

We describe the use of an adult cystoscope to extract a coin with the help of a Foley catheter passed alongside which permits safe extraction under vision (Fig. 24.5).

The offending object usually lodges at one of the anatomical esophageal constrictions, the cricopharyngeus, aortic indentation, or at the lower end. If retrieval is difficult, pushing the foreign body into the stomach usually permits passage through the gastrointestinal tract with the administration of laxatives to help it along. A Foley catheter with its bulb inflated after passage distal to the object is a very simple and useful tool to extract objects which are not easily grasped or snared and if an endoscope is not available. The bulb can be filled with radio opaque contrast material to permit extraction under fluoroscopy if the object is metallic.

Esophageal Foreign Bodies in Adults

The debilitated elderly, and those predisposed to esophageal obstruction with esophageal strictures and reflux esophagitis, are those who present with esophageal obstruction. A bone or a large piece of ingested meat is the usual offender, but there can be a variety of other objects in those with psychiatric illness. In the elderly, dentures have also been swallowed unwittingly and these do present a formidable challenge to the endoscopist and are probably best handled at higher centers. They may require exploration if lodged further along the GI tract, as in the distal ileum. Quite often, the foreign body may have passed into the stomach leaving an ulcer or abrasion in the esophagus which mimics the symptoms from an obstructed foreign body. An X-ray or CT scan can provide definition, if the object is radio-opaque. Endoscopic visualization can lay the suspicion of a lodged foreign body to rest. Any object less than 5 cm in diameter will usually continue its journey through and out of the gastrointestinal tract. Pins, razor blades, and needles can perforate the esophagus spontaneously or during extraction. Tri-prong graspers, the trapezoid snare, and rat tooth forceps are very useful in a variety of foreign bodies. The Foley catheter is also an excellent option to extract obstinate objects resisting capture or grasp. The procedure can be performed under sedation in a cooperative patient, but a combative or restive patient is best intubated to permit protection of the airway and easy retrieval. The overtube is protective of the esophagus during extraction of a sharp object.

Foreign Bodies in Ear or Nose

The remote surgeon is often presented with a plethora of objects that have been thrust into various orifices by children as young as 6 months to 12 years of age. Erasers, beads, legumes, nuts, and sharp objects such as pins, paper clips, and needles have all been introduced into nostrils and ears. Flying insects may also decide to enter the auditory canal, to the great discomfiture of the individual.

The child may present to emergency room either calm and quiet or irritable and cranky. Otoscopic examination or examination of the nasopharynx usually permits visualization of the offending object, and though the temptation to reach out and attempt removal is tantalizing, it must be overcome and retrieval must be performed under sedation. Attempting to remove the object without sedation will only cause the child to jerk and move, complicating the situation with dislodgment and bleeding driving the object deeper into the orifice. A quiet child, good light, and suction are prerequisites for a painless extraction. The application of gentle suction often moves the object upward permitting it to being grasped and removed with a mosquito clamp. Though a variety of spoons, forceps, and probes are available for this purpose, the humble Kelly clamp is sufficient to grasp and extract the object. Vegetable matter tends to swell and fragment. A scoop may come in handy for this situation. A bead with a hole often resists grasp, revolving within the cavity. Getting one limb of the clamp into the central hole or using a probe positioned within the central hole permits extraction. Insects can be drowned with saline and then grasped and extracted. It is unwise to try to irrigate the object out, particularly nuts or legumes because they will swell and then be removable only with difficulty under general anesthesia.

Prior to extracting foreign bodies in the nasopharynx, packing the throat under sedation is important, because the object could be pushed from the nasopharynx into the oropharynx during the attempt and then be aspirated, which will convert the benign procedure of the removal of a foreign body from the nose into the critical extraction of the foreign body from the trachea or bronchus!

Lymph Node Biopsies

Swellings in the neck form a significant proportion of patients presenting to the outpatient department. The different diagnoses present a plethora of conditions, each to be assessed clinically and investigated with appropriate imaging. Neck masses may be approached considering their chronology of appearance and their location. That helps classify disease into congenital, inflammatory, traumatic, or neoplastic headings, which are baskets that permit narrowing down the differential diagnosis by the conduct of a good history and clinical examination. These are cheap and time-tested techniques of whittling down the differentials yet this is also a fading art with the advent of advanced and expensive imaging, often unavailable to the rural surgeon. The details of this are beyond the scope of this chapter which will mainly focus on the approach to lymph nodes in various triangles of the neck. One should remember that following trauma, a small pseudoanurysm of a vessel in the neck can mimic a lymph node without obvious pulsations. An

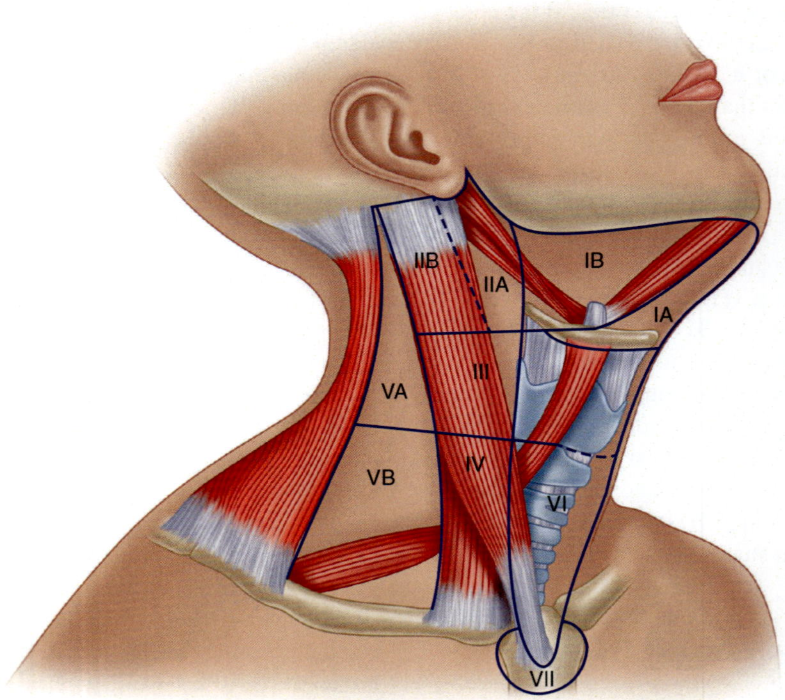

Fig. 24.6 Anatomy of the distribution of the lymph nodes of the neck: a guide to biopsies

ultrasound, when available, can be very helpful in the diagnosis (Fig. 24.6).

Lymph node swellings are very common in all ages. Mothers bring their toddlers worried about swellings in the submandibular or jugulodigastric location that have appeared coincident with a sore throat, or tonsillitis. Older children can present with nodes in the post-auricular or post-occipital location coincident with ear discharge and otitis media. At a later age, dandruff is often the culprit for nodes in level Va, in the preening adolescent or even up to middle age. A good shampoo is often curative. Most of these nodes are below 2 cm in size, discrete, well defined, non-tender, and mobile. In low- and middle-income countries, tuberculosis is ubiquitous and forms up to 30% of all extrapulmonary disease. These nodes tend to be larger and firmer and coalesce prior to caseating and becoming fluctuant. They may be accompanied by night sweats and fever. Lymphomas lurk in the shadows of these nodes, so a good histopathological diagnosis is vital prior to the initiation of treatment. Being described as rubbery and discrete are not enough to differentiate them from the nodes of tuberculosis. Infectious mononucleosis, brucellosis, tularemia, HIV, and parasitic infections are other causes. Tuberculous nodes in the neck can caseate and burst, leaving a potential nonhealing sinus. Histopathology from these nodes can still be obtained by curetting them and suturing the skin closed. The administration of appropriate antituberculous medication can prevent the formation of a sinus. A 6-month course is often curative. Resistant nodes that do not regress in 6 months need to be biopsied again, sent for culture sensitivity, and may need change of the treatment regime to a drug-resistant regime with culture-sensitive medicines. On rare occasions, obstinate nodes may need a modified nodal neck dissection, which decreases the burden of disease and permits clearance of the neck. This may be approached like a neck dissection exempting the jugular vessels but removing all gross nodal disease.

The traditional investigative approach to a lymph node swelling in the neck is to approach it with a fine needle. This may suffice when positive, but its yield is often inconclusive and does not provide additional material for subsequent culture-sensitive tests. Our preference is to subject suspicious swellings to a traditional biopsy which provides adequate preserved tissue for the pathologists, often located many miles away.

Though an excision biopsy of the node is most satisfying when the entire node is removed for examination, it is wise to err on the side of caution and settle for an incision wedge biopsy for nodes in levels approaching the base of the neck or along the carotid sheath, particularly if the node is partially submerged behind the clavicle. A suture taken through the substance of the node provides for traction and permits easy dissection (Fig. 24.7).

Biopsy of nodes in levels IV or IIB should only be attempted cautiously in the operating theater with a senior attending available for the instant need to convert to general anesthesia and undertake a major procedure if any major bleeding is encountered. It is wiser to settle for a good incision biopsy rather than ambitiously embark on an excision biopsy and get into trouble for very little gain. We have had to resect the clavicle to control bleeding from the subclavian vein and have also had to establish vascular control of the internal jugular vein on occasion. Thus, the lowly lymph node biopsy is not to be underrated.

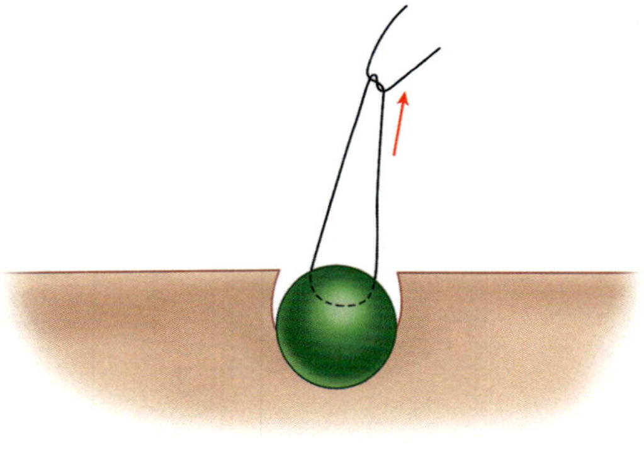

Fig. 24.7 Suture taken through the node and used for traction during dissection

Difficult Airway and Access

The pediatric and adult airway can present formidable challenges to the general surgeon in remote and rural locations, far away from specialized help and instrumentation.

The Pediatric Airway

The neonatal airway can be a challenge, but it can be usually intubated with careful positioning in "sniffing position," a good laryngoscope, and an endotracheal tube of the appropriate size. The formula gestational weeks/10 and the formula (age/4 + 4) usually works for the neonatal and pediatric age group, respectively. Typically, a 2.5 tube is appropriate for infants <1 kg weight, a 3.0 tube for infants weighing 1–2 kg, a 3.5 tube for infants 2–3 kg, and a 3.5 or 4.0 tube for infants over 3 kg. The appropriate size for larger children can be calculated using the formula of (age/4 + 4) for uncuffed tubes and (age/4 + 3) for cuffed tubes. Eyeballing the little finger permits an approximation for the size of the appropriate endotracheal tube. The approximate depth of insertion of the endotracheal tube from the middle of the upper lip in centimeters can be calculated as (weight in kg + 6 cm). The straight blade laryngoscope is usually sufficient, in combination with a good suction at hand.

The laryngeal mask airway is an excellent alternative in the patient with a non-intubatable airway. It provides the ability to ventilate adequately for shorter procedures. The size can be read off the chart in Table 24.1.

Bag mask ventilation is a short-term option with the disadvantage of gastric distension despite presence of a nasogastric tube and failure to protect the airway from aspiration. An I-gel LMA has an inbuilt aspiration channel to prevent this.

Table 24.1 LMA sizing

LARYNGEAL MASK AIRWAY SIZING

L.M.A Size	Patient Size
1	Neonates/Infants < 5 kg
1.5	Infants 5-10 kg
2	Infants/Children 10-20 kg
3	Children/Small adults 30-50 kg
4	Adults 50-70 kg
5	Large adult >70 kg

Tracheostomy in children is rarely indicated and beset with the danger of tracheomalacia or stricture formation in the period following post-decannulation.

The Adult Airway

Elective surgery can provide the luxury of pre-anesthetic estimation of airway difficulty using the Mallampati classification [9](Fig. 24.8).

Those with a short thyromental distance or wide neck allow the operator to be forewarned and therefore forearmed. An endotracheal bougie is inexpensive and should be present in all remote and rural theatres, since it permits the endotracheal tube to be railroaded into the trachea with minimum fuss. For the anterior larynx not permitting entry of the tip of the bougie, an ordinary bronchoscope or even a flexible endoscope can be adapted to permit visual intubation along the side or with the endotracheal tube preloaded onto the scope prior. An ingenious system has been devised by one hospital using a mobile phone with a camera attached to the tip of a laryngoscope [10].

Ludwig's angina, extensive facial trauma, suprathyroid injury, and severe glottic edema and spasm all transform an elective situation into an emergent one to achieve control of the airway, and it is in these situations that a needle or surgical cricothyroidotomy becomes life-saving. This is a relatively easy procedure that permits easy surgical access to the airway through the cricothyroid membrane which can been accessed with a broad gauge needle or with serial dilators that permit passage of a small size endotracheal tube as a temporizing airway.

Tracheostomy: The traditional tracheostomy though described as an emergency and life-saving procedure should be probably undertaken in a semi-elective setting, after already having access in some fashion to the airway by one of the above methods. Beating the life clock in rushing through an emergency tracheostomy, without prior airway access, makes for a lot of confusion, with possibilities of overt bleeding and damage to neck structures, all the time beset with the possibility of hypoxic brain damage or, even worse, with death. Airway access, surgical assistance, good positioning, good light, suction, a responsible person at the head end controlling the airway, and a sedated patient are ideal elements for an uneventful tracheostomy. Post-procedure, care should also be taken to deflate the bulb periodically to prevent tracheal erosion and also avoid overfilling the bulb to avoid anterior displacement of the balloon and occlusion of the tip. When connected to a ventilator circuit, undue traction on the tracheostomy during the first 48 h while turning the patient or if the patient becomes combative can predispose to sudden extubation. Replacement of the tube within the first 24 hours post-procedure can be harrowing.

Immobilization of the Neck

Cervical injuries are the insidious cause of mortality and long-term incapacitation, often the cause of the "second accident" due to unpro-

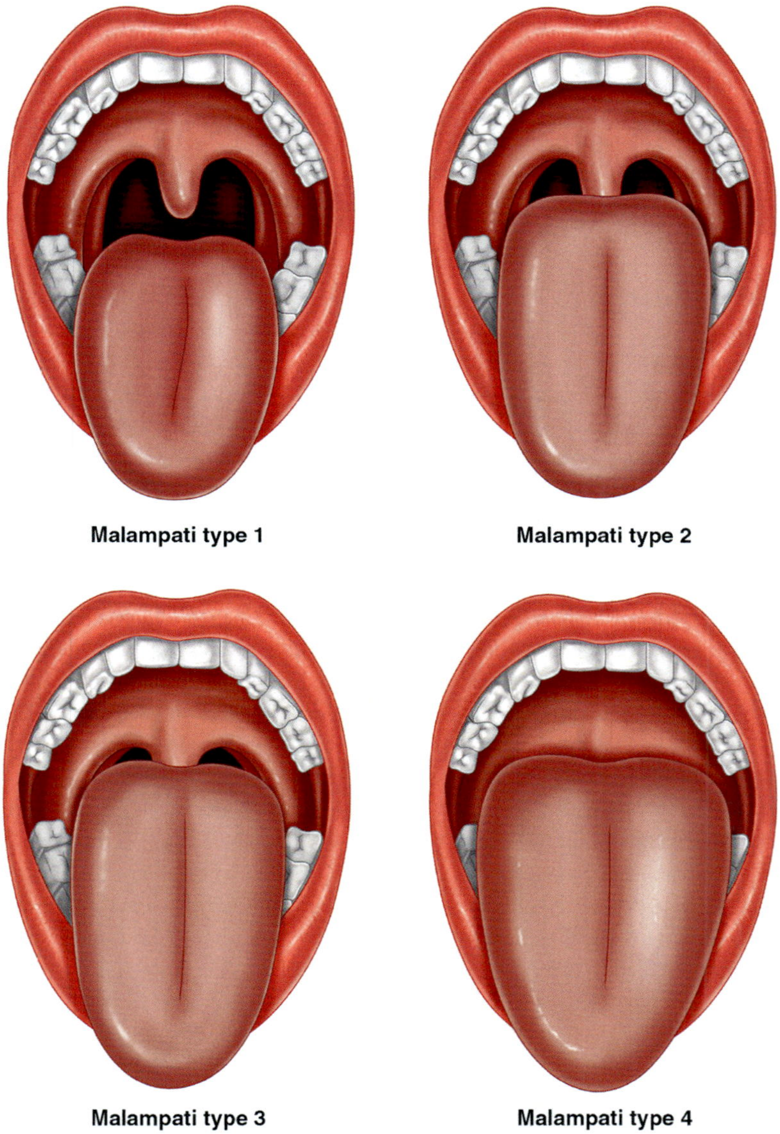

Fig. 24.8 The Modified Mallampati classification

tected transfer of the injured accident victim, both outside and within the hospital setting. Protection of the cervical spine is not universal as yet in the initial management of the injured patient worldwide, both in pre-hospital and hospital settings. A community will do well to train its populace in BLS inclusive of safe transfer of the injured patient hospital to mitigate the lifelong consequences of injury to the cervical spine.

In our hospital we had made simple backboards of plywood covered with Rexene and with handles along the edges and made them available to the local taxi drivers, accompanied with instruction on safe transfer (Fig. 24.9). This has decreased the incidence of post-accident spinal injuries being brought to the hospital and protected the injured spine. We describe simple pre-hospital alternatives for immobilization and transfer which could be implemented in low-resource settings.

Pre-Hospital Measures

Different cultures have varied community responses to the acutely injured patient. In India, an invariable community response is to pour water down the throat of the injured patient, douse his face and simultaneously yank the victim to his or her feet notwithstanding the degree of injury, with the intent that if the victim stands up, everything will be well. These are interventions that are mentioned to be condemned. The EMS medical service is often nonexistent in the third world, more so in the remote or rural third world. Permitting the patient to remain recumbent, ensuring an adequate airway and utilizing locally available materials as a backboard can be both life and spine saving during transfer, as opposed to being transported hammock style in a blanket or slung over the back or in the arms of a bystander. A door frame, planks nailed together, or even a "charpai" or woven bed frame can all serve as safe alternatives to the commercial "backboard." Two padded bricks, bunched clothes, or sandbags (if available) can serve to stabilize the head, being secured with a cloth sash, or the belt of a gentleman. This level of health awareness has not as yet trickled down to the grass roots.

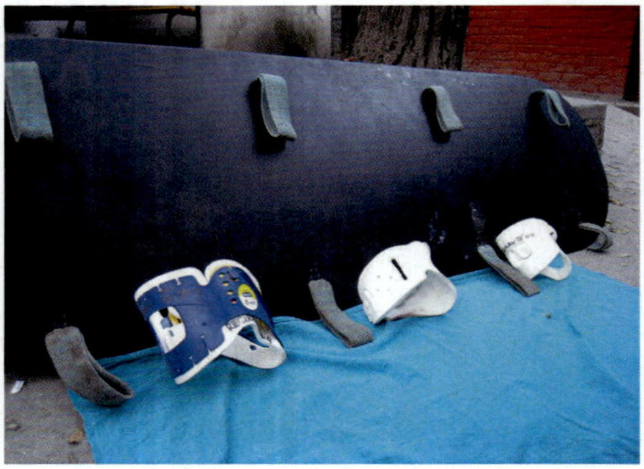

Fig. 24.9 Indigenous plywood backboard and cervical collars

Hospital Measures

The approach to trauma has now been systematized and protocolized, and there should be little excuse for deviating from it. The approach, whether ABC or CAB, demands the placement of a cervical collar of the appropriate size as part of the "A." Cervical collars are now easily available commercially as are backboards. However, we still utilize our indigenous plywood backboards which have served us well at a fraction of the cost. Children involved in motor vehicle accidents should not be exempt from this treatment, given the incidence of SCIWORA (spinal cord injury without radiologic abnormality). The NEXUS guidelines [11] serve a practical standard for the requirement of neck stabilization. Radiologic exclusion of cervical injury can be established by standard cross-table lateral X-rays or a CT scan if available. Inebriated and unconscious patients always need a collar till the spine is cleared.

Cervical injuries are to be classified as stable and unstable injuries. All of them will need transfer to a service which can stabilize the spine operatively. This can be difficult, particularly in instances of Jeffersons fracture or Jones fracture, or clay shoveler's fracture. A halo traction device is not easy to replicate unless available. Crutchfield tongs and traction are an alternative, but they make transfer over mountain and uneven roads difficult. We have found stabilizing the sides of the head with sandbags and strapping the forehead onto the backboard effective in the transport of the acutely injured cervical injury.

Injuries to the Neck

Vignette

A 32-year-old male was brought to the emergency room with history of having attempted sui-

cide by slitting his throat with a knife. On examination he was conscious, with a 7 cm laceration on his anterior neck which was bubbling with blood. The carotids on either side were intact. He was taken up for surgery and intubated on the table, and an infrathyroid tracheal laceration was found and repaired with Prolene sutures. Postop airway was established with a tracheostomy established distal to the laceration. He did well on postoperative follow-up and was decannulated later (Fig. 24.10).

Blunt injury predisposes to large hematomas, tracheal injury, and soft tissue injury, with bleeding into the spaces of the neck which in turn can cause respiratory compromise. Most blunt injury can be treated conservatively after ensuring there is no airway compromise. Emergent intubation followed by a tracheostomy may be required if there is airway compromise. The investing layer of cervical fascia provides a closed space and will result in respiratory distress if there is ongoing bleeding into the space. Most hematomas will settle with conservative management provided anticoagulants are not on board and there is no vessel wall transection.

Direct sharp injury will result in dramatic and profuse bleeding, which has to be controlled surgically. Pre-hospital control may be established by direct compression if the bleeding is venous or the placement of hemostats when available if the bleeding is arterial. Tracheal injuries can cause bubbling respiration through the injured segment. It is best to let them bubble and breathe till they reach the hospital rather than try to attempt any control of such an injury on the field, unless there is occlusion of the airway. Concurrent spinal injury is to be kept in mind, both during transport and during early resuscitation. A cervical collar may restrict access to the bleeding area or may not be practical in such a setting, when spinal stabilization should be ensured by alternative means of sandbags and strapping to a board.

Ideally, all vascular injuries to the neck should be managed in the operating theater under general anesthesia, with good light, suction, vascular instruments, and blood at hand. All components may not always be available. The dictum of "proximal and distal control" cannot be overemphasized in the management of these vascular injuries. Lacerations in the vessels can be repaired with partial isolation of the vessel with a curved Satinsky clamp. There may not be time to ensure a continuity of the circle of Willis, but if the carotid on one side is beyond repair or grafting, a CT angio should preclude ligation of the carotid vessels. Extracranial injury can usually be controlled. A Foley catheter introduced into the rent and gently withdrawn with the bulb inflated serves well to permit visibility and control and plan a repair in an otherwise bloody field (Fig. 24.11).

A snugger can be devised (Fig. 24.12) with a length of wire with a loop at its tip retractable through a cut length of nasogastric tube or infant feeding tube. A suture or a thin rubber vessel loop

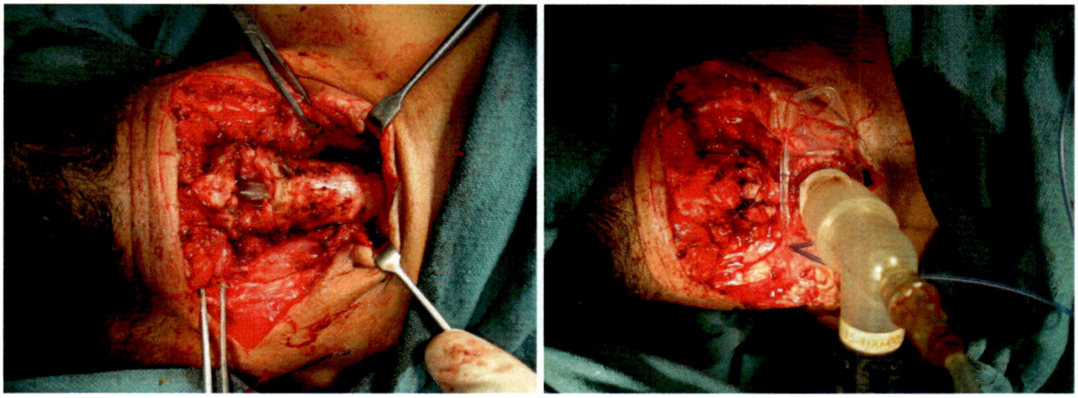

Fig. 24.10 The neck is particularly susceptible to both blunt and sharp injury

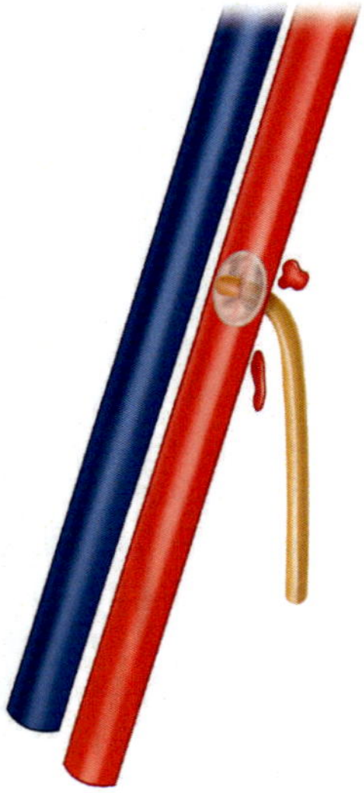

Fig. 24.11 Use of a Foley catheter to staunch arterial bleeding

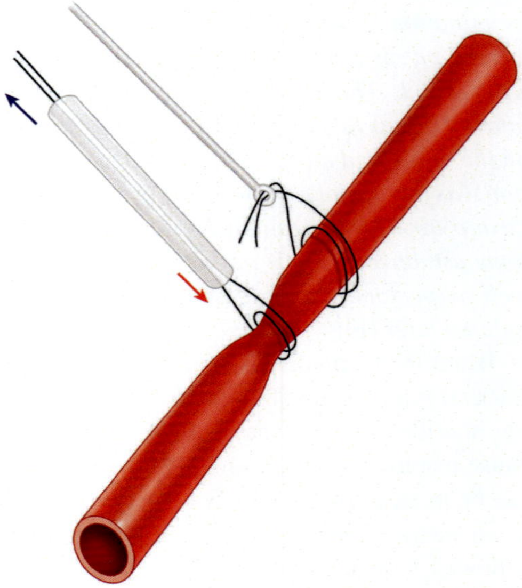

Fig. 24.12 A snugger made with a segment of a nasogastric tube and wire to control arterial bleeding

is doubly passed around the vessel and then extracted through the length of nasogastric tube using the wire loop passer. This can be used to permit atraumatic occlusion of the vessel for proximal control. A mosquito clamp secures the tension at the proximal end of the cut length of nasogastric tube.

Segmental loss of tissue from the side of a vessel can be repaired with a vein graft harvested from the saphenous vein, eminently serviceable as a vein graft. Arterial repair with loss of tissue or length will necessitate use of prosthetic graft material and postoperative anticoagulation.

In remote regions, the access to digital subtraction angiography and embolization and coiling is not usually available. The surgeon bears the responsibility to control and staunch the bleeding with what measures he or she has available.

Injury to the Trachea

Tracheal injuries are best repaired primarily, using nonabsorbable sutures of Prolene, approximating the tracheal rings. A tracheostomy may be performed proximally or distally to permit airway access and control. Tissue loss from the trachea is challenging, and the rent may be converted into a tracheostomy if the rent occurs in second to fourth tracheal rings. Larger tissue loss may require the use of prosthetic material as Teflon, or a vascularized graft. Healing without stenosis is the ultimate aim, because tracheal stenosis is quite challenging to deal with, as is tracheomalacia induced by trauma and the consequence of repair. Tracheomalacia is particularly challenging in the pediatric population.

Injury to the Thyroid

The thyroid can be salvaged by debriding devascularized tissue and obtaining hemostasis. Debridement can follow the guidelines for hemithyroidectomy or lobectomy, ensuring hemostasis by the ligation of the vessels feeding the appropriate vascular territory, whether it be the superior or inferior thyroid arteries. Removal of the thyroid while protecting the recurrent laryngeal nerves and the parathyroids may be very difficult following an injury and should be avoided if possible.

Injury to the Esophagus

Injuries to the esophagus are challenging and usually require primary repair if the rent is small and the duration from injury to repair is brief. Repair can be done using nonabsorbable Prolene sutures or Vicryl sutures. A feeding gastrostomy allows the wound to heal without the interference of the passage of food. Injuries that have a delayed presentation or injuries with tissue loss are best temporized by a cervical esophagostomy, feeding gastrostomy, and subsequent reconstruction with a gastric pullup using a thoracic or a retrosternal approach and anastomosis in the chest or neck, respectively.

Conclusion

We have tried to summarize only the urgent management of a number of emergent problems in the neck that present with relatively high frequency to a nonspecialist surgeon in the underserved environment. Care of patients under those conditions sometimes requires ingenuity and originality, as well as knowledge of basic anatomy and physiology to apply basic surgical skills to solve or temporize a dangerous medical problem. All the problems mentioned are more difficult to manage in infants and children than in adults because of frequent lack of appropriate instruments and of potential physiologic instability. This is partially compensated by more rapid healing and rehabilitation following injuries. This chapter addresses a few management options and "tricks"; it requires the use of ancillary specialist text or digital media for detailed information regarding specific surgical issues that may arise.

References

1. Fitzpatrick PC, Guarisco JL. Pediatric airway foreign bodies. J La State Med Soc. 1998;150(4):138.
2. Committee on Injury, Violence, and Poison Prevention. Prevention of choking among children. Pediatrics. 2010;125(3):601.
3. Tan HK, Brown K, McGill T, Kenna MA, Lund DP, Healy GB. Airway foreign bodies (FB): a 10-year review. Int J Pediatr Otorhinolaryngol. 2000;56(2):91.
4. Zhijun C, Fugao Z, Niankai Z, Jingjing C. Therapeutic experience from 1428 patients with pediatric tracheobronchial foreign body. J Pediatr Surg. 2008;43(4):718.
5. Tang LF, Xu YC, Wang YS, Wang CF, Zhu GH, Bao XE, Lu MP, Chen LX, Chen ZM. Airway foreign body removal by flexible bronchoscopy: experience with 1027 children during 2000-2008. World J Pediatr. 2009;5(3):191–5. Epub 2009 Aug 20
6. Limper AH, Prakash UB. Tracheobronchial foreign bodies in adults. Ann Intern Med. 1990;112(8):604.
7. Uyemura MC. Foreign body ingestion in children. Am Fam Physician. 2005;72(2):287.
8. Athanassiadi K, Gerazounis M, Metaxas E, Kalantzi N. Management of esophageal foreign bodies: a retrospective review of 400 cases. Eur J Cardiothorac Surg. 2002;21(4):653.
9. Samsoon GL, Young JR. Difficult tracheal intubation: a retrospective study. Anaesthesia. 1987;42:487.
10. Dr. Arpit Mathew, Mr. Jeremiah Naveen Joseph, Madhipura Christian Hospital, Personal communication.
11. Hoffman JR, Wolfson AB, Todd K, et al. Selective cervical spine radiography in blunt trauma: methodology of the Na- tional emergency X-radiography utilization study (NEXUS). Ann Emerg Med. 1998;32(4):461–9.

How to Manage Thoracic Surgical Problems in Low- and Middle-Income Countries

25

Warren D. Widmann

The greatest wealth is health.
– Virgil, 70–19, BCE

Abbreviations

HIC	High-income countries
LMICs	Low- and middle-income countries
RTAs	Road traffic accidents

Introduction

The role of thoracic surgical interventions at the local level in LMICs is very limited because of the lack of trained personnel, the absence of the basic infrastructure (clean water, electricity, oxygen, anesthetists, and staff) to support advanced interventions, and the lack of financial resources to purchase diagnostic and therapeutic supplies. Accordingly, we will not focus on the underlying socioeconomic changes needed to improve global health but rather on what can be done at the present time using the limited resources in LMIC [1].

We will address appropriate interventions that are feasible given limited resources—appropriate meaning both effective and practical. In the absence of personnel trained in advanced thoracic surgical skills, including general surgeons, in regions lacking advanced diagnostic and therapeutic equipment, what can the basic healthcare workers and general surgeons do to lessen the burden of the common thoracic surgical conditions in LMIC?

W. D. Widmann (✉)
Surgical Education, State University of New York Downstate Health Sciences University, Brooklyn, NY, USA

Trauma

It is widely recognized that trauma is a huge cause of morbidity and mortality in LMICs. The deaths from trauma exceed the combined total of deaths from HIV/AIDS, TB, and malaria. Most of the world's trauma deaths occur in LMICs. What are the treatable thoracic injuries?

Loss of Consciousness with Loss of Airway/Endoscopy

A common cause of death from trauma is the loss of the airway with resultant hypoxemia. This occurs most often in association with road traffic accidents (RTAs) in LMIC. Traumatic brain injury with loss of consciousness results in the tongue falling back obstructing the airway in the recumbent victim. Hypoxemia and death follow.

M. A. Hardy, B. R. Hochman (eds.), *Global Surgery*, https://doi.org/10.1007/978-3-031-28127-3_25

The estimated frequency of death from this mechanism is about 30% [2].

Diagnosis of Airway Obstruction

In any patient who does not respond to verbal stimulation and is not breathing, there may be gurgling sounds with attempted inspiration or a total lack of any air exchange. There may be cyanosis on checking the mucous membranes or skin. There will be no motion of the chest wall and no breath sounds on auscultation of the chest.

Treatment of Airway Obstruction Due to Loss of Consciousness

The rescuer must assume airway obstruction, and after checking for any foreign material in the mouth with a finger swipe, the airway must be opened. In the unconscious patient, the tongue falls backward into the hypopharynx. The head-tilt-chin-lift maneuver that is used when loss of consciousness is due to a medical condition is shown in Fig. 25.1.

Treatment of Airway Obstruction Due to Loss of Consciousness in Trauma Patients

In cases where there is any history of trauma and loss of consciousness, airway obstruction occurs by the same mechanism as in medical causes of unconsciousness. The floppy tongue falls backward. However, performing the head-tilt-chin-lift maneuver is fraught with danger. Head trauma and loss of consciousness is associated with cervical spine injury in 15% of cases. The rescuer must assume there is concomitant instability of the cervical spine and that the head tilt maneuver may convert a partial spinal cord injury to a complete spinal cord injury. The proper maneuver in all trauma cases is the jaw-thrust maneuver as shown in Fig. 25.2.

Endoscopy for Intubation

When used appropriately the head-tilt-chin lift or the jaw-thrust maneuvers may reestablish a patent airway, but for continued maintenance of the airway in the unconscious patient, endotracheal intubation is needed. Tracheal intubation in the

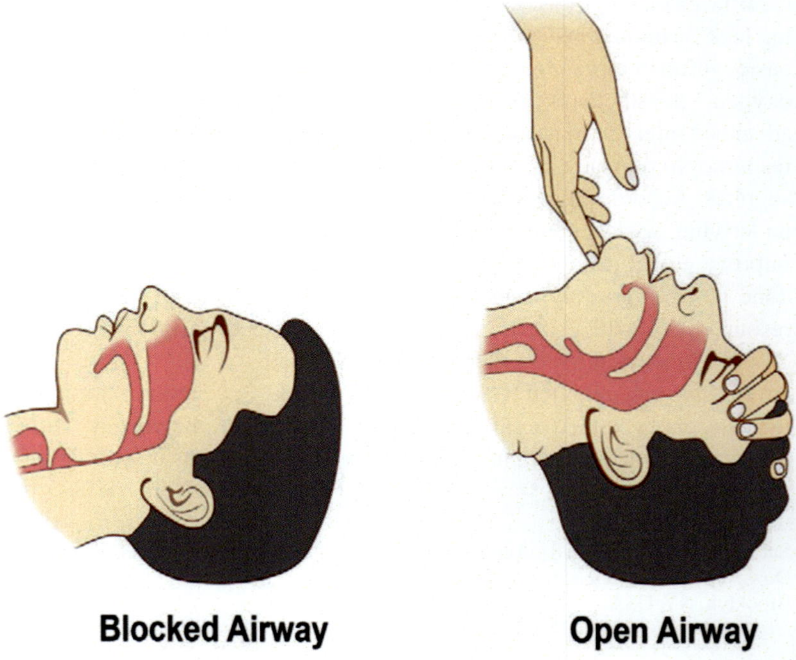

Fig. 25.1 By tilting the head backward and hyperextending the neck while simultaneously using the other hand to lift the chin upward, the tongue is pulled forward and the airway is opened. This procedure *should not be used in cases of trauma*

unconscious patient does not require administration of drugs. In the field or in the clinic, this is best performed using a battery-powered laryngoscope. The operator must know the basics—there are two types of blades used for laryngoscopy to expose the larynx and the vocal cords by lifting the epiglottis anteriorly (ventrally).

When using the curved blade (Macintosh), the blade is inserted into the vallecula just to the left side of the epiglottic fold, and the operator lifts the back of the tongue upward. The fold of tissue holding the epiglottis to the base of the tongue thus pulls the epiglottis ventrally exposing the vocal cords and the operator can pass the endotracheal tube between the vocal cords inserting the tube beyond the teeth to the 22–26 cm markings on the tube. The balloon on the tube is inflated. The tube is secured in place with tape, and the patient can then be ventilated with the operator breathing directly into the tube but preferably with use of an AMBU bag connected to the endotracheal tube. There should be symmetrical chest wall rise with squeezing the AMBU bag, and the operator can listen to the chest on each side to hear breath sounds. The luxury of measuring end-tidal carbon dioxide may not be available in the field in LMICs.

When the operator uses the straight blade (Miller) for laryngoscopy, the tip of the blade is inserted just under the epiglottis, and then the epiglottis and tongue are directly lifted anteriorly (ventrally) to expose the vocal cords. Figure 25.3 shows the proper placement of the laryngoscope blades.

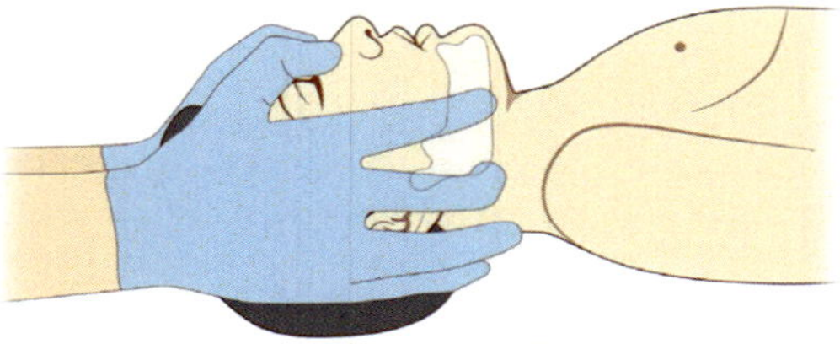

Fig. 25.2 In unconscious trauma patients, the rescuer must keep the head in the neutral position while performing the jaw-thrust. The steady traction by both thumbs and ring and little fingers keeps the head in the neutral position while the index and middle fingers pull upward on the mandible moving the tongue forward and opening the airway

Advanced Endoscopy (Bronchoscopy)

Both in the field and in the station hospitals/clinics in LMICs, the support for advanced endoscopy is lacking. Clean water, reliable electricity, expensive instruments, and trained personnel are usually not available. However, should endotracheal intubation fail, the airway can be established in emergencies by performing a cricothyroidotomy as described later in this chapter.

Tension Pneumothorax

A tension pneumothorax is the result of a progressive buildup of air within the chest cavity

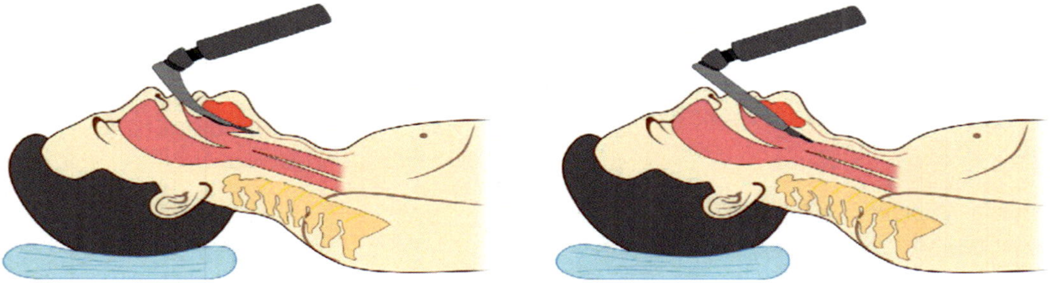

Fig. 25.3 Notice that when using the curved blade (Macintosh), the tip is inserted into the vallecula, just to the side of the epiglottis and that lifting the blade anteriorly (ventrally) will lift the epiglottis (shown in white) giving the operator a view of the vocal cords and trachea. When using the straight blade, notice that the operator has lifted the epiglottis directly

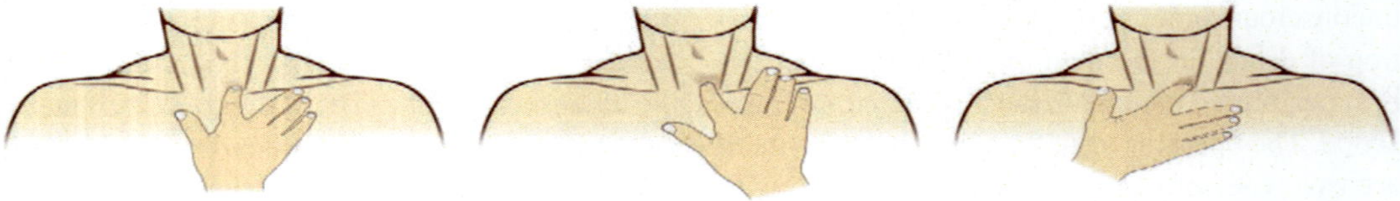

Fig. 25.4 The examiner uses the right-hand index finger to palpate the space between the trachea and the head of the clavicle on each side. The fingertip should easily enter the space on each side. In the presence of tracheal deviation, there will be an easily felt discrepancy with the trachea shifted away from the side with the tension pneumothorax. Additionally, the examiner might notice jugular venous distention in obstructive shock

caused by leakage of air from the lung into the pleural space (most commonly) or by entry of air into the chest through an open wound of the chest wall during inspiration and then the air getting trapped by closure of the opening during exhalation. In either case, as intrathoracic pressure builds up, the lung on the side of the injury progressively collapses while the pressure within the pleural cavity increases. As the intrathoracic pressure increases, return of blood to the heart decreases and obstructive shock and death ensue.

How Can you Diagnose a Tension Pneumothorax?

Let's start with the injured patient with rib fractures. The sharp fractured ribs can lacerate the lung with resultant leakage of air into the pleural cavity. The mechanism of injury in LMIC most commonly would be RTA. The history of RTA, the presence of pain localized to the chest wall, shortness of breath, tachycardia, and dyspnea are clues. In LMIC we do not have readily available XRAY machines. We do have physical examinations available! Diminished breath sounds are the hallmark for a pneumothorax—along with a loss of tactile fremitus. With a tension pneumothorax, there will be a shift of the mediastinum away from the injured side. A simple palpation of the trachea can help secure the diagnosis, as shown in Fig. 25.4.

How Do you Treat a Tension Pneumothorax?

Immediate Decompression Is the First Step The traditional approach until recently was needle decompression by puncturing the chest wall with a needle in the second intercostal space approaching in the midclavicular line. Recent data shows that decompression on the first needle pass was not achieved in many patients and that approaching initially transaxillary in the third, fourth, or fifth interspace anterior axillary line was more likely to be successful on the first needle pass. All that is needed is a basic skin prep and a needle or needle catheter. Two approaches are shown in Fig. 25.5.

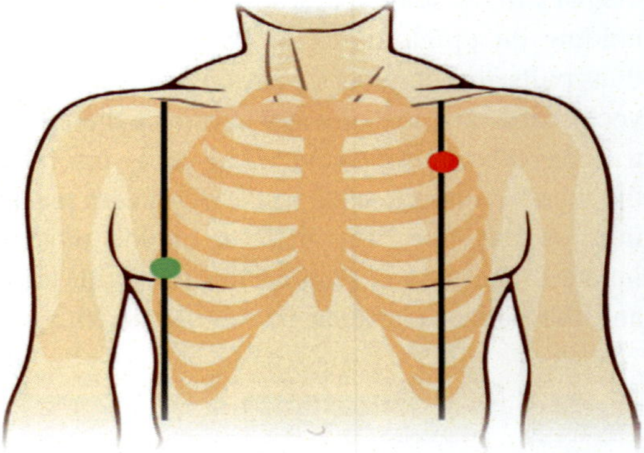

Fig. 25.5 After cleansing the chest wall, the anterior puncture site uses the angle of Louis (the junction of the manubrium with the body of the sternum) and the level of the second rib as a landmark. The needle can be inserted in thin individuals at the lower aspect of the second interspace which is easily determined by palpation just below and lateral to the angle of Louis, making the insertion in the midclavicular line to avoid hitting the internal thoracic artery and close to the top of the third rib to avoid hitting the main intercostal artery, nerve, and vein which run in a groove close to the inferior border of each rib (as shown in red dot)

Alternatively, in obese and muscular patients, the preferred approach would be puncture at the anterior axillary line (which is at the lateral border of the easily felt pectoralis major muscle) gaining entry through the third, fourth, or fifth interspace avoiding the axillary hair and again staying close to the superior edge of the rib to avoid the main intercostal artery, nerve, and vein (as shown in green dot).

Once decompression of the pleural cavity has been achieved, the obstructive shock has been relieved, but there is now a collapsed lung on the injured side needing re-expansion.

How Can a Collapsed Lung be re-Expanded?

The traditional approach for getting the lung re-expanded is for a chest tube to be inserted and put to a controlled suction device. There may be no available controlled suction in LMIC. At best, a packaged sterile chest tube can be inserted, and at worst one can use a urethral catheter with two extra holes cut out. Size 28 has been shown to be as effective as the larger sizes and causes less pain. In the absence of available controlled suction, an improvised Heimlich valve can be applied which allows for exit of air from the chest cavity without reentry as the improvised valve closes.

Procedural Steps in Chest Tube Insertion

Basic supplies needed are antiseptic solution for cleansing the operative site, some sterile towels to create an operative field, sterile gloves for the operator, local anesthetic, needles, syringes, sterile scalpel, sterile hemostats or Kelly clamps, sterile chest tube size 28 or a sterile flexible length of plastic tubing of equivalent size, 2–0 silk sutures to close the wound and secure the chest tube in place, a needle holder, scissors, gauze pads for dressing, adhesive tape, and an improvised Heimlich valve which can be made from the finger of a sterile glove. With the patient recumbent and the arm tucked behind the head, the operative field is prepped (Fig. 25.6). After the prep, local anesthetic is injected (Fig. 25.7).

The chest cavity is entered by blunt dissection with the Kelly clamp angled superiorly to allow the chest tube to be "tunneled up" to the interspace above the incision. Thus, as shown in Fig. 25.8, two interspaces required numbing, the lower interspace of the incision and the upper interspace for tube insertion both require injection of local anesthesia.

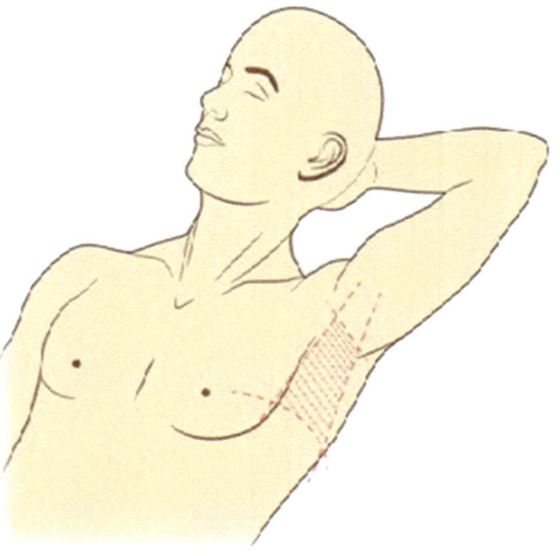

Fig. 25.6 The safe area for chest tube insertion is outlined below. Going too far cranially risks injury to the subclavian artery, vein, and brachial plexus; in addition, too far caudally risks injury to the heart, spleen, and stomach on the left side and injury to the liver on the right side

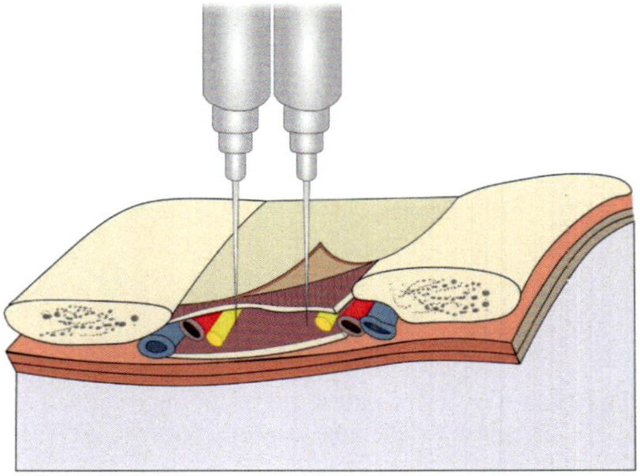

Fig. 25.7 The main intercostal nerve runs in a groove behind the lower border of the rib. An additional branch runs along the upper border of the rib. Both sites require injection. The interspace below the site for chest tube insertion is anesthetized because that is where the incision will be made. The interspace above the incision is anesthetized because that is the interspace through which the chest tube will be inserted

The initial dissection is done with the Kelly clamp, and the tract enlarged sufficiently to allow insertion of the index finger, following which the

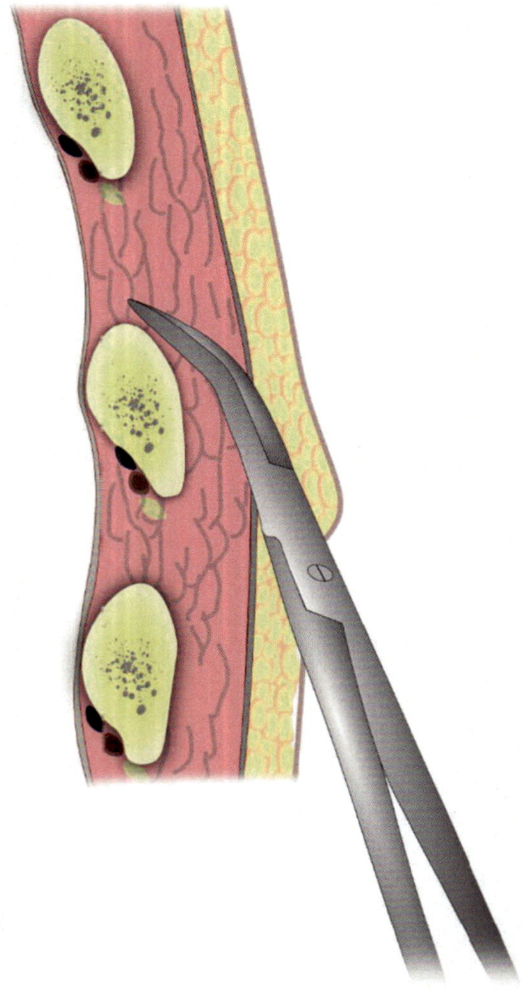

Fig. 25.8 The lower interspace of the incision and the upper interspace for the tube insertion both require injection of the local anesthetic

chest tube is grasped between the jaws of the Kelly clamp and inserted into the chest cavity, as shown in Fig. 25.9.

The chest tube insertion site should be closed medial and lateral to the tube to prevent air from being sucked into the chest through the incision. These sutures also serve a "stay" sutures by anchoring the chest tube to the skin closure, as shown in Fig. 25.10. The stay sutures have an "air knot" placed about 1 cm after tying the suture to close the skin and then that suture is wrapped tightly around the chest tube and firmly tied so that the chest tube cannot be accidentally pulled out. By placing one suture medially and one suture laterally and securing them to the chest tube, they help to make the chest tube "stay" in place (Figs. 25.10 and 25.11).

Without a Controlled Suction System, how Will Air Escape from the Pleural Cavity and the Collapsed Lung Get Re-Expanded?

A Heimlich valve can be made simply by tying a condom or even the cut-off finger of a used glove to the end of the chest tube. A slit is cut into the distal end of the floppy attached "valve." With each inspiration the floppy condom/glove finger collapses on itself preventing air from being sucked into the chest. With each expiration as air pressure is increased within the chest, gas will bubble out. Lung re-expansion can be facilitated by having the patient cough (Fig. 25.12).

There is no agreement among thoracic surgeons about the best way to remove the chest

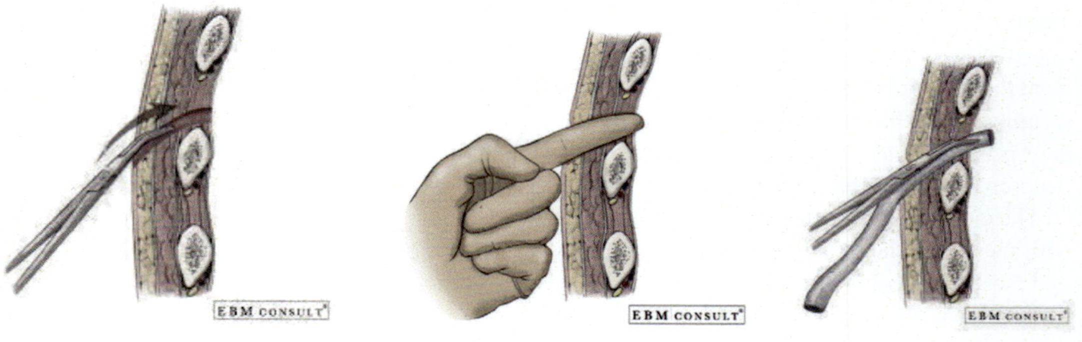

Fig. 25.9 After the incision is carried down to the fascia of the intercostal muscles in the interspace below the site of planned entry into the pleural cavity, a Kelly clamp is used to bluntly dissect upward, and once the pleural cavity is entered, the tract is enlarged to allow passage of the operator's index finger to confirm that there are no local adhesions. The chest tube is grasped by the Kelly clamp and then the clamp and tube are inserted angled superiorly

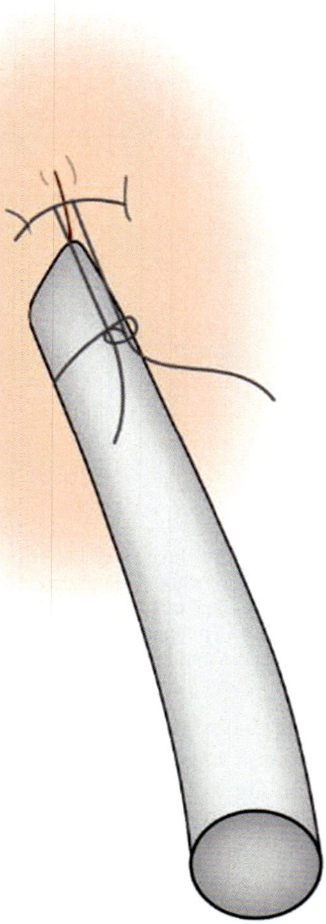

Fig. 25.10 The stay sutures shown are used to close the skin incision and have an initial "air knot" against which the tube is tightly tied

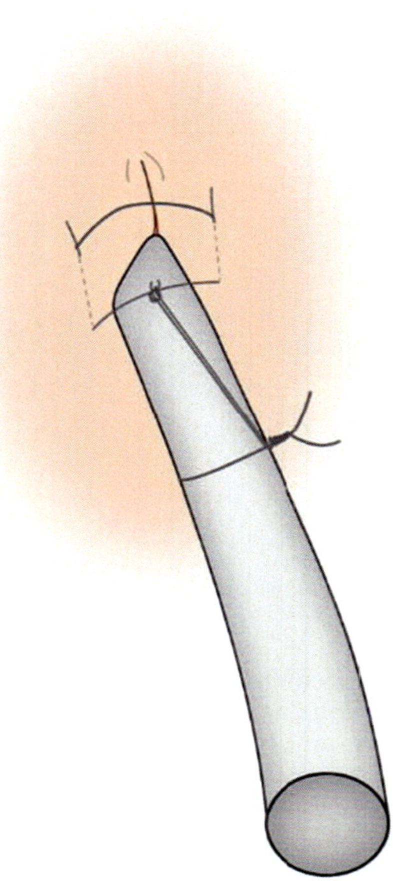

Fig. 25.11 Additionally, a "U" stitch is placed. It is not fully tied close to the skin. A single throw is placed against the chest tube and its ends will be tied around the chest tube well away from the stay sutures. The purse string "U" suture is left long. When the chest tube is no longer needed, the stay sutures are cut freeing the tube and the "U" stitch is tied promptly as the chest tube is rapidly withdrawn preventing air from being sucked into the chest when the chest tube is removed

tube once the lung is expanded, whether with the patient at full inspiration or full expiration. The author's preference is full inspiration with cutting of the stay sutures just proximal to the air knot with rapid removal and tying of the purse string suture followed by placing an occlusive dressing over the site.

Open Chest Wound/Sucking Chest Wound

While rib fractures may cause a simple pneumothorax or a tension pneumothorax, collapse of a lung with or without tension physiology may result from an external penetrating wound with atmospheric air gaining entry into the chest cavity. With each inspiration, air is "sucked" into the chest and it may or may not exit during expiration. If it does not exit, tension may develop with resultant obstructive shock.

Diagnosis of an Open Chest Wound/Sucking Chest Wound

The history of trauma and the physical examination make this diagnosis. If the lung has been injured, bloody froth may bubble in and out of the wound with inspiration and expiration.

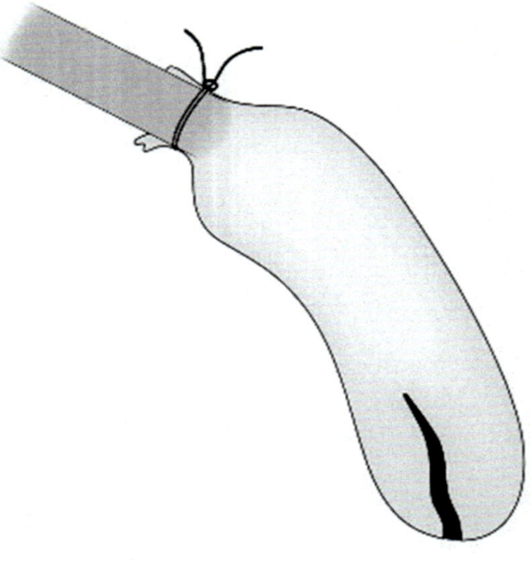

Fig. 25.12 An improvised Heimlich valve can be made easily by cutting a slit in a condom or a glove finger and fastening it to the end of the chest tube

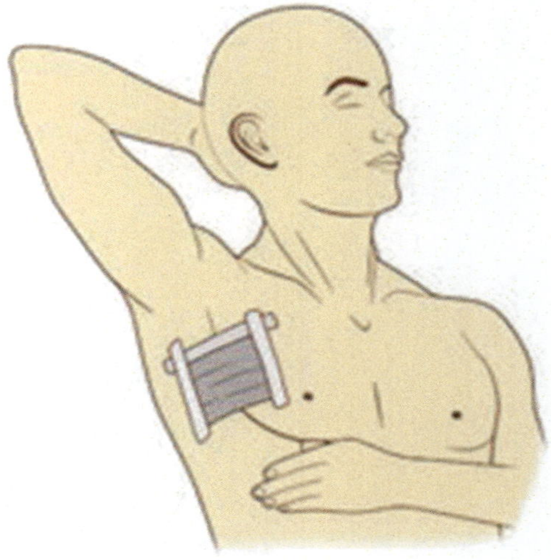

Fig. 25.13 The three-sided application of tape over cellophane or any other clean impermeable flexible material allows for escape of air from the chest without air getting sucked back in. Ongoing internal bleeding may require fluid or blood administration if available

Management of an Open Chest Wound/ Sucking Chest Wound

The management of this type of injury is quite simple. An occlusive dressing is applied and taped only on three sides as shown in Fig. 25.13. Most penetrating chest wounds do not require surgery for control of bleeding. Thoracotomy may be a very difficult, if not dangerous, option in LMIC. Fortunately, it is rarely needed for penetrating chest trauma. The best course of treatment is to get the patient to a major LMIC facility that can safely perform open chest surgery if there is continued bleeding.

Flail Chest

Road traffic accidents (RTAs) and falls may produce multiple rib fractures, and especially when serial ribs are broken at two sites, the chest wall becomes unstable with a resultant inward collapse of the chest wall on inspiration and then outward bulging on expiration. There is lessened air entry into the lungs, and respiratory insufficiency with hypoxia and hypercarbia develops.

The diagnosis is readily made by the history of trauma, and examination shows the paradoxical caving in of the chest wall with inspiration and bulging out with expiration. Bony crepitus may be felt. The patient will be anxious and tachypneic. Pain is severe. While the ideal treatment would be intubation and ventilator support, along with pain relief by a high epidural catheter, these modalities are rarely available in LMIC.

Management of a Flail Chest

In LMIC the practical approach is to stabilize the chest wall with a tight dressing being careful to avoid restricting motion of the opposite side of the chest. Pain relief by intercostal nerve block with local anesthetics is preferable to narcotic medication which may suppress the ventilatory drive. Figure 25.14 shows such a dressing using expandable elastic wrapping. If possible, the dressing should be taped only to the midline to avoid restricting the opposite chest wall motion. If available, plastic IV fluid bags can be taped on instead of bulky gauze material to compress and stabilize the chest wall.

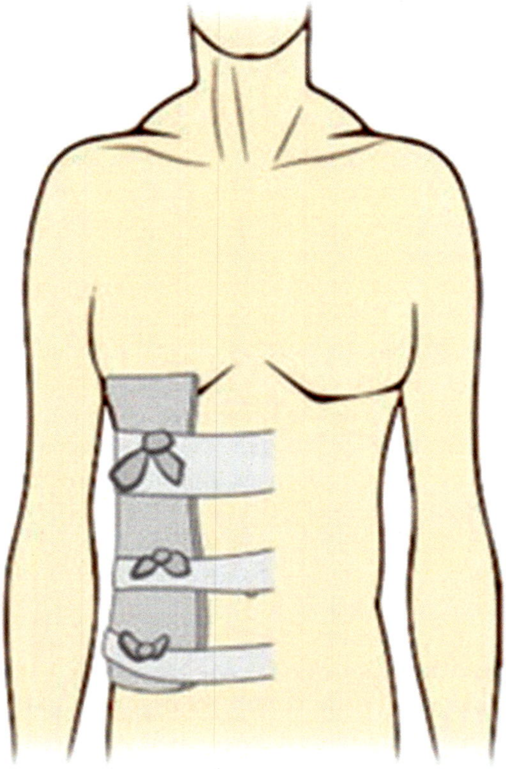

Fig. 25.14 The flail segment of the chest should be splinted by a bulky dressing with care to avoid restriction of the opposite side of the chest. Pain medication is needed, and coughing is encouraged

Thoracic Infections

The complications of pulmonary infection may lead to empyema, a buildup of pus within the pleural cavity. This can be the result of bacterial pneumonia or tuberculosis. Undrained, sepsis and septic shock may be fatal. In LMIC patients typically present with advanced stages of empyema with thick intrathoracic pus. Tuberculous effusions are most common. Echinococcal effusions may also occur.

The diagnosis is made from the history of fever, cough, and sputum production, and it is confirmed by physical examination showing diminished breath sounds on the affected side, with dullness to percussion, and loss of tactile fremitus. Weight loss and dehydration are common findings. Chronicity suggests tuberculous empyema.

While combined medical management with appropriate antibiotics and chest drainage is needed, the appropriate means for determining the exact organisms involved (bacteriologic identification) and then antibiotic sensitivity profiling for selecting the appropriate antibiotic treatment program may be lacking in a station hospital in LMIC. However, usually a microscope and an incubator are available. A smear of the sputum with acid-fast stain may confirm diagnosis of TB. Cultures should be sent to the major hospital in the area, preferably along with the patient for more precise and effective care. Basic supplies of antibiotics are frequently lacking for empiric therapy and may require sending the patient's family to obtain them. Additionally, chest tube drainage is most effective when instituted while the empyema fluid is "thin," that is, not thick/viscous and will drain out from the chest without suction. Further, with patients presenting with advanced disease, the underlying lung may have become encased in a thick, fibroinflammatory "peel" and not re-expand. Such cases need operative decortication or combined enzymatic lysis, modalities beyond local treatment in a station hospital in LMIC. Almost all LMICs have regional facilities with such capabilities for treatment of tubercular and non-tubercular empyema [3]. However, in most station hospitals or rural clinics in LMICs, the only treatment readily available is chest tube drainage, with possible diagnosis and antibiotic treatment only until the patient can be transferred to an appropriate facility.

Airway Obstruction by Infection/ Foreign Bodies

The airway can become obstructed by aspiration of foreign bodies most typically aspirated food and by infection both bacterial and viral. Complete obstruction rapidly results in anoxic death. If the airway is not completely obstructed, the patient may be brought to medical attention.

Diagnosis of Airway Obstruction

The history of eating and talking with a mouth full of food followed by gasping and coughing sometimes associated with a loss of the ability to speak and with concomitant pointing to the neck by the patient is the classical presentation. On examination with a stethoscope or simply by listening to the chest by placing the examiners' ear directly on the chest wall, there may be localized wheezing or diminished sounds on just one side if the material is blocking just one major bronchus, but most commonly the food or other foreign materials are lodged just at or above the vocal cords, and breath sounds are diminished on both sides. Stridor is common when the vocal cords are inflamed by bacterial or viral infection.

Management of Airway Obstruction

Ancillary personnel should be trained in the simple potentially life-saving maneuvers that may aid the patient's ability to cough out the foreign material. The simplest means of increasing intrathoracic pressure to expel foreign material is by forceful slapping the patients back between the scapulae. A more advanced and more effective maneuver is the Heimlich maneuver, in which the operator gets behind the victim, and with one hand formed into a fist and placed in the subxiphoid region, the other hand overlying that hand, and then both are forcefully pulled into the victim's upper abdomen. The sudden increase in intraabdominal pressure is transmitted through the diaphragm, and the resultant elevated intrathoracic pressure may be sufficient for the impacted foreign material to be dislodged and coughed out, as shown in Fig. 25.15.

When the Heimlich maneuver is not successful with repeated thrusts, the traditional approach in medical facilities when patients are stridulous would be to perform endotracheal intubation with laryngoscopy and bronchoscopy for removal of any foreign material. Such an approach requires trained personnel, available instruments, and resources (electricity) to utilize endoscopic removal. Lacking these in an LMIC facility, the next step should be performance of a cricothyroidotomy.

Cricothyroidotomy

When the airway cannot be cleared by back-slapping or the Heimlich maneuver, the next

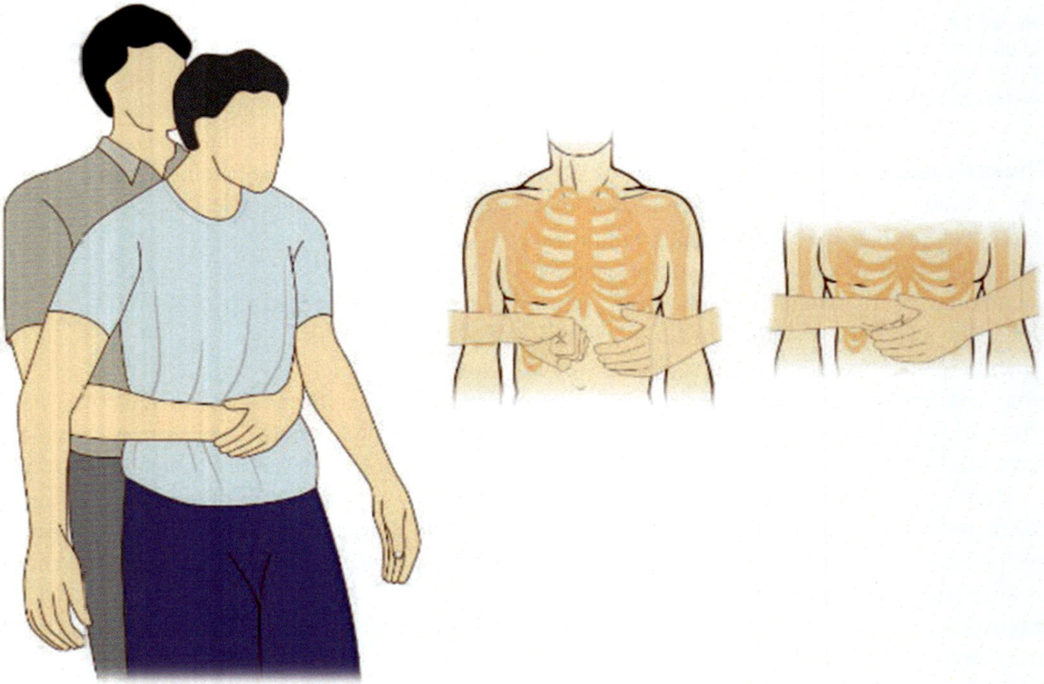

Fig. 25.15 As shown, the Heimlich maneuver requires just one trained person and no additional equipment

step when bronchoscopy cannot be done for various reasons, relief of obstruction must be done by performing the simplest, fastest opening of the airway **below the larynx**. The equipment needed is minimal and the simplicity of cricothyroidotomy makes it feasible for medical personnel other than trained general or thoracic surgeons to perform the procedure safely. The anatomic features of the neck dictate that tracheostomy is a more advanced procedure, fraught with more bleeding and need for more equipment. To perform a tracheostomy may require more equipment and more surgical skill as the isthmus of the thyroid is in the operative field, bleeding is more of a concern, and the time required is more than for a cricothyroidotomy. Figure 25.16 shows that there are no significant structures in front of the cricothyroid membrane, while the thyroid can cover tracheal rings and make rapid bloodless approach to the tracheal lumen difficult. The quickest and least bloody access to the cricothyroid membrane is by a vertical midline incision. There is no need for sophisticated specialized tubes to be inserted. Any hollow tube suffices, as shown in Fig. 25.17.

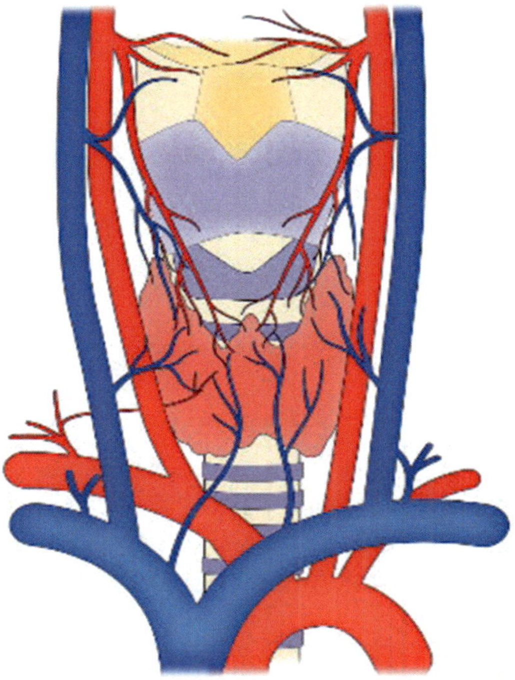

Fig. 25.16 The larynx and just inferior to it the cricoid cartilage can be felt easily. Note that the very vascular thyroid gland covers much of the proximal trachea below the cricoid cartilage

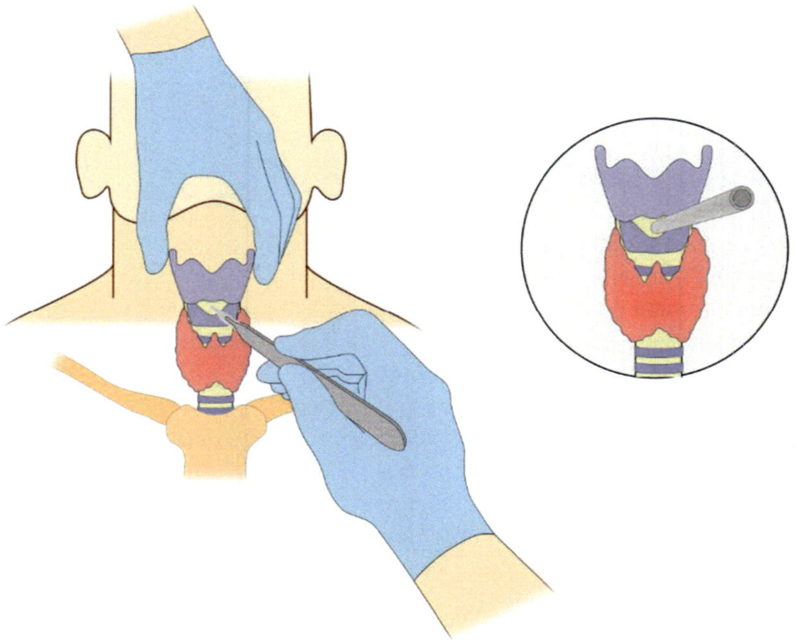

Fig. 25.17 The vertical skin incision should be 2–3 cm long. A Kelly clamp or hemostat can be used to spread the skin and subcutaneous tissue laterally, and then a horizontal incision is made in the underlying cricothyroid membrane. The opening can be dilated with a clamp, and any type of hollow tube can be used to establish the airway

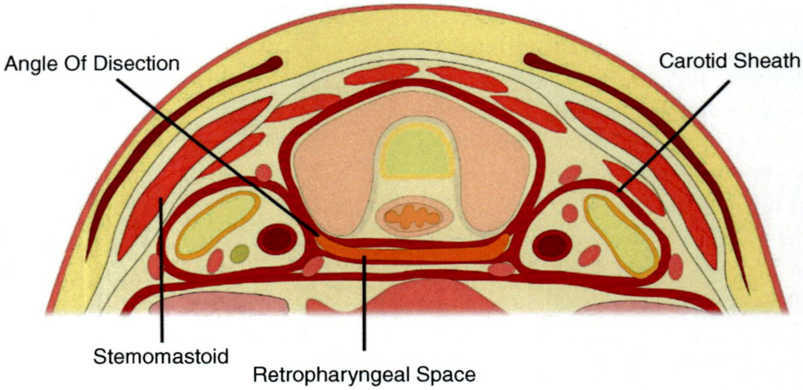

Fig. 25.18 Under local anesthesia after making an incision anterior to the right or left sternocleidomastoid muscle and extending it through the underlying platysma muscle, dissection is bluntly continued anterior to the carotid sheath and dorsal to the thyroid gland. This leads to the posterior (retropharyngeal) visceral space involved in descending cervical mediastinitis. Soft drains are then inserted

Esophageal Injuries: Mediastinitis

Penetrating neck wounds may injure the proximal esophagus and produce mediastinitis. Similarly, neglected dental and tonsillar infection may cause descending mediastinitis. In LMIC non-major hospitals, the only treatment practical and safe for the patient would be transcervical drainage by a longitudinal incision anterior to the sternocleidomastoid muscle (Fig. 25.18). Transcervical drainage can be performed using local anesthesia and requires minimal instruments beyond scalpel, Kelly clamps, and soft drainage tubes [4].

Chest Wall Burns

While most trauma especially road traffic accidents (RTAs) affect men, in LMIC burns are more common among women due to their predominant engagement in cooking [5]. Chest wall full-thickness burns may result in formation of a restrictive eschar which impairs ventilation. Providing the patient has been able to take sufficient fluids by mouth and not succumb to "burn shock" given such a patient, escharotomy is the appropriate treatment. Since full-thickness burns result in an insensate eschar, anesthesia is not needed. Incisions must be made to allow relief of the chest constriction. The typical incisions needed are shown in Fig. 25.19.

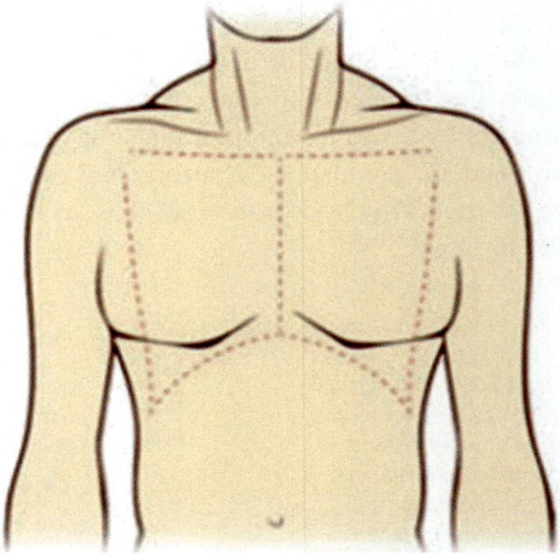

Fig. 25.19 The incisions allow the constricted chest wall to regain motion. Insensate skin and subcutaneous tissue can be incised down to the fascia with little bleeding

Cardiac Injuries

Cardiac injuries can result in cardiac tamponade or exsanguination into the pleural cavity. If patients survive with cardiac tamponade and are able to present to a basic clinic in LMICs, facili-

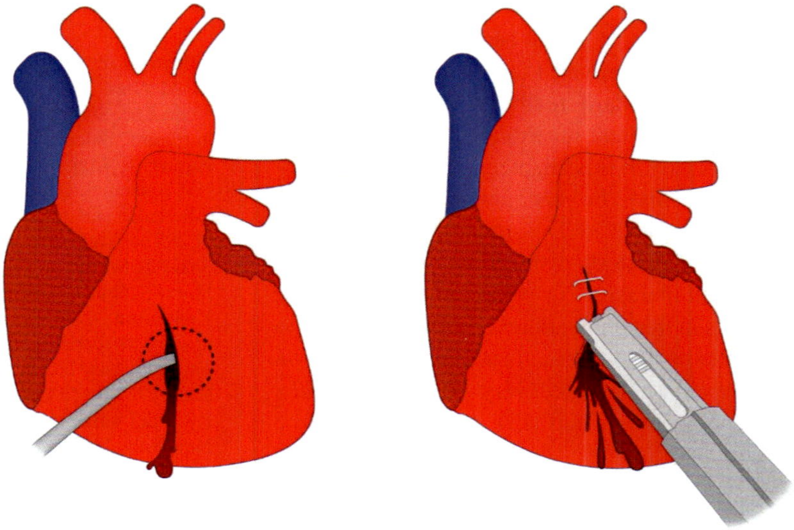

Fig. 25.20 Damage control techniques in Cardiac Trauma. In cardiac injuries extending through the endocardium a Foley catheter can be inserted into the wound, inflated, and gently retracted to achieve hemorrhage control. Skin staples may be used to close the cardiac wound

ties will not likely have staff sufficient to perform emergency left anterior lateral thoracotomy and decompression of the tamponade. For such a procedure, anesthesia staff, nursing personnel, surgical equipment, and then postoperative care are not available. Trained physicians may be able to perform subxiphoid decompression of the pericardium as an alternative approach. Along with the inability to provide operative care for traumatic cardiac injuries, treatment of congenital heart disease and acquired heart disease remain beyond the scope of available care in other than in major health centers in some LMICs. These efforts are frequently strengthened by collaboration under mutual agreements with visiting cardiac surgery NGOs from high-income countries (HICs) such as the USA or Sweden.

The possibility of saving a patient with a stab wound of the heart is highly unlikely in a rural station hospital in LMICs. If the diagnosis appears clear by physical examination or ultrasound, an attempt at repair of the hole in the heart may be tried (Fig. 25.20). An anterolateral left thoracotomy is needed in the fifth interspace, and once the hole is found, bleeding may be controlled with a finger or Foley catheter. The cardiac wound can be closed using skin staples. Blood replacement must follow, and the patient must be evacuated to the nearest major facility if they are to survive.

Summary

At the current time, the thoracic procedures most likely to be performed and to meaningfully save lives in LMIC are for trauma victims and for those suffering from infectious pleural effusions. Securing an airway, treating a pneumothorax, and draining the chest are basic procedures that can be performed with a minimum of supplies and not needing readily available complete operating room infrastructure, including staff, supplies, equipment, and anesthesiologists. There remain a vast number of conditions needing thoracic surgical care for congenital and acquired diseases of the chest that remain untreated—most notably pediatric cyanotic heart conditions and adult malignancies. Because of the infrastructure needed to support major thoracic and cardiac operations, basic structural changes in LMICs need to be either supported or initiated before those conditions can be treated effectively and successfully in many LMICs. Basic training for the procedures discussed in this chapter can be performed with the limited resources in rural station hospitals in LMICs at the current time and should be a part of global health initiatives.

The reader is advised to seek further information from standard textbooks of surgery and from the websites, regarding the problems discussed briefly in this chapter and any other problems that may be encountered during daily practice in LMICs. This includes treatment of unusual respiratory distress syndromes associated with parasitic or viral infections. Other chapters in this book address problems related to diseases of the thorax including chapters on trauma (Chap. 14), recovery room (Chap. 12), operating room (Chap. 13), and injuries of the neck (Chap. 24).

References

1. Lebenthal A, von Holzen U. Adult chest surgery. 2nd ed. McGraw-Hill Education; 2015. p. 366–80.
2. Khan RM, Sharma PK, Kaul N. Airway management in trauma. Indian J Anaesthesia. 2011;55:463–9.
3. Kumar A, Lingaraju CV, Pulle MV, Asaf BB, Puri HV, Bishnoi S. Comparison of outcome of surgery for tubercular and nontubercular empyema: an analysis of 285 consecutive cases. Lung India. 2021;38:514–9.
4. Sakai T, Matsutani N, Iito K, Mochiki M, Mineda J, Shirai S, Kanaoka R, Yamamuchi Y, Saito Y, Sakao Y, Kawamura M. Deep cervical and paratracheal drainage for descending mediastinitis. Asian Cardiovasc Thoracic Ann. 2020;28:29–3.
5. Smiley KE, DeBas HT, deVries CR, Price RR. Schwartz's principles of surgery. 11th ed. New York; 2019. 2077-2112

26 How to Manage Conditions of the Stomach in Low- and Middle-Income Countries

Philip Vareed Alexander and Myla Jacob

Nothing can be done without hope and confidence.

– Helen Keller

Abbreviations

EGD	Upper endoscopy
GI	Gastrointestinal
IV	Intravenous
LMICs	Low- and middle-income countries
NCCN	National Comprehensive Cancer Network
NDMA	N-nitrosodimethylamine
NSAIDS	Non-steroidal anti-inflammatory drugs

Endoscopy

Upper GI endoscopy is an essential part of the armamentarium of the surgeons in LMICs. Besides being confronted with the chameleon of epigastric discomfort and pain, the sinister spectre of upper gastrointestinal haemorrhage requires life-saving intervention, particularly when the next port of referral is many hours away. Endoscopic training is being increasingly incorporated into the syllabus of the general surgeon, and rightfully so, but this is not yet quite universal. Short courses in endoscopy being made available to the general surgeon will be invaluable in widening his repertoire, and those planning to serve in LMICs should learn it. Colonoscopy is one step further in the interventional skill required of the remote rural surgeon, but is more demanding in terms of training, and skill and experience. Chapter 10 addresses the approach to organizing an effective endoscopy program in LMICs.

Heartburn

Heartburn, or upper abdominal discomfort and pain, is reportedly more common in the Western world (10–20% prevalence) than in Asia (5% prevalence) [1], but is a very common presentation to both the outpatient clinic and the emergency room. What is more sinister is that it can camouflage life-threatening conditions, like acute myocardial infarctions, pancreatitis, ruptured aortic aneurysms, or duodenal ulcer perforations, and even severe cholecystitis. Failure of subsidence of pain to routine measures should raise the index of suspicion and the search for these lethal

P. V. Alexander (✉)
Lady Willingdon Hospital, Manali, India

M. Jacob
Christian Medical College Vellore, Vellore, Tamil Nadu, India

M. A. Hardy, B. R. Hochman (eds.), *Global Surgery*, https://doi.org/10.1007/978-3-031-28127-3_26

lurkers. While endoscopy is not really indicated emergently in such situations, it is reassuring to schedule a routine endoscopy as part of a weekly list for patients whose pain does subside and whose symptoms do not merit further emergent treatment.

All upper GI bleeds for any reason merits an endoscopy emergently or electively. Emergent endoscopic skills in the face of active and violent bleeding require teamwork inclusive of the anaesthetist and theatre staff who need to be trained in what is expected of them, and conversant with the steps to be followed with an operating room on standby. This presents a challenge in any circumstance, particularly so in a resource-poor environment. In any emergent trauma or crisis, the first chance is often the best chance to surmount the situation. If the surgeon is not confident of being ably equipped to undertake this challenge, timely resuscitation and referral may be the wiser alternative.

Endoscopy in GERD

Endoscopy is indicated in patients with symptomatic GERD to evaluate alarm features. The alarm features are detailed in Table 26.1. Endoscopy is also indicated if "Barrett's" oesophagus is suspected on the basis of suspicious four-quadrant oesophageal biopsy.

Gastritis

Gastritis is a common melting pot for a variety of conditions. Inclusive of gastropathy (epithelial damage and regeneration without inflammation), the presence of inflammation in the stomach lining presents a blurred criterion that has resulted in a plethora of systems to grade gastritis. It is also divided into acute or chronic by chronology of symptoms and type of inflammatory cells present. Concerns regarding a progression to malignancy imbue the interpretation of these biopsies. Endoscopically the lack of rugae, increase in vascularity, superficial erosions, and ulcerations are well-described features that surprisingly do not always have a strict correlation with the histopathologic extent of disease or the severity of symptoms. Multiple biopsies from four quadrants and the incisura help the pathologist's interpretation. Chromoendoscopy can be performed quite easily to help identify aberrant mucosa. The dyes commonly used are methylene blue for absorptive epithelium (such as Barrett's oesophagus), Lugol's iodine for squamous epithelium, and toluidine blue for oesophageal malignancies.

Endoscopic screening for detection of gastric cancer on a community level is found to have worth in communities with a high predilection for gastric malignancy but is of doubtful value in other communities [2]. Any suspicious area encountered upon endoscopy should be mandatorily biopsied.

Table 26.1 Alarm features in patients with symptoms of GERD

- New onset of dyspepsia in patient ≥60 years
- Evidence of gastrointestinal bleeding (haematemesis, melena, haematochezia, occult blood in stool)
- Iron deficiency anaemia
- Anorexia
- Unexplained weight loss
- Dysphagia
- Odynophagia
- Persistent vomiting
- Gastrointestinal cancer in a first-degree relative

Gastric Ulcers

Gastric ulcers may be symptomatic or quiescent till they present with complications; 70% may be asymptomatic [3] and 43% to 87% with bleeding ulcers may have no antecedent symptoms [4]. Older patients or those on non-steroidal anti-inflammatory drugs may first present with complications [5]. Previous history of *Helicobacter pylori* infection is a red flag. Of those who are symptomatic with upper abdominal pain, 80% would have an ulcer [5]. Prepyloric and duodenal ulcer pain may be differentiated by the relationship to meals; prepyloric and antral ulceration cause pain and duodenal ulcers occur typically 5–6 h post prandially [6]. Acid reflux symptoms and feeling of bloating may accompany these symptoms in up to 47% of the time [5].

The common complications of ulcers are bleeding, perforation, fistulation, and gastric outlet obstruction when an ulcer is unattended to. Perforations are usually anteriorly placed and are cataclysmic events necessitating emergent surgical intervention. The incidence of perforations [7] is described as being anywhere between 2% to 10%; this has decreased with liberal use of H2 blockers and proton pump inhibitors which usually are not readily available in LMICs. Haemorrhage, if posterior, is a profuse life-threatening event mandating emergent intervention. Less profuse bleeding also necessitates endoscopic examination and non-operative intervention if possible.

The diagnosis of ulcer disease is primarily endoscopic. All ulcers should be four quadrant biopsied if they have the following features suspicious of malignancy; raised edges, ulcers more than 1 cm in diameter, and friable mass lesions, with altered morphology of the adjoining mucosa are features that must alert the endoscopist to a malignancy. Only in areas with a low prevalence of gastric cancer is there a role of not taking biopsies from an innocuous ulcer that does not have suspicious features. *H. pylori* testing should be routine in all patients with ulcer disease. A "test and treat" policy may be more cost-effective, but in areas of high incidence of *H. pylori* with symptoms, the reverse "treat and test" policy may be justified.

Perforation

The typical "air under the diaphragm" is found in only15% of all duodenal perforations. Late presentations may seal off the perforation and permit absorption of the air, whereas very early perforations may not permit visualization on radiography. The rare posterior perforation may permit air to outline the right heart border or highlight the medial cardiophrenic angle. CT scan findings may show a mucosal discontinuity or demonstrate a mucosal outpouching of an ulcer crater extending through variable thickness of the gastric wall [8].

Fistulation

Fistulation into a perivisceral abscess cavity, including the lesser sac, or into adjacent coelomic cavities can result in biliary enteric fistulae that present with chronic symptoms [9] or with acute life-threatening symptoms if blood vessels are breached [10], such as the pancreatico- or gastroduodenal artery.

The treatment of ulcer disease, unless complicated, is primarily medical. Eradication of *H. pylori* yields higher healing rates [11] and lower recurrence rates [12]. Discontinuing NSAIDS, continuing proton pump inhibitors for 2 weeks for uncomplicated ulcers and up to 12 weeks for complications usually permits healing and prevents recurrences. Continuation of NSAID use, if mandated, is to be considered with concurrent use of proton pump inhibitors to prevent recurrences.

Bleeding

Patients who present with upper gastrointestinal haemorrhage are best managed algorithmically (see Fig. 26.1). All patients who present with bleeding whether profuse and fresh, or altered blood with melena per rectum, are first resuscitated with two large bore IV cannulae, nasogastric tube in situ, and Foley catheter in situ and admitted to a high dependency or intensive care unit. Labs are procured for haematocrit and for cross matching blood wherever the facilities exist. Using matched family donors urgently is an option that should be exercised if necessary. A good history and examination can differentiate the probability of the aetiology of haemorrhage being either variceal or non-variceal. If non variceal, all patients who remain tachycardic and unstable require endoscopy. The patients who stabilize with intravenous proton pump inhibitor therapy may be endoscoped electively.

On endoscopy the stigmata of recent haemorrhage and the Forrest classification [13] which stratifies severity of upper GI bleeding according to the endoscopic findings and thus permits decisions to intervene or follow up [14]. Actively

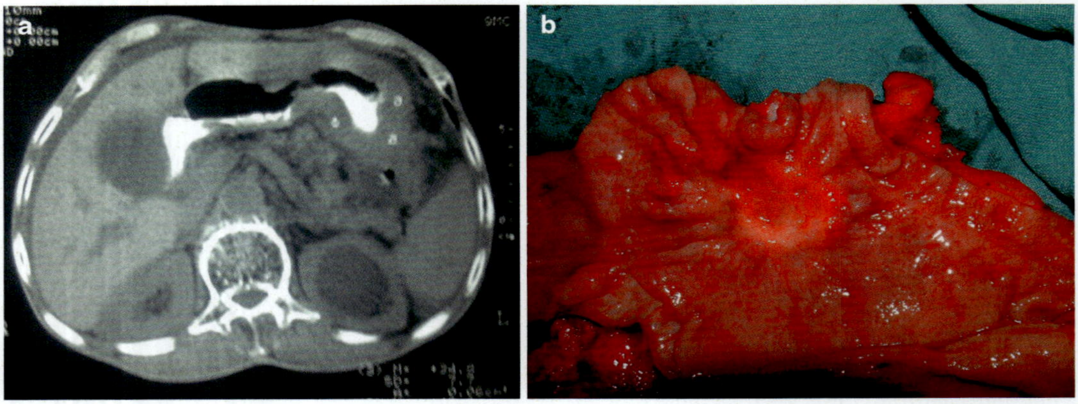

Fig. 26.1 (**a**, **b**) Gastric carcinoma: (**a**) CT view with large defect; (**b**) gross pathologic specimen

bleeding or oozing ulcers, or those with a visible vessel or clot, need intervention to control bleeding and prevent a rebleed while those with flat pigmented spot or clean ulcer base do not. Intravenous proton pump inhibitors and tranemexic acid prior to endoscopic intervention and adequate preparation for the endoscopy are vital in remote locations distant from tertiary help in LMICs.

The endoscopic intervention of bleeding ulcers should not be undertaken lightly. It is best conducted in the main operating theatre and not in an adjacent endoscopic suite, with the patient intubated to protect the airway and avoid aspiration of blood. A good working endoscope with clear air and water channels is mandatory and so is a team practised and well versed in the steps of intervention since the procedure is dependent on multiple operators, one to manoeuver the endoscope and another to man the injection cannula. Banding is the procedure of choice, but not many peripheral centres may possess the technology or expertise to permit banding. Injection sclerotherapy is the next best alternative, using a sclerosant agent, or absolute alcohol. The injection of cyanoacrylate glue will require disposable cannulae and practised assistants to permit execution without the glue solidifying in the cannula itself. Intralesional or perilesional techniques may be used depending on the choice of the endoscopist and findings at the time of endoscopy. A relay of pre-loaded syringes with saline permits quick flushing of blood and visualization of the source of bleeding in an otherwise bloody field. Post sclerotherapy observation in a high dependency unit with blood cross matched and at hand is ideal for the next 72 hours prior to discharge. Large (>1 cm) ulcers in the stomach are best biopsied to rule out malignancy or biopsied at a later elective sitting. Bleeding from posterior ulcers involving the gastroduodenal artery can be torrential and difficult to control endoscopically. Advanced centres can use the thermal gold electrode coagulation or clips to attain haemostasis, but these measures are not available easily in LMICs in remote regions. When the arterial bleeding cannot be controlled, the procedure can be converted into an open procedure, and the artery approached with an anterior duodenotomy and controlled with a horizontal mattress stitch, being careful not to take sutures too deep to involve the common bile duct.

Other common causes of non-variceal bleeds are outlined in Table 26.2.

Stress ulcerations can be very troublesome in patients who are admitted to the intensive care unit and be hypotensive as a result of multiple ulcerations in the stomach, extending into the GI tract. The treatment is primarily medical and supportive. Less severe stress ulcerations may not be diagnosed, and endoscopy is challenging with the patient on multiple inotropic supports and on assisted ventilation.

Mallory-Weiss tears occur at the gastroesophageal junction as a result of violent retching, usually in alcoholics. While this bleeding is usually self-limiting, it could result in massive haemorrhage needing endoscopic intervention.

Table 26.2 Causes of non-variceal upper GI haemorrhage

• Gastric and/or duodenal ulcers
• Severe or erosive gastritis/duodenitis
• Severe or erosive oesophagitis
• Stress ulceration
• Portal hypertensive gastropathy
• Angiodysplasia (also known as vascular ectasia)
• Mallory-Weiss syndrome
• Mass lesions (polyps/cancers)
• No lesion identified (10–15% of patients).
• Dieulafoy lesion
• Gastric antral vascular ectasia
• Haemobilia
• Hemosuccus pancreaticus
• Aortoenteric fistula
• Cameron lesions
• Ectopic varices
• Iatrogenic bleeding after endoscopic interventions

Vascular ectasias and Dieulafoy lesions are sinister causes that may be difficult to diagnose, presenting with massive haemorrhage causing hypotension. Endoscopy during an active bleeding episode is the best chance at finding them because the vessel retracts when the patient is stable or the bleeding is quiescent. Dieulafoy lesions are usually in the territory of the left gastric artery, and recurrent and troublesome bleeding without visualization of the culprit vessel may validate the role of prophylactic ligation of the left gastric artery to prevent further rebleeds.

Large (>1 cm) bleeding gastric ulcers especially in an elderly patient will need wide excision of the ulcer at the least and an antrectomy or subtotal gastrectomy at best, due to the possibility of a malignancy. Endoscopic control of the bleeding and biopsy followed by subsequent definitive management is the safer alternative, decreasing the morbidity and mortality of attempting resection emergently in an unstable patient.

Perforation

Gastric and duodenal perforations are very common presentations in LMICs, though literature has reported decrease in incidence with the wide use of proton pump inhibitors [15]. Presenting with the classic history of the sudden onset of upper abdominal pain "like a bolt from the blue", it is still a contender in the causes of the acute surgical abdomen in LMICs. Duodenal perforations are more common than gastric perforations, and large gastric ulcer perforations, especially in the elderly, may be manifestations of a malignancy lurking in the ulcer, thus requiring definitive management rather than just a closure of the perforation. The Modified Roscoe Graham omental patch technique is the time tested procedure of choice for the perforated duodenal ulcer, where a strip of vascularized omentum is used to seal the perforation with three retaining sutures of silk, followed by subsequent *H. pylori* eradication therapy on follow-up. Large perforations may still permit this technique to be used by first tying the suture to permit approximation and then applying the omentum over it.

A chronic scarred and deformed duodenum or a very large perforation may be better served by converting the perforation into a pyloroplasty, with or without a vagotomy. Posterior duodenal perforations are rare and difficult to diagnose with the absence of free air under the diaphragm. Suggestion of this perforation may be found by noticing air outlining the right border of the heart or when the left cardiophrenic angle is outlined by air. Intraoperative injection of sparkling water may be done to note the air bubbles (better than methylene blue which discolours the whole field. Kocherization of the duodenum, and closure of the perforation with or without an omental patch, is the treatment of choice. Posterior ulcers are more prone to bleed than perforate. Follow-up endoscopy to document healing of the ulcer is rarely indicated, but measures to avoid reinfection with *Helicobacter* such as boiling the drinking water and avoidance of smoking are simple measures to prevent recurrence [16].

Bezoars

Bezoars are an uncommon cause of gastric outlet obstruction when patients who are mentally challenged compulsively swallow foreign bodies, hair, or vegetable matter that conglomerates in the stomach into a bezoar. Vegetable matter bezoars (phytobezoars) and hair bezoars (trichobezoars) often have long tails that may enter and populate the proximal jejunum. A variety of other swallowed objects may constitute foreign body bezoars. Endoscopic diagnosis and surgical removal via an anterior gastrotomy is the treatment of choice. Psychiatric and psychologic assistance postoperatively is mandatory to address the root cause of the problem.

Gastric Cancer

Epidemiology and Demographics

Gastric cancer is a sleeper. Investigations after the onset of symptoms usually reveal widespread disease. Screening programs in high-risk countries permit early detection and treatment. High-risk areas may condense into geographical regions even within countries. The ubiquitous banner of "gastritis" camouflages and permits insidious growth of the carcinoma till it presents itself as unresectable or metastatic. 25% of these patients would have had a history of ulcer disease in the past, and the relationship with *H. pylori* infection charts a pathway from gastritis to transformation into carcinoma.

Gastric cancer is the fifth most common cancer and the third leading cause of cancer-related mortality after lung and colorectal cancers, contributing to more than one million cases per year [17]. Gastric cancer incidence rates increase with increasing age and are twofold to threefold higher for men than women [18]. Gastroesophageal junctional and proximal gastric cancers have greatly increased while distal lesions have decreased. Early diagnosis of gastric cancer is difficult because most patients are asymptomatic in the early stage. Adenocarcinoma is the most common malignancy affecting the stomach. It accounts for 90% of malignant tumours found within the stomach; and the rest include lymphomas, carcinoids, and gastrointestinal stromal tumours.

Distal gastric cancers are more common in developing countries and in the lower socio-economic groups. Environmental factors like chronic infection with *H. pylori* are the main cause of gastric cancer, accounting for approximately 90% of distal gastric cancer cases worldwide [19]. Dietary substances such as nitrates and nitrites and, in particular, N-nitrosodimethylamine (NDMA) have increased the risk of gastric cancer. NDMA occurs in dietary foods as a food additive often used in processed meats and is a potential carcinogen [20]. Proximal tumours are predominating in developed countries, among whites, and in higher socio-economic classes; the major risk factors for proximal cancers are gastroesophageal reflux disease and obesity [21]. Smoking increased the risk of gastric cancer, especially for proximal gastric cancers, and the magnitude of risk linearly increases with number of cigarettes per day and duration of smoking [22]. An excess body mass index (over 25 kg/m^2) has a 1.13 odds ratio of developing cancer [23]. The strength of the association increased with increasing BMI. There is also an increased risk of gastric cancer with high alcohol consumption. Risk of gastric cancer is up to tenfold higher in persons with a family history of gastric cancer [24] and in those who have had previous gastric resection or duodenal bypass with reflux of bile or pancreatic secretions [25]. Chronic atrophic gastritis with pernicious anaemia and adenomatous polyps, but not hyperplastic, have significant malignant potential.

History

A significant number of patients with gastric cancer have a history of gastric ulcer.

Overt or occult gastrointestinal bleeding, with haematemesis or melaena, is seen in one fifth of the patients who may present to the hospital with anaemia. Abdominal mass is the most common physical finding in advanced disease. Many of the patients may present with signs or symptoms of distant metastatic disease. The most common sites of metastatic disease are the liver, the peritoneal surfaces, and para-aortic lymph nodes and less commonly, ovaries in female patients, the brain, bone, lungs, and soft tissue. Common presenting symptoms, besides gastritis, are weight loss, anaemia, and epigastric pain. Melaena is often noticed but ignored. Dysphagia occurs in proximal and oesophagogastric junction carcinoma. Early satiety and nausea are also symptoms that lurk for a while prior to presentation.

Physical Examination

A palpable mass is indicative of disease that has already spread locally or systemically. Distant spread to ovaries, liver, or to distant organs may also be the primary presentation of gastric carcinoma. Metastases to the left supraclavicular node (Virchow's node), umbilicus (Sister Mary Joseph's nodule), or the axilla (Irish node) may be detectable signs on general physical examination. Jaundice from the liver metastases, ascites, and gastric outlet obstruction are also late presenting features. Jaundice is occasionally seen with locally advanced distal tumours with periportal lymph nodes causing biliary obstruction. Very rarely, direct infiltration of gastric cancer to the transverse colon resulting in gastrocolic fistula, patient presents with feculent vomiting or passage of recently ingested material in the stool. Often, infiltration into the pancreas causes severe back pain. More subtle presentations of a coincident paraneoplastic process may be with acanthosis nigricans pigmentation in skin folds, polyarteritis nodosa or microangiopathic haemolytic anaemia, membranous nephropathy, diffuse seborrheic keratosis (Leser Trelat sign), or hypercoagulability (Trousseau syndrome). Peritoneal spread can present with an enlarged ovary (Krukenberg tumour) or a mass in the cul-de-sac on rectal examination (Blumer's shelf). Presence of ascites can also be the first indication of peritoneal carcinomatosis.

Investigations

A patient with suspected gastric malignancy warrants the following investigations.

Liver function tests, creatinine, chest X-ray, and upper GI endoscopy which is the primary modality of investigation of any suspected gastric cancer is an upper GI endoscopy (OGD), which allows the direct visualisation and identify the location of lesion and biopsies can be taken as required. Gastroscopy is recommended for any patient with new-onset dysphagia or aged >55 years with significant unintentional weight loss, epigastric pain, or reflux.

The traditional barium meal with follow through has now largely been replaced by endoscopy and the CT scan, both of which are able to provide diagnosis, histopathologic evidence, and capability of staging the extent of the disease at presentation [26]. Barium studies have a limited role in identifying the gastric lesions; sensitivity is as low as 14% in identifying early gastric cancers. Linitis plastica is the only variety of carcinoma best diagnosed by barium meal examination, which is capable of demonstrating the "leather bottle" stomach.

Contrast-enhanced computed tomography (CECT): CT scan of the abdomen and pelvis provides information about the primary tumour, local extent of the lesion, and distal metastatic findings such as ascites, peritoneal metastases, liver metastases, and peri-gastric and distant nodal disease. However, CT imaging cannot reliably detect subcentimetre lymph nodes, solitary liver, and lung metastasis smaller than 5 mm and depth of tumour invasion.

MRI scans should be reserved to confirm liver metastasis.

18-fluorodeoxyglucose positron emission tomography scan (PET scan): It is reserved for patients with equivocal findings of possible metastasis on CECT scan. However, diffuse or mucinous gastric tumours are not FDG avid. The sensitivity of PET scanning for peritoneal carcinomatosis is only approximately 50 percent [27].

Gastric carcinoma may present in a variety of morphologies at endoscopy. The characteristic large friable ulcer with overhanging ulcer edge margins is easily biopsied for conformation. Any large gastric ulcer merits a biopsy since the wide based flat ulcer or mucosal thickening may also bely the insidious growth of gastric carcinoma. The biopsy technique of taking multiple (as many as 7) biopsies increases the yield of diagnosis rather than relying on a few samples of seemingly representative specimen.

Staging and Treatment

The Japanese classification has gradually given way to the universal AJCC/IUCC TNM classification system, as the treatment of this disease has now changed to incorporate neoadjuvant chemotherapy. The treatment of this disease can be divided into the treatment of early disease, locoregional disease, or systemic disease as described below. The details of adjuvant therapy are not discussed here since these require patient management in a centre where specialized cancer is practised. We focus in this chapter primarily on urgent care of patients with gastric cancer.

Staging Laparoscopy

Staging laparoscopy is performed to detect occult peritoneal dissemination in physically fit patients who appear to have locoregional disease in staging investigations, who are considered for neoadjuvant chemotherapy followed by curative resection. If staging indicates need for neoadjuvant chemotherapy, patient should be transferred to an oncology center.

Staging

- TNM staging of gastric cancer AJCC eighth Edition: Table 26.1.
- Initial preoperative staging work up enables patients to be classified into three clinical stage groups:
  1. Localized cancer (stages cTis or cT1a).
  2. Locoregional cancer (stages cT1b–cT4a; cM0).
  3. Metastatic cancer (stage cT4b; cM1).
- Carcinoma stomach treatment flow chart: Image 1.

Role of Perioperative Nutrition

In patients with proximal gastric cancers who have dysphagia should have preoperative nasogastric feeding and distal tumours with gastric outlet obstruction should have nasojejunal feeding till the time of surgery. There is no role of perioperative total parenteral nutrition (TPN). Immune nutrition may be useful in reducing the postoperative morbidity but has no impact on mortality.

Peri-Operative Chemotherapy/Neo-Adjuvant Chemotherapy

Peri-operative chemotherapy further treatment of localized gastric cancer has been the standard of care in many countries after the significant major clinical trials (MAGIC, FNCLOC, EORCC) which showed statistically significant improvement in terms of 5-year and overall survival as compared to the surgery alone patients [28]. The two main benefits of peri-operative chemotherapy are down staging of disease for surgical resection and to prevent micro metastasis. Detailed discussion of the types of pre- and post-operative chemotherapy for gastric cancer is beyond the scope of this book, and the reader is advised to consult recent standard textbooks and the literature on this subject.

Adjuvant chemotherapy in patients with locally advanced disease without any metastasis who underwent radical gastrectomy with D2 lymphadenectomy, adjuvant chemotherapy had significant benefit disease-free survival and overall survival [29].

Surgery

Peri-operative chemotherapy has made significant disease regression in locally advanced gastric adenocarcinoma. En block resection of primary tumour along with regional lymph node resection remains the cornerstone of therapy. The decision of total or subtotal gastrectomy depends on the location, extent, and histology of the tumour with lymphadenopathy. Surgical resection includes resection of primary tumour with the tumour-free margins of at least 4 cm with adequate lymphadenectomy (minimum 16 nodes) to ensure optimum curative resection.

Tumour located in the antrum and lower 2/3 of the stomach can be treated with subtotal gastrectomy, while tumours located in the proximal or upper third of the stomach and type III Siewert gastroesophageal junction tumour and gastric tumour with linitis plastica will require more extensive resection, including total gastrectomy.

Lymphadenectomy

Although there is no worldwide consensus on the extent of lymphadenectomy, traditionally in East Asia and Japan, D2 lymphadenectomy is practised, and this is an extensive and aggressive lymphadenectomy. However, D1+ lymphadenectomy which includes peri-gastric lymph nodes and nodes along coeliac artery and its branches, is generally recommended in the West and is associated with low postoperative morbidity and mortality.

Reconstruction

After subtotal or total gastrectomy, reconstructive procedure is determined based on the surgeon's individual experience. There is a lack of evidence for the best optimal reconstruction procedure in the available literature. Roux-en-Y jejunal reconstruction with gastrojejunostomy and jejunojejunostomy, 40 to 60 cm below the GJ to avoid bile reflux, is the most frequently performed procedure worldwide (Fig. 26.2).

Follow-Up

At present, the National Comprehensive Cancer Network (NCCN) guidelines on follow-up and surveillance of gastric cancer recommends a history and physical every 3–6 months for 1–2 years, followed by every 6–12 months for 3–5 years, and then annually. Investigations including complete blood count (CBC), creatinine, liver function tests, and radiological imaging are recommended; in addition, the NCCN also recommends monitoring for nutritional deficiency (e.g. B12, calcium, and iron) in surgically resected patients. Upper GI endoscopy surveillance at least every 2 years is recommended in higher-risk populations, inpatients with other underlying disorders that increase risk, like intestinal metaplasia or dysplasia, and in patients with closed resection after total or subtotal gastrectomy [30].

Palliation

Best Supportive Care

The main focus for patients who are too frail to have chemotherapy or surgical excision, or those who have unresectable disease and/or metastatic disease, is to relieve their symptoms and support them and their families through a terminal illness. Nausea and vomiting is treated with anti-emetics such as granisetron and ondansetron. Poor appetite may respond to steroids such as dexamethasone.

In locally unresectable, metastatic gastric cancers with obstruction, bleeding, perforation, and pain, a palliative resection or a gastrojejunostomy is advised if it can be tolerated. There is no role for lymphadenectomy or multiorgan resection, liver resection, or peritoneal cytoreduction for metastatic disease. There is no survival benefit

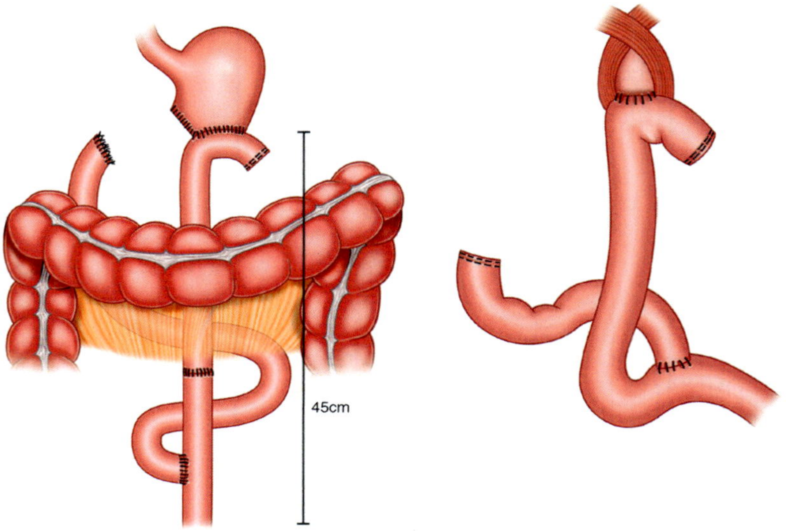

Fig. 26.2 Reconstruction after subtotal gastrectomy and total gastrectomy

related to palliative gastrectomy. Patients with gastric outlet obstruction who have persistent vomiting may benefit from the endoscopic placement of a self-expanding metallic stent, although the results are unpredictable. Palliative chemotherapy is recommended in fit patients with metastatic and unresectable disease. Bleeding from advanced gastric tumours can be troublesome and can be greatly reduced by a short course of external beam radiation.

Prognosis

Overall 5- year survival rates for stomach cancer are 32%; if the tumour hasn't spread outside the stomach (localized), 70%; and if tumours have spread to nearby lymph nodes or structures outside the stomach (regional), 32%. In metastatic disease, 5-year survival is as low as 6% [31].

Treatment of Recurrent Disease

Patients with recurrent disease should be evaluated to distinguish isolated locoregional recurrence should be evaluated for disease control using surgery, chemotherapy, radiotherapy, or a combination of the above. Patients who are not suitable or unfit for definitive treatment and with distant metastases should be treated symptomatically.

References

1. Dent J, El-Serag HB, Wallander MA, Johansson S. Epidemiology of gastro-oesophageal reflux disease: a systematic review. Gut. 2005;54(5):710.
2. Dan YY, So JB, Yeoh KG. Endoscopic screening for gastric cancer. Clin Gastroenterol Hepatol. 2006;4(6):709.
3. Lu CL, Chang SS, Wang SS, Chang FY, Lee SD. Silent peptic ulcer disease: frequency, factors leading to "silence," and implications regarding the pathogenesis of visceral symptoms. Gastrointest Endosc. 2004;60(1):34.
4. Wilcox CM, Clark WS. Features associated with painless peptic ulcer bleeding. Am J Gastroenterol. 1997;92(8):1289.
5. Barkun A, Leontiadis G. Systematic review of the symptom burden, quality of life impairment and costs associated with peptic ulcer disease. Am J Med. 2010;123(4):358.
6. Kang JY, Yap I, Guan R, Tay HH. Acid perfusion of duodenal ulcer craters and ulcer pain: a controlled double blind study. Gut. 1986;27(8):942.
7. Chung KT, Shelat VG. Perforated peptic ulcer—an update. World J Gastrointest Surg. 2017;9(1):1.
8. Tonolini M, Ierardi AM, Bracchi E, Magistrelli P, Vella A, Carrafiello G. Non-perforated peptic ulcer disease: multidetector CT findings, complications, and differential diagnosis. Insights Imaging. 2017;8(5):455. Epub 2017 Jul 4
9. Van Steenbergen W, Ponette E, Marchal G, Fevery J, De Groote J. Distal common bile duct stenosis secondary to benign duodenal ulceration: report of a case. Gastrointest Radiol. 1990;15(3):215.
10. Odze RD, Bégin LR. Peptic-ulcer-induced aortoenteric fistula. Report of a case and review of the literature. J Clin Gastroenterol. 1991;13(6):682.
11. Leodolter A, Kulig M, Brasch H, Meyer-Sabellek W, Willich SN, Malfertheiner P. A meta-analysis comparing eradication, healing and relapse rates in patients with Helicobacter pylori-associated gastric or duodenal ulcer. Aliment Pharmacol Ther. 2001;15(12):1949–58.
12. Ford AC, Delaney BC, Forman D, Moayyedi P. Eradication therapy in Helicobacter pylori positive peptic ulcer disease: systematic review and economic analysis. Am J Gastroenterol. 2004;99(9):1833–55.
13. Forrest JA, Finlayson ND, Shearman DJ. Endoscopy in gastrointestinal bleeding. Lancet. 1974;2(7877):394.
14. Katschinski B, Logan R, Davies J, Faulkner G, Pearson J, Langman M. Prognostic factors in upper gastrointestinal bleeding. Dig Dis Sci. 1994;39(4):706.
15. Bashinskaya B, Nahed BV, Redjal N, Kahle KT, Walcott BP. Trends in peptic ulcer disease and the identification of helicobacter pylori as a causative organism: population-based estimates from the US Nationwide inpatient sample. J Glob Infect Dis. 2011;3(4):366–70.
16. Bellack NR, Koehoorn MW, MacNab YC, Morshed MG. A conceptual model of water's role as a reservoir in helicobacter pylori transmission: a review of the evidence. Epidemiol Infect. 2006;134(3):439. Epub 2006 Mar 2
17. Bray F, Ferlay J, Soerjomataram I, Siegel RL, Torre LA, Jemal A. Global cancer statistics 2018: GLOBOCAN estimates of incidence and mortality worldwide for 36 cancers in 185 countries. CA Cancer J Clin 2018;68(6):394–424. doi:https://doi.org/10.3322/caac.21492.
18. Gastric cancer: overview. Gastroenterol Clin N Am. 2013;42:211–7.
19. Correa P. Helicobacter pylori and gastric carcinogenesis. Am J Surg Pathol. 1995;19(Suppl 1):S37–43.
20. Tricker AR, Preussmann R. Carcinogenic N-nitrosamines in the diet: occurrence, formation, mechanisms and carcinogenic potential. Mutat Res. 1991;259:277–89.

21. Catalano V, Labianca R, Beretta GD, Gatta G, de Braud F, Van Cutsem E. Gastric cancer. Crit Rev Oncol Hematol. 2009;71:127–64.
22. Praud D, Rota M, Peluchi C, et al. Cigarette smoking and gastric cancer in the Stomach Cancer Pooling (StoP) Project. Eur J Cancer Prev. 2018;27:124–33.
23. Bae J-M. Body mass index and risk of gastric cancer in Asian adults: a meta-epidemiological meta-analysis of population-based cohort studies. Cancer Res Treat. 2020;52:369–73.
24. Han X, Xiao L, Yu Y, et al. Alcohol consumption and gastric cancer risk: a meta-analysis of prospective cohort studies. Oncotarget. 2017;8:83237–45.
25. Namikawa T, Kitagawa H, Iwabu J, Okabayashi T, Kobayashi M, Hanazaki K. Tumors arising at previous anastomotic site may have poor prognosis in patients with gastric stump cancer following gastrectomy. J Gastrointest Surg. 2010;14:1923–30. https://doi.org/10.1007/s11605-010-1298-4. [PubMed]
26. Dooley CP, Larson AW, Stace NH, et al. Double-contrast barium meal and upper gastrointestinal endoscopy. A comparative study. Ann Intern Med. 1984;101:538.
27. Gertsen EC, Brenkman HJF, van Hillegersberg R, et al. 18F-Fludeoxyglucose-positron emission tomography/computed tomography and laparoscopy for staging of locally advanced gastric cancer: a multicentre prospective Dutch Cohort Study (PLASTIC). JAMA Surg. 2021;156:e215340.
28. Yang Y, Yin X, Sheng L, Xu S, Dong L, Liu L. Perioperative chemotherapy more of a benefit for overall survival than adjuvant chemotherapy for operable gastric cancer: an updated meta-analysis. Sci Rep. 2015;5:12850. https://doi.org/10.1038/srep12850.
29. Paoletti X, Oba K, Burzykowski T, et al. For the GASTRIC (Global Advanced/Adjuvant Stomach Tumor Research International Collaboration) group. Benefit of adjuvant chemotherapy for resectable gastric cancer: a meta-analysis. JAMA. 2010;303:1729–37.
30. NCCN Clinical practice guidelines in oncology (NCCN guidelines): gastric cancer. Natl Comp Cancer Netw Available at: http://NCCN.org.
31. Gastric Cancer, Version 2.2022. NCCN clinical practice guidelines in oncology. J Natl Compr Cancer Netw. 2022;20:2. (jnccn.org)

How to Diagnose and Manage Acute Abdomen and Intra-Abdominal Infections in Low- and Middle-Income Countries

27

Mark A. Hardy and Christine Yang

The man who asks a question is a fool for a minute, the man who does not ask is a fool for life.

– Confucius

Abbreviations

AA	Acute appendicitis
ADA	Adenosine deaminase
ATT	Anti-tuberculosis therapy
CT	Computerized tomography
DEC	Diethylcarbamazine
GITB	Gastrointestinal tuberculosis
HICs	High-income countries
IAI	Intra-abdominal infection
ICU	Intensive care unit
ID	Infectious disease
LMICs	Low- and middle-income countries
MDA	Mass drug administration
MDR	Multidrug resistant
PPD	Purified protein derivative skin test
SES	Socio-economic status
SOFA	Sequential (sepsis-related) Organ Failure Assessment
USG	Ultrasonography

M. A. Hardy (✉) · C. Yang
Department of Surgery, Columbia University Vagelos College of Physicians and Surgeons, New York, NY, USA
e-mail: mah1@cumc.columbia.edu; cy2634@cumc.columbia.edu

Introduction and Background

Acute abdomen and intra-abdominal infections (IAI) are surgical emergencies commonly encountered in both HICs and LMICs, and a major cause of non-traumatic deaths in LMICs. Several studies have shown that operations for IAIs account for approximately 11–12% of surgeries in LMICs. In a recent review, Sartelli et al. reported that of 989 operations at one LMIC hospital, 299 (30.2%) were explorations for acute abdomen. In that group, the male to female ratio was 4.1:1, and patient ages ranged from 15 to 95 years [1]. In another series of 3114 surgical patients in Ghana [2], (male-female ratio 2:1 and similar age range to that in Sartelli's series), the most common indications for surgery were acute appendicitis (22.4%), typhoid ileal perforations (16.2%), acute intestinal obstruction (12.6%), gastroduodenal perforations (11.0%), non-specific abdominal pain (9.8%), abdominal injuries (8.3%), and acute cholecystitis 102 (3.2%), with a surprisingly similar incidence of sigmoid volvulus and small bowel obstruction (whereas HICs encounter small bowel obstruction far more frequently than sigmoid volvulus), and a relative paucity of diverticular and neoplastic indications

M. A. Hardy, B. R. Hochman (eds.), *Global Surgery*, https://doi.org/10.1007/978-3-031-28127-3_27

for surgery, both of which are seen frequently in HICs. Of all patients who underwent surgery, 7.4% died, most postoperatively. Half of those who died experienced a delay of 3 or more days in presenting to the hospital, and most deaths occurred after emergency colon resection (26%) or closure of gastroduodenal perforation (23.7%). Late presentation was associated with increased mortality.

In all reports and our experience from LMICs, the most common presenting symptoms of patients with abdominal surgical problems were, not unexpectedly, abdominal pain, distention, and vomiting, and associated signs were abdominal tenderness, rebound tenderness, guarding, and pain on coughing and walking or jumping. Acute appendicitis remains the leading cause of acute abdomen globally. Approximately one-third of the patients prompting surgery for acute abdomen in LMICs were 20–40 years of age, and of those, half had acute appendicitis. There is little doubt that intra-abdominal infections (IAIs) are a serious source of morbidity and mortality throughout the world, both in LMICs and HICs [3]

Over the last 15 years, the outcomes of IAI have improved with early recognition and better use of antibiotics and supportive intensive care to treat sepsis. It has become obvious that early recognition, removal of the offending source by drainage or operation, appropriate selection of antibiotics, along with resuscitation and stabilization of the patient have resulted in better outcomes in all environments, and the resources to implement these strategies are therefore critical. Surgical sepsis continues to have high mortality, and early recognition and treatment of acute abdomen and IAI remains the main therapeutic goal for these patients to survive. Many organizations have published guidelines outlining the clinical management of IAIs [4, 5], and we will draw on many to summarize the important lessons in this chapter. The most recent one consists of recommendations to clinicians, jointly completed by a group of international and national societies, for reasonable approaches to the management of IAIs.

Principles of Diagnosis

The diagnosis of acute abdomen and IAIs relies primarily on history and physical exam. Patients present generally with pain, tenderness that is localized to the source of infection, fever, increased white blood cell count with a shift to the left, sometimes tachycardia, and hypotension if dehydrated sufficiently. If the delay is long enough, the patient may present in greater distress and show signs of end-organ hypoperfusion including oliguria and confusion. Adequate detection of the source through exam, cultures, or imaging which can then guide targeted treatment is essential to minimize complications [6, 7]. Ultrasound (USG) and computed tomography (CT) have both been used over the last two decades as imaging tools to complete the clinical assessment of patients with IAIs. While CT has higher sensitivity, USG is far more universally accessible, and, when performed by a trained clinician, can be very valuable in detecting perforations and collections. It is now generally recommended to use USG as the initial diagnostic study following physical examination, and if that is inconclusive, to resort to CT if that is available. As soon as the diagnosis of an acute abdomen with IAI is made, management includes appropriate selection of antibiotics and additional source control as needed via percutaneous or operative drainage and/or removal.

Principles of Management (Fig. 27.1)

The most important tenet in the management of an acute abdomen, with or without IAI, is to control the source of the problem. If the problem is mechanical obstruction, then the obstruction has to be decompressed via nasogastric tube (for small bowel), colonoscopy (for volvulus), or reduction and repair (for hernia). If the problem is bleeding or bowel ischemia, then bleeding needs to be halted, normal blood flow restored to the bowel, and dead bowel resected. If the problem is perforation, then the leaking viscus needs to be drained and potentially resected (for

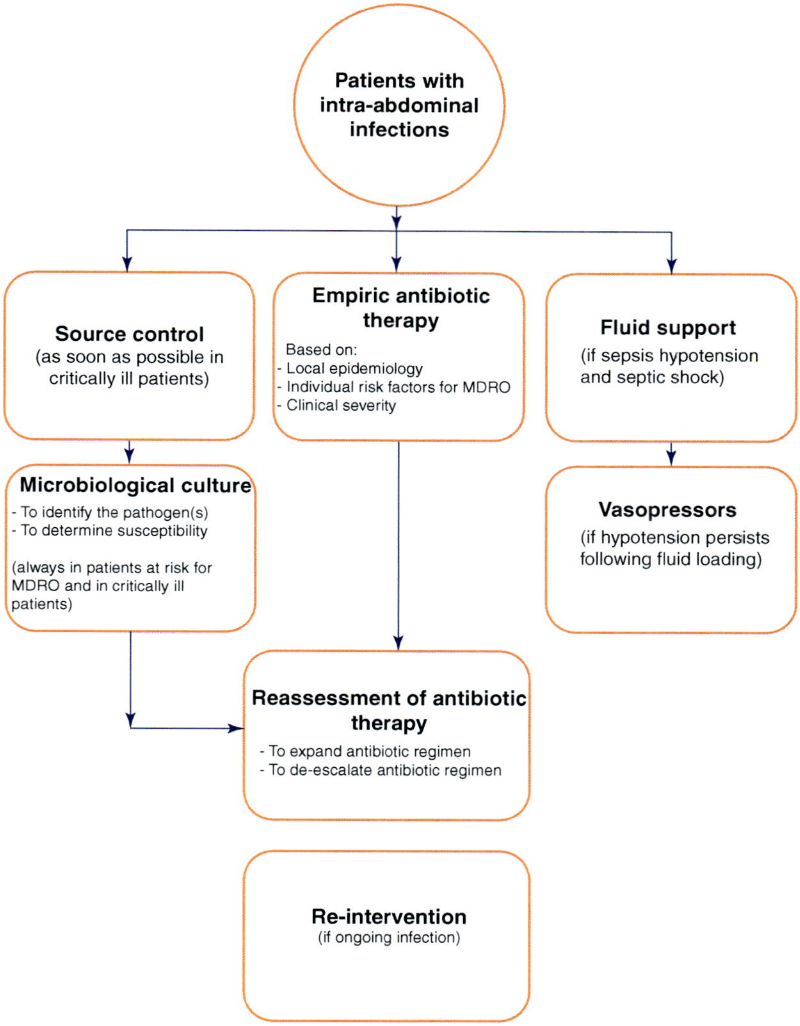

Fig. 27.1 Principles of management (Ref. [1])

appendicitis, small bowel perforation, or diverticulitis) or repaired (for gastroduodenal ulcer). If the underlying diagnosis is uncertain but an abscess is found, drainage may be necessary. Throughout this period, while diagnosis is made and initial treatment started, the patient must be resuscitated with intravenous fluid therapy to account for fluid losses incurred from limited intake exacerbated by losses from vomiting and/or diarrhea. Resuscitation should be guided primarily by the goal of achieving and maintaining euvolemia with normal blood pressure and urine output [8, 9]. For any acute abdomen with IAI, broad-spectrum antibiotics should accompany, if not precede, source control. The antibiotics should be selected based on the most likely bugs in the presumed source and then adjusted based on culture data revealing specific bugs and drug sensitivities. When formal cultures cannot be obtained, gram stain can be a helpful starting point in tailoring antibiotic regimens. Antibiotics alone can be an effective means of achieving source control in some patients with contained localized IAI. This has recently gained popularity in HICs in treating acute appendicitis; however, we do not recommend this approach in situations where follow-up of the patients may be inadequate or infeasible.

The rules of IAI source control outlined by Sartelli et al. [1] and Fig. 27.1 are the following: "(First) Time, Totalization, Technique, and (Second) Time." The first time refers to the starting time of treatment. Each hour in delaying the first time equates to a negative risk factor for patient outcome. Totalization refers to removal of any infectious source and related devitalized tissues, including ischemic bowel, and washing out any purulent material from the abdominal cavity. The "second time" refers to timing of any additional surgical drainage or debridement, which may be scheduled or "on demand" depending on the patient's clinical symptoms and physiological stability. Non-operative percutaneous drainage of abscesses under USG guidance requires skilled personnel generally found only at tertiary centers. Some general surgeons are now trained in these skills and can successfully drain abdominal and extraperitoneal abscesses in selected patients. Surgery remains the most reliable therapeutic intervention to control surgical infections, as it allows the opportunity to both drain collections and identify and directly treat the underlying source of the infection. Traditionally, extensive irrigation of the peritoneal cavity with saline is used prior to closing an infected abdomen, but this practice has been recently questioned in favor of targeted focal irrigation. Primary closure of the abdominal wound following peritonitis has also been debated over the years for fear of major wound infection with subsequent sepsis and large hernia. We advise in most instances to close the fascia with absorbable sutures and leave the skin and subcutaneous tissue open and allow it to granulate with daily packing or the use of a negative pressure-based temporary closure device. Since the commercial vacuum dressings are quite expensive, it is possible to make one as described by Campbell et al. [10]. They use the top of a Porto-Vac closed drainage container, slice off the top and simply place it on the center of the abdominal dressing or wound packing, before the top Opsite is placed over the whole abdomen (Fig. 27.2). This was originally designed when the abdomen was left open to avoid a compartment syndrome with edematous bowel or in cases of trauma or ischemic bowel when re-exploration is indicated. Such vacuum-assisted closure of the open abdomen is very useful and inexpensive in LMICs. Leaving an abdomen open, which could otherwise be closed primarily, introduces risks of excessive fluid and electrolyte loss and intestinal fistula and is recommended only for very specific situations where re-exploration is indicated within 48–72 h of index exploration. In these circumstances, if an open abdomen is too complex to manage, one could also temporarily close skin directly with a running monofilament suture without closing fascia.

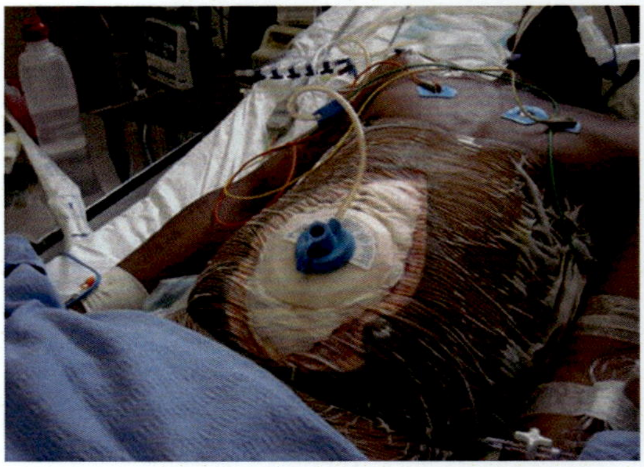

Fig. 27.2 The top of Porto-Vac container top over the wound covered with Opsite to allow vacuum suction

The Use of Antibiotics

Antibiotics should be used as soon as a treatable infection has been recognized or if there is a high degree of suspicion of an infection. Appropriate use of antibiotics may be difficult, and consultation with an ID expert can help avoid under- or over-use and thereby optimize quality clinical care while avoiding antibiotic resistance. While uncomplicated IAIs, such as uncomplicated appendicitis or cholecystitis, require as little as a single preoperative dose of antibiotics, complicated IAIs may require a short 4–7 day course of antibiotic therapy after operation or drainage is performed. It has been previously shown that patients with complicated IAI did as well with a 4-day course of antibiotics as those maintained for a longer time as long as the source was successfully treated [11].

However, if the infection is ongoing, individualized judgment must be made regarding continued use and type of antibiotics. Since patients with IAI are usually started on empiric antibiotics, these agents ought to be deescalated based on the findings of cultures obtained during drainage or exploration. Cultures typically require up to 48–72 h before a specific answer is available. Empiric antibiotic therapy should include agents with activity against aerobic Gram-negative bacteria (e.g., Enterobacteriaceae), aerobic streptococci, and also obligate enteric anaerobic organisms found in the gastrointestinal tract. In selected patients, such as diabetics or immunosuppressed patients, additional antimicrobials such as antifungals may be indicated. Similarly, patients with increased risk of tuberculous or parasitic exposure may require antimicrobials accordingly. Microbiologic results obtained during interventions may be based on Gram stain if no microbiology laboratory is available on site. Even when cultures need to be sent away to a microbiology laboratory and results are delayed, the results remain informative in adjusting antibiotics to prevent overtreating the patient with ineffective antibiotics. Attention must be paid to the local existing endemic conditions and resistance epidemiology and the clinical condition of the patients. Surgeons must be aware that drug pharmacokinetics may be altered significantly in critically ill patients particularly as they are high risk for multisystem organ dysfunction, and adjustments may have to be made in dose, frequency, and method of administration depending on the daily changing situation. It may be sometimes wiser to administer an antibiotic continuously rather than intermittently, as is usually done, to achieve higher and more effective serum levels and reach therapeutic serum levels more effectively.

Patients who don't appear to be improving after 5–7 days following drainage or operation while on appropriate antibiotics should have further work-up to determine if they need a change in their antibiotics or reinvestigation for an inadequately controlled or new source. It is beyond the purpose of this chapter to discuss the worldwide recent problems with expansion of resistant microorganisms. Even response to common sources of IAIa, like *E. coli* and other Enterobacteriaceae, have now sometimes become resistant to fluoroquinolones, which were previously very effective. Assistance by a local ID expert, by telephone or virtually as necessary, is not only desirable but strongly recommended in difficult situations. As we will discuss later in this chapter, specific antibiotics for some of the fungal, parasitic, and unusual IAIs encountered primarily in LMICs (e.g., typhoid, TB, schistosomiasis) require specific regimens which may include several agents at the same time. Management of these diseases will most strongly benefit from the advice of a local ID expert.

Management of Sepsis

Sepsis is a dreaded complication of acute abdomen with IAI. It is a systemic inflammatory response to infection and can result in multiorgan dysfunction leading to death if unrecognized or untreated. Sepsis may be part of a patient's initial presentation, or can occur at any stage in the patient's clinical course, even after what is considered a successful drainage or exploration. Sepsis is the main cause of death in patients with acute abdomen with IAI with severe sepsis in 27.8%, and septic shock in 67.8% of those who die [1]. The pathophysiology of sepsis is directly related to the endotoxins of both Gram-negative and Gram-positive organisms. This is well described by Levy and colleagues [12], but its detailed discussion is beyond the scope of this chapter. The definition of sepsis has changed over the years, most recently defined as life-threatening organ dysfunction caused by a dysregulated host response to infection [1]. Septic shock is sepsis with circulatory dysfunction wherein vasopressors are required to maintain a mean arterial pressure of 65 mm Hg or greater and serum lactate, a marker of organ perfusion, is elevated despite adequate fluid resuscitation. Prognostication of sepsis is most closely captured by trends in a patient's Sequential (sepsis-related) Organ Failure Assessment (SOFA) score, which includes mean arterial pressure, Glasgow coma scale score, and several lab values. An increase of

2 or more points is associated with a mortality >10%, while those patients who have septic shock incur a mortality rate of 40%. The quick-SOFA (qSOFA) score, which is based simply on respiratory rate, mental status, and systolic blood pressure, is an aptly named way to quickly identify patients at risk of poor outcomes from sepsis [1, 12–14].

The progression of sepsis is characterized by relative hypovolemia in the setting of myocardial depression along with inappropriate vasodilatation and capillary leakage with consequently decreased venous return to the heart. The release of inflammatory cytokines in response to infection drives this entire dysregulated response, which in turn increases oxygen demand and eventually precipitates tissue hypoxia, end-organ hypoperfusion, and if sustained then ultimately multiorgan failure.

The mainstay of sepsis management, in addition to targeted treatment of the source of infection with antibiotics and drainage or removal as indicated, is fluid resuscitation to improve circulating blood flow and support cardiac output, followed by vasopressor support to augment vascular tone. When the overall metabolic demand from this process exceeds a patient's innate ability to ventilate themselves, intubation and ventilator support may be necessary. Such management requires trained staff and an intensive care unit (ICU), which may require transfer to a tertiary facility if not locally available.

Since hypotension is the most common indicator of sepsis, initial resuscitation with crystalloid infusion is critical to restoring perfusion and oxygenation of various organs. This should not be based on preset protocols but on patient-specific evidence of preserved end-organ function including mentation, urine output, and vital signs (heart rate, blood pressure, respiratory rate, oxygen saturation). Once resuscitative efforts are established, urgent surgical intervention should be undertaken as indicated, and resuscitative efforts continued intraoperatively and postoperatively. In the process of fluid resuscitation, one must be aware of the possibility of generating bowel edema and abdominal compartment syndrome, pulmonary edema, and respiratory failure. To avoid this, when adequate resuscitation has been achieved as evidenced by no further improvement in vital signs with fluid boluses, the treatment strategy should transition to use of vasoactive agents rather than additional fluid to maintain organ perfusion. Vasoactive agents require close monitoring and titration, preferably in an ICU setting.

Vasopressor Agents

Vasopressor and ionotropic agents are critical to management of progressive sepsis in IAI, in addition to antibiotics, fluid replacement, and intervention to remove the offending causative source. They should be available, or be made available, at all local, regional, and tertiary hospitals. The most common catecholamine agents available are phenylephrine (alpha), norepinephrine (alpha and beta-1), and epinephrine (alpha and beta. They have somewhat different effects on alpha- and beta-receptors, but may be carefully substituted for each other to maintain vasoconstriction and thereby increase blood pressure to organ perfusion levels. Since beta-receptors act mainly on cardiac contractility and chronotropy and may cause vasodilatation, norepinephrine (noradrenaline), which has far more alpha-1 activity than beta-1 activity, is the drug of first choice to bolster blood pressure without increasing myocardial demand. Vasopressin, which contracts vascular smooth muscle and functions as an antidiuretic hormone, is the second line agent for blood pressure augmentation, though this agent may be less readily available. Other vasopressors used instead of norepinephrine include dopamine; however norepinephrine is more efficacious than dopamine and may be more effective for reversing hypotension in patients with septic shock [15]. Also, dopamine is more likely to cause tachycardia and arrhythmias as it is a beta-1 agonist at moderate doses.

Epinephrine (adrenaline) has essentially similar activity on alpha-1 and beta receptors and therefore functions as both a vasopressor and an inotrope. It is the agent of choice after norepinephrine and vasopressin if the patient continues to require blood pressure support and has evidence of cardiac dysfunction. Adrenaline infusions are readily available in LMICs and much less expensive than noradrenaline. Since they have equivalent vasopressor effect to noradrenalin and are more available, they are used more often in local LMICs hospitals as a first-line pressor despite the fact that they are more likely to cause tachyarrhythmias. Dobutamine, another inotropic agent, has far greater beta than alpha activity and therefore increases heart rate and cardiac output but given its beta-2 activity can cause peripheral vasodilatation, making it a less desirable agent for inotropy in an already hypotensive patient. Dobutamine can also cause undesirable tachyarrhythmias.

Sepsis secondary to acute abdomen with IAI has come under better control in LMICs with the greater availability in the last decade of antibiotics and vasopressors, even in local hospitals. However, morbidity and mortality from sepsis secondary to acute abdomen with IAI remains significant, second only to pneumonia. Lack of ICUs for close monitoring and adequately trained staff to perform timely surgical interventions for source control continues to delay progress in this field in many LMICs.

Complications of Management of Acute Abdomen

Complications encountered following operative interventions on patients who present with an acute abdomen are numerous and depend on many factors discussed previously.

The average age of patients presenting with an acute abdomen in many studies was between 25 and 35 years of age (range 15–95) and males predominated at a ratio of 2:1 to 4:1. The most common diagnosis in most studies was appendicitis accounting for almost 50% of cases followed by small bowel obstruction (16%), sigmoid volvulus (12.7%), and perforated ulcer (4.3%) [16]. In smaller studies appendicitis was less frequent and only 10% while the most frequent cause of peritonitis was perforation due to typhoid [17]. Incidence of perforation from diverticulitis or colon cancer was rare. It appears that in Africa middle-aged and older people have a much lower incidence of colon cancer, diverticulitis, or even appendicitis than those living in HICs. This has been thought to be due to three times higher ingestion of dietary fiber in SSA as compared to people in HICs who eat over-processed foods. About one-third of patients undergoing operations for peritonitis and acute abdomen, including volvulus, colon, and peptic perforations, developed post-operative complications. The most frequent were wound infections in about 20% of patients and pneumonia in approximately 10% in several series. Post-operative mortality varied widely among several reports from 6% to almost 14% [16–18]. It was frequently associated with bowel perforation and delay in diagnosis and treatment that may have been due to lack of trained surgeons and facilities and then complicated by delay in transfer to a tertiary center. The main cause of death in all series was sepsis or hypovolemic shock which could have been prevented by early diagnosis and adequate ICU management (if an ICU was available). The main factors associated with the relatively high morbidity and mortality following exploration for acute abdomen appear to be (1) age of the patient >65; (2) a delay in diagnosis >72 h; (3) a delay in surgical intervention >48 h; (4) diagnosis of peritonitis; (4) duration of operation >2 h; and (5) major spillage during exploration [18]. Three of these causes, 2, 3, and 4 can be modified and are preventable by organization of public awareness campaigns to prompt rapid consultation in the event of acute abdominal pain and the improvement in surgical staffing, providing of adequate equipment and supplies to local and regional health facilities, and facilitating transport of the sickest patients to tertiary hospitals and well-equipped ICUs.

Acute Abdomen and Peritonitis

Acute abdomen and peritonitis are among the main causes of non-trauma surgical emergencies in many centers worldwide and in many instances require more surgical interventions than trauma

[19]. The proportion of non-trauma surgical emergencies is reported to be between 30% and 57% [19, 20] with more than half requiring surgical intervention. This pattern is determined by both the country and rural vs. urban sites and continues to change as a result of environmental factors. Acute appendicitis which was thought to be infrequent among Africans is now the most common cause of acute abdomen in West Africa while diverticulitis which was also rarely seen among the elderly has become more common in the growing urban areas. This is thought to be related to increased intake of a refined fiber-depleted diet which encourages formation of fecaliths which obstruct the appendix and diverticula by slow moving feces [21].

With the growing incidence of emergent abdominal surgical non-trauma IAIs needing exploration, facilities for patients needing emergency care in LMICs were found to be inadequate in most reports. Frequently, more than half the patients who needed surgical intervention needed to be transferred to another facility, thus increasing delay in treatment and leading to complications and fatalities. The general impression has been that greater attention should be paid to the expansion, staffing, and provision of needed equipment and supplies of emergency surgical services to the increasing number of patients in LMICs. Deficiencies in surgical manpower and financial support, as well as the lack of basic laboratory and blood banking services coupled with difficulties in procuring materials required for resuscitation and surgery, are the main problems that account for the delay and increased morbidity and mortality [19, 20]. The main reasons for deaths from acute abdomen and/or peritonitis in many previous studies focused on late presentation, having spent considerable time in another hospital and difficulty with transfers, inability to carry out required investigations, and failure to have needed immediate surgical intervention.

Appendicitis

Epidemiology

Acute appendicitis (AA) remains the most common abdominal surgical emergency and cause for IAI worldwide and in LMICs. It has been shown that one-third of these cases were thought to be complicated [1]. Although in the past acute appendicitis had a low rate in SSA, Asia, and Latin America, it appears now to be increasing, both because of better records probably because of environmental changes and change in diet.

Diagnosis

Diagnosis is based primarily on clinical history and findings familiar to all medical students and surgeons and will not be detailed here except to say that it is the "great mimic" and may be easily confused with other IAIs. Attempts have been made to differentiate complicated (retrocecal, perforated) from uncomplicated acute appendicitis without much success except for a CT scan which is rarely available in LMICs. USG has been successfully used to identify appendicitis, especially in pregnant women and may be also useful to differentiate between complicated and uncomplicated appendicitis. Imaging may show increased diameter and wall thickness of the appendix, appendicolith (may be also seen on abdominal X-ray), local abscess, and fluid around the appendix.

Management

All general surgeons are very familiar with management of acute appendicitis, and this chapter will focus on it only briefly since it is most common, and its treatment has changed over the years in HICs but not in LMICs. Although in HICs, laparoscopic appendectomy has become the standard of care, this is not practical nor indicated at this time in LMICs because of lack of staff training and of laparoscopic equipment which is expensive. Treatment of uncomplicated, non-perforated appendicitis with antibiotics alone has recently gained popularity in HICs. Although it is tempting to use it in LMICs, it should be avoided since it requires close follow-up and laboratory support which the infrastructure in most LMICs rarely permits. Delay in presentation, in diagnosis, and in operation contribute to high morbidity and significant mortality. The estimated rate of perforation occurring at a higher rate primarily in the younger and older age groups has been 16–40% in most studies from LMICs.

Postoperative antibiotics are not needed if the appendix is not perforated, but should be used for 4–7 days if a peri-appendiceal abscess or perforation is present, under which circumstances the small wound may be left open above the closed fascia and packed to avoid wound infection.

Cholecystitis

Epidemiology

Cholelithiasis is a common disease worldwide but is very rare in Africa (less than 5%) and infrequent in China and Asia (about 5–10%), while in HICs it is about 8% in men and 16 + % in women [22]. The pathophysiology and diagnosis should be very familiar to most medical students and is very familiar to most physicians and to all general surgeons. Acute cholecystitis is related to cholelithiasis in most instances (more than 90%). In LMICs it may also occur in many cases with obstruction of the cystic duct by a helminthic infection (ascariasis) which may lead to perforation or gangrene of the gall bladder.

Diagnosis

Diagnosis of acute cholecystitis is made on clinical basis and is well known to all trained surgeons and needs not to be repeated here. The characteristic right upper quadrant pain provoked by fatty fired foods with Murphy's sign, belching, nausea, occasional vomiting, and fever with leukocytosis are only some of the characteristic basic clinical findings. The diagnosis is confirmed by findings of stones, pericydtocholic fluid, and distention of the gallbladder with thickening of the wall on an USG.

Management

First-line treatments include fasting, intravenous fluids, antibiotics, and analgesia. Percutaneous cholecystectomy under USG is a safe alternative to cholecystectomy for very ill and/or septic patient who may be unfit to undergo surgery or where the infrastructure for operation is inadequate. Gallbladder perforation or gangrenous cholecystitis require emergent interventions and are life-saving. Urgent cholecystostomy (percutaneous transhepatic gallbladder drainage) with or without delayed laparoscopic cholecystectomy appears to be the correct clinical approach for those not fit for surgery, or for those who fail to improve after 2–3 days of antibiotic treatment.

Effective treatment is almost always surgical within 24–48 hours but can be delayed and postponed with judicious use of antibiotics. This is dangerous in diabetic or immunosuppressed or elderly patients where the gall bladder can become gangrenous and rupture resulting in a major complication and frequently death. The timing of cholecystectomy continues to be debatable. When elective, the operation should be done under optimal conditions. In HICs the new standard of care for cholecystectomy is laparoscopic intervention, but in many LMICs it remains an open approach due to inadequate laparoscopic training and expertise and the lack of expensive equipment.

Cholangitis

Epidemiology

Acute cholangitis results from biliary obstruction combined with bacterial infection in the bile either by ascent from the intestine or from the venous portal system. It usually starts following choledocholithiasis and blockage of the common bile duct (CBD) which may also be blocked by tumor or parasites (vide infra). It is not uncommon in LMICs but the record of cases is poor and unreliable. Its incidence parallels that of cholelithiasis at a much lower frequency in LMICs than in HICs.

Diagnosis

Clinical findings associated with acute cholangitis include abdominal pain, jaundice, fever (Charcot's triad), and rigor and may mimic acute cholecystitis when the common bile duct is compressed by a distended gall bladder. The disease is also charcterized by Charcot's triad of right upper quadrant pain, fever, jaundice and rigors; this has been expanded to Reynid's pentad with addition of hypotension (shock) and confusion. Diseases which should be differentiated from acute cholangitis are acute cholecystitis, gastric and duodenal ulcer, acute pancreatitis, acute hepatitis, and septicemia of other origins as well as hepatic abscess, and right lower lobe pneumonia. Laboratory data show elevated white count and abnormal liver function test with elevated bilirubin and enzymes and alkaline phosphatase. Blood cultures are also helpful for severity assessment, as well as for the selection of antimicrobial drugs. Plain X-ray may demonstrate free air, pneumobilia, and ileus. Abdominal ultrasound (US) and abdominal computerized tomography (CT) with intravenous contrast are very helpful studies in evaluating patients with acute biliary tract disease. Since CT may not be available, USG must demonstrate the presence of biliary obstruction and its level as well as the cause of obstruction which is usually a gallstone and rarely stricture or tumor. In LMICs it may be one of the parasites that infect the liver such as *Ascaris*, or one of the liver flukes.

Management

Patients with acute cholangitis are at risk for developing severe infection that can be fatal unless appropriate medical care is provided at an early stage. Prompt treatment with appropriate antibiotics (blood culture) and acute care in an ICU is mandatory. The best treatment is decompression by biliary endoscopy and removal of obstructing stone or biopsy of any mass and placement of a stent to keep the duct open and draining. If the stone is large, endoscopic sphincterotomy can be done. This requires special expertise and experience which can usually be found only at the tertiary hospital. If an open drainage must be done because of no available expertise the simplest procedures such as T-tube placement without choledocholithotomy should be done as a temporary solution in unstable patients to avoid a prolonged operation. Whenever possible, definitive elimination of the biliary obstruction should be the goal of surgery. Once this is accomplished, a cholecystectomy should be performed after the patient recovers from sepsis and is stable to avoid further stones from that source. Emergent drainage is essential for severe cases, whereas patients with moderate and mild disease should also receive drainage as soon as possible if they do not respond to conservative treatment, and their condition has not improved. Biliary drainage can be achieved via three different routes/procedures: endoscopic, percutaneous transhepatic, and open methods. Drainage of the CBD without delay has resulted in reduction of morbidity and mortality from acute cholangitis. However, it remains a life-threatening disease.

Diverticulitis

Etiology

Diverticular disease has been considered a "disease of the western civilization" [1] due to the fact that the incidence and prevalence of diverticular disease differ more than 20–40-fold between high- and low-risk populations, and tend to be more common in high-income countries, where Westernized lifestyles prevail, than in low-income countries. It is especially rare among the native black population in rural Africa where a high intake of dietary fiber has been associated with a reduced risk of diverticular disease in several studies. Although it was previously reported that diverticular disease was unknown in black Africans, it has been noted recently that the incidence has increased in the cities. The disease manifestations range from localized diverticular inflammation best treated with intravenous and oral antibiotics to perforation and fecal peritonitis which requires colon resection. It is therefore recommended that the index of suspicious for diverticular disease of the colon and its complications should also increase.

Diagnosis

Localized inflammatory diverticular disease manifests itself with low-grade fever and tenderness over the site of inflammation, on the left or right lower quadrant. On the right the differential diagnosis must include appendicitis. It may be accompanied by diarrhea. Diarrhea may be melanotic or even bloody if there is diverticular bleeding which may be intermittent and copious. History of similar recurrent episodes increase the probability of diveticulitis, especially if there is a history of a previous barium enema or CT scan that may have shown diverticular disease.

Elevated white count with a shift to the left accompanies the pain which is most significant if there is a walled off perforation with an abscess. This is best demonstrated with a CT scan and may be detected with an USG.

Management

This subject is extensively covered in standard surgery textbooks and is presented here for the sake of completion since it is still relatively rarely seen urgently with an acute abdomen in LMICs and is well recognized by surgeons in HICs. The management of left- and right-sided perforations or bleeding is all too familiar to western-trained surgeons despite their differences in the choice of operative procedure in the emergent situation – resection with or without colostomy. Implications of colonic re-anastomoses have been attractive, but the incidence of leaks and anastomotic breakdowns by inexperienced staff has led to wound infections and fatalities. This suggests that the use of diversion may be more prudent. The management of perforated diverticulitis has recently changed dramatically, due to better radiological imaging and the availability of non-surgical treatment options by percutaneous drainage and laparoscopic resections. This kind of approaches is only possible in select tertiary centers in LMICs where such patients should be transferred for optimal treatment.

Sigmoid Volvulus

Epidemiology

Sigmoid volvulus is the commonest cause of large bowel obstruction in many regions of the world, and in some LMICs it is second only to acute appendicitis as a cause of acute abdomen. In Ethiopia it is the most common cause for intestinal obstruction. In Africa it is 4 to14 times more common in men than in women, and majority of them are older than 60 years of age [23]. The etiology is unknown but it has been suggested in the past that dietary habits, cultural stool withholding behavior, and chronic constipation can lead to a redundant sigmoid which can twist along its narrow mesenteric base.

Diagnosis

The chief complaint is abdominal pain and inability to defecate and pass flatus, and the physical finding is marked abdominal distention. About a quarter to half of the patients are first seen with an acute abdomen after a delay in arriving at the hospital which ranges sometimes up to 5 days during which they may take local remedies, if the transport from distant rural areas in an LMIC is intermittent or unavailable. In one study representative of findings in Ethiopia, but also found in Pakistan and Uganda, one-half to two-thirds of the patients developed gangrenous bowel which carries a far worse prognosis despite prompt operative intervention. Flat and upright X-ray of the abdomen is usually a sufficient imaging study to visualize sigmoid volvulus, with its typical bird's beak sign, in LMICs where CT scans are rarely available in smaller than regional hospital.

Management

The primary treatment for almost all the patients around the world is derotation in the very early stage with subsequent elective resection, and most often in LMICs where delay predominates, primary resection and anastomoses. The overall mortality of 4.5% to 18% [23] is highly dependent on the delay between onset of symptoms and intervention. Non-operative treatment of viable bowel may be a better treatment for older frail patients and emergent surgery can be made semi-elective. Without surgery however, recurrence rate is very high, almost 50%, and many patients refuse surgery after being relieved with decompression. The highest mortality occurs when gangrenous sigmoid is resected and a primary anastomosis is performed when compared to those who have viable bowel. This suggests that resection with Hartmann's pouch following resection for gangrenous bowel is generally underutilized. The main factors associated with mortality and with main complications of wound infection and sepsis are duration of illness, being female because they appear to ignore symptoms longer, and most importantly, primary resection and anastomoses in face of gangrenous bowel.

Abdominal Emergencies of Parasitic and Uncommon Origin

Abdominal emergencies of parasitic origin although relatively infrequent do present to the emergency room at sufficient rate in LMICs not only to be aware of them but to be able to diagnose and treat them. Although the incidence of parasitic infections is decreasing in LMICs due to improved sanitation, access to portable water and availability of potent antibiotics, peritonitis secondary to ruptured liver amebic abscess or typhoid perforation should remain part of the differential diagnosis of all acute abdomen in LMICs, while gastrointestinal tuberculosis (GITB) should be high on the differential list for abdominal pain or appendicitis. Many of these parasitic infections may not initially require surgical intervention. Pre-operative diagnosis could lead to a non-operative management that may be associated with better prognosis by being treated with appropriate antibiotics. The following is a brief summary of the most common parasitic and less common diseases that require diagnosis and treatment of an acute abdomen.

Intestinal Tuberculosis

Epidemiology

Intestinal TB accounts for 11–16% of cases of extra-pulmonary TB, and accounts for 1–3% of all TB cases worldwide. It most commonly affects the ileocecal region, but can involve any part of the GI tract. There is unclear association of GI TB with sex predisposition or age of the patient, but GI TB is commonly seen in populations with lower socio-economic status (SES), and is associated with illiteracy, malnutrition, and co-infection with HIV/AIDS. Although the prevalence rate of GITB is rare in LMICs, it is 20 to 50 times greater than in HICs and should be looked for. Surgery which should be avoided, once done, could show the effect on more than one organ and reveal tuberculous granulomas, which would prompt a more specific treatment of these patients.

Diagnosis

Diagnosis of abdominal TB is often delayed because the clinical presentation is often atypical. Important part of it includes clinical suspicion on the basis of relevant history or risk factors for prior TB. The most common signs and symptoms are abdominal pain or distention, ascites, and intestinal obstruction. Other common complaints include fever, weight loss, melena, abdominal mass, diarrhea or bowel obstruction, and anorexia [24]. A family history may not be evident, and some patients may not manifest any symptoms of GITB. Symptoms depend on the site of involvement and may include clinical manifestations of intestinal ulcero-constrictive disease, adjacent tissue involvement, or chronic inflammation. High-risk populations for tuberculous peritonitis include Asians, American Indians, alcoholics, chronic ambulatory peritoneal dialysis patients, and AIDS patients. Definitive diagnosis can usually be made by laparoscopic guided peritoneal biopsy.

There is no gold standard for diagnosis of intestinal TB, which is usually made from a combination of imaging (CT scans) for extent and type of GI TB, alongside clinical signs and laboratory findings. A high erythrocyte sedimentation rate, anemia, hypoalbuminemia, and leukocytosis raise suspicion for GITB. Purified protein derivative skin test (PPD) which is readily available in LMICs and interferon-gamma release assay like T-spot test (not generally available in LMICs) can be positive in 50–80% of patients, but negative results do not exclude GITB. Mycobacterium-specific testing modalities for GITB such as quantiferon testing or PCR assays have high specificity but low sensitivity and may not be practical in LMIC. Adenosine deaminase (ADA) levels in ascitic/peritoneal fluid may serve as a good diagnostic marker. Finally, empirical anti-tuberculosis therapy (ATT) may be used when clinical suspicion is high and has been proposed as a diagnostic criterion; there is no recommendation on when to discontinue ATT if used as a diagnostic therapeutic trial. GITB is often confused with Crohn disease and has been known to mimic esophageal cancer, esophageal ulcers, gastric ulcers, gastric cancer, colorectal cancer, and sarcomas, or other acute infections such as appendicitis, colitis, acute cholecystitis, and necrotizing fasciitis. Intestinal sarcoidosis is commonly confused for GITB, and even on biopsy the two conditions may be difficult to differentiate. PCR testing for *M. tuberculosis* is highly specific for GITB, with specificity of 95% and can be used for differentiation.

Management

GITB generally responds to standard anti-TB drugs, and early initiation of ATT with high clinical suspicion significantly reduces morbidity and mortality. The recommendation is the same as for pulmonary TB, a 6-month therapy with standard regimen of isoniazid, rifampicin, pyrazinamide, and ethambutol 3x weekly for the first 2 months, and isoniazid and rifampin for an additional 4 months. Full recovery is sometimes difficult to assess but can be generally seen in 2 months. Those with disseminated disease may require prolonged therapy. Surgery is only used in patients unresponsive to anti-TB therapy or for complications such as strictures or obstruction and for misdiagnosis of appendicitis. In one series of 96 patients with abdominal TB [25], 70 (72.90%) were admitted as acute intestinal obstruction and 22 (22.9%) with acute diffuse peritonitis. The emergency bowel resections in 74 of these patients were for 34 ileocecal masses, 16 strictures, 10 perforations, and 10 adhesions. Acute intestinal obstruction was the main acute presentation in this report from 2006, and although the incidence of GITB in LMICs has decreased since then, following milk pasteurization in some areas and improved public health measures, GITB remains a significant surgical/medical problem in LMICs.

Complications

Common complications following treatment are upper and lower GI bleeding, fistula, stricture, intussusceptions, perforation, anemia, and malnutrition with weight loss or vitamin deficiency. ATT often results in drug-induced liver injury requiring discontinuation and/or change.

Typhoid

Epidemiology

There are an estimated 11–20 million cases of typhoid worldwide each year, with approximately 8–15 million cases in LMICs. Typhoid is most commonly found in developing areas in Southeast Asia or Africa, primarily in Central Africa, India, Pakistan, or Bangladesh, and it is also found less commonly in East Asia, South America, and in the Caribbean. The risk of typhoid is high in populations with high poverty, inadequate sanitation, or lack of access to clean food and water, as well as in vulnerable groups such as children.

Diagnosis

The incubation period is 6–30 days from exposure, with gradual onset of increasing fatigue and fever. Other signs and symptoms of typhoid commonly include prolonged high fever that peaks in the late afternoon or evening, fatigue, headache, nausea, abdominal pain, constipation, or diarrhea. Less commonly, patients present with abdominal distention, hepatosplenomegaly, myalgia, dry cough, sore throat, or a transient, maculopapular rash on the trunk. Signs and symptoms appear gradually and can be confused with malaria; typhoid can be clinically suspected when patients are in areas where typhoid is endemic when there is a lack of response to antimalarials. Left untreated or even ineffectively treated, typhoid is often fatal, sometimes with recurrent intestinal perforations after an original operation and/or with late symptoms of delirium and "typhoid state" (lying motionless and exhausted) [26].

Patients with typhoid will have bacteremia, and the gold standard test for typhoid is positive multiple blood cultures since a single culture is positive in only 50% of cases. Multiple cultures from a large volume of blood and bone marrow cultures can increase the sensitivity and diagnostic yield and partially neutralizing the antibiotic effect. Serologic tests and stool and urine cultures have lower diagnostic yield, and are not substitutes for blood cultures.

Management

Typhoid responds well to antibiotic therapy, and fluoroquinolones are empirically effective in adults. Cephalosporins and other newer antibiotics may be preferred now since a resistance of typhoid to fluoroquinolones is emerging in endemic regions. Azithromycin needs to be reserved for multidrug-resistant (MDR) typhoid and should not be used empirically. Treatment should be initiated as soon as possible, even before results of blood culture are available either with oral cefixime 400 mg q12hr or IV ceftriaxone 1 gm q12hr or 2 gm q24 hr. If there are any signs of complications or no clinical improvement after 5 days of treatment with PO cefixime and blood culture results and sensitivities are available, it is prudent to give a new antibiotic intravenously. Recommended therapy depends on the type of typhoid and its sensitivity. For non-resistant typhoid, fluoroquinolones for 14 days are effective and cephalosporins should be de-escalated to first-line antibiotics. Chloramphenicol (50 mg/kg in 4 doses), trimethoprim sulfamethoxazole (4–20 mg/kg in 2 doses), or ampicillin/amoxicillin (75–100 mg/kg in 4 doses) are also effective. For multidrug-resistant typhoid third-generation cephalosporins for 14 days should be used. For extensive drug-resistant typhoid (XDR), fin a clinically stable patient azithromycin with 1gm loading dose, followed by either 500 mg or 1gm PO q24hr for 7–10 days depending on patient's weight (<60 kg vs >60 kg).

There are also two vaccines available, but they are generally not available in many endemic countries and do not have a long-lasting effect.

Ileal perforations occur frequently in children and young adults where the diagnosis is delayed because they may be treated for malaria for more than a week before being diagnosed properly when they present with peritonitis and with septic shock. After initial resuscitation with IV fluids, antibiotics, nasogastric decompression, and blood transfusion if necessary, they are explored and the area of perforation is usually resected followed by re-anastomoses followed by copious irrigation of the abdomen with warm saline. Search for more than one perforation is mandatory. Re-exploration may be necessary to look for a new perforation if patient is not improving in 3–5 days. Occasionally a right hemicolectomy is necessary or a tube ileostomy if the patient cannot tolerate the operation. Patients who present early have a mortality of about 10% while those who present late with an abdomen filled with pus and intestinal content have a mortality of 20–50% depending on the length of the delay and of post-operative ICU care and sensitivity to the antibiotics. Typhoid remains a dangerous and frequently fatal disease [27].

Complications

Complications occur in 10–15% of patients, particularly those who have been ill for more than 2 weeks. The most common complication is GI bleeding, usually slight bleeding but can be rapidly fatal depending on location. Intestinal perforation is the most serious complication, requiring surgery, and occurs in 1–3% of patients, manifesting with worsening abdominal pain, and sign of septic shock with hypotension and with acute abdomen. Neuropsychiatric presentations, such as reduced level of consciousness or encephalopathy, severe agitation, or delirium, are also common in certain countries. Relapse occurs in 5–10% of patients 2–3 weeks after resolution of symptoms, though the relapse is usually less severe than initial disease. Relapse must be differentiated from reinfection before treatment.

Dysentery

Dysentery can either be bacillary dysentery, caused by *Shigella* bacteria, or amoebic dysentery, caused by *Entamoeba histolytica.*

Amoebic Dysentery (Amoebiasis)

Amoebic dysentery is most common in tropical areas with poor sanitation, and only 10–20% of people infected become sick. An estimated 500 million people are infected worldwide, with between 40,000 and 100,000 deaths. It is endemic in tropical areas, particularly in developing parts of Central and South America, Africa, and Asia [28].

Bacillary Dysentery (Shigellosis)

Bacillary dysentery has approximately 188 million cases annually worldwide and 164,000 associated deaths. Globally, shigella is the second most common cause of diarrheal deaths. Prevalence of dysentery is generally highest in children aged 1–4 years in LMICs, and peaks between 18 and 23 months of age [28]. Since it is spread by fecal contamination of food and water, dysentery often appears as an epidemic in impoverished areas with poor sanitation, overcrowding, or refugee populations. Since 1991, there have been dysentery epidemics in Angola, Burundi, Malawi, Mozambique, Rwanda, Tanzania, Democratic Republic of the Congo, and Zambia.

Diagnosis of Dysentery

The incubation period depends on the pathogen, generally around 1–4 days, with approximately 50% of detected shigella infections being asymptomatic and up to 90% of *E. histolytica* infections being asymptomatic. Early clinical presentation commonly includes fever, headache, anorexia, and vomiting, followed by abrupt onset of watery diarrhea. Often, it resolves within 3–7 days and symptoms are mild in healthy individuals. Progression to dysentery is generally marked by frequent, small stools with blood or mucus in nearly half of cases of *Shigella* diarrhea. At this point, patients commonly present with fever, lower abdominal cramps, rectal pain, tenesmus, bloody stool, and especially dehydration. Persistent diarrhea associated with malnutrition is the leading cause of death among children. Dysentery is often confused with other causes of diarrhea such as bacterial enteritis and non-typhoidal salmonella, which differ from *Shigella* by an abrupt onset, more than four frequently bloody stools per day, no vomiting at onset, and fever. The diagnosis can also be confirmed by the identification of the parasite in fresh stool specimens, ulcer scrapings, and on rectal biopsy.

The current gold standard for diagnosing dysentery is rectal swab and conventional bacterial culture showing evidence of dysentery-causing *Shigella* or amoeba. Bacterial culture provides information on antibiotic susceptibility to dictate treatment. Fecal leukocytes can also help differentiate dysentery from other diarrheal diseases, but are not sufficient replacement for bacterial culture. In amoebiasis the typical punched-out ulcer is almost diagnostic on sigmoidoscopy, and these may be found throughout the colon. Amoebic dysentery is commonly confused with other parasites under a microscope, such as non-pathogenic *Entamoeba dispar* which is 10 times more common. Unfortunately, most laboratories are unable to differentiate between *E. histolytica* and *E. dispar*.

Management of Bacterial Dysentery

Current treatment guidelines endorse oral ciprofloxacin as first-line therapy for bacterial dysentery, and parenteral ceftriaxone for severe disease. In children, oral ciprofloxacin 15 mg/kg twice daily for 3 days, or in case of severe disease, parenteral ceftriaxone followed by oral for 10–14 days. For adults, first-line therapy is oral ciprofloxacin 500 mg once a day for 3 days or for severe disease, parenteral ceftriaxone for 3 days IV or IM. If there is no improvement after 48 hours of antibiotics, therapy needs to be adjusted according to susceptibility. Second-line therapy with β-lactams, cephalosporins, and azithromycin is appropriate in regions where ciprofloxacin resistance is high.

Management of Amoebic Dysentery

Treatment of amoebiasis in tissue is treated with nitroimidazoles, such as metronidazole, tinidazole, or nitazoxanide, dehydroemetine, or chloroquine. These should be given 3× a day for 5–10 days. Amoeba infection of the lumen is treated with diloxanide furoate or iodoquinoline, though it may require a combination of medications for effective treatment. First-line recommended therapy is metronidazole (500–750 mg for 5–10 days for adults, 35–50 mg/kg per day divided into 3 doses for 10 days). There is toxicity associated with nitroimidazoles and concern for development of resistance [29].

The general surgeon is likely to be faced with complications arising from amoebiasis wherever he works in LMICs. Amoebic colonic ulcers heal with a thin scar but may appear as pseudopolyps and rarely go on to form an amoebic granuloma in the cecum or rectosigmoid and confuse the surgeon. Amoebic abscess may occur in the lung, pleura, even in the brain, but it is most common in the liver which they invade from the colon via the portal vein and are found most commonly in alcoholics. When operation is considered in a patient who has amoebiasis, pre-operative treatment of the disease should be done if at all possible. Colon resection should be avoided because the bowel is very friable, and diverting ileostomy may be sufficient for amoebic colitis. Perforation is rare and the signs of peritonitis may be masked, and it may be diagnosed primarily by free air on repeated abdominal films in a patient who is getting worse on antibiotics. If a bowel resection is done at any point, a diverting colostomy or ileostomy is almost mandatory because intestine infested with amoeba does not heal well and breakdown of the anastomosis is common. The mortality following colonic resection in fulminant amoebic colitis is high. Occasionally perforation is multiple, especially if antibiotic treatment has been delayed. Hemorrhage from an ulcer that invades an artery is very rare, and treatment should consist of blood replacement and embolization by interventional radiologist, and avoiding exploration that carries a very high mortality. Amoeba can locate in the appendix and mimic appendicitis leading to a very difficult appendectomy with friable bowel which may require exteriorization of the cecum. Colonic lesions can occasionally lead to strictures and rarely fistulae. Amebic liver abscess is caused by extraintestinal spread of *Entamoeba histolytica*. It is usually diagnosed from imaging, and the gold standard of treatment is metronidazole. Only about 15% of cases require percutaneous drainage. The prognosis is good, with almost universal recovery.

Complications

Common complications include dehydration, liver abscess, post-infectious arthritis (joint pain, inflammation, and stiffness), and hemolytic ureic syndrome, a rare complication of *Shigella*. Bacteremia is a common complication in young children under the age of 5, as well as leukemia reaction in children between 2 and 10 years old. The most common neurological symptom is generalized seizures, which leads to increased mortality. Dysentery can result in colon perforation (primarily in infants or malnourished patients), intestinal obstruction, toxic mega colon, prostates (in infants and young children), dermatitis, or even acute myocarditis.

Ascaris

Epidemiology

Worldwide, ascariasis, caused by the parasitic worm *Ascaris lumbricoides*, infects approximately 807 million to 1.2 billion people in the world with more than 60,000 deaths annually and contributes significantly to the burden of parasitic diseases worldwide. *Ascaris* survives best in warm, humid areas and is endemic to tropical and subtropical areas of East Asia, China, sub-Saharan Africa, and Latin America, particularly in areas with poor sanitation, or in regions where human feces is often used as fertilizer.

Diagnosis

People with ascariasis often have no symptoms other than malnutrition, or mild symptoms such as abdominal discomfort or pain, nausea, vomiting, bloating, and diarrhea. In children, ascariasis may present with growth retardation. Severe infection depends on the passage of larvae; ascaris larvae in the lungs can cause Loeffler syndrome (pneumonitis and eosinophilia, with wheezing, dyspnea, hemoptysis, and fever), whereas ascariasis migration to the biliary or pancreatic system can cause cholecystitis, cholangitis, pancreatitis, volvulus, appendicitis, and intussusceptions. Spontaneous resolution is possible, as the adult parasite lives on average for 1 to 2 years, and cannot multiply in the human host, after which it dies and is eliminated through the digestive tract.

The best diagnostic test is a stool exam for ova, which look like large oval brown trilayered eggs and parasites. However, eggs will not appear in stool until a month to 40 days after infection, and if one is infected with a male worm, there will be no eggs in the stool. Patients may also notice a worm in their stool or cough one up and make their own diagnosis.

Management

Ascaris infection responds well to antihelminthic therapy, with a single-dose treatment of albendazole of 400 mg resulting in over 95% cure rate and reduction in eggs. Medical therapy should be repeated after 1–3 months, to target larvae that have matured to adulthood. Second-line treatment is mebendazole 100 mg 2× a day for 3 days, or 500 mg as a single dose. For pregnant patients, pyrantel pamoate 11 mg/kg up to 1 g is recommended, and second-line therapy is 50 mg/kg/day piperazine for 5 days. Children should also have vitamin A supplementation. If a patient presents with active parasite migration through the lungs, medical therapy is contraindicated due to increased risk of pneumonitis. It is common for patients to be reinfected especially with no change in location, hygiene habits, or health education. Since *Ascaris* can invade various organs, treatment is directed to those organs, such as removal for appendicitis or cholecystitis.

Complications

Complications of ascariasis result from parasite migration, and children are more likely to have complications than adults. Common complications are rectal bleeding, hepatobiliary disease, and pancreatic pseudocyst. Depending on worm burden, heavy ascariasis may cause intestinal blockage and perforation.

Filariasis

Epidemiology

Filariasis is caused by parasitic roundworms called filariae that dwell in blood and tissue spread by mosquitoes. Lymphatic filariasis, also known as elephantiasis, is the most important and common filarial disease, infecting 120 million people with approximately a billion people at risk for infection. 70% of cases are found in India, Nigeria, Bangladesh, and Indonesia, though the parasite is endemic in around 80 tropical and subtropical countries in Central Africa, the Middle East, Southeast Asia, and coastal South America. The main pathogen is *Wuchereria bancrofti*, comprising 90% of cases, with the remaining mostly due to *Brugia malayi*. In many countries, men are much more susceptible to filariasis, possibly due to women's mode of dress being more covered and protected from infective mosquito bites.

Diagnosis

From infection by mosquito bite, it may take anywhere from 4 weeks to 16 months or longer for clinical manifestation to occur. More than half the patients with filariasis appear asymptomatic, despite hidden lymphatic damage, and the duration without symptoms is linked directly to the patient's immune competence. Filariasis is characterized by acute, episodic attacks of lymphadenitis and lymphangitis, with fever and malaise, lasting 3–15 days. There may also be lumps in subcutaneous tissue, breasts, or testicles. These acute inflammatory episodes, due to the parasite invading lymph nodes, prevent lymph flow and result in painful lymphatic trunks with red streaks in the skin, and swelling for several days, usually isolated to a single limb.

Filariasis is difficult to diagnose and relies on history of exposures in an endemic area.

The standard method is identifying microfilariae by microscopic exam of a thick blood smear obtained at night since microfilariae exhibit nocturnal periodicity and are only detected circulating in the blood at night. Serologic assays can be used but are frequently negative because of the timing of the infection. Recently, ultrasonography has been used to visualize adult worms of *W. bancrofti* even in asymptomatic males with microfilaremia. A highly sensitive antigen detection assay, the Alere Filariasis Test Trip is now available and recommended for mapping, monitoring, and transmission assessment of *W. bancrofti* independent of periodicity. This is, however, not applicable for *B. filariasis* or the other less common pathogens.

Management

The WHO recommends mass drug administration (MDA) of a preventive chemotherapy strategy, by an annual dose to an entire at-risk population, to reduce the density of microfilariae in the bloodstream and prevent spread to mosquitoes for long-term eradication of filariasis. A combination of diethylcarbamazine citrate (DEC) (6 mg/kg), ivermectin (200 mcg/kg) and albendazole (400 mg) as a single dose can clear almost all microfilariae in the blood within a few weeks. 17 countries have successfully implemented MDA and eliminated filariasis as a public health threat (Cambodia, Egypt, Kiribati, Maldives, Malawi, Marshall Islands, Palau, Sri Lanka, Thailand, Togo, Tonga, Vanuatu, Vietnam, Yemen, Niue, Wallis and Futuna, and the Cook Islands).

The goals of therapy are to kill the adult worms and slow the progression of disease, as well as manage the morbidities and complications. The medical therapy of choice is diethylcarbamazine citrate, which can target both the adult worm and the microfilaria. DEC has a potent and selective effect on microfilaria, allowing them to be phagocytosed by tissue fixed monocytes, starting with a low dose to decrease risk of adverse effects with a gradual increase in frequency and dose for 4–21 days [30]. Concurrent corticosteroid treatment should be considered to minimize allergic reaction to the disintegration of microfilaria. Other medical therapy includes ivermectin or suramin, which causes tonic paralysis in nematodes. Mebendazole or flubendazole also work to kill or immobilize the parasites, which are then cleared from the gut. Lymphatic damage is irreversible, so early diagnosis and prevention of progression of disease are crucial. Exercise and elevating affected limbs relieve the symptoms. Filariasis-associated adenolymphangitis is treated with repeated courses of DEC, but the late phase of chronic disease is not affected by DEC. Surgery is necessary for hydrocele [31].

Complications

Severe disease manifests with painful and visible disfigurement including acute dermatolymphangioadenitis (ADLA) and elephantiasis, referring to gross enlargement of the body, particularly the limbs. Male urogenital disease such as hydrocele and lymph scrotum have been reported, concurrent with other symptoms due to filarial abscesses in the genital area, which swell until rupturing. Tropical pulmonary eosinophilia rarely occurs as an extreme immune response, characterized by high eosinophil count, asthma-like attacks, splenomegaly, and restrictive lung disease.

Schistosomiasis

Epidemiology

Schistosomiasis is a parasitic disease caused by trematode worms, commonly *Schistosoma mansoni*, *S. haematobium*, or *S. japonicum*, that infects approximately 250 million people worldwide causing around 25,000 to 200,000 deaths globally per year. Freshwater snails release the larvae, and people become infected on skin contact with infected usually still water, with adult worms living in the blood vessel releasing eggs. It is endemic to tropical and subtropical regions, particularly agricultural or fishing populations or areas without adequate sanitation or access to clean water, with more than 200 million cases in Africa, particularly sub-Saharan Africa. There is also considerable morbidity in the Middle East, South America, and Southeast Asia. Adolescents have the highest intensity of infection by wading and swimming in still waters and are targets for screening and mass drug administration campaigns.

Diagnosis

About 60% of infected patients are symptomatic, but only 10% result in serious disease requiring treatment. Adult worms in the blood vessels are relatively harmless – the only clinical manifestations are terminal dysuria, hematuria, and rarely dysentery. The symptoms can be divided into three phases: acute disease, subacute disease, and chronic disease. In acute disease, clinical manifestation is a sudden presentation with a swimmer's itch or cercarial dermatitis (a local inflammatory, itchy, maculopapular skin eruption is evident at the site of cercarial penetration), bronchopneumonia, myalgia, and Katayama syndrome (a delayed hypersensitivity reaction that coincides with worm maturity, characterized by fever, arthralgia, and vasculitic skin eruption). Acute symptoms usually resolve spontaneously after 2–10 weeks, but can progress to weight loss, dyspnea, diarrhea, toxemia, hepatosplenomegaly, and widespread rash. In the subacute phase, species- and organ-specific lesions form in certain organs depending on egg location, leading to granulomatous, cell-mediated inflammation in affected organs. In chronic disease, fibrosis replaced granulomas, leading to reduction of symptom severity, though urinary, hepato-intestinal, cardio-pulmonary, or ectopic clinical manifestations may persist. Morbidity is generally more aggressive in the chronic phase after healing, and the most serious manifestations, namely, fibrotic lesions, glomerulonephritis, amyloidosis, and bladder or rectal malignancy, usually occur many years after initial infection and treatment.

Symptoms depend on inflammation secondary to schistosomiasis in either intestinal, hepatosplenic, or urogenital locations. Intestinal schistosomiasis manifests as abdominal pain, diarrhea, blood in stool, and hepatomegaly, associated with fluid accumulation in the peritoneal cavity. Hepato-splenic schistosomiasis manifests as hepatic fibrosis and portal hypertension, which occasionally lead to the development of esophageal varices, ascites, delayed growth, and severe anemia. Urogenital schistosomiasis is characterized by hematuria, increased frequency of micturition, and dysuria. Untreated urogenital schistosomiasis leads to fibrosis of the bladder and ureter, and possibly the kidney in advanced cases. Women, particularly in communities where women do household chores in unclean bodies of water, may develop urogenital schistosomiasis with genital lesions, vaginal bleeding, pain during intercourse, and vulvar nodules. In men, urogenital schistosomiasis causes pathological degradation of urogenital structures leading to infertility and other long-term consequences [32].

Schistosomiasis is diagnosed by stool or urine sample and identification of parasite eggs during active or late chronic infection, though during acute infection the low worm burden makes these methods relatively ineffective. Acute infection with its mild symptoms is often confused for malaria, salmonellosis, or acute hepatitis. Intestinal schistosomiasis can be detected in stool samples using the Kato-Katz technique to identify eggs. For urogenital schistosomiasis, the gold standard is a filtration technique using nylon, paper, or polycarbonate fibers. In regions where *S. mansoni* is endemic, the circulating cathodic antigen (CCA) test is an appropriate alternative. PCR-based detection of parasite DNA in stool and urine and ultrasonography for pathological changes are also used in high-resource areas for higher sensitivity but are frequently not available in LMICs.

Management

The gold standard and mainstay of medical treatment is oral praziquantel 20 mg/kg PO TID for 1 day (at intervals of 4–6 hours), which is effective against all 6 types of *Schistosoma* adult worms, and safe in children over the age of 4 and pregnant women after the first trimester. Adverse effects are minimal, nausea, itch and rash, and likely due to immune response to dying and dead worms. If there is a co-infection of schistosomiasis with *T. solium* (pork tapeworm), praziquantel can induce seizures, cerebral infarction, or permanent eye lesions. The limitations of praziquantel are that reinfection is common, and drug tolerance is of increasing concern. There is also a MAD campaign to eradicate schistosomiasis, with an annual single dose of praziquantel in endemic populations targeting adolescents that has been effective in China and Egypt. However, limitations of praziquantel and concerns of relying on a single drug impede scalability and efficacy of this campaign. In spite of a decrease in prevalence of hepato-splenic schistosomiasis thanks to mass-treatment with praziquantel, severe cases of portal hypertension are not exceptional due to esophageal varices. Operative interventions may be indicated for portal hypertension with a spleno-renal shunt or splenectomy. In Brazil hepatosplenic schistosomiasis is a serious clinical presentation of this disease, associated with splenomegaly, liver fibrosis, and portal hypertension, and is responsible for approximately 7% of schistosomotic patients. The surgical treatment of portal hypertension in schistosomotic deals with preserved hepatic function as compared to cirrhosis, and therefore decompression of portal vein might interfere with hepatic function. Recent focus therefore has been on splenectomy, division of the left gastric vein, devascularization of great gastric curvature, and postoperative endoscopic variceal sclerosis, as a surgical option to esophageal varices in hepatosplenic schistosomiasis [33]. In urogenital involvement cystoscopy may be indicated with irrigation and fulguration as necessary and stenting of the ureter in rare cases.

Complications

Complications include infertility, spontaneous abortion, and urinary tract obstruction leading to ESRD and bladder cancer, commonly squamous cell carcinoma. Chronic inflammation results in complications such as anemia of chronic disease, malnutrition, and growth retardation or failure to thrive. Patients with schistosomiasis are also susceptible to co-infection with other parasitic, bacterial, or viral infections endemic in the area, particularly HPV, Hepatitis B and C, and HIV.

Conclusion

In this chapter we have briefly summarized the difficult problem of diagnosing and managing patients with acute abdomen and IAI in LMICs primarily because of frequently deficient infrastructure. This includes shortage of trained staff in local and sometime in regional hospitals, difficulties and delays in transferring patients to regional or tertiary health facilities when needed, and lack of appropriate equipment, instruments, supplies, and medications at the local hospitals and even at regional hospitals. This chapter initially proposes in general terms the best ways to address these problems before proceeding to describe briefly the epidemiology, diagnosis, and management of very common general surgical conditions with which every general surgeon in LMICs or in HICs must become well acquainted. The chapter then describes in greater detail the most common parasitic, protozoan, and bacterial causes of acute abdomen and IAI in LMICs with which local general surgeons are much more familiar than the visiting surgeons or residents from HICs. The chapter also emphasizes the collaboration between local and visiting surgeons at the level of surgical and medical health care delivery while maintaining the teaching and learning communication that care of patients with IAIs and acute abdomens engenders.

References

1. Sartelli, et al. World J Emerg Surg. 2021;16(49):16–49. https://doi.org/10.1186/s13017-021-00387-8.
2. Ohene-Yeboah M. Acute surgical admissions for abdominal pain in adults in Kumasi, Ghana. ANZ J Surg. 2006;76(10):898–903. https://doi.org/10.1111/j.1445-2197.2006.03905.x.
3. Sartelli M, Abu-Zidan FM, Catena F, Griffiths EA, Di Saverio S, Coimbra R, et al. Global validation of the WSES sepsis severity score for patients with complicated intraabdominal infections: a prospective multicenter study (WISS study). World J Emerg Surg. 2015;10(1):61. https://doi.org/10.1186/s13017-015-0055-0.5.
4. Mazuski JE, Tessier JM, May AK, Sawyer RG, Nadler EP, Rosengart MR, et al. The surgical infection society revised guidelines on the management of intra-abdominal infection. Surg Infect. 2017;18:1–76.
5. Chow AW, Evans GA, Nathens AB, Ball CG, Hansen G, Harding GK, et al. Canadian practice guidelines for surgical intra-abdominal infections. Can J Infect Dis Med Microbiol. 2010;21(1):11–37. https://doi.org/10.1155/2010/580340.
6. Sandell E, Berg M, Sandblom G, Sundman J, Fränneby U, Boström L, et al. Surgical decision-making in acute appendicitis. BMC Surg. 2015;15(1):69. https://doi.org/10.1186/s12893-015-0053-x.
7. Solomkin JS, Mazuski JE, Bradley JS, Rodvold KA, Goldstein EJ, Baron EJ, et al. Diagnosis and management of complicated intra-abdominal infection in adults and children: guidelines by the Surgical Infection Society and the Infectious Diseases Society of America. Surg Infect. 2010;11:79–109.
8. Marshall JC, al Naqbi A. Principles of source control in the management of sepsis. Crit Care Clin. 2009;25(4):753–68.,viii-ix. https://doi.org/10.1016/j.ccc.
9. Sartelli M, Catena F, Abu-Zidan FM, Ansaloni L, Biffl WL, Boermeester MA, et al. Management of intra-abdominal infections: recommendations by the WSES 2016 consensus conference. World J

Emerg Surg. 2017;12(1):22. https://doi.org/10.1186/s13017-017-0132-7.9.08.001.
10. Campbell AM, Kuhn WP, Barker P. Vacuum-assisted closure of the open abdomen in a resource-limited setting. S Afr J Surg. 2010;48(4):114–5.
11. Sawyer RG, Claridge JA, Nathens AB, Rotstein OD, Duane TM, Evans HL, et al. Trial of short-course antimicrobial therapy for intraabdominal infection. N Engl J Med. 2015;372(21):1996–2005. https://doi.org/10.1056/NEJMoa1411162.
12. Levy MM, Fink MP, Marshall JC, Abraham E, Angus D, Cook D, et al. 2001. SCCM/ESICM/ACCP/ATS/SIS international sepsis definitions conference. Crit Care Med. 2003;31(4):1250–6. https://doi.org/10.1097/01.CCM.0000050454.01978.3B.
13. Singer M, Deutschman CS, Seymor CW, et al. The third international consensus definitions for sepsis and septic shock (Sepsis-3). JAMA. 2016;315(8):801–10. https://doi.org/10.1001/jama.2016.0287.
14. Ferreira FL, Bola DP, Bross A, Melot C, Vincent JL. Serial evaluation of the SOFA score to predict outcome in critically ill patients. JAMA. 2001;286(14):1754–8. https://doi.org/10.1001/jama.286.14.1754.
15. Levy MM, Evans LE, Rhodes A. The surviving sepsis campaign bundle: 2018 update. Intensive Care Med. 2018;44(6):925–8. https://doi.org/10.1007/s00134-018-5085-0.
16. Hagos M. Acute abdomen in adults: A two year experience in Mekelle, Ethiopia. Ethiop Med J. 2015;53(1):19–24.
17. Magagi IA, Adamou H, Habou O, Magagi A, Halidou M, Ganiou K. Urgences chirurgicales digestives en Afrique subsaharienne : étude prospective d'une série de 622 patients à l'Hôpital national de Zinder, Niger [digestive surgical emergencies in sub-Saharan Africa: a prospective study of a series of 622 patients at the National Hospital of Zinder, Niger]. Bull Soc Pathol Exot. 2017;110(3):191–7. https://doi.org/10.1007/s13149-016-0499-9. French. Epub 2016 Jun 14.
18. Bang GA, Bwelle Moto G, Chopkeng Ngoumfe JC, Ekani Boukar YM, Tientcheu Tim F, Savom EP, Essomba A. Complications des prises en charge chirurgicales des abdomens aigus non traumatiques d'origine digestive à l'hôpital central de Yaoundé, Cameroun (novembre 2019 - juillet 2020) [complications of surgical management of non-traumatic acute abdomens of digestive origin at the Yaoundé central hospital, Cameroon (November 2019 - July 2020)]. Med Trop Sante Int. 2021;1(4):mtsi.2021.99. https://doi.org/10.48327/mtsi.2021.99. French. PMID: 35685854; PMCID: PMC9128490
19. Mofikoya BO, Enweluzo GO, Tijani KH, Ogunleye EO, Kanu OO. Emergency surgical services in a sub-Saharan African country: can we meet the needs? Eur J Sci Res. 2010;43:265–71.
20. Ibrahim NA, Oludara MA, Ajani A, Mustafa I, Balogun R, Idowu O, Osuoji R, Omodele FO, Aderounmu AO, Solagberu BA. Non-trauma surgical emergencies in adults: Spectrum, challenges and outcome of care. Ann Med Surg (Lond). 2015;
21. Walker AR. Diet and bowel diseases–past history and future prospects. S Afr Med J. 1985;68:148–52. https://doi.org/10.1016/j.amsu.2015.09.004. 14;4(4):325-30. PMID: 26566434; PMCID: PMC4600937
22. Reshetnyak VI. Concept of the pathogenesis and treatment of cholelithiasis. World J Hepatol. 2012;4(2):18–34. https://doi.org/10.4254/wjh.v4.i2.18.
23. Mulugeta GA, Awlachew S. Retrospective study on pattern and outcome of management of sigmoid volvulus at district hospital in Ethiopia. BMC Surg. 2019;19(1):107. https://doi.org/10.1186/s12893-019-0561-1. PMID: 31399131; PMCID: PMC6688328
24. Al-Zanbagi AB, Shariff MK. Gastrointestinal tuberculosis: A systematic review of epidemiology, presentation, diagnosis and treatment. Saudi J Gastroenterol. 2021;27(5):261.
25. Ohene-Yeboah M. Case series of acute presentation of abdominal TB in Ghana. Trop Dr. 2006;36(4):241–3. https://doi.org/10.1258/004947506778604643.98-2003
26. Butler T. Treatment of typhoid fever in the 21st century: promises and shortcomings. Clin Microbiol Infect. 2011;17(7):959–63.
27. Ugochukwu AI, Amu OC, Nzegwu MA. Ileal perforation due to typhoid fever—review of operative management and outcome in an urban Centre in Nigeria. Int J Surg. 2013;11(3):218–22. https://doi.org/10.1016/j.ijsu.2013.01.014. Epub 2013 Feb 9
28. Shirley DA, Farr L, Watanabe K, Moonah S. A review of the global burden, new diagnostics, and current therapeutics for amebiasis. InOpen forum infectious diseases 2018 Jul (Vol. 5, No. 7, p. ofy161). US: Oxford University Press.
29. Henry FJ. The epidemiologic importance of dysentery in communities. Rev Infect Dis. 1991;13(Supplement_4):S238-44.
30. Biritwum NK, de Souza DK, Marfo B, Odoom S, Alomatu B, Asiedu O, Yeboah A, Hervie TE, Mensah EO, Yikpotey P, Koroma JB. Fifteen years of programme implementation for the elimination of Lymphatic Filariasis in Ghana: impact of MDA on immunoparasitological indicators. PLoS Negl Trop Dis. 2017;11(3):e0005280.
31. Medeiros ZM, Vieira AV, Xavier AT, Bezerra GS, Lopes MD, Bonfim CV, Aguiar-Santos AM. Lymphatic filariasis: a systematic review on morbidity and its repercussions in countries in the Americas. Int J Environ Res Public Health. 2021;19(1):316.
32. Lo NC, Bezerra FS, Colley DG, Fleming FM, Homeida M, Kabatereine N, Kabole FM, King CH, Mafe MA, Midzi N, Mutapi F. Review of 2022 WHO guidelines on the control and elimination of schistosomiasis. Lancet Infect Dis. 2022;
33. Ferraz AA, Bacelar TS, Silveira MJ, Coelho AR, Câmara Neto RD, de Araújo Júnior JG, Ferraz EM. Surgical treatment of schistosomal portal hypertension. Int Surg. 2001;86(1):1–8.

How to Diagnose and Manage Anorectal Disorders in Low- and Middle-Income Countries

28

Connie Hong-Hung Keung

A good leader inspires people to have confidence in the leader, a great leader inspires people to have confidence in themselves.

– Eleanor Roosevelt

Abbreviations

AIN	Anal intraepithelial neoplasia
DRE	Digital rectal exam
HIV	Human immunodeficiency virus
IBD	Inflammatory bowel disease
LMICs	Low- and middle-income countries
SCC	Squamous cell carcinoma
TB	Tuberculosis

Introduction/Background

Anorectal problems, while not often discussed due to their location, can often seriously affect patients and cause severe pain and discomfort. They can be debilitating for patients as they often do not know where to seek help. The breadth of issues can range from benign pathology to malignancies and from an anal itch to life-threatening disease. A good understanding of the anatomy and common problems will allow a surgeon to bring comfort, healing, and recovery for these patients.

C. H.-H. Keung (✉)
Indiana University School of Medicine, Department of Surgery, Indianapolis, IN, USA

Principles of Diagnosis

With experience, a surgeon will be able to formulate and narrow the differential diagnosis by obtaining a focused history and asking pertinent questions about the patient's symptoms. While there are many additional tests that can be performed, the diagnosis and treatment algorithm can be initiated soon after obtaining a complete history and performing a complete physical examination, not confined only to the anus and rectum. A good history supplemented by a confirmatory physical examination is essential to diagnose anorectal issues [1].

History and Physical Examination

The patients' histories of their anorectal symptoms are very important and the highlights are outlined below.

M. A. Hardy, B. R. Hochman (eds.), *Global Surgery*, https://doi.org/10.1007/978-3-031-28127-3_28

Pain: Its important characteristics are (1) dull vs. sharp, (2) associated with bowel movement, and (3) persistent or intermittent.

Bowel habits: (1) Constipation vs. diarrhea, (2) straining, (3) duration on the toilet.

Mass: (1) Fixed vs. mobile, (2) location, (3) bleeding.

Protrusion: (1) Piles vs. circumferential protrusion, (2) reduction (spontaneous, manual, persistent).

Bleeding: (1) Copious vs. smear, (2) bright red vs. melena, (3) with bowel movement vs. spontaneous.

Mucus or discharge: (1) Continuous or intermittent, (2) foul smelling, clear, or purulent.

Pruritus: (1) Certain time of day/night, (2) associated with BM, (3) associated with specific foods.

Physical Examination may be foreign to a patient and needs to be proposed and approached carefully. Assurances and explanation of the examination is very important so that the patient can anticipate all the steps of the investigation. There are three potential positions for the examination of the anorectum: prone, knee-chest or jackknife, or left lateral decubitus positions (Fig. 28.1). The ideal exposure is in one of the prone positions as that provides optimal exposure. However, this position may be limited by the patient's comorbidities, specifically joint issues limiting pressure on the knees. It is also not desirable in elderly patients with cardiac or pulmonary problems. Aside from assurance, careful explanation of each step of the examination must be done as part of the consent process. The examination includes (1) external inspection, (2) digital rectal exam (DRE), and (3) anoscopy.

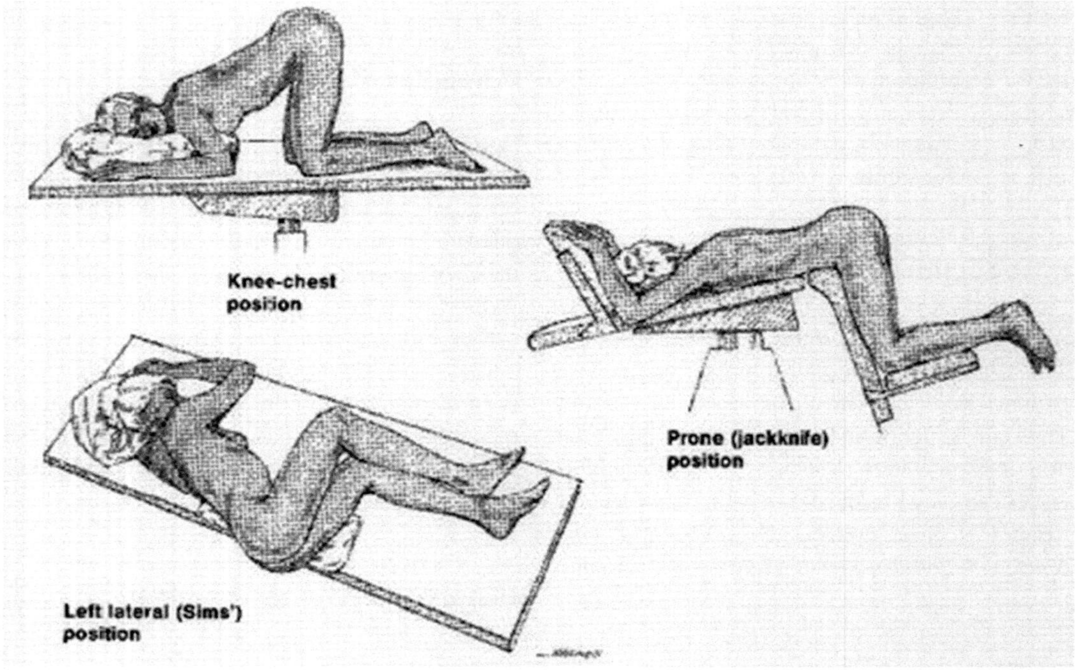

Fig. 28.1 Positions for anoscopy and for colonoscopy. *Source: Corman's Colon and Rectal Surgery, online at* https://abdominalkey.com/evaluation-and-diagnostic-techniques*by Abdominal Key - Fastest abdominal insight engine. Evaluation and Diagnostic Techniques. Denoya PT and Corman ML*

Principles of Management

Hemorrhoids

Patients often blame all anorectal problems on hemorrhoids (Fig. 28.2). While there are other pathologies, hemorrhoids do account for one of the most common surgical problems of the anorectum. Hemorrhoids are normal anatomic structures. They are vascular cushions that assist with continence. They are often located in standard locations: left lateral, right posterior, and right anterior positions. The blood supply is the superior hemorrhoidal artery and drainage is through the inferior, middle, and superior hemorrhoidal veins. There have been many postulations as to why hemorrhoidal disease arises; often cited are excessive straining (as with persistent constipation) or pressure from above (as in portal hypertension in cirrhosis). A study in northwest Ethiopia found that constipation and obesity contributed to increased odds of having hemorrhoidal problems requiring surgical attention [2]. Hemorrhoidal pathologies can be divided between external hemorrhoids and internal hemorrhoids. External hemorrhoids often cause pain, discomfort, and an acute bulge at the anal verge. These are located below the dentate line. Although internal hemorrhoids often protrude on straining and bleed, they originate above the dentate line. Internal hemorrhoids are classified in four stages (see Table 28.1). Physical examination begins with inspection, then DRE, and anoscopy.

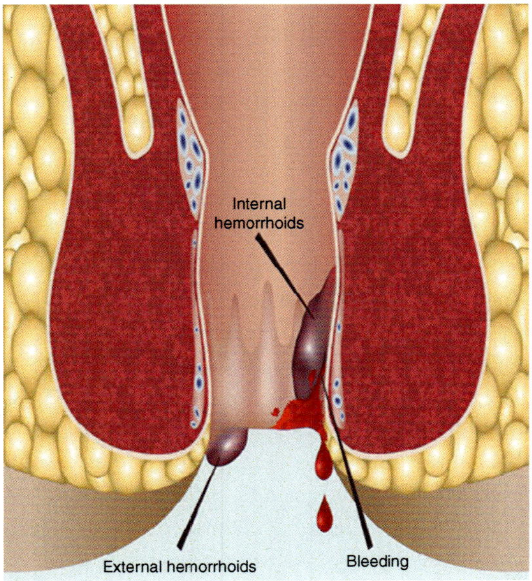

Fig. 28.2 Locations of internal and external hemorrhoids. *Source: GOGRAPH 370 Hemorrhoid. Clip Art | Royalty Free*

Table 28.1 Hemorrhoids/piles—"Goligher grading"

Stage I	No protrusion of hemorrhoids which remain above the dentate line
Stage II	Protruding hemorrhoids below the dentate line that spontaneously reduce
Stage III	Protruding hemorrhoids, possible to push back in manually
Stage IV	Protruding hemorrhoids that cannot be pushed back in manually anymore

External hemorrhoids can be detected on external examination. The small mass (generally not larger than 1–2 cm) must be differentiated between acute vs. resolving thrombosis. Acute thrombosed hemorrhoids are extremely tender and examination should be concluded at this point. Patients can often have patulous tags around the anal verge, indicating history of thrombosis in the past, and these should not be operated on. In the case of a thrombosed hemorrhoid, patient level of discomfort and pain as well as the duration of symptoms will dictate the type of intervention. Perianal pain is worst about 72 hrs following thrombosis, and will begin to improve after that, especially if sitz baths are instituted. Before 72 hours, excision of the clot is recommended as long as the patient does not have portal hypertension. Therefore, if the patient's symptoms are improving after 3 days, it is advisable to allow spontaneous resolution with no intervention other than sitz baths for comfort. If an excision is indicated, it can be performed in the office under local anesthesia. Incision of the overlying skin of the thrombosed hemorrhoid permits evacuation of the clot. The skin should not be reapproximated. Pressure can be applied to the area to control oozing and application of Monsel's solution or silver nitrate [3].

Internal hemorrhoids can sometimes be palpated on DRE; however this is not reliable as even pathologically enlarged hemorrhoids are vascular cushions which can be easily compressed by finger pressure and may feel "normal" on DRE. It is still important to perform DRE as other pathological findings can mimic hemorrhoidal findings and need to be ruled out.

Anoscopy is the defining test for internal hemorrhoids with the assurance that the anal canal is examined circumferentially. Depending on the skill of the anoscopist and the tolerance of the patient, this maneuver may require insertion of the anoscope a few times. Internal hemorrhoids above the dentate line should be examined for their size and documented for their mucosal irritation or bleeding. It is also important to determine the extent of any prolapse after asking the patient to Valsalva during anoscopy. This may provide an improved sense of the severity of the disease.

Rectal bleeding can often be attributed to hemorrhoids, but in addition the patient may harbor a more concerning diagnosis while presenting with concomitant hemorrhoids. A complete family history and careful review of systems may help to indicate the need for further testing, such as a colonoscopy, to rule out more proximal colonic and rectal pathologies such as a malignancy. In 2017 health-seeking behaviors were evaluated in Nigeria, and many physicians attributed rectal bleeding to hemorrhoids and failed to refer patients for colonoscopy which suggested a need for stronger educational programs about colorectal cancers [4].

Management of hemorrhoids should first begin with careful review of lifestyle habits and recommendations for modifications to decrease strain in the anorectum. Optimizing stool bulk and consistency with fiber supplementation is essential. Careful discussion on fiber amount (25 to 30 g a day) and type of diet is important. In addition, patients should be advised to spend as little time sitting on the toilet as possible (no sitting and reading). For discomfort, sitz baths 2–3 times/day for 10–15 min may alleviate any acute pain. Trial of these lifestyle modifications can be done for 2–3 months, followed by discussion of any symptom improvements.

If patients remain symptomatic, then other options may be pursued. There are numerous approaches available for further interventions to manage internal hemorrhoids. These include sclerotherapy, infrared photocoagulation, rubber band ligation, or excisional hemorrhoidectomy.

Rubber or plastic band ligation can be done in the office and is suggested for grade I to grade III hemorrhoids. This should be performed in a patient who is awake. The patient is placed in position, and the hemorrhoid is either grasped or suctioned through an anoscope; then a device will deploy a rubber band to noose the internal hemorrhoid (Fig. 28.3). The patient may feel pressure or dull discomfort, but should not experience any sharp pain. If there is pain, the rubber band is below the dentate line and the band should be removed. It is recommended to place no more than 3 bands in one sitting so as to avoid anal stenosis [3]. The delivery instrument metal or plastic (Fig. 28.4) is reusable and affordable and the rubber or plastic bands are very inexpensive.

Operative excisional hemorrhoidectomy can be performed by using several different techniques. Most commonly used presently are either the open (Milligan-Morgan) technique or the closed (Ferguson) technique. Both techniques follow the same principles of excision. An elliptical incision is made starting in the perianal margin; the hemorrhoidal tissue is then dissected off the underlying internal sphincter muscles. The internal apex is then suture ligated. In a closed technique, the ligating suture is then used to approximate the edges of the excision. In an open technique, suture ligation alone is done and the edges of the excision are not reapproximated.

Anal Fissures

An anal fissure is a tear in the epithelium of the distal anal canal. This is often the result of anal trauma secondary to a large hard bowel movement. The tear, or the fissure, persists due to sphincter hypertonicity. The most common position of an anal fissure is in the posterior location. Vascular studies have demonstrated relative ischemia in this location, and supports postulations that there is relative ischemia in the posterior midline location of the anus.

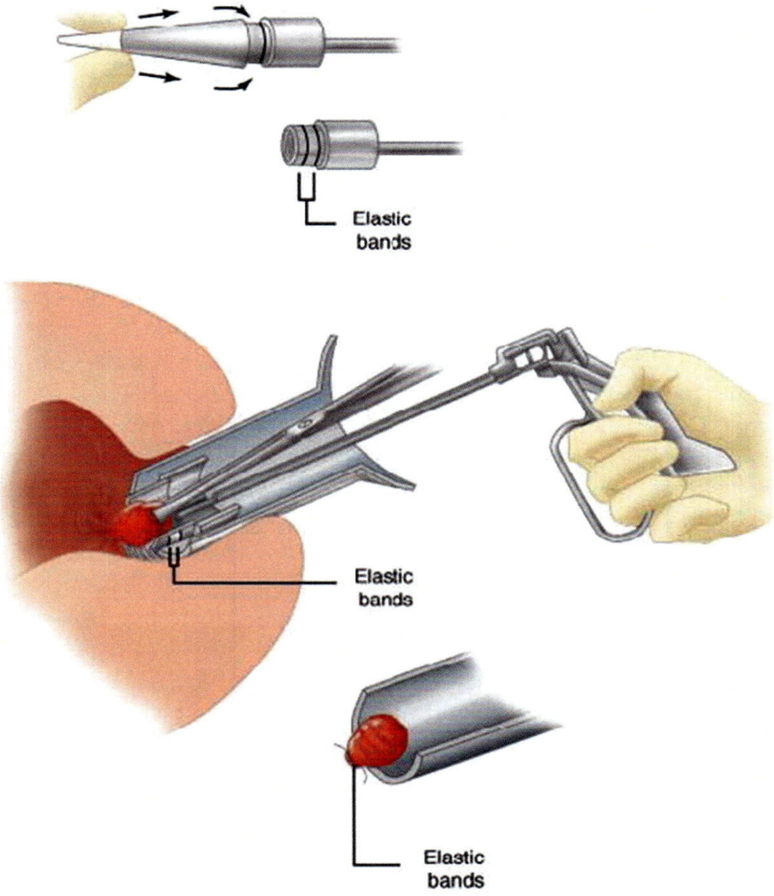

Fig. 28.3 Application of a plastic band to an internal hemorrhoid. *Source: Sabiston Textbook of Surgery, 17th Ed. Nelson, H, Chapter 49, p.1493, Fig.7 (Elsevier)*

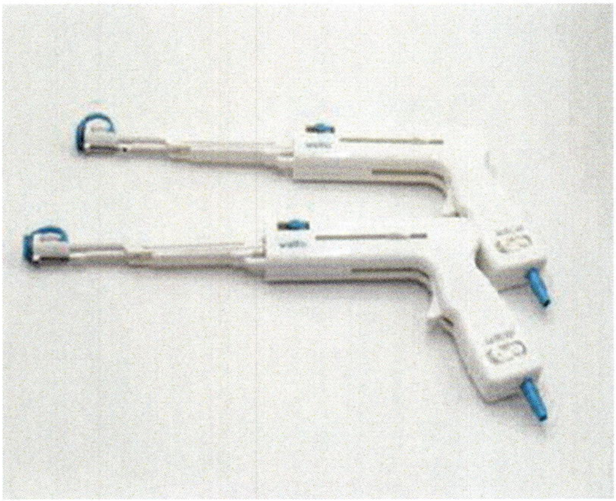

Fig. 28.4 Disposable ligators for application of the rubber band *(photo courtesy of MA Hardy)*

History of a fissure usually includes an initial sharp pain on defecation that can last a few hours after toileting. This is the most characteristic complaint of a patient with an anal fissure and is diagnostic. The pain has also been described as burning or tearing of the skin, followed by muscle spasm in the region. Due to the tear in the epithelium, there can be some bleeding from the region of the fissure. Patients can report fear can report fear or anxiety about going to the bathroom to pass the next bowel movement due to the anticipated severity of pain.

Physical examination is often limited only to the external inspection, as the pain from the fissure limits a useful DRE or anoscopy unless the patient is anesthetized. Frequently external inspection with gentle spreading of the anal verge will reveal a disruption in the anal epithelium confirming the diagnosis of an anal fissure. At this point the exam is complete and focus should be geared towards several treatment options. After the healing of the fissure, it is important to conduct a full examination, including DRE and anoscopy, to ensure that there are no other pathologic lesions that may contribute to the patient's symptoms and presentation. If this is not possible, then an examination under anesthesia is warranted to complete the evaluation. Chronic fissures have a sentinel skin tag that can be readily seen during the external examination in the office. There is often an anal papilla that can also be visualized on anoscopy [3].

Typical presentations for fissures include the anterior or posterior positions. If a fissure is located in the lateral position, either right or left anus, suspicion should be raised for other pathologies. Fissures can be divided into acute fissures (<6 weeks) and chronic fissures (>6 weeks). Most acute fissures heal with lifestyle modifications such as fiber supplementation and sitz baths. Chronic fissures generally do not heal spontaneously, and therefore treatment is geared towards addressing hypertonicity of the sphincter muscles. Topical ointment to the perianal region of nitroglycerin, diltiazem, or nifedipine has been shown to be effective in the treatment of chronic fissures. Due to the vasodilatory effects of these drugs, patients should be cautioned about headaches and/or dizziness after their application. These drugs may be used only with caution in patients with cardiac or valvular diseases.

After the failure of lifestyle modifications and of the use of topical vasodilators, options include the use of Botox injection or sphincterotomy. Botox injections may be prohibitively expensive and therefore not appropriate for use in low- and middle-income countries (LMICs). Recurrence rates with Botox injections are higher than the successes of complete healing achieved with sphincterotomy. Sphincterotomy, which involves cutting of the internal sphincter, results in >90% resolution of fissures depending on the technique. This method may, however, result in incontinence in up to 30% of patients. Sphincterotomy should be approached with caution, especially in women who may have experienced peripartum trauma from vaginal delivery [3].

Anorectal Abscess and Fistulas

Prevalence of fistula-in-ano was the leading cause of perianal admission at a referral hospital in Addis Ababa, accounting for 43% of admissions [5].

While abscesses may seem like a basic surgical issue, thorough understanding of the anal anatomy (Fig. 28.5) will allow a surgeon to successfully drain perianal and perirectal abscesses. The majority of such abscesses originates from cryptoglandular tissues. These glands are located at the dentate line, and their obstruction leads to abscess formation in the potential spaces that surround the anorectum. These spaces include perianal, ischiorectal, intersphincteric, and supralevator locations (Fig. 28.5). The most common site of infection is the perianal space while the supralevator space abscesses are relatively rare. When the abscess spreads circumferentially, it results in a horseshoe abscess located in the deep post anal space [1].

Patients usually present with fever, perianal pain, and swelling in the perianal region. It is

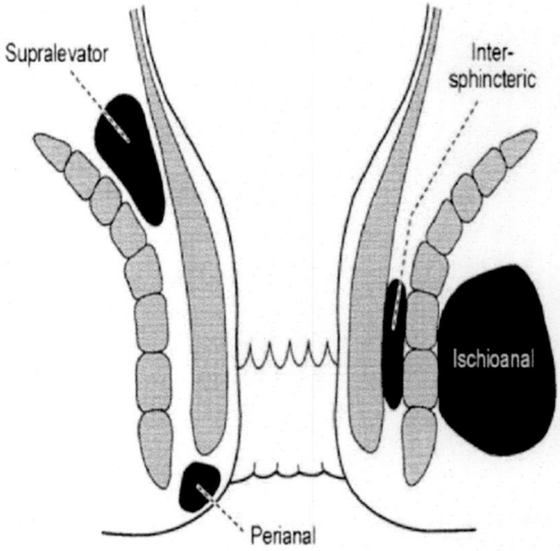

Fig. 28.5 Various perianal spaces for abscesses and fistulas

important to note that supralevator and intersphincteric abscess may not have external manifestations on physical examination and are more difficult to diagnose. A digital rectal exam for tenderness is important to rule out these locations for potential abscesses although at times, this may cause significant discomfort and even extreme tenderness. Ischiorectal and perianal abscesses will often present as a swelling with fluctuance adjacent to the anal verge or within the anal margin [1].

The urgent treatment for an anorectal abscess is incision and drainage. After preparation of the area with a betadine scrub, local anesthesia is injected circumferentially around the abscess. After the apex of the abscess is identified, a cruciate incision may be made and then the edges are removed to create adequate opening for drainage. In order for the wound edges not to coapt, resulting potentially in recurrence or inappropriate drainage, the edges must be kept wide apart. For ischiorectal abscesses which can be a few centimeters from the anal verge, the center of the incision should be placed as close to the anal verge as possible. This will then decrease the potential length and tortuous nature of a subsequent fistula. Horseshoe abscesses require drainage of the post anal space since the origin of this type of abscess is an intersphincteric infection. In those cases, the internal sphincter muscle often needs to be divided and separate counter incisions need to be made over each ischiorectal fossa.

Fistulotomy is often discouraged at the same time as incision and drainage. This is due to the acute inflammation in the potential operative field, and fear that attempts to find a fistula will create false passages and more trauma to the perianal region. Therefore localization of fistulas should be delayed till after the acute inflammation and infection has been controlled [1].

Severe necrotizing soft tissue infections are relatively rare, but progression of an undiagnosed and untreated anorectal abscess may frequently lead to generalized septicemia, including Fournier's gangrene which may be fatal. Such patients often present with sepsis and even shock. They must be aggressively resuscitated while initial surgical treatment must focus on wide local debridement to excise all necrotic tissue and to limit the spread of infection.

Fistulas usually form following an anal gland infection or abscess which burrows to the outside of the skin as it communicates with the inside of the rectum. Fistulas are classified based on their relationship to the anal sphincter complex and result because of an abnormal connection between two distant epithelial surfaces (Fig. 28.6). The majority of anorectal fistulas result from cryptoglandular pathology while less than 10% originate from inflammatory bowel disease (IBD), anal fissures, and tuberculosis (TB).

The diagnosis of fistulas is made by physical examination. Sometimes this may have to be done under sedation in order to find the internal opening with the aid of probes. Goodsall's rule (Fig. 28.7) while not always predictive, can help guide location of the internal opening. The rule suggests that if an imaginary transverse line was drawn to divide the anus, external os found anteriorly will tract radially internally. External openings posteriorly will drain to the posterior midline. Careful DRE may lead to the internal defect by careful palpation of the anoderm. Examination under anesthesia will help to definitively locate the fistula tract and permit to make decisions on next treatment steps. If no fistula is found, then MRI and fistulography may be useful diagnostic adjuncts if they are available; if not, repeat examination may be informative.

Treatment of fistulas has two goals. First, control of inflammation/sepsis. Second, closure of the tract while preserving continence and muscle integrity. This is frequently a two-step process with the first step being frequently done at the first examination which results in the definite diagnosis. At the time of the anorectal examination under anesthesia, after the fistula tract has been identified, a seton (heavy silk, #2) or preferably a vessel loop (thin rubber) can be placed through and through the fistula tract (Fig. 28.8). This should be loosely tied to itself in order to remain in place without cutting through the tract. Placement of the seton prevents recurrence of the

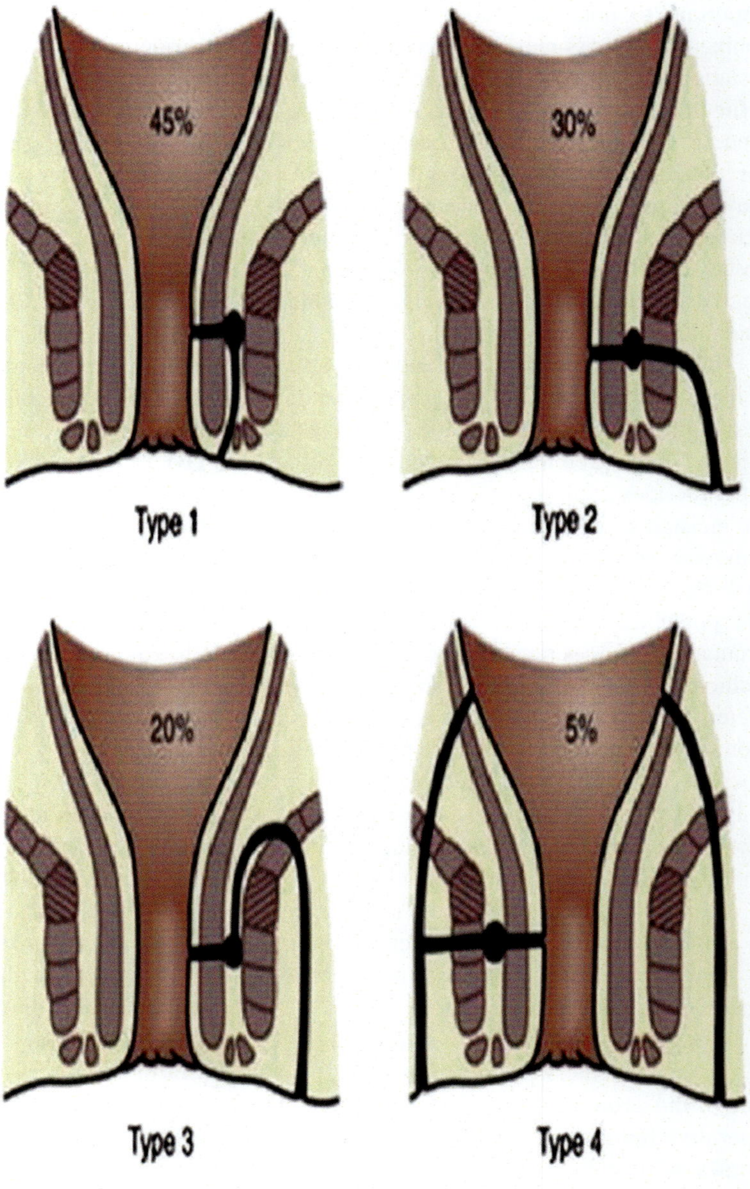

Fig. 28.6 Classification of fistulas. 1. Intersphincteric; 2. Transsphincteric; 3. Suprasphincteric; 4. Extrasphincteric. *Source: Sneider EB & Maykel JA. Anal abscess and fistula. Gastroent. Clin. Of NA, 2013 (Figs. 2 & 3), Publ. Elsevier*

abscess and permits appropriate fibrosis of the tract. Approximately 8 weeks are allowed for fibrosis to occur and then the fistula is reevaluated for the second step procedure. In the second step, three options are available to the surgeon to obliterate the fistula tract: (1) fistulotomy, (2) ligation of intersphincteric tract, or (3) rectal mucosal advancement flap [3].

Fistulotomy should be reserved for those who have minimal muscle involvement. The tract is then opened widely, the edges are marsupialized, and the tract is allowed to granulate and heal by secondary intention.

In ligation of intersphincteric fistula tract, the intersphincteric groove is identified and a 3–4 cm incision made over this plane. A probe is passed through the fistula. Dissection is then carried down toward the fistula with the probe assisting in the identification of the tract along its whole length. A right angle clamp is then used to circumferentially isolate the fistula within the groove. The probe is removed and ligation of the tract is done with 2-0 vicryl sutures on both sides (ends) and the fistula is then sharply divided between the suture ligatures. The intersphincteric plane is then approximated, first at the muscular layer and then at the skin level.

Endorectal advancement flap is coverage of the internal opening with healthy anorectal mucosa. The fistula tract is identified with a probe. Dissection is initiated 1 cm distal to the internal os and a curvilinear broad based flap partial or full thickness is raised about 3–4 cm. Once the flap is made, the opening within the muscle layer is closed with a 3-0 suture. The distal portion of the flap is then trimmed including the internal opening. The flap is then sutured to the distal wound edge. This procedure should be performed primarily by those who have done this before and are already familiar with the technique and should be reserved for fistulas which have recurred.

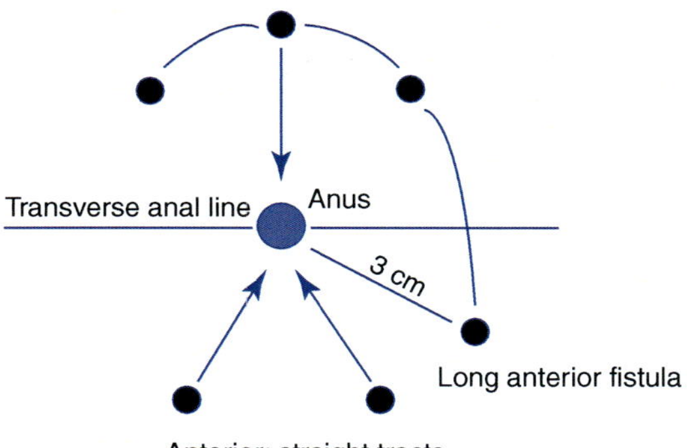

Fig. 28.7 Goodsall's rule. *Source: Feingold, D.L., Kiely, J.M. (2019). Cannot Find Internal Opening of Fistula-in-Ano. In: Lee, S., Steele, S., Feingold, D., Ross, H., Rivadeneira, D. (eds) Colorectal Surgery Consultation. Springer, Cham.* https://doi.org/10.1007/978-3-030-11181-6_27

Complex fistulas can become recurrent despite multiple attempts at closure. Such recurrent fistulas and those related to specific etiologies, such as rectourethral, rectovaginal, or malignant fistulas, may require a transabdominal approach to resolve. In those cases, occasionally a more proximal stoma may be needed to divert the flow of stool to control the fistula and allow appropriate repair and healing [3].

Anorectal Infections

Anorectal infections are frequent in LMICs and can be unfamiliar to physicians in HICs. There are infectious etiologies that may cause colitis and extend distally into the rectum or others that are specific pathogens associated with proctitis. The infectious colitis specific pathogens are covered separately in Chap. 27 about

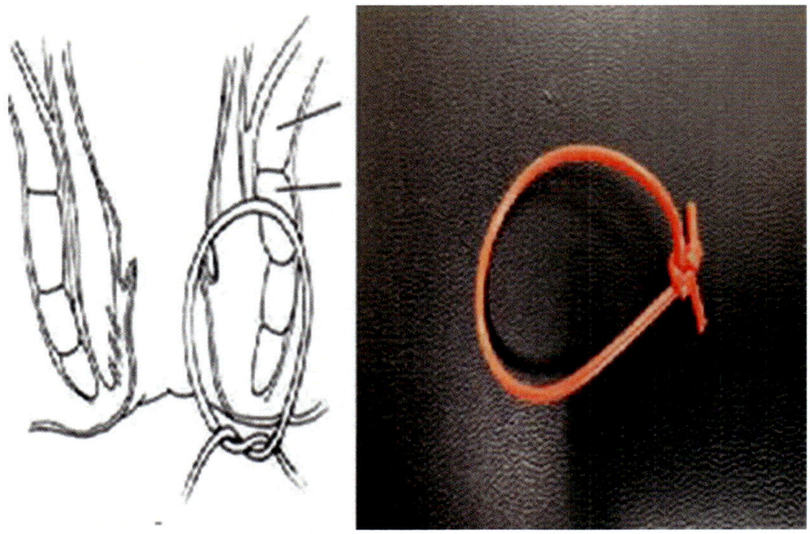

Fig. 28.8 Seton placement using a soft vessel loop. *Source:* www.drmaherabbas.com, *courtesy of Maher A. Abbas, MD, FACS, FASCRS, Post Anorectal Surgery Care*

the acute abdomen. Focusing on proctitis-specific pathogens, one must be alert to a patient's sexual history and risk factors for transmission. Treatment of potential contacts must be considered. Other potential anorectal infections include HPV, HIV/AIDS, molluscum, lice, scabies, or TB.

Proctitis is the inflammation of the rectum. Patients will complain of anorectal pain, tenesmus, and discharge. This can often be confused with inflammatory bowel disease so a careful history must be obtained including a sexual history. Please see Table 28.2 for the list of pathogens and their recommended treatment. The exact diagnosis is frequently unclear so workup must begin with anal swabs for culture (HSV, chlamydia, and gonorrhea). This should be done prior to lubrication or DRE. Treatment is started empirically with broad antiviral drugs and antibiotics. This can be narrowed as culture results return (Fig. 28.9).

Human papillomavirus (HPV) (condylomas) has approximately 40 subtypes with only some that cause condylomas (type 6 and 11) and others that are associated with possible precursors to anal malignancies (type 16 and 18). Many of these patients have a sexual history of anal receptive intercourse. HPV is also frequently associated with HIV so HPV proctitis should trigger further investigations for HIV since both are found in the same high-risk groups. The goal of treatment of HPV is primarily to treat the symptoms of HPV since the warts can often self-resolve. Treatment options for warts include home-based treatment regimens or surgical management. Home-based regimens include applications of podofilox, imiquimod, or sinecatechins. Surgical treatments are usually reserved for those with extensive burden of warts. Options include excision/cautery, cryotherapy, or provider application of trichloroacetic or bichloroacetic acid. HPV is closely associated with precursor lesions to squamous cell

Table 28.2 Anorectal bacterial pathogens, presentation, and treatment

Pathogen	Presentation	Testing	Treatment	Notes
Syphilis	Papules	RPR, Darkfield examination	PCN 2.4million units IM × 1	Latent syphilis has systemic presentation
HSV	Vesicles	NAAT, culture, serologic testing	Valganciclovir 1 g po bid × 10 days	Counsel, educate, and treat partner
Chancroid	Deep painful ulcer with lymphadenopathy	NAAT, culture	Azithromycin 1 g po × 1	Counsel, educate, and treat partner
Donovanosis	Painless nodules that develop into ulcer	Difficult to culture, Donovan bodies on tissue crush biopsy	Azithromycin 1 g po >3 weeks	Treat till all lesions are healed
Lymphogranuloma venereum (LGV)	Anal pain, discharge, tenesmus	NAAT	Doxycycline 100 mg bid × 21 days	Retest in 3 months after treatment; all partners within 60 days should be treated as well

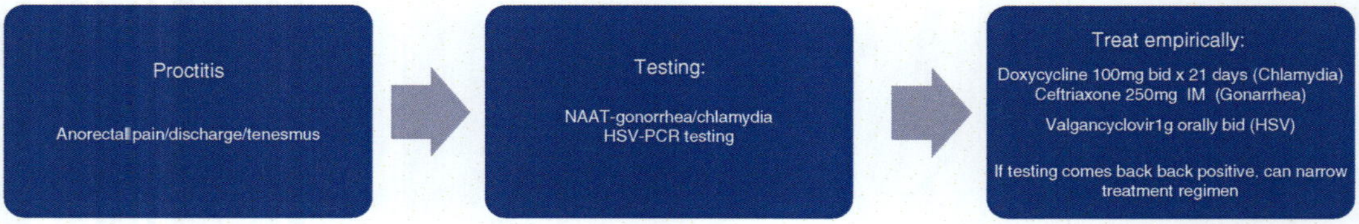

Fig. 28.9 Proctitis management

carcinoma. It is uncertain whether these lesions are causative for squamous cell carcinoma and therefore some advocate destruction of these precursor lesions with serial high resolution anoscopy exams and cauterization to prevent progression to cancer. Others argue that there is a low risk of developing anal cancer and do not support serial exams and ablation of these lesions. When available, the HPV vaccine should be administered to everyone prior to the initiation of sexual activity. A study performed in female sex workers in Ibadan, Nigeria, found the prevalence of HPV infection to be as high as 88% in the vulva, 84% in the cervix, and 75% in the anus. Development of cervical cancer is also known to be associated with HPV infections and patients should have annual Papanicolaou smears. There is little doubt that all high-risk populations should urgently be vaccinated against HPV to at least prevent continued transmission [6]. There are bivalent vaccines that focus on oncogenic subtypes and there are quadrivalent vaccines whose major protection is against HPV 6, 11, 16, and 18. These vaccines could probably reduce significantly the risk of anal cancers. Unfortunately, the vaccines are still not readily available worldwide and especially in LMICs.

HIV/AIDS may present initially with anorectal issues such as a fissure; therefore suspicion should be high dependent on patient risk factors and presentation. Another manifestation of HIV/AIDS could be an anal ulcer, abscess, or fistula. Ulcers are often more proximal than the common fissures. Fissures infected with HIV/AIDS may present in an atypical position and may therefore be difficult to locate and track.

Molluscum contagiosum can also present initially in the perianal region. Diagnosis is often made by visual confirmation as molluscum have characteristic features. These include papules that have waxy domes with an umbilication centrally. If there is uncertainty and a PCR test is available, it should be done (it may not be available on site). The disease is persistent in immunocompromised patients and treatment is similar to genital warts. Imiquimod can be applied topically, or these lesions can be removed surgically by excision, cautery, or cryotherapy.

Pubic lice is caused by the parasite *Pthirus pubis*. Transmission is usually from a close contact which may be sexual or just from sheets or mattresses as it jumps from one patient to the next one. Recommended treatment is permethrin 1% cream or pyrethrins 0.3%/piperonyl butoxide 4% cream. Sheets/linens/clothing must also be treated in hot water.

Scabies is caused by the mite *Sarcoptes scabiei.* Skin contact is required for transmission as mites do not jump. Mites burrow in folds/webs/creases and burrow into skin. They can mimic a pruritic rash in the groin or buttock region. Diagnosis is often by visualization and can be confirmed by skin scrapings. Treatment is with topical permethrin 5% cream. Oral regimen with ivermectin can be used as either first or second line of treatment. Like with lice, sheets/linens/clothing must be treated in hot water and heat dried to eradicate the mites [3].

Tuberculosis, among its many presentations, can also initially present as an anal lesion. It is rare that it is confined to the anus and therefore full systemic workup needs to be initiated. The initial presentation of anal TB can vary from ulceration to fissures, to fistulas. High suspicion for tuberculosis should be considered if anorectal treatment of a lesion is refractory to standard treatments. To confirm the diagnosis of anal TB, a scraping of the lesion should be examined with acid-fast stain of a smear and/or biopsy of the lesion or PCR. Anal TB can also often mimic anal malignancies by not responding to treatment. While it has been reported that anal TB is rare and accounts for only 1% of all GI-related TB cases [7], a recent study which evaluated pus/samples taken from anorectal abscess/fistulas revealed that TB was found in 13.7% of patients' samples by GeneXpert testing [8]. Treatment of anorectal TB includes standard anti-TB therapy. In cases of anorectal obstruction by inflammation and stenosis, a temporary diverting stoma should be created and reversed after remission of TB and of obstruction.

Anal Cancer

Workup of anal cancer consists of diagnosis, staging, and then treatment planning. The etiology of anal cancer appears to be due to HPV infection. The progression is thought to be HPV infection (subtypes 16 and 18) leading to dysplasia resulting in anal intraepithelial neoplasia (AIN). AIN then progresses to anal squamous cell carcinoma. This pathway from virus leading to neoplasia is especially concerning in immunocompromised individuals. These and high-risk patients (men who have sex with men, MSM) should be monitored more carefully for anal cancer. With the prevalence of HIV/AIDS in some LMICs, specifically in sub-Saharan Africa, this specific population should be counseled and monitored for these issues.

Squamous cell carcinoma (SCC) is the most common malignancy of the anal canal and anal region while adenocarcinoma is very rare. The incidence of anal carcinoma was relatively rare in LMICs at approximately 3% of malignancies in the past, but it has increased significantly with the increased incidence of HIV/AIDS as outlined above. The symptoms can mimic many of the conditions that have been described above and include pain, anal mass, bleeding, change in bowel habits and narrow stools, and sometimes a feeling of fullness in the rectum. The diagnosis starts with DRE and progresses to anoscopy and colonoscopy with biopsies of the lesion. Blood tests and total body CT scan should be performed to rule out metastases. In the past, treatment of anal SCC consisted of surgical resection, sometimes abdominoperineal resections, or for smaller tumors of 1 cm or less wide local excision. There is now a debate as to the correct course of action for anal intraepithelial neoplasia. While some advocate for no intervention and simply observation for mild dysplasia, others advocate for treatment of even mild dysplasia with surgical excision and/or cautery. Effective treatment of AIN includes ablation with electrocautery; this can be aided with high resolution anoscopy to specifically target areas of dysplasia. This should be done for moderate- and high-grade dysplasia. It is important to be mindful of not excising and cauterizing too much anal tissue as this may lead to anal stricture and stenosis. Serial exams and observations are required every 3–6 months of serial evaluations [3].

If left untreated, moderate- and high-grade dysplasia can progress to anal cancer. Presentation is often anal pain and bleeding. Examination will reveal a mass which should be biopsied. Initial workup should also include a careful physical examination with abdominal examination inclusive of inguinal node examination. Anoscopy can sometimes be limited due to pain from the malignant lesion. Therefore, examination under anesthesia may be warranted to fully appreciate the extent of the tumor and permit a biopsy. It is important to document the size of the lesion prior to biopsy and the location in relation to anal verge (distance), presence within the anal canal, and/or location in the anal margin.

Biopsy is important as even unsightly masses may not be cancer. Buschke-Lowenstein tumors are such an example. Similar in etiology from anal carcinoma, the pathogen is HPV virus and progression is from small condylomata acuminata to a large cauliflower like lesion. As opposed to anal carcinoma, treatment management is surgical excision alone [9].

Anal squamous cell carcinoma, after diagnosis, needs appropriate staging with CT of the chest/abdomen/pelvis to rule out its extent and any metastasis. HIV testing and cervical evaluation (pap smear) should be pursued to perform a comprehensive workup. Case discussion regarding treatment plan should be done in conjunction with oncology and radiation oncology. For small select cases of anal margin cancers (tumor size less than 1 cm and no involvement of sphincter musculature), surgical excision alone can be curative.

Most recent approach to the treatment of large tumors with local invasion has focused on the use of chemoradiation which has revolutionized the treatment of SCC as it has improved local recurrence rates as well as survival. It rarely requires colostomy which is frequently not accepted by patients in LMICs. Since the number of cases of anal cancer is on the rise in Africa, especially in HIV infected women where it is 3.9 to 30 per million, as well as men, greater attention than ever should be focused on early diagnosis of any anal complaints and on prevention by vaccination against HPV.

Anal melanoma is another neoplasia within the anorectal region that has poor prognosis. It represents 1–4% of all anorectal malignancies, and therefore it should be included in the differential diagnosis. Lesions are often pigmented or present as an ulceration. There is often distant metastatic disease at the time of diagnosis so the discussion is usually geared towards palliation rather than cure [3].

Anal adenocarcinoma accounts for 3% of anal cancers. These are treated like rectal adenocarcinoma and should be staged similarly. Like rectal cancers, treatment discussion and plan should be done in a multi-disciplinary fashion with oncology and radiation oncology [3].

Especially in late presentation of anorectal malignancies, it is important to address the urgent issues of prognosis and complications of treatment prior to discussion of cure or therapy. Anal neoplasia can potentially fistulize leading to infections (GU/GYN), obstruct, or bleed causing severe anemia. These acute issues must be addressed initially while the oncologic workup proceeds simultaneously. These problems may imply diversion with an ostomy for obstructions or fistulas that cause sepsis. Transfusions may be needed to replete blood loss for anemia. It is most important that at these late stages, the futility of cure and discussions of palliative goals should be discussed with patient and their family.

Since anal cancer does not require emergency treatment, patients who are discovered to have it should be promptly transferred to tertiary centers where surgical and medical oncology teams may apply the latest modalities of treatment.

Conclusion

This chapter offers a brief review of the urgent surgical anal problems that a general surgeon is likely to face in LMICs, both in the clinic and in the emergency room. Most of these conditions are not life threatening and can be treated successfully, once properly diagnosed. The diagnosis can be sometimes confusing and the surgeon must be very aware that benign diagnoses such as hemorrhoids may be masking a more dangerous diagnosis such as a malignancy. Most of the infectious problems can be treated successfully if the infectious agent is properly identified. The discomfort of pain, disturbed bowel movements, and occasional anal bleeding can be frequently relieved by office or outpatient procedures performed under local anesthesia. Other problems, like abscesses, may require hospital admissions, drainage, and intense course of antibiotics to avoid occasional death from septicemia. The high frequency of anal pathology makes this type of surgical care urgently needed in LMICs as it is in HICs. Although the incidence of anal malignancies is much lower in LMICs than in HICs, it is on the rise and is frequently associated with HPV and HIV. The modern treatment of these malignancies is still best practiced in tertiary centers in LMICs and it is strongly recommended that once diagnosed, patients be referred there where chemoradiation therapy can be applied and selective surgical procedures can be performed by experts.

References

1. Wexner, S.a.B., D, Fundamentals of Anorectal Surgery. 1998. https://www.amazon.com/Fundamentals-Anorectal-Surgery-David-Beck/dp/0702023663.
2. Kibret AA, Oumer M, Moges AM. Prevalence and associated factors of hemorrhoids among adult patients visiting the surgical outpatient department in the University of Gondar Comprehensive Specialized Hospital, Northwest Ethiopia. PLoS One. 2021;16(4):e0249736.
3. Steele S. The ASCRS manual of colon rectal surgery. 2019. https://www.amazon.com/ASCRS-Manual-Colon-Rectal-Surgery/dp/303001164X/ref=asc_df_303001164X/?tag=hyprod-20&linkCode=df0&hvadid=333072128347&hvpos=&hvnetw=g&hvrand=452502010252282729&hvpone=&hvptwo=&hvqmt=&hvdev=c&hvdvcmdl=&hvlocint=&hvlocphy=9021556&hvtargid=pla-649739926449&psc=1.
4. Alatise OI, et al. Health-seeking behavior and barriers to Care in Patients with Rectal Bleeding in Nigeria. J Glob Oncol. 2017;3(6):749–56.
5. Ashebir DZ, Gebreselassie HA. Pattern and outcome of colorectal and perianal surgery in a Referral Hospital, Addis Ababa, Ethiopia. Ethiop J Health Sci. 2021;31(5):985–92.
6. Morhason-Bello IO, et al. Oral, genital and anal human papillomavirus infections among female

sex workers in Ibadan, Nigeria. PLoS One. 2022;17(3):e0265269.
7. Malikowski T, et al. Tuberculosis of the gastrointestinal tract and associated viscera. J Clin Tuberc Other Mycobact Dis. 2018;12:1–8.
8. Garg P, et al. Diagnosis of anorectal tuberculosis by polymerase chain reaction, GeneXpert and histopathology in 1336 samples in 776 anal fistula patients. World J Gastrointest Surg. 2021;13(4):355–65.
9. Kadouri Y, Nouini Y. Buschke-Lowenstein tumor. Pan Afr Med J. 2020;36:359.

How to Manage Hernias in Limited-Resource Settings

29

Imad Aljabban and Zachary Gleit

Success is not the key to happiness. Happiness is the key to success. If you love what you are doing, you will be successful.

– Albert Schweitzer

Abbreviations

CT	Computed tomography
LMICs	Low- and middle-income countries
MRI	Magnetic resonance imagining
US	Ultrasonography
WHO	World Health Organization

Introduction

The anterolateral abdominal wall is a complex structure involved in a myriad of functions, including protecting the abdominal viscera from injury, trunk mobility, ventilation, and regulation of intra-abdominal pressure. Abdominal wall hernias are protrusions of abdominal contents through the musculofascial layers of the abdominal wall and represent one of the most common problems encountered by the general surgeon. In this chapter, we will limit our discussion to the most common kinds of groin (inguinal and femoral) and ventral abdominal (primary and incisional) hernias. Diaphragmatic, lumbar, spigelian, obturator, and other rare abdominal wall hernias are beyond the scope of this discussion.

Hernias are often diagnosed by physical exam, but in some instances ultrasonography (US) or computed tomography (CT) may be useful in further characterizing anatomy and hernia contents, presence of bowel obstruction, and potential bowel compromise. Indications for repair of hernias include pain or discomfort, and the treatment or prevention of conditions associated with acute incarceration—namely, strangulation and obstruction. Techniques for repair are varied, including open and laparoscopic approaches, with or without mesh prostheses.

Availability of hospital resources has the potential to impact modalities of diagnosis and treatment significantly. Surgeons in some low- and middle-income countries (LMICs) often lack the equipment necessary to adequately diagnose and provide a durable repair of abdominal wall

I. Aljabban
Post-Graduate Residency Fellow, Department of Surgery, NY Presbyterian Hospital,
New York, NY, USA
e-mail: ia2444@cumc.columbia.edu

Z. Gleit (✉)
Department of Surgery, Columbia University Vagelos College of Physicians & Surgeons,
New York, NY, USA
e-mail: zlg1@columbia.edu

M. A. Hardy, B. R. Hochman (eds.), *Global Surgery*, https://doi.org/10.1007/978-3-031-28127-3_29

hernias. Here we will discuss the barriers providers face in LMICs and methods that may be employed for optimal repair. Some of the limitations that the surgeon faces in LMICs when it comes to the diagnosis and repair of abdominal wall hernias include availability of diagnostic imaging, laparoscopic equipment, and prosthetic mesh.

Imaging

The first-line modality for the diagnosis of abdominal wall hernias is careful physical examination, which is sufficient in most cases. The patient should be evaluated while supine and standing. A Valsalva maneuver may be useful in demonstrating the hernia. Physical exam may need to be supplemented if the hernia is small or subtle, or if the exam is limited by the patient's body habitus (obesity) or difficulty in cooperating with the physical exam. In these cases, US is a sensitive diagnostic tool in identifying the hernia defect [1]. When US is non-diagnostic, cross-sectional imaging (CT) can be used.

Lack of imaging availability in LMICs may be due to the cost of equipment, lack of resources for maintenance, and limited availability of trained technicians to perform imaging studies. However, compared to CT and magnetic resonance imaging (MRI), US is safe, inexpensive, and mobile. In a study conducted in Rwanda, Noble et al. demonstrated that a short training program led to the successful uptake of US by hospital clinicians in limited-resource environments, with acceptable accuracy and a significant impact on clinical decision-making [2]. The World Health Organization (WHO) estimated that nearly 50% of LMICs did not have access to US in 1997, but evidence suggests that US availability and usage has increased significantly in the last decade [3]. Although US has become increasingly less expensive, lack of sonography training continues to be a major reason for underutilization [4].

When US is non-diagnostic, CT may be useful for diagnosis and operative planning for abdominal wall hernias. Indeed, in high-income countries (HIC), CT is often the imaging modality of choice for investigation of ventral hernias, but CT is much less available in LMICs: there is one CT scanner per 25,000 people in HIC, but only one per 1.7 million people in LMICs [5].

Laparoscopy

Modern surgical techniques for ventral and groin hernia repair include robotic and laparoscopic ("minimally invasive") approaches in addition to open approaches. In ideal circumstances, the surgical approach is individualized to each patient. Laparoscopic and robotic repairs have advantages that potentially include easier recovery, lower risks of chronic pain, better visualization of abdominal wall and hernia anatomy, and lower risks of wound complications related to large open wounds. However, robotic and laparoscopic repairs require surgical expertise, and equipment and instruments that may not be available in limited-resource environments. In addition, laparoscopic and robotic hernia repairs typically require general anesthesia, which can often be avoided for the repair of groin hernias and small ventral hernias. General anesthesia itself is associated with significant resource demands and expense. Because of the resource requirements of minimally invasive surgery, minimally invasive techniques are beyond the scope of this chapter.

Availability of Mesh

Over the last four decades, hernia repairs involving the use of synthetic mesh have largely supplanted non-mesh repairs, except for small primary ventral hernias. In multiple contexts, mesh has been shown to decrease recurrence rates substantially, and some data suggest that mesh repairs are associated with more-rapid recovery. Although simple polypropylene mesh implants are fairly inexpensive by the standards of HIC, with estimates ranging as low as $40–50 for typical implants [6], healthcare expenses are frequently paid out-of-pocket in LIC, where many live on less than $2 per day [7]. For this reason, cheaper alternatives to commercial mesh have been investigated and will be discussed later in his chapter.

Historically and prior to the availability of synthetic mesh, complex procedures involving muscle and fascial flaps were advocated for hernia repair. We do not advocate these repairs in limited-resource settings, since we think that surgical expertise for these unusual procedures is likely less available than mesh. In emergency settings, the use of temporizing procedures (such as primary repair or soft-tissue closure, with the expectation of a hernia recurrence) until adequate resources are available is more prudent than attempting a complex repair with a high failure rate and a significant likelihood of making subsequent repair more complicated.

Less expensive alternatives to commercially produced mesh have been studied, mainly in the setting of inguinal hernia repair. The use of mosquito netting, discussed below, has been especially well-investigated, but there are very limited data regarding its use other than for inguinal hernias.

Observation Vs Repair

Estimates of the risk of acute incarceration for ventral and inguinal hernias vary, but this risk is likely to be low, less than 3% at 5 years for incisional hernias [8] and less than 3% at 7 years for small inguinal hernias [9]. Risk of hernia-related emergency is related to the site and size of the hernia, so it is difficult to generalize, and clinical judgment is appropriate.

Though several studies have supported the idea that observation of small, asymptomatic or minimally symptomatic inguinal hernias is a safe strategy, there are also abundant data suggesting that the crossover rate from observation to operative repair is high. Fitzgibbons et al. reported that nearly a third of men initially pursuing a strategy of watchful waiting with regard to their minimally symptomatic inguinal hernias crossed over to the repair group within 2 years, generally because of an increase in pain [10]. With longer follow-up, the authors reported a nearly 70% crossover rate after 7 years [9]. Thus, although repair of small inguinal hernias is rarely urgent, a planned repair is generally appropriate.

Similar outcomes have been demonstrated with regard to minimally symptomatic ventral hernias. In a retrospective study with more than a thousand patients, 19% and 16% of patients with incisional and umbilical/epigastric hernias (respectively) who were initially asymptomatic elected to have surgery over a period of 5 years. However, when comparing readmission, reoperation, and overall mortality, there was no difference between the cross-over group and those who elected to have surgery initially [11], again suggesting that there is generally little urgency to repair.

In non-urgent settings, abdominal binders are simple and inexpensive and can offer palliation of reducible ventral hernias by reducing the discomfort associated with visceral bulging and by providing stability to the abdominal wall. They may be especially useful when temporizing is desirable – for instance, if timing is inconvenient or suitable resources are temporarily unavailable. Their efficacy is dependent on the ability to find a binder that provides suitable support to the area of herniation without migrating on the abdominal wall. They are mainly helpful when the patient is active, and they need not be worn during times of rest or recumbency. Binders are likely to be of less use in chronically incarcerated ventral hernias.

Similarly, a hernia belt or truss may be helpful to treat the symptoms of inguinal hernia when surgery is to be deferred, though some evidence suggests that only a minority of patients will achieve symptom control [12]. Attention to fit is important, and patients should be instructed on how to wear them; in particular, a truss should be donned when the hernia has been reduced, and the part of the truss that supports the hernia must be accurately located near the external inguinal ring in order to provide appropriately localized pressure.

Groin Hernias

Inguinal hernia repairs are among the most common surgical procedures performed worldwide. It has been estimated that more than 25% of men will undergo inguinal hernia repair during their lifetimes [13], and inguinal hernia repair is thought to be the most common surgical procedure worldwide. Femoral hernias are far less common than inguinal hernias, and they are more common in women than in men. Numerous techniques for inguinal hernia repair have been developed, and these can generally be performed under local anesthesia in outpatient settings. Of note, most modern guidelines recommend mesh techniques [14]. Especially in non-specialist hands, mesh repairs have been shown to have lower recurrence rates with at least comparable risks of chronic pain and very low risks of other complications. However, commercially produced mesh may not be readily available in LIC, and, as mentioned above, it can be expensive (in excess of $100 according to one report) [7].

The Shouldice repair is the best-studied modern non-mesh technique for inguinal hernia repairs. It involves a multi-layer repair of the inguinal floor, starting with incision of the inguinal floor and release of the cribriform fascia inferior to the inguinal ligament, providing mobility to the external oblique aponeurosis. The inguinal floor is repaired in two overlapping layers, by sewing the two divided flaps of the inguinal floor/transversalis fascia to the conjoined tendon/internal oblique aponeurosis and to the shelving edge of the inguinal ligament respectively. This repair of the floor is then imbricated by approximating the external oblique aponeurosis to the conjoined tendon/internal oblique aponeurosis, again in two overlapping layers. In experienced hands and appropriately selected patients (generally excluding recurrent hernias or scrotal hernias), some studies have reported recurrence rates comparable to those associated with open mesh repairs. However, other studies have failed to confirm these results, and meta-analyses suggest that recurrence rates are worse with the Shouldice repair than with mesh repairs, though better than with traditional non-mesh repairs [15].

In 2001, Dr. Mohan Desarda published a technique for non-mesh inguinal hernia repair that seems to be simpler than the Shouldice repair [16]. It involves creating a pedicle of external oblique aponeurosis that is then sutured to the inguinal ligament inferolaterally and to the conjoined tendon/internal oblique aponeurosis superomedially. The external oblique pedicle is sewn in a similar fashion to that in which mesh is sutured over the inguinal floor in a Lichtenstein repair. Although data are more limited than for the Shouldice repair, studies have reported recurrence rates that are similar to those following a Lichtenstein mesh repair, even with long-term follow-up [17]. As with the Shouldice repair, however, patient selection may be important; in particular the external oblique aponeurosis has to be intact and strong enough to permit a durable reinforcement of the inguinal floor. To date, there are no studies that directly compare the Desarda and Shouldice techniques.

The Lichtenstein mesh inguinal hernia repair is generally regarded as the standard against which other open inguinal hernia repairs are measured. It is a straightforward procedure, in which a synthetic mesh bridge is placed across the inguinal floor and sewn to the shelving edge of the inguinal ligament inferolaterally and to the conjoined tendon/internal oblique aponeurosis superomedially. Mosquito netting has been studied as a replacement for commercially produced mesh for this procedure. It is cheap and widely available, and it is similar to commercially produced mesh in construction and makeup. It is often made of polymers (especially nylon, polyester, and polyethylene) that are used in surgical implants. Several studies over the last 25 years have investigated the use of mosquito netting in place of commercially available mesh for groin hernia repair, without evidence of worse outcome in short-term or even long-term follow-up [18]; however long-term data are limited. Of note, however, different mosquito netting products are made of different materials and are not subject to the same quality-control and reporting regimens associated with commercially available hernia mesh. Attention must be paid to adequate sterilization and, of course, only mosquito netting that is not impregnated with insecticide should be used.

Femoral hernias are much rarer than inguinal hernias and hence are less well-studied. Both mesh and non-mesh repairs have been described.

A modification of the Shouldice repair incorporating Cooper's ligament into the inguinal floor reconstruction addresses both inguinal and femoral hernias. Similarly, the Lichtenstein repair can be modified to include Cooper's ligament rather than the inguinal ligament inferomedial to the femoral vein, thereby closing the femoral canal.

Ventral Hernias

Ventral hernias are hernias that occur on the anterior or ventral surface of the abdomen. They may be further subdivided into primary and incisional hernias. Primary ventral hernias occur spontaneously without prior surgical trauma to the abdominal wall in their vicinity, and they may be either congenital or acquired. The most common primary ventral hernias are umbilical and epigastric hernias; they have a high prevalence in the population (in excess of 20% of the population in one screening study [19]). Incisional hernias are related to the failure and breakdown of abdominal wall closure following abdominal surgical incisions and have been estimated to occur in about 10% of patients following midline laparotomy [20].

Primary ventral hernias are almost always in the midline (spigelian hernias, which are rare and will not be discussed here, are a notable exception). Incisional hernias can occur at any site of incision but are also most common in the midline. Perhaps the most effective intervention to decrease the health-care burden of incisional hernias is proper surgical technique to prevent their occurrence to begin with. Minimizing the use of midline incisions when feasible is one way to accomplish this: the risk of incisional hernia after midline laparotomy has been estimated to be 11%, and less than half that if a transverse incision is used [21]. Similarly, the use of nonabsorbable or slowly absorbable suture instead of rapidly absorbable suture has been shown to decrease the risk of subsequent incisional hernia [21]. Finally, when midline incisions are used, a small-bite closure technique has been shown to decrease the rate of hernia formation significantly (from 21% to 13% in one randomized trial [22]); with this technique, a relatively fine (2-0) suture is used to take fascial bites of 5 mm every 5 mm, rather than taking larger bites with more travel and a larger-caliber suture.

For epigastric and umbilical hernias up to 2 cm in diameter, primary repair is associated with a relatively low recurrence rate (8% in one study of small umbilical hernias [23]), though even for these small hernias, this risk of recurrence is more than twice the recurrence risk when mesh is used. Small, primary hernias can generally be repaired under local anesthesia. For larger hernias and for almost all incisional hernias, the recurrence risk for non-mesh repairs is unacceptably high (22% for umbilical hernias larger than 2 cm in the afore-mentioned study [23], and 33% for incisional hernias according to a Cochrane review [24]). Multiple techniques for mesh repairs of ventral hernias have been described, including inlay (within the peritoneal cavity), preperitoneal, retromuscular, and onlay techniques.

Unlike for inguinal hernias, mosquito netting in place of commercially produced mesh has not been well studied in the setting of ventral hernias, perhaps because incisional and large primary ventral hernias are much less common than inguinal hernias. We are aware of one case series describing the use of mosquito netting in this setting, but follow-up was short [25]. In principle, the experience in the setting of ventral hernias might not be expected to be significantly different than that for inguinal hernias. However, ventral hernia repair may require a significantly larger mesh patch than is necessary for inguinal hernias, and the risk of surgical-site complications (seromas and infections, in particular) is significantly higher for large ventral hernias. Thus, the experience with ventral hernias might differ from that noted with inguinal hernias.

Different forms of myofascial release have been described to provide increased mobility to the abdominal wall to permit primary repair for midline hernias and theoretically avoid the use of mesh. The underlying principle is that if the fascia and muscle layers are separated from each other, the rectus muscles can be advanced to midline, allowing restoration of the midline and linea alba. This can be done with an anterior or posterior/transversus abdominis component release. Anterior component separation has been particularly described as a technique to avoid the use of mesh and may be useful when mesh is unavailable or the surgeon chooses to avoid it. Anterior component separation can result in 20 cm of mobilization of the rectus muscles. The procedure involves creating a subcutaneous flap over the external oblique past the linea semilunaris. An incision is made in the external oblique aponeurosis just lateral to the linea semilunaris, and the external oblique aponeurosis is separated from the underlying internal oblique muscle. Incising the posterior rectus sheaths medially, at the margins of the hernia on each side, creates additional mobility, allowing for midline approximation with reduction in tension [26]. However, this technique and posterior component separation (involving division of the transversus abdominis muscle and dissection between this divided muscle and the more-superficial muscle layers) are generally combined with mesh reinforcement when possible. Recurrences following myofascial release procedures are difficult to repair, and we therefore do not advocate these non-mesh approaches except in extenuating circumstances. Again, in urgent circumstances, it is often preferable to perform a simpler temporizing procedure (such as primary closure or soft-tissue closure) with a plan to fix a likely recurrence under optimal circumstances in the future.

Conclusion

Hernias are the most common healthcare challenge requiring surgical expertise worldwide. Most hernias can be repaired with minimal demands for extensive surgical or anesthetic resources or need for advanced expertise. Mesh repairs have revolutionized the surgical approach to hernia repair and are widely advocated for most hernia repairs. Though commercially produced mesh is comparatively expensive, cheap replacements for mesh (namely, mosquito netting) have been extensively used and studied. For uncomplicated groin hernias and small ventral hernias, non-mesh techniques exist, with acceptable reported outcomes.

References

1. Simons MP, et al. International guidelines for groin hernia management. Hernia. 2018; https://doi.org/10.1007/s10029-017-1668-x.
2. Shah SP, et al. Impact of the introduction of ultrasound services in a limited resource setting: rural Rwanda 2008. BMC Int Health Hum Rights. 2009; https://doi.org/10.1186/1472-698X-9-4.
3. Stewart KA, et al. Trends in ultrasound use in low and middle income countries: a systematic review. Int J MCH AIDS. 2020; https://doi.org/10.21106/ijma.294.
4. Shah S, et al. Perceived barriers in the use of ultrasound in developing countries. Crit Ultrasound J. 2015; https://doi.org/10.1186/s13089-015-0028-2.
5. Hricak H, et al. Medical imaging and nuclear medicine: a lancet oncology commission. Lancet Oncol. 2021; https://doi.org/10.1016/S1470-2045(20)30751-8.
6. Alkhoury F, Helton S, Ippolito RJ. Cost and clinical outcomes of laparoscopic ventral hernia repair using intraperitoneal nonheavyweight polypropylene mesh. Surg Laparosc Endosc Percutan Tech. 2011; https://doi.org/10.1097/SLE.0b013e3182139602.
7. Löfgren J, et al. A randomized trial of low-cost mesh in groin hernia repair. N Engl J Med. 2016; https://doi.org/10.1056/nejmoa1505126.
8. Dadashzadeh ER, et al. The risk of incarceration during nonoperative management of incisional hernias. Ann Surg. 2022; https://doi.org/10.1097/SLA.0000000000003916.
9. Fitzgibbons RJ, et al. Long-term results of a randomized controlled trial of a nonoperative strategy (watchful waiting) for men with minimally symptomatic inguinal hernias. Ann Surg. 2013; https://doi.org/10.1097/SLA.0b013e3182a19725.
10. Fitzgibbons RJ, et al. Watchful waiting vs repair of inguinal hernia in minimally symptomatic men: a randomized clinical trial. J Am Med Assoc. 2006; https://doi.org/10.1001/jama.295.3.285.
11. Kokotovic D, Sjølander H, Gögenur I, Helgstrand F. Watchful waiting as a treatment strategy for patients with a ventral hernia appears to be safe. Hernia. 2016; https://doi.org/10.1007/s10029-016-1464-z.
12. Law NW, Trapnell JE. Does a truss benefit a patient with inguinal hernia? BMJ. 1992; https://doi.org/10.1136/bmj.304.6834.1092.
13. Primatest P, Goldachre MJ. Inguinal hernia repair: incidence of elective and emergency surgery, readmission and mortality. Int J Epidemiol. 1996; https://doi.org/10.1093/ije/25.4.835.
14. The HerniaSurge Group. International guidelines for groin hernia management. Hernia. 2018; https://doi.org/10.1007/s10029-017-1668-x.

15. Amato B, et al. Shouldice technique versus other open techniques for inguinal hernia repair. Cochrane Database Syst Rev. 2009; https://doi.org/10.1002/14651858.CD001543.pub3.
16. Desarda MP. Inguinal herniorrhaphy with an undetached strip of external oblique aponeurosis: a new approach used in 400 patients. Eur J Surg. 2001; https://doi.org/10.1080/110241501750243798.
17. Mitura K, et al. Desarda technique as a valuable alternative for inguinal hernia patients refusing mesh implantation: long-term results fifteen years after a pure tissue repair in 198 patients. Mini-invasive Surg. 2021; https://doi.org/10.20517/2574-1225.2021.19.
18. Patterson T, et al. A systematic review and meta-analysis of the post-operative adverse effects associated with mosquito net mesh in comparison to commercial hernia mesh for inguinal hernia repair in low income countries. Hernia. 2017; https://doi.org/10.1007/s10029-017-1608-9.
19. Bedewi MA, et al. Prevalence of adult paraumbilical hernia. Assessment by high-resolution sonography: a hospital-based study. Hernia. 2012; https://doi.org/10.1007/s10029-011-0863-4.
20. Biceknbach KA, et al. Up and down or side to side? A systematic review and meta-analysis examining the impact of incision on outcomes after abdominal surgery. Am J Surg. 2013; https://doi.org/10.1016/j.amjsurg.2012.11.008.
21. Le Huu Nho R, Mege D, Ouaïssi M, Sielezneff I, Sastre B. Incidence and prevention of ventral incisional hernia. J Visc Surg. 2012; https://doi.org/10.1016/j.jviscsurg.2012.05.004.
22. Deerenberg EB, et al. Small bites versus large bites for closure of abdominal midline incisions (STITCH): a double-blind, multicentre, randomised controlled trial. Lancet. 2015; https://doi.org/10.1016/S0140-6736(15)60459-7.
23. Kaufman R, et al. SMesh versus suture repair of umbilical hernia in adults: a randomised, double-blind, controlled, multicentre trial. Lancet. 2018; https://doi.org/10.1016/S0140-6736(18)30298-8.
24. Den Hartog D, et al. Open surgical procedures for incisional hernias. Cochrane Database Syst Rev. 2009; https://doi.org/10.1002/14651858.CD006438.pub2.
25. Dubey V. Use of sterilised nylon mosquito net mesh in incisional hernias. Int J Pharma Bio Sci. 2014;
26. Vargo D. Component separation in the management of the difficult abdominal wall. Am J Surg. 2004; https://doi.org/10.1016/j.amjsurg.2004.08.051.

How to Diagnose and Treat Benign and Malignant Diseases of the Breast in Low- and Middle-Income Countries

30

Soji F. Oluwole and Olakunle O. Oluwole

Often we look so long at the closed door that we do not see the one that has been opened for us.

– Helen Keller

Abbreviations

AI	Aromatase inhibitor
ALND	Axillary lymph node dissection
DCIS	Ductal carcinoma in situ
ER	Estrogen receptor
FNA	Fine needle aspiration
HER	Human epithelial growth factor receptor
HR	Hormone receptor
LCIS	Lobular carcinoma in situ
LMICs	Low- and middle-income countries
MRI	Magnetic resonance imaging
PR	Progesterone receptor
SERM	Selective estrogen receptor modulator
SLNB	Sentinel lymph node biopsy
USG	Ultra-sonography

S. F. Oluwole (✉)
Emeritus Professor of Surgery, Columbia University College of Physicians & Surgeons, New York, NY, USA

Harlem Hospital Center, New York, NY, USA

Cancer Control Center of Harlem, New York, NY, USA

Obafemi Awolowo University, Ile Ife, Nigeria

Old Tappan, NJ, USA
e-mail: so5@columbia.edu

O. O. Oluwole
Old Tappan, NJ, USA

Introduction

Breast diseases, both benign and malignant, are major public health problems encountered in general surgical practices worldwide, especially in low- and moderate-income countries (LMICs). Breast cancer is the most common female cancer worldwide and second leading cause of female cancer death in the USA [1]. Increased awareness of the disease in the wealthy countries and promising new approaches to screening that include mammography and magnetic resonance imaging-targeted biopsy have led to the detection of early-stage breast cancer in women with non-palpable abnormalities [2]. This has not been true in most LMICs because of lack of sufficient number and kind of equipment, and lack of education about the seriousness of the problem. Since the presence of any breast mass raises the question of cancer, it is important to understand the statistical relationship between a variety of benign and malignant lesions of the breast.

M. A. Hardy, B. R. Hochman (eds.), *Global Surgery*, https://doi.org/10.1007/978-3-031-28127-3_30

Despite recent innovative advances in the detection, treatment, and chemoprevention of breast cancer, frequently not readily available in LMICs, surgery remains the cornerstone for most women diagnosed with this disease [3]. Reported reduction in breast cancer deaths among women in the USA and Europe has been attributed to early disease diagnosis, surgery, and systemic chemotherapy [4]. The early excision of ductal carcinoma in situ might also have reduced the incidence of invasive carcinoma [5]. In LMICs early diagnosis continues to be difficult, especially in the rural areas.

Anatomy

The details of the anatomy of the female breast may be found on Google or in most anatomy books. Of importance is that the breast consists of 15 to 20 lobes, each has its duct which opens through a small orifice onto the nipple. The areola, nipple, and mouth of the lactiferous ducts are covered by squamous epithelium. Blood supply to the breast arises from three main sources, namely, branches of the axillary artery, perforating branches of the internal mammary artery, and lateral branches of the posterior intercostal arteries. The venous drainage of the breast follows the course of the arterial supply. As described by Haagensen [6], the lymphatic drainage of the breast comprises 6 main groups of axillary lymph nodes and the internal mammary lymph node group. The important nerves encountered during breast surgery consist of (1) long thoracic nerve of Bell which innervates the serratus anterior; (2) the thoracodorsal nerve supplies latissimus dorsi (its injury causes winged scapula syndrome); and (3) the other nerves are primarily sensory and are third and fourth branches of the cervical plexus and the thoracic intercostal nerves which supply the skin of the upper part of the breast and the lower part of the breast, respectively, while branches of the second intercostal nerve supply the medial aspect of the upper half of the arm.

Hormonal Regulation of the Breast

Figure 30.1 illustrates interaction of a number of hormones that are responsible for the development, function, and maintenance of the female mammary gland during puberty, pregnancy, and lactation. Of interest is that manipulation of these hormones is actively utilized in the treatment of breast cancer.

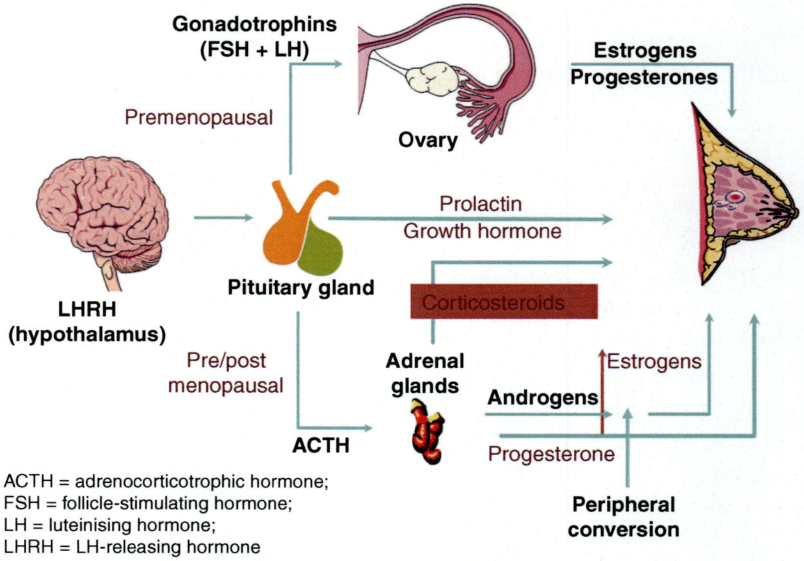

Fig. 30.1 Hormones regulating the breast

Estrogen and progesterone promote the growth of some breast cancers, which are called hormone-sensitive (or hormone dependent) breast cancers. Breast cancer cells contain proteins called hormone receptors (estrogen receptors (ERs) and progesterone receptors (PRs)) that become activated when hormones bind to them. The activated receptors cause changes in the expression of specific genes, which can stimulate cell growth.

Tumor cells that contain estrogen receptors are called estrogen receptor positive (ER positive), estrogen sensitive, or estrogen responsive. Similarly, tumor cells that contain progesterone receptors are called progesterone receptor positive (PR positive). Breast tumors that contain estrogen and or progesterone receptors are called hormone receptor positive (HR positive). Most ER-positive breast cancers are also PR positive. Breast cancers that lack ER are called ER negative, and if they lack both ER and PR they may be called HR negative. Approximately 67% to 80% of breast cancers in women are ER positive [7]. Additionally, 90% of breast cancers in men are ER positive and approximately 80% are PR positive [8].

Evaluation of the Breast

History

The goal of breast evaluation is to determine if a patient who presents with a breast problem/complaint has normal physiologic breast variations, clearly defined benign disorder, or possibly malignant disease. This involves taking a thorough medical history from a patient who may be frightened because of the fear of having breast cancer. Careful questioning will reassure the patient, give her confidence, provide important diagnostic information, and result in a good doctor-patient relationship.

The history usually starts with the patient's presenting symptom(s) which is frequently a breast mass in 70–90% of cases while 5% present with pain [9]. Presentation with nipple discharge is higher in benign lesions (5%) than in malignant disease (1.8%). Other presenting symptoms include breast enlargement or swelling, skin retraction/dimpling, nipple retraction, ulceration or itching, and an axillary mass. Unlike white women in the USA and in Europe, many women in LMICs, especially in Africa, present with foul smelling, fungating, and ulcerated mass [10]. History also includes answers to questions related to breast diseases like age, reproductive history, family history of breast disease, previous history of hormonal replacement therapy, and radiation to chest wall (Table 30.1).

Table 30.1 Relevant history of common breast problems

Start with risk assessment:
• Age
• Personal history of breast disease
• Family history of breast cancer
• Early menarche and late menopause
• Parity and age at delivery of first child
• Hormone replacement therapy
• Oral birth control
• Hereditary cancer syndrome, e.g., BRCA
• Obesity
• Radiation exposure

Note that >75% of women with newly diagnosed breast cancer have no identifiable risk factors

Breast Examination

Inspection of the breast is done in supine and upright positions. This will demonstrate the breast size, shape, asymmetry, skin or nipple retraction (dimpling), skin edema (peau d'orange), erythema, and skin distortion. Breast palpation will confirm skin or nipple retraction, breast discharge on squeezing, and presence of a mass or masses. The axilla is examined for palpable lymph nodes which may be soft, mobile, and normal as opposed to large, firm, hard, or fixed nodes suggestive of malignancy.

Screening and Diagnostic Mammography

Mammography Has become a useful tool for breast screening and diagnosis. It is available only in large/tertiary medical centers in LMICs and almost never in district hospitals in rural areas.

With the hypothesis that early detection will improve outcome, medical screening of asymptomatic, apparently healthy women for breast cancer is very desirable but not readily available in LMICs. Mammographic screening in the detection of breast abnormalities reduces breast carcinoma mortality by nearly 40% with a 30% increase in overall survival. The most frequently diagnosed carcinoma by mammography is ductal carcinoma in situ (DCIS). Utilization of mammographic screening leads to reduction of the size of invasive breast cancer due to early detection [5]. Women who fail to comply with annual mammography, the usual finding in LMICs, develop large breast cancers, 50% of which are invasive tumors compared to smaller size tumors found in the regularly screened women. Since screening mammography saves lives, it would be important to add such a modality to healthcare in underserved rural areas in LMICs.

Guidelines for mammographic screening are uncertain in LMIC settings. In wealthy countries, there is no reported beneficial effect of screening mammography in young women under 40 with no known risk factors for breast cancer. For women age 40 years and older who are at average risk for breast cancer, recommendation is for annual clinical breast examination and annual mammography.

Apart from screening, mammography in symptomatic patients is to detect synchronous non-palpable lesions in the ipsilateral or contralateral breast. Figure 30.2 is the magnification view of diffuse, pleomorphic, clustered microcalcifications suspicious for malignancy confirmed by the stereotactic biopsy of this lesion. It is reported that 15–30% of non-palpable lesions detected on mammogram that are biopsied are malignant. This approach is facilitated by the use of standard reporting system recommended by the radiologist, with numerical risk assessment from 0 (inadequate study) to 5 (highly suggestive of malignancy, action required).

Ultrasonography (USG) has the advantage of being more available in LMICs and being easy to use in the clinic. It is, however, limited by the experience of the operator. Ultrasound employed as an adjunct to mammography is especially useful in a dense breast and is very effective in the differentiation between cystic and solid masses and in guidance to biopsy. In contrast to benign masses with sharp, well-defined edges, malignant masses have irregular margin (Fig. 30.3a, b, c). USG can show a mass within a cyst in the rare case of intracystic carcinoma.

Magnetic Resonance Imaging (MRI) Is infrequently found in LMICs and is expensive. MRI is another modality of breast imaging that employs magnetic and radio frequency fields to visualize intravenously administered

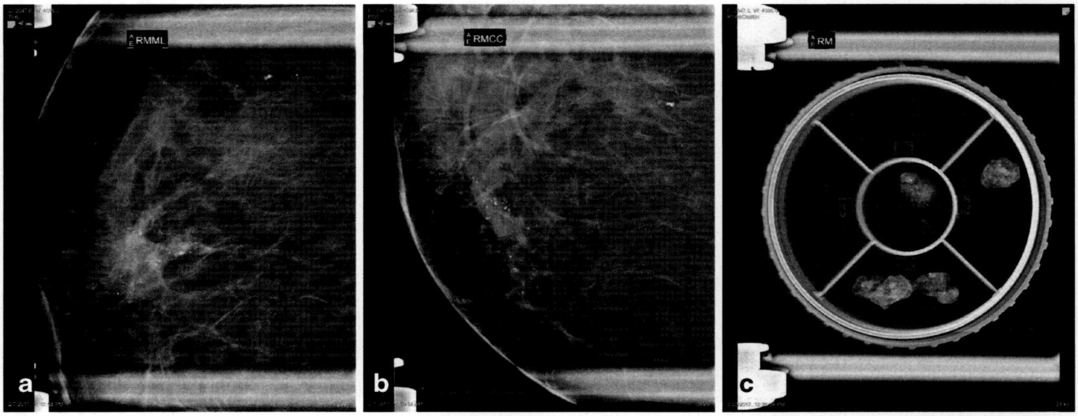

Fig. 30.2 Magnification right craniocaudal view showing extensive clusters of microcalcifications for which core needle biopsy was done. Histology was DCIS (**a**) Right breast mediolateral view showing microcalcifications. (**b**) Right breast craniocaudal view showing microcalcifications. (**c**) Stereotactic core needle biopsy specimen

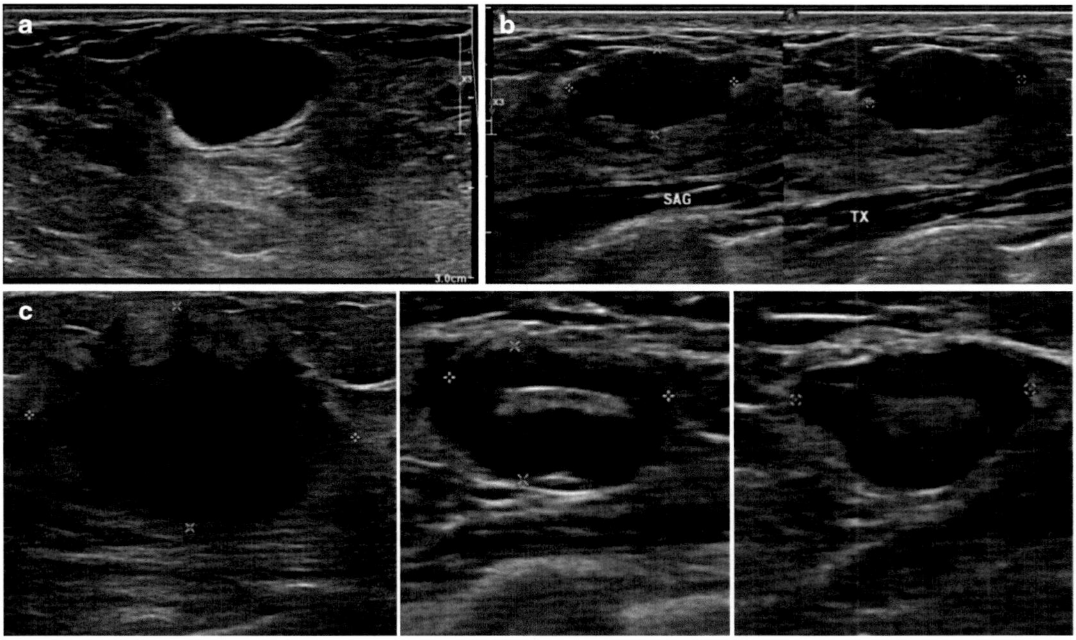

Fig. 30.3 Real-time ultrasound of the right breast showing: (**a**) Anechoic, smooth-walled mass which is a simple cyst. (**b**) A well demarcated and hypoechoic mass which is fibroadenoma. (**c**) A spiculated mass in left breast which on core needle biopsy demonstrated infiltrating ductal carcinoma

Gadolinium-DTPA in enhanced breast lesions due to increased blood flow and capillary permeability. It is 100% sensitive in determining invasive breast cancer and the sensitivity is not impaired by dense parenchyma. It can detect cancers not detected by mammography.

Breast Biopsy

Fine needle aspiration (FNA) is performed in the clinic under USG guide to aspirate cyst or biopsy a mass. One uses a 1.5 inch, 22-gauge needle attached to a 10 or 20 milliliter syringe. A clear straw-colored aspirate is discarded while cloudy or bloody fluid aspirated from a cyst is sent for cytology. The material is smeared on microscope slides that are air dried or fixed with 95% ethanol before being sent for cytology.

Vacuum assisted USG-guided core needle biopsies are performed in the clinic. Unlike FNA, it is uncomfortable and a 14-gauge needle is used and the syringe is connected to a vacuum automated device. The piece of tissue obtained is put in formalin and sent for histological exam and immunohistochemistry.

Stereotactic core needle biopsy is performed as an outpatient procedure in the radiology department for non-palpable lesions like microcalcifications (Fig. 30.2). It is either performed guided by mammography or by MRI. It is usually done under local anesthesia because it is very uncomfortable. Accuracy of this technique is 96–100%.

Open surgical biopsy may be the method of choice in District Hospitals in LMICs where mammography or MRI machines are not available. It is an invasive procedure performed under local anesthesia in the operating room using sterile conditions. It gives the surgeon the opportunity to obtain an adequate tissue sample for histologic evaluation and diagnostic genetic testing which is available only in major academic centers in LMICs.

Benign Breast Disease

The breast is a physiological dynamic structure with cyclical variations where aberrations of normal development and involution may account for many, if not all, benign breast disorders (Table 30.2). Such disorders receive less attention than breast cancer despite reports showing that benign breast disease is an important risk factor for breast cancer. Women with nonproliferative lesions, proliferative findings but no atypia, and those with atypical hyperplasia have a relative risk of breast cancer of 1.27, 1.88, and 4.24, respectively. Classification of benign lesions is based on whether the biopsy is proliferative, non-proliferative atypia on histology with atypia being the most worrisome.

Fibrocystic breast disease is a nonspecific disorder which occurs in response to cyclic hormonal stimulation of the breast. It has been described as chronic cystic mastitis, fibrocystic changes, or cystic mastopathy. Patients may present with breast pain (mastodynia), breast mass, or nipple discharge. Patients are reassured that there is no evidence of cancer and some might need treatment for mastodynia.

Cyclical mastalgia [Mastodynia] is a common presentation in women with benign breast disease. Pain usually correlates with menstrual cycle, waxes and wanes, and is usually bilateral. The breast exam confirms tender, nodular breasts. Mastalgia is caused by either increased estrogen or decreased progesterone production, abnormal prolactin secretion, or psychogenic disorder. Pain relief is dependent on the use of any of the following: diuretics, progesterone, anti-estrogen (tamoxifen), antigonadotrophin suppression (danazol), or essential fatty acid (primrose).

Cysts are an aberration of normal lobular physiology and can be single or multiple. The common presenting symptom is a breast mass which may be palpable and well demonstrated on USG (Fig. 30.3a). Patients can be safely observed if the cyst is small or aspirated with a fine needle when it is large. Cytological examination should be obtained when the fluid is bloody but is not

Table 30.2 Pathogenesis of Benign breast diseases

Physiologic state of breast	Normal	Benign disorder	Benign disease
Development	Duct development Lobular development Stromal development	Nipple inversion Fibroadenoma Adolescent hypertrophy	Mammary fistula Giant fibroadenoma
Cyclical change	Hormonal activity Epithelial activity	Mastalgia & nodularity Benign papilloma	
Pregnancy & lactation	Epithelial hyperplasia Lactation	Blood stained discharge Galactocele	
Involution	Ductal involution Lobular involution Involutional epithelial hyperplasia	Duct ectasia, Nipple retraction, Cysts, Sclerosing adenosis, Hyperplasia & Micropapillomatosis	Periductal mastitis, Suppuration, Lobular & ductal hyperplasia, Atypia

useful if it is clear. Cystic lesions do not need excisional biopsy unless the fluid is bloody, the cyst persistently refills X 3, or there is a residual mass after aspiration.

Fibroadenoma is the most common breast lesion in nulliparous adolescents and young women. The peak age incidence of the disease is 16–25 years [10]. Of interest is the finding that fibroadenoma is more frequent than fibrocystic disease and cancer in blacks in the USA [9], Africa [10], and the West Indies [11]. In contrast, the order of occurrence of breast neoplasm in a predominantly white population is fibrocystic disease, cancer, and fibroadenoma [6]. Fibroadenoma generally presents as either a painless, enlarging breast mass or multiple unilateral or bilateral breast masses in 15% of patients [9]. It is easily distinguished from a cyst with breast USG (Fig. 30.3). The mass is usually observed and not excised in women under 30 years of age unless it rapidly enlarges or becomes painful which may occur with pregnancy. If the cytology report is not diagnostic on the FNA of the mass, an excisional biopsy is performed.

Fibroadenoma may grow in size and become giant fibroadenoma which is referred to as cystosarcoma phyllodes (Fig. 30.4). A few may fill up the breast and mastectomy may be indicated.

Galactocele is a breast cyst filled with milk and is frequently seen during lactation or after cessation of breast feeding. The patient presents with a breast mass which is most often painful. USG delineates the mass and mammography is rarely indicated. Treatment is needle aspiration of the cyst containing milk.

Sclerosing adenosis: Is a benign condition that is easily confused with breast cancer on mammography because its appearance is similar to that of radial scar. The recommended treatment is excisional biopsy.

Intraductal papilloma may be solitary or multiple and frequently presents with a history of spontaneous nipple discharge. The discharge can be serous, blood-tinged, or bloody. The lesion can be demonstrated on ductogram and is treated with excisional biopsy. Solitary papilloma does not increase the risk of breast cancer like multiple or diffuse papillomatosis [6].

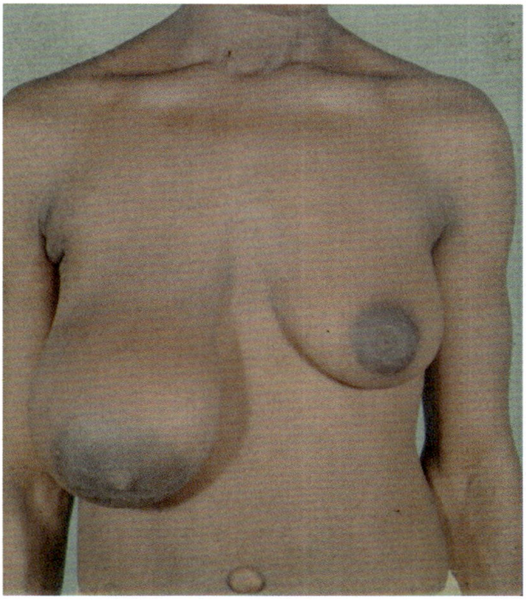

Fig. 30.4 A 26-year-old Nigerian woman with a right breast cystosarcoma phyllodes

Atypia can be ductal or lobular hyperplasia and is only an incidental pathological finding without clinical and mammographic features. Atypia carries a risk factor of 4–5 for breast cancer compared to the general population. It is treated by needle localization and excisional biopsy.

Lobular carcinoma in situ (LCIS) is also an incidental pathological finding that lacks clinical and mammographic features. It is an uncommon disorder that has a high (8–10) risk factor for development of bilateral breast cancer. Women with LCIS are closely monitored with digital breast exam every 4–6 months and mammography 12 to 18 months. Bilateral prophylactic mastectomy is an alternative treatment for women who are unwilling to take the risk of developing breast cancer.

Disorders of the nipple are identified by nipple discharge which may be physiological or pathological. The discharge may be milky, serous, greenish, blood tinged, or bloody. Only bloody nipple discharge raises the question of neoplastic disease while the others are associated with lactation, prolactinoma, and fibrocystic disease. All patients with nipple discharge are evaluated with USG and mammography. It is recommended that the draining duct in women with bloody nipple discharge be excised for histological examination for intraductal papilloma or cancer.

Other benign lesions of the nipple include nipple inversion which is congenital and nipple retraction which may be caused by duct ectasia, cancer, or previous surgery. Accessory nipples are almost always benign.

Breast Infection

Breast Infection Can Occur during Lactation or May be Spontaneous

Lactational Breast Abscess The incidence of pyogenic breast abscess is high in Africa where breast feeding is commonly practiced until the child is 2–3 years old [10]. The infection starts as a localized area in the breast that becomes painful, red, tender, and indurated. When the patient is seen early, the infection can be treated with antibiotics, suspending breast feeding on affected breast, and observation. Occasionally, acute mastitis may progress into an abscess. The patient presents with fever and a warm, tender, fluctuant mass in the breast. The abscess is usually secondary to cracked nipple or breast engorgement at weaning. The abscesses are peripherally located and can be treated with antibiotics and repeated needle aspirations. Incision and drainage may be necessary to drain and debride necrotic tissue in large abscesses which when neglected are associated with overlying skin necrosis.

Nonlactational or spontaneous breast abscess begins as a tender periareolar mass that frequently has a high incidence of recurrence. The initial treatment is incision and drainage with antibiotics to clear the surrounding cellulitis. The antibiotic of choice is based on previous culture studies, and if the infection becomes recurrent, the treatment requires excision of the diseased ducts.

Malignant Breast Diseases

Despite new approaches to breast cancer screening that includes the use of molecular markers and magnetic resonance imaging, breast cancer remains the most frequently diagnosed cancer in women worldwide, and the second most common cause of cancer deaths in the USA. The female to male incidence ratio is 99 to 1. The breast cancer mortality rate continues to decline. The mortality rate in the USA is 40% higher in blacks compared to whites (28.4 vs 20.3 deaths per 100,000) [12]. This disparity is more pronounced among African American women who are younger than 50 years in whom mortality is 77% higher compared to white women. Use of race/ethnicity in our discussion is a sociopolitical construct without any anthropologic implications. A Black or African American is a person who has origins in any black racial groups of Africa. A White is a person having origins in any of the original peoples of Europe, the Middle East, or North Africa.

Breast Cancer Risk Factors

Although the identification of the BRCA1/BRCA2 and PALB2 gene mutations has contributed greatly to understanding the cause of familial forms of breast cancer in 5–10% of breast cancer risks, we still do not have explanation for all the causes of the remaining 90% of sporadic breast cancer. It is estimated that 20–30% of sporadic breast cancers are familial. And it is hypothesized that most sporadic breast cancers are likely to be polygenetic disorders involving multiple genes. A number of studies have recently shown that sporadic breast cancer is closely related to duration of exposure of the breast to estrogens [13]. In general, the risk factors leading to the development of breast cancer include:

- **Family history of breast cancer:** 5–10% of breast cancers are associated with proven genetic predisposition for the disease, while 20–30% have a strong family history of breast cancer. The markers in high-risk families include involvement of multiple generations and first degree relatives, occurrence in premenopausal women, and history of bilateral breast disease and ovarian cancer.

- **Personal history of breast cancer:** A woman with history of cancer in one breast is more likely than the general population to develop a new cancer in the contralateral breast.
- **Benign breast disease:** Atypical hyperplasia and lobular carcinoma in situ increase the risk of breast cancer.
- **Overexpression of estrogen receptors:** Overexpression or exposure of the receptors to estrogen in normal breast epithelium augments [13] the risk factor for breast carcinoma in the following settings: (1) older age; (2) early age menarche; (3) nulliparity; (4) late age of first full term pregnancy; (5) breast feeding; (6) overweight and morbid obesity; (7) post-menopausal hormone therapy; (8) use of oral contraceptives; (9) later age at menopause; (10) number of years since last birth; (11) increased interval between menarche and birth of first child; and (12) years of education (may delay child birth).
- **Inherited germline mutations (BRCA1/2, PALB2, and BRIP1/MCPHI)** are associated with 5–10% of breast cancers. Women with BRCA 1/2 mutations have up to 85% risk of developing breast cancer during their lifetime. The majority of these women develop cancer before the age of 50 years. Additionally, cancers in women with BRCA 1/2 mutation are aggressive and display high histologic grade, triple negative, and HER2/Neu immunophenotype. And these women are at high risk of developing ovarian cancer. Men with BRCA mutation are at high risk of developing breast and prostate cancer [14]. Besides BRCA, mutations in PALB2, BRIP1/MCPHI, RAD51C and RAD41D, and others are associated with hereditary breast cancer. Of note, PALB2 mutation is also associated with pancreatic cancer while BRIPI/MCPHI mutation is associated with ovarian cancer.
- TP53 mutation (Li-Fraumeni syndrome) is very rare and increases incidence of hereditary breast cancer in less than 1% of women.
- **Radiation exposure** for treatment of other diseases during the first three decades of life is strongly linked to breast cancer.

Breast Cancer Biological Characteristics

Recent advances in clinical practice, radiology, immunohistochemistry, and molecular biology have shed some insight in the development of cancer. A review of the literature indicates that hormonal receptors, genetic mutations, irradiation, and other factors increase breast cancer risk in women. This complex subject is extensive and is only briefly discussed here.

Molecular Subtypes

Historically, female breast cancer mortality has a bimodal age distribution with early and late age at diagnosis. Early age breast cancer is hormone-dependent and the peak age incidence is at 50, whereas the second breast cancer type is hormone-independent and has a peak incidence at age 60 [7]. Recently, use of immunohistochemistry has shown that the etiologies of these two age based groups of breast cancer are different. They can be further separated into four molecular subtypes according to hormone receptor expression (HR) and/or human epidermal growth factor receptor 2 (HER2/Neu also referred to as ERBB2) expression. The molecular subtypes are referred to as luminal A {HR+/HER2-), luminal B (HR+/HER2+), HER2 enriched (HR-/HER2+), and triple negative (HR-/HER2-). These are significant for the choice of hormonal and/or chemotherapy.

Incidence rates for triple-negative breast cancer subtype with the worst prognosis are twice as high among black women compared to white women [7, 12]. In Blacks, incidences of HR+/HER2+, HR-/HER2+, and triple-negative subtypes are significantly higher than in non-Hispanic white women. Compared to non-Hispanic white women, Asian/Pacific Islander women have higher incidence of HR-/HER2+ but lower incidences of HER+/HER2- and triple-negative subtypes.

Histological grades rely on degree of tumor differentiation varying from well differentiated to undifferentiated. Tumors with a high grade are aggressive and have poor prognosis. The recent cohort study by Kong et al. [15] demonstrates that the frequency of various histological grades of breast cancer varied significantly by race/ethnicity. In Blacks, while the incidences of grade I and II are lower than in non-Hispanic white women, grade III incidence is higher. Similarly, the incidences of grades I and II are significantly lower in Asian/Pacific Islander, Hispanic white women, and American Indian/Alaskan native women compared with non-Hispanic white women.

Histologic Types Cancer cells may be in situ or invasive depending on violation of the basement membrane. Breast cancer can either be carcinoma in situ when the cancer cells are confined to the ducts and alveoli or invasive carcinoma when the malignant cells have violated the basement membrane and spread to the surrounding stroma.

- **Ductal carcinoma in situ (DCIS)** was originally termed intraductal carcinoma and was treated like invasive breast cancer. The widespread use of mammography after 1969 has led to the diagnosis by mammography in 90% of DCIS which appear as heterogeneous, faint, and linear oriented calcifications on mammogram (Fig. 30.2) and present with a palpable mass in only 10% of patients. Clustered microcalcifications that suggest malignancy leads to core needle biopsy and subsequent treatment with needle localization and excisional biopsy. Currently, treatment for DCIS is wide local excision with clear margins followed with radiotherapy. After treatment, there is a 30% risk of developing invasive carcinoma at the site of excision and also a 30% lifetime risk of bilateral breast invasive cancer.
- **Invasive breast carcinoma** can arise from either the ductal or lobular components of the breast. Nearly 75% of invasive cancer is of ductal origin while lobular carcinoma constitutes 10–15%.
- **Invasive lobular carcinoma** is rarely palpable and unlikely to be visualized on mammography because it does not form microcalcifications. It has a higher incidence of bilaterality, multifocality, and multicentricity compared to invasive ductal carcinoma and has indistinct margins.
- **Invasive ductal carcinoma** usually presents as a hard, palpable mass which shows irregular margin on USG (Fig. 30.3c), spiculated mass or aggregates of micro calcifications on mammography. The other variants of invasive ductal carcinoma are medullary carcinoma (4%), tubular carcinoma (2%), mucinous carcinoma (2%), and papillary carcinoma (2%). Regardless of race/ethnicity, invasive ductal carcinoma is the most common pathological pattern found among all patients. Non-Hispanic white women have a higher proportion of lobular carcinoma and tubular adenocarcinoma than Black, Asian/Pacific Islander, Hispanic white, and American Indian/Alaskan native patience [15].
- **Paget's disease of the nipple** is a form of extensive DCIS which may be associated with invasive carcinoma. Patient usually presents with chronic nipple eczema with or without erosion. Palpation may reveal a mass. The diagnosis is confirmed on fine needle aspiration (FNA). Treatment necessitates excision of the nipple-areola complex.

Breast Cancer Staging and Survival

Staging describes the extent of spread of the disease at time of diagnosis. It is a useful tool in determining the choice of therapy and in predicting prognosis of the disease. The American Joint Committee on Cancer (AJCC) TNM Staging is based on the extent of the primary tumor (T), absence or presence of regional lymph node involvement (N), and absence or presence of distant metastasis (M). Once the TNM are determined, a stage of I, II, III, or IV is assigned, with stage I being early and stage IV being advanced disease (Table 30.3). The overall 5-year survival rate for women with breast cancer in the USA is 98% for stage I, 92% for stage II, 75% for stage III, and 27% for stage IV [12]. Unfortunately many breast cancers in LMICs present late and are stage IV, sometimes fungating.

Table 30.3 TNM stage grouping for breast cancer

*T1 includes T1mic.

Stage grouping			
0	Tis	N0	M0
I	T1*	N0	M0
IIA	T0	N1	M0
	T1*	N1	M0
	T2	N0	M0
IIB	T2	N1	M0
	T3	N0	M0
IIIA	T0	N2	M0
	T1*	N2	M0
	T2	N2	M0
	T3	N1	M0
	T3	N2	M0
IIIB	T4	N0	M0
	T4	N1	M0
	T4	N2	M0
IIIC	Any T	N3	M0
IV	Any T	Any N	M1

Breast cancer prognostic factors previously emphasized primarily the presence or absence of metastasis in draining axillary lymph nodes. However, the recent use of immunohistochemical tests to evaluate tumors has led to the discovery of tumor characteristics that significantly correlate with disease-specific survival. Such characteristics include histologic grade, hormonal receptors, HER2/Neu, TP53, BRCA, cyclin DI, cyclin D2, and cyclin E expression [12, 15]. Compared to post-menopausal women, young breast cancer patients have tumor characteristics associated with poor prognosis. Young women with tumors expressing HR -/HER2 + and high cycling level are associated with aggressive cancer, early locoregional recurrence, and death [16].

Breast Cancer Treatment

The objective of breast cancer treatment is threefold, namely, eradication of locoregional disease, prevention of locoregional recurrence, and achievement of disease-free survival. Taking into account age, tumor size, stage, and other tumor characteristics (histologic grade, receptor status, and tumor subtype) as well as patient preference, treatment may involve lumpectomy (wide local resection of tumor with clear margin), total mastectomy (surgical removal of all breast tissue), subcutaneous mastectomy (surgical removal of all breast tissue but preserving the nipple-areolar complex), and modified radical mastectomy (surgical removal of the breast combined with axillary lymph nodes dissection). Treatment may include radiation therapy, chemotherapy (before and/or after surgery), and hormonal therapy (tamoxifen, aromatase inhibitors), or targeted therapy (like Trastuzumab for HER2+ tumors). Two or more modalities of treatments are used in combination. In the USA, a multidisciplinary approach is used for making the appropriate decision on the treatment of choice for all cancer patients and this is encouraged in LMICs whenever possible. Breast cancer cases are presented at tumor board comprising surgical, medical, radiation, and nursing oncologists, pathologists, radiologist, psychologist/psychiatrist, nurse practitioner, tumor registrar, patient navigator, social worker, and quality assurance representative. Ideally, such tumor boards should be organized in many tertiary hospitals in LMICs.

Surgery for early breast cancer aims for breast-conserving surgery or lumpectomy (wide local tumor resection with free margin). This is usually combined with radiation therapy for stages I and II tumor. Lumpectomy with irradiation has been shown to give similar survival rates with mastectomy (modified radical mastectomy). The 5-year survival for breast stages I and II without lymph node involvement is 98% for either breast conserving-surgery with irradiation or mastectomy. If the cancer has spread to regional lymph nodes, the 5-year survival is 84%. 10-year survival for stages I and II tumor is 80% [17].

- **Surgical axillary staging for stages I, IIA, IIB, and IIIA (T3NIM0):** Breast-conserving surgery and irradiation have become the recommended treatment for stages I and II tumor. **Sentinel lymph node biopsy (SLNB) and axillary lymph node dissection (ALND)** have been employed to ascertain whether cancer has spread beyond breast tissue. Lymph nodes draining the tumor site are identified by lymphatic mapping using radioisotope (Technetium-99 sulfur colloid) or isosulfan blue injected intradermally into the subareolar area in close proximity to the tumor. If cancer cells are present in the sentinel lymph node, ALND is performed to determine if cancer cells are present in the nodes. Indications for SLNB include (1) men with breast cancer; (2) multicentric or multifocal disease; (3) patients undergoing neoadjuvant chemotherapy; (4) elderly patients; (5) T1-T2 tumors; and (6) DCIS treated with mastectomy. Contraindications for SLNB are (1) T4 tumors, (2) clinically and/or FNA positive lymph node, (3) pregnancy, (4) inflammatory breast cancer, and (5) local recurrence.
- **Locoregional Treatment of Clinical Stages I, IIA, or IIB disease or T3 N1, M0:**
  Early breast cancer with negative axillary lymph nodes (AL N) is treated with lumpectomy with surgical axillary staging (SLNB) combined with whole breast radiation. Radiation fields are increased for 1–4 or more positive LN. Additionally, it is recommended that radiation therapy follow chemotherapy when chemotherapy is indicated. For large T2 or T3 tumors, it is suggested that patients be considered for neoadjuvant chemotherapy prior to breast-conserving surgery or total mastectomy as indicated. When total mastectomy is the treatment of choice, it is recommended that radiation therapy should include the chest wall and all the regional LN fields. It is a common practice that radiotherapy should follow chemotherapy when chemotherapy is indicated.
- **Systemic adjuvant treatment for pT1, pT2, pT3, pN0/pN1mi, and HER2+ disease**:
  Treatment includes lumpectomy and radiation of whole breast and regional lymph nodes followed by adjuvant hormonal therapy, adjuvant chemotherapy, and Trastuzumab for women with $T < 0.5$. However for $T > 0.6–1.0$ cm, and for positive lymph nodes with $T > 1.0$ cm, patients should have adjuvant chemotherapy combined with Trastuzumab followed by hormonal therapy after surgery.

If the cancer is HER2-negative for patients with pT <0.5 cm, pNO only hormonal therapy after surgery is used, but those with $T > 0.5$ cm are treated with both adjuvant hormonal therapy and chemotherapy as are those with positive nodes.

Stage IV (any T, any N, M1): disease may not be cured but treatment may prolong life and improve quality of life if such advanced cancer is treated with hormonal therapy for HR-positive tumors and chemotherapy for HR-negative tumors. In the developing countries where patients present late with large, fungating, ulcerated, disfiguring lesions (Fig. 30.5), treatment with a combination of "toilet" mastectomy followed by radiotherapy, chemotherapy, or hormonal therapy may be beneficial.

Factors that Favor Breast-Conserving Surgery (Lumpectomy) over Mastectomy Include (1) location and size of tumor favorable for good aesthetic result; (2) unifocal tumors; (3) problems with general anesthesia; and (4) patient preference.

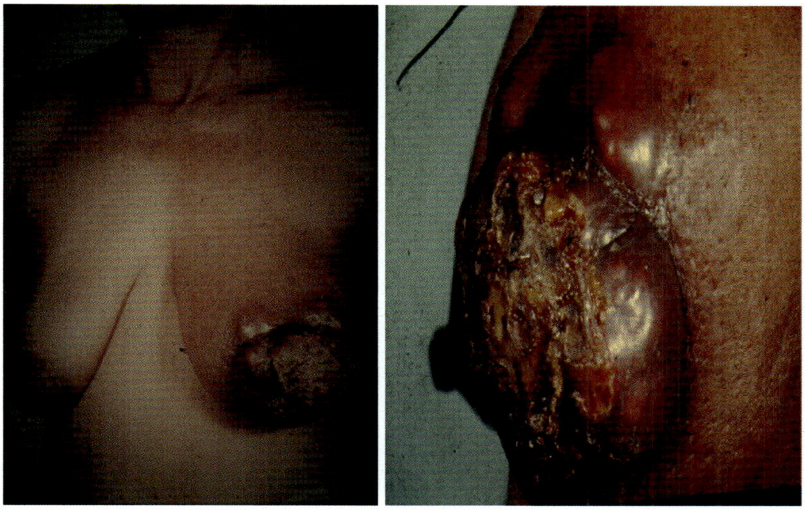

Fig. 30.5 Advanced left breast carcinoma in a Nigerian woman

Factors Favoring Mastectomy over Breast-Conserving Surgery for Operable Breast Cancer Include (1) multifocal or multicentric lesions; (2) inability to achieve negative margins after reexcision; (3) medical contraindications to radiation therapy; (4) unfavorable tumor-to-breast ratio; (5) patient preference; (6) anticipated difficulty with follow-up especially in LMICs; (7) previous breast or chest therapeutic irradiation; and (8) early in pregnancy (first and second trimesters).

Systemic adjuvant chemotherapy is the administration of cytotoxic agents after primary surgery for early-stage breast cancer. It is designed to eliminate or delay the recurrence of clinically occult micrometastatic disease that eventually leads to treatment failure. Details of management of chemotherapy are beyond the scope of this book and should be sought in most recent literature and textbooks on this subject.

Neoadjuvant chemotherapy is being increasingly used in patients with operable breast cancer, either to improve the likelihood of breast-conserving surgery or to attain pathologic complete response. Neoadjuvant therapy may also predict the subsequent response to the same agent. Agents that have been evaluated in neoadjuvant therapy include taxanes (paclitaxel, docetaxel), doxorubicin/cyclophosphamide (AC), aromatase inhibitor (letrozole, anastrozole, and exemestane), and targeted agents (Trastuzumab).

Adjuvant radiotherapy for early breast cancer augments disease-free survival after lumpectomy because breast irradiation controls subclinical residual tumor. Additionally, radiation to chest wall and regional lymph nodes decreases locoregional disease recurrence. Indications for radiation therapy include both post wide excision for DCIS and post wide excision (lumpectomy) for early stage invasive cancer, as well as post mastectomy in high-risk women (T3–4, nodal involvement, high histologic grade, HR-negative, and HER2/Neu over expression) and especially in inflammatory breast cancer.

Adjuvant hormonal therapy that either interferes with estrogen-mediated signaling pathways or interrupts the synthesis of estrogen has become an integral part of the management of hormone-dependent breast cancer. These include selective estrogen receptor modulator (SERM) and aromatase inhibitors (AI).

Selective estrogen receptor modulators (SERM) commonly used are tamoxifen and raloxifene. Tamoxifen is a compound with both estrogen-like and anti-estrogen properties (SERM). It has been demonstrated to reduce the risk of developing cancer in the contralateral breast in ER-positive early breast cancer patients by 45–55% over 10 years after treatment [18]. Additionally, tamoxifen is synergistic with chemotherapy in improving disease-free survival and is effective in treating advanced disease. Tamoxifen therapy is associated with side effects that include increased risk of endometrial cancer and thromboembolism; however its use has also been shown to improve lipid profile, preserve mineral bone density, and decrease the incidence of hip and spine fractures [18]. Tamoxifen is a first-line hormonal therapy for premenopausal women with or without ovarian suppression for at least 5 years. Following 5 years of adjuvant tamoxifen therapy, a second course of tamoxifen or aromatic inhibitor is recommended because it further improves disease-free survival.

Aromatase inhibitors (AI) (anastrozole, letrozole, and exemestane) block the conversion of androgens to estrogens in breast tumors, fat, muscle, and liver. AI reduces the stimulatory effects of estrogens on breast tumors by suppressing the formation of estrogens in all women, particularly post-menopausal women who depend on this source of estrogen. Therefore, AI has superior outcomes compared to tamoxifen use in post-menopausal women [18]. It is the recommended hormonal therapy for post-menopausal women with ER-positive breast cancer. The first dose is given for 5 years and this is followed by additional 5 years which has been shown to lower risk of relapse and also reduce cancer-related mortality.

Trastuzumab therapy for HER+ tumors is used since these are relatively resistant to certain types of chemotherapy. Trastuzumab improves the outcome of patients with HER2-positive invasive stage II or III breast carcinoma. It is also efficacious in the treatment of metastatic HER2+ breast cancer when combined with chemotherapy especially docetaxel. With combined treatment, women with HER2 overexpressing metastatic breast cancer showed a 20% decrease in relative risk of death. Unfortunately Trastuzumab therapy is associated with 0.5 to 1% cardiac toxicity [19].

Breast Cancer Prevention

The fear of developing breast cancer with its consequences has raised the question of how can women with a family history or in the high-risk group with genetic predisposition prevent breast cancer. Currently the risk reduction strategies include regular surveillance, prophylactic mastectomy, oophorectomy or both, and chemoprevention. The two strategies that have proven to reduce the risk of breast cancer in high-risk patients are prophylactic mastectomy and use of chemopreventive drugs [18, 20].

Prophylactic mastectomy is indicated in women with genetic predisposition, women with one breast cancer, and women with atypia, LCIS, and DCIS. Prophylactic bilateral total mastectomy prevents breast cancer in young women with BRCA1/2 mutations [20]. Since cancer of the ovary is associated with BRCA mutation, it is recommended that such patients should consider simultaneous bilateral mastectomy and oophorectomy. Recently, younger women under 40 years are more eager to choose prophylactic mastectomy for reasons that include their reluctance to undergo radiation therapy, fear of recurrence, and a desire for aesthetic appearance. It is strongly recommended that all these patients undergo counseling before the surgical procedure. Consideration for prophylactic mastectomy in women with unilateral breast cancer includes (1) genetic predisposition, (2) diffuse microcalcifications, (3) LCIS, (4) large breast which is difficult to evaluate, (5) history of LCIS followed by invasive breast cancer, and (6) atypical hyperplasia.

Chemoprevention drugs such as adjuvant tamoxifen have been shown to reduce the risk of new cancer in the contralateral breast by 47–55% in women 49 years or younger and by 55% in women age 60 and older [21]. Women with atypical hyperplasia experienced an 86% risk reduction. Similarly, raloxifene study in post-menopausal women with osteoporosis has shown a 76% reduction in relative risk for invasive breast cancer [21]. The use of tamoxifen and raloxifene prophylactically showed an equal (50%) reduction in the risk of developing invasive breast cancer. There is not enough data yet to support the use of tamoxifen for the prevention of breast cancer in patients with genetic mutations.

Racial Disparities in Breast Cancer Outcomes

In recent years, breast cancer prognosis has improved. Whereas the incidence of the disease is higher in whites compared to blacks, the mortality rate is higher in black women than in white women [12, 16]. This has been attributed to many factors, primarily in LMICs, that include poverty, lack of health awareness, later stage at diagnosis, socioeconomic status, and various barriers to healthcare. In wealthy countries, there are problems of higher prevalence of obesity and comorbidities, disparity in treatment, type of insurance, and unfavorable biologic characteristics of the tumor. More recently, biologic factors have been shown to influence the prognostic disparities in breast cancer [22].

Influence of Unfavorable Tumor Biologic Characteristics on Survival

It is difficult to compare the disparities from data in wealthy countries with lack of data from LMICs. Interestingly, the younger age distribution seen among African American women in the USA is similar to the finding that 57% of the women with breast cancer in Nigeria were younger than 50 years at diagnosis [10]. Of note is the finding that young premenopausal women develop a more aggressive, larger breast tumor with higher histologic grade, which are ER negative and have more lymph node metastasis [16]. All these findings are associated with poor prognosis.

Another unfavorable factor is the advanced tumor stage at diagnosis in black women both in wealthy countries [5] and in LMICs [10]. This has been shown in the studies from Nigeria where 81% of the patients presented with stages III and IV disease [10, 23]. Non-Hispanic Black women have a significantly higher T4-sized tumors and stage IV disease than non-Hispanic white women [15]. These findings demonstrate that early breast cancer diagnosis in African American women lags behind that of white women and that also appears to be the case in Nigeria and Sub-Saharan Africa (SSA).

In terms of hormonal markers, African American women have many more ER-negative tumors than white women [12], and ER-negative expression is an adverse prognostic factor that is associated with poor survival.

Breast cancer subtypes are also strongly influenced by race and menopausal status; the highest prevalence of basal-like and lowest prevalence of luminal A tumors were observed among premenopausal African American breast cancer patients [15]. The basal-like/triple-negative cancers exhibit aggressive features that include high proliferative index, high histologic grade, high nuclear grade, and frequent TP53 mutation [16]. Compared to US-born blacks, the prevalence of the triple-negative tumor is 47% lower in women born in East Africa but only 8% lower in West Africa-born blacks [12]. Higher incidence of triple-negative cancer is associated with poor breast cancer survival in blacks.

By histologic grade, African American women have most commonly grade 3 breast cancer (45.2%) while grade 2 is the most frequently seen breast cancer grade in non-Hispanic white women (43.3%) [12]. Thus, African American women have more aggressive tumors associated with poorer prognosis.

Although BRCA 1&2 identification has contributed greatly to understanding the cause of hereditary breast cancer risk among white women, the prevalence of mutations among African American women and blacks in Africa has not yet been well studied.

Barriers to Healthcare in African American and Blacks Worldwide

African American women and black women in Africa and the Caribbean Islands with breast cancer are more likely to die from the disease than women of any other race or ethnicity. The higher breast cancer mortality among black women compared to non-Hispanic white women in the USA is due to a myriad sociocultural, economic, behavioral, environmental, and educational factors. The major healthcare barriers to breast cancer include:

1. **Poverty:** Many patients especially the poor and uninsured meet significant barriers to obtaining timely healthcare in medically underserved communities in the USA [5] and even more so in LMICs; these barriers include, but are not limited to, financial income, communication, and healthcare. Poor people, particularly in LMICs, face substantial obstacles to obtaining cancer care and often do not seek care if they cannot pay for it. Poverty is commonly associated with low educational level, substandard living conditions, inadequate social support, unemployment, and diminished access to healthcare. Poverty does not only impede access to the healthcare system, it is associated with cofactors that can negatively affect outcomes, such as comorbidities, lack of breast health awareness, and mistrust and misunderstanding of the system.
2. **Breast cancer screening:** Randomized controlled trials of mammography screening have shown that regular screening significantly improves breast carcinoma outcome due to detection of the disease at an early stage [4, 5]). Unfortunately, the vast majority of women in the developing countries [10, 23] present with late stage disease compared to non-Hispanic white women [24]. The most dramatic effect of mammography screening is the marked reduction in the size of invasive tumors associated with an increase in the percentage of breast conserving surgery in screened patients.
3. **Disparities in treatment:** Compared to whites, black women are more likely to have a delay in recall for abnormal mammography studies and also for initiating therapy for breast cancer diagnosis [22]. They also have a higher incidence of misuse of treatments. Similarly, African American breast cancer patients suffer from racial disparity in the underuse of appropriate adjuvant chemotherapy. And they have less access to timely and high-quality care and treatment [25]. Data on this subject for patients in LMICs is scarce and is urgently needed.
4. **Comorbidity:** There is a preponderance of morbidity among African American women compared to whites. It is unknown whether this is true for patients in LMICs. The major problems have been morbid obesity, hypertension, and diabetes mellitus [24]. More women die of competing comorbidities than of breast cancer among African Americans and it is unknown for patients in LMICs.
5. **Insurance and cost-related barriers to cancer care:** Paying for the costs of treatment should not be a concern with diagnosis of cancer, but for many, it becomes an important issue. For many cancer patients, financial barriers delay or limit access to treatment and supportive services both in the USA and more so in SSA, and for almost all patients, cancer treatment presents a significant burden. Lack of access to healthcare, regardless of reason, adversely affects cancer care.

Intervention to Correct Breast Cancer Disparities

African American women and women who live in LMICs are more likely to develop and die from breast cancer than any other racial and ethnic groups. This section discusses some of the plans that can improve or eliminate the observed disparities in breast cancer outcome.

Patient Navigation Program

Patient navigation has evolved as a strategy to improve outcome in vulnerable populations by eliminating barriers to timely diagnosis and treatment of cancer patients. The Harlem Hospital patient navigation model established in 1990, where this author (S.F.O.) was a former director, is comprised of a team of lay and professional patient navigators that collaboratively assist patients from initial screening through diagnosis, treatments, and follow-up care [5, 26]. It is a patient-centered model that provides one-on-one assistance to any patient with a positive finding in order to diminish and eliminate barriers to treatment. Additionally, there is an outreach component of the program which promotes cancer prevention and encourages appropriate cancer screening for detection, diagnosis, and treatment. The program's intervention is to promote and support community (and could be country) based patient navigation particularly among the poor who experience barriers to breast healthcare. The Harlem Hospital experience over 10 years showed improvement in survival rate from 39% prior to patient navigation to 70% after 10 years of navigation based on earlier detection and earlier intervention [5, 26].

How does the patient navigator help patients?

Through one-on-one contact, the patient navigator has been trained to work with the patients to help them solve problems and overcome barriers that might keep them from getting the care they need. A navigator knows the healthcare system and the community of patients served. They can communicate with the patients and patients' caregiver(s) while anticipating and solving problems to clear the path from timely diagnosis and treatment through to resolution. No woman should present with advanced stage breast cancer at diagnosis because of barriers to obtaining prompt medical care, especially those living in rural areas, as they do now in most LMICs. None should go untreated, irrespective of their socioeconomic status or should be forced to spend more time fighting their way through the healthcare system than fighting their disease.

A review of breast cancer in Nigeria suggests that the patient navigation model described above that includes both lay and professional navigators may be optimal to help patients in the LMICs. Although breast cancer in Nigeria is the most frequently diagnosed cancer in women, 5-year survival for all stages is 10–15% [10, 23] compared to 87% for American women [12]. This disparity in survival rates is due to late stage presentation which is very common in all LMICs. This has been attributed to poverty, lack of transport, fatalism about cancer, alternate care, communication and information barriers, and medical system barriers [27]. In most hospitals in LMICs, there are no facilities for mammographic screening. It is inconceivable but true, that other LMICs, like Nigeria with its manpower and financial resources, have not developed a National Health Policy on prevention, early detection, diagnosis, and treatment of breast cancer that includes cancer education and outreach programs to fight the dreadful effects of the disease. This is why a Patient Navigator System is sorely needed in most, if not all, LMICs. Such a program will raise public awareness of early detection, prevention, and treatment of cancer, coordinate education and screening programs to increase early detection, develop culturally sensitive outreach programs and educational materials, establish a Physician education program, including courses and credits for clinical oncologists as well as non-cancer clinician, and develop regional and national tumor boards that hold conferences to ensure standardized treatment.

Tumor Board and Coordination of Treatments

Breast cancer management is a multidisciplinary team of care providers comprising surgical, medical, and radiation oncologist, oncology nurse, social worker, psychologist, navigator, and tumor registrar. Unfortunately, most hospitals in the rural areas, especially in the LMICs, have no functioning tumor board. Since the healthcare delivery system in such hospitals is suboptimal, breast cancer patients are better referred to tertiary teaching hospitals from the rural district general hospitals. A way of improving care for all women, particularly recovering from primary surgery, is to ensure that triage to medical oncology is successfully accomplished. Reducing such missed opportunities to facilitate oncology referrals and enabling receipt of appropriate adjuvant chemotherapy has the potential to reduce racial disparities in treatment.

Use of Information and Communication Technology (ICT)

ICT offers a great opportunity to electronic health records, telemedicine, clinical decision-making, and links among professionals and between professionals and patients. This is particularly important in the developing countries where communication and information barriers contribute to poor patient outcome. This is discussed in greater detail in Chaps. 8 and 12. The government can afford to make available to the healthcare providers in rural hospitals the network facilities for virtual care. Telemedicine will give healthcare providers in primary care facilities the opportunity to consult with specialists in tertiary teaching hospitals either in their home countries or in specialist hospitals abroad (Europe, the USA, and Middle East). Virtual consultations/conferences will improve patient outcomes in vulnerable communities by integrating ICT with physician expertise, and collaborating with existing global healthcare.

Breast Cancer During Pregnancy and Lactation

Although breast cancer during pregnancy or lactation is very rare, it is still the most common malignancy in pregnant women and occurs at a rate of 1 in 3000 pregnancies [28]. It constitutes 0.9–2.8% of all breast carcinomas in white women [6] compared to 4.3% in Nigerian women [10]. The mean age of pregnant white women with breast cancer is 33.4 years compared to 28.8 years in Nigerian women. Again pregnant women in Nigeria present with late stage disease. The disease is a challenge to patients and physicians due to difficulties encountered with diagnosis and treatment. Breast palpation is difficult because of breast engorgement. Diagnosis of breast masses during pregnancy is made with USG and core needle biopsy since mammography is contraindicated. Treatment is based on tumor stage and the trimester of pregnancy. The protocol for management is based on modification of the multidisciplinary management recommended by Keleher et al. [28] and differs for each trimester of pregnancy. The pregnancy is terminated if axillary nodes are positive in the first trimester; otherwise the patient is treated with MRM or breast-conserving surgery for stages I and II cancer with continuation of pregnancy. In the second trimester decision is more difficult and patient has to decide about continuation of pregnancy as chemotherapy is used for all stages. In the third trimester, the pregnancy is continued and standard therapy is used with chemotherapy. Chemotherapy used in pregnancy that is considered to be relatively safe is a combination of 5-fluorouracil, doxorubicin, and cyclophosphamide (FAC).

Male Breast Disease

The male breast is a rudimentary structure composed of small glands with fibrous tissue and periductal fat. The common disorders of the male breast are gynecomastia and carcinoma.

Gynecomastia

Gynecomastia is hypertrophy of the breast due to excessive development of the male mammary glands. It can be seen in boys at puberty or in old men. Gynecomastia can be unilateral but is often bilateral in most patients. There is also a fibrous form which is comprised of dense cellular connective tissue with fewer ducts. Gynecomastia is usually evaluated with palpation for presence of masses and ultrasonography for confirmation of a mass and for FNA. Mammography is recommended when there is suspicion for malignancy.

Causes of gynecomastia include chromosomal abnormality (Klinefelter's syndrome), endocrine dysfunction, or exogenous hormonal use. Occasionally, gynecomastia may result from use of exogenous hormones or medications (cimetidine, digoxin, etc.)

Treatment is either surgical or pharmacological. Surgical treatment can be liposuction or subcutaneous mastectomy. Pharmacological treatment includes endocrine therapy using antiestrogens (tamoxifen, clomiphene, and danazol).

Male Breast Carcinoma

Breast cancer is a rare disease in men and constitutes less than 1% of the total breast cancer cases worldwide. Male breast cancer incidence for all breast cancer cases varies wildly between geographical regions with a 12% incidence in Uganda compared to 2% in Nigeria and less than 1% in white men in the USA [8]. This geographic incidence rates are likely partially due to inadequate data collection and to lack of awareness of the disease in men which leads to diagnosis at a late stage which adversely affects its prognosis. The diagnostic work up for male breast cancer consists of USG, mammography, and FNA biopsy.

Risk factors for male breast cancer include age, BRCA 1/2 mutation, PALB2, Klinefelter's syndrome, exogenous estrogen or progesterone use, obesity, and chest wall radiation [29]. In contrast to female breast cancer, males have a much higher percentage of hormone receptor positive tumors but significantly lower HER2 over expression. Staging of male breast carcinoma is the same as that of women using the TNM system. More than 40% of men with breast cancer present with stage III and IV disease [8].

Surgical options for men with early stage breast cancer are either MRM or breast-conserving surgery. Stages 1 IB, III, and IV are treated with modified radical mastectomy followed by chemotherapy, radiotherapy, and/or hormonal therapy for ER-positive tumors like in women. Men who develop metastatic disease respond well to endocrine therapy. The overall survival is worse in men than in women. Prognosis of male breast cancer in node positive patients is very poor.

References

1. Siegel RL, Miller KD, Fucks HM, Jemal A. Cancer statistics, 2022. CA Cancer J Clin. 2022;72:7–33.
2. Nelson HD, Fu R, Cantor A, et al. Effectiveness of breast cancer screening: systematic review and meta-analysis to update the 2009 U.S. Preventive services task force recommendations. Ann Int Med. 2016;164:244–55.
3. Woolam GL. What's new in breast cancer surgery? CA Cancer J Clin. 2000;50:276–8.
4. Henney JE, Devita VT Jr. The evolution of primary multimodality treatment in resectable breast cancer. Cancer. 1980;46:999–1008.
5. Oluwole SF, Ali AO, Adu A, et al. Impact of a Cancer screening program on breast cancer stage at diagnosis in a medically underserved urban community. J Am Coll Surg. 2003;196:180–8.
6. Haagensen CD. Diseases of the breast. 3rd ed. Philadelphia: WB Saunders Co.; 1986.
7. Kohler BA, Sherman RL, Howlader N, et al. Annual report to the nation on the status of cancer, 1975–2011, featuring incidence of breast cancer subtypes by race/ethnicity, poverty, and state. J Natl Cancer Inst. 2015;107(6):adj048.
8. Rudlowsky C. Male breast cancer. Breast Care (Basel). 2008;3(3):183–9.
9. Oluwole SF, Freeman HP. Analysis of benign breast lesions in Blacks. Am J Surg. 1979;137:786–9.
10. Oluwole SF, Fadiran OA, Odesanmi WO. Diseases of the breast in Nigeria. Br J Surg. 1987;74:582–5.
11. Raju GC, Naraynsingh V. Benign breast disease in West Indian population. Br J Surg. 1985;72:17–8.
12. Desantis CE, Ma J, Gaudet MM, et al. Breast cancer statistics, 2019. CA Cancer J Clin. 2019;69:438–51.
13. Comings DE, Gade-Andavolu R, Cone LA, et al. A multigene trial for the risk of breast carcinoma. Cancer. 2003;97:2160–70.
14. Newman B, Mu H, Buthler LM, et al. Frequency of breast cancer attributable to BRCA1 in a population-based series of American women. JAMA. 1998;279:915–21.
15. Kong X, Liu Z, Cheng R, et al. Variation in breast cancer subtype incidence and distribution by race/ethnicity in the United States from 2010 to 2015. JAMA Netw Open. 2020;3(10):e2020303. doi2020303.
16. Li Y, Lu S, Zhang Y, et al. Loco-regional recurrence trend and prognosis in young women with breast cancer according to molecular subtypes: analysis of 1099 cases. World J Surg Oncol. 2021;19:113.
17. Jacobson JA, Danforth DN, Cowan KH, et al. Ten year results of a comparison of conservation with mastectomy in the treatments of stage I & stage II breast cancer. N Engl J Med. 1995;332:907–11.
18. Vogel VG. Breast cancer prevention: a review of current evidence. CA-Cancer J Clin. 2000;50:156–70.
19. Dang C, Guo H, Najita J, et al. Cardiac outcomes of patients on adjuvant weekly paclitaxel and trastuzumab for node negative HER2 positive breast cancer. JAMA. 2016;2(1):29–36.
20. Meijers-Heijboer H, van Geel B, van Putten WLJ, et al. Breast cancer after prophylactic bilateral mastectomy in women with BRCA1 or BRCA2 mutation. N Engl J Med. 2001;345:159–63.
21. Kissinger LS, Harris R, Woolf SH, et al. Chemoprevention of breast cancer: a summary of the evidence for US preventive services task force. Ann Intern Med. 2002;137:59–67.
22. Daly B, Olopade OI. A perfect storm: how tumor biology, genomics and healthcare delivery patterns collide to create a racial survival disparity in breast cancer and proposed interventions for change. CA Cancer J Clin. 2015;65:221–38.

23. Adesunkanmi ARK, Lawal OO, Adelusola KA, et al. The severity, outcome and challenges of breast cancer in Nigeria. Breast. 2006;15:399–409.
24. Tammemagi CM, Nerenz D, Neslund-Dudas C, et al. Comorbidity and survival disparities among black and white patients with breast cancer. JAMA. 2005;294:1765–72.
25. Bikell NA, Wang JJ, Oluwole S, et al. Missed opportunities: racial disparities in adjuvant breast cancer treatment. J Clin Oncol. 2006;24:1357–62.
26. Freeman HP, Rodriguez RL. History and principles of patient navigation. Cancer. 2011;117:3539–42.
27. Oluwole S. Strategic vision for health care development in Nigeria. In Adegoke OS, et al Ed. developing a road map for the rapid technological and industrial development of Nigeria (Part 1): Proceedings of the second forum of Laureates of the Nigerian National Order of Merit 2008; p167–177.
28. Keleher AJ, Theriault RL, Gwyn KM. Multidisciplinary management of breast cancer concurrent with pregnancy. J Am Coll Surg. 2001;194(1):54–64.
29. Ruddy KJ, Winer EP. Male breast cancer: risk factors, biology, diagnosis, treatment, and survivorship. Ann Oncol. 2013;24:1443.

How to Provide Acute Burn Care in Low- and Middle-Income Countries

31

Cameron Gibson, Meghan Hoyle, and James Gallagher

Do not worry if others do not understand you. Instead worry if you do not understand others.

– Confucius

Abbreviations

ATLS	Advanced Trauma Life Support
GBR	Global Burn Registry
HICs	High-income countries
LD50	Lethal dose of 50%
LMICs	Low- and middle-income countries
LR	Lactated Ringers
TBSA	Total body surface area
WHO	World Health Organization

C. Gibson (✉)
UCHealth Burn and Frostbite Center, University of Colorado Anschutz Medical Campus, Aurora, CO, USA
e-mail: cameron.2.gibson@cuanschutz.edu

M. Hoyle
North Colorado Medical Center, Greeley, CO, USA
e-mail: meghan.hoyle@bannerhealth.com

J. Gallagher
William Randolph Hearst Burn Center, New York-Presbyterian Weill Cornell Medical Center, New York, NY, USA
e-mail: jag9027@med.cornell.edu

Introduction

While the incidence of burns has decreased over the past few decades in high-income countries (HICs), burn injury continues to plague low-resource settings. Worldwide, burns represent the fourth most common type of traumatic injury and are a common cause of severe disability and death in low- and middle-income countries (LMICs) [1]. With over 11 million burn injuries and >250,000 deaths annually (>90% of which occurred in LMICs), burns represent a significant burden on the healthcare system [2]. The economic impact is also disproportionately severe due to the high incidence of disability related to even minor neglected burns.

The unfortunate reality is that the true impact of burn injuries may be underrepresented because there is a paucity of epidemiological data from LMICs. In order to address this problem, the WHO created the Global Burn Registry (GBR) in 2018 which collects burn data using a standardized form on a publicly available platform. Utilization of the GBR has been sporadic with LMICs and underrepresented compared to HICs [3]. Regardless of what platform is used, any

M. A. Hardy, B. R. Hochman (eds.), *Global Surgery*, https://doi.org/10.1007/978-3-031-28127-3_31

effort to improve burn care in LMICs needs to begin with an accurate data collection which should be an integral part of any international collaborative effort.

Burn care at the local level is likely to be different from one country to another, and even between different regions of a country. It is important to realize that the vast majority of patients will present days, weeks, or even months after the burn occurred, having cared for the burn at home using potentially harmful remedies, ointments, and potions. Without a dedicated ward, which is rare in LMICs, burn patients are often scattered throughout the medical and surgical wards rather than cohorted. Nearly all mission style trips in plastic and reconstructive burn surgery will focus on congenital (cleft lip) or acquired (contracture) surgical backlog rather than on hospitalized acute burn patients. In most underserved areas hospitalized acute burn patients will fit into one of five groups (Table 31.1).

The first group is patients whose burns have fully re-epithelialized and no longer have any open wounds, but for some reason have not been discharged for reasons that may be difficult to determine. Understanding why they are not discharged can provide valuable insight into the system that is being visited. The second group is patients with burn injuries who are unlikely to require surgery for best outcome but need ongoing inpatient care for medical management, wound care, and/or pain control. The third group is patients with a surgical need (infected eschar, chronically granulating wounds or contracture with or without open wounds, and the rare early smaller third degree burn, etc.) who are deemed medically stable for surgery (Fig. 31.1). This is your target surgical group if your outreach includes acute surgical burn care. The fourth group is patients who have a surgical need but are not medically stable or cannot safely undergo surgery at their stage of healing. The final group is patients with a non-survivable burn injury. This

Table 31.1 Types of burn patients

Types of Burn Patients	
I	Fully healed, can be *medically* discharged
II	Patient with burn that does *not* require skin grafting but requires inpatient care (e.g. large partial thickness burns)
III	Medically stable patient with burn requiring skin grafting surgery
IV	Medically ***unstable*** patient with burn requiring skin grafting surgery
V	Non-survivable burn injury, palliative care recommended

group can sometimes be difficult to determine because it is dependent upon the resources available locally, regionally, and nationally. While the LD50 for burn injuries in HICs is ~65–70% TBSA, the LD50 can be 30–40% or lower in LMICs [4]. A common mistake that HIC surgeons make when working in LMICs is to categorize patients into group 3 or 4 who really fit into group 5, or try to apply sound principles of care used in HICs that may not be available or safe in LMICs. Having a clear understanding of your local resources – what is possible medically/surgically and what is not – will prevent one from miscategorizing a patient and potentially causing undue harm.

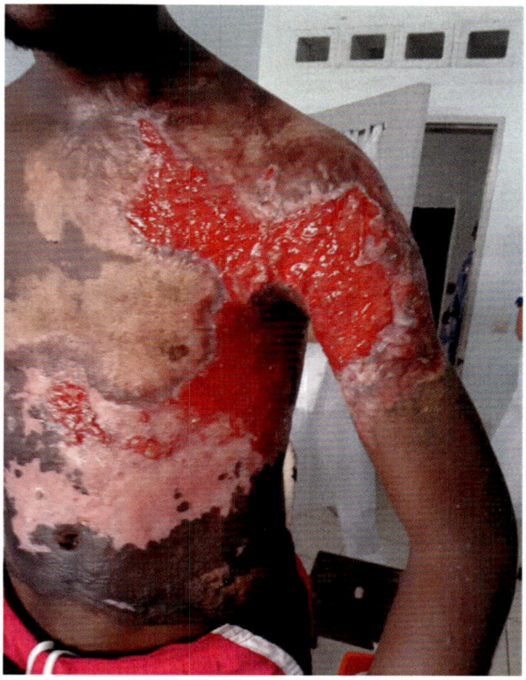

Fig. 31.1 Example of a category 3 patient – partially healed burn wound with healthy granulation tissue ready for skin grafting

The work of global surgery can be broadly grouped into three pillars: clinical care, education, and capacity building. A true "global surgeon" works in all three, although a given trip or intervention may have a primary focus on only one or two. Each of these pillars has unique issues for burn surgeons (Fig. 31.2). For instance, you may determine that the staff at the hospital is well educated on burn care and has the necessary basic tools, but the surgical backlog, urgent cases, and limited OR time are burdening the healthcare system so much that patients are having to wait weeks or months to undergo skin grafting or scar contracture release. In fact, burn reconstructive surgery alone accounts for almost 50% of surgical backlog cases in LMICs [5]. This backlog has been the main focus of mission style global outreach programs and, if done well, including teaching, can help to ease the surgical burden of the local teams (i.e., "give a man a fish"). Alternatively, one may find that the local staff has only rudimentary knowledge of appropriate burn care and very limited ability to provide surgical burn care. Therefore, focus needs to be on education prevention, first aid, acute burn care, teach principal skills for basic skin grafting, scar contracture prevention, etc. (i.e., "teach a man to fish"). Or perhaps the local team in LMIC has the know-how and simply needs the pre-requisite tools to start skin grafting, in which case your focus should be primarily on partnership and on capacity building (i.e., "give the man a fishing rod so he can ACTUALLY fish"). In each one of

Fig. 31.2 Pillars of the "Global Burn Surgeon"

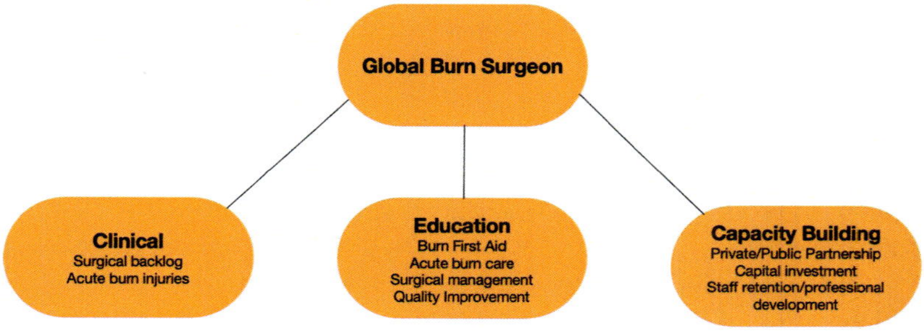

Clinical Site Visit

Staffing

Surgical capacity/capabilities for burns

Wound care supplies

Pharmacy

Protocols/Processes specific to burn patients

IT infrastructure

Prevention/Outreach

Community beliefs and practices

Burn first aid training

Governance

NSOAP

Ministry of Health—local and national

Local NGO's

Data Management

Local/national registries for trauma/burns

WHO Global Burn Registry

Fig. 31.3 Suggested topics that should be included in a needs assessment survey on burn care in a specific country or region. NSOAP, National Surgical, Obstetric and Anesthesia Plan; NGO, non-governmental organization; WHO, World Health Organization

these scenarios, asking questions, listening, and collaborating is critical to determine how best to help. Decisions on the degree of commitment going forward, and on how one can integrate and work together with other surgical disciplines to elevate the surgical capacity of the community must be primary goals of the visiting team. Long-term partnership by a visiting organization from a HIC to help form a stable burn team and burn unit creates a home for future mission trips and enables the local burn teams to provide acute burn care and more fully address the needs of its current patients.

Preparation

Prior to a visit – whether for burns or any other specialty, as has been defined in previous chapters – the visiting individual or team need to determine the extent and nature of planned work. Is this a one-off medical mission trip or will there be future trips to the same facility or region? Is the team's focus purely clinical or is there an educational component? Have leaders or "local champions" on the ground been identified that wish to collaborate with the team? What sort of follow-up will the patients have once the team has left? Answering these and many other important questions prior to departure will ensure a successful and effective visit and, most importantly, that no unintended harm comes to the healthcare professional or their patients that one partners to help.

If the team is looking to develop a long-term collaboration with a health center, it is important to start with an assessment of the current state of burn care in the locality. A needs assessment will help determine the strengths and weaknesses of the local healthcare system and guide future interventions. Figure 31.3 recommends specific topics that should be addressed in a needs assessment survey; however this list represents a minimum that should be included and recommend tailoring your survey to address the realities on the ground. Answers to survey questions as well as interviews with stakeholders (patients, medical staff, local/regional/national health officials) should guide the nature of your work. Ultimately, any intervention needs to be driven by local stakeholders as this leads to enduring change that will be durable beyond the visits and financing from outside the host country.

Prehospital Burn Care

Prevention

Most burns are avoidable accidental injuries, and the best prehospital treatment for a burn is prevention. Compared to other injuries, burns on average are more costly, labor-intensive, and have significantly longer length of stays. As countries develop, technology and safety protocols improve, leading to fewer burn injuries. This is evident in HICs where the incidence of burn injuries has been decreasing for several decades. It is strongly recommended that any long-term intervention or collaboration should include a prevention outreach component. As the old adage goes, "an ounce of prevention is worth a pound of treatment."

Burn First Aid

Prehospital care for burn injuries including first aid is essential. Done properly it will decrease the depth of burn injury and lessen infection and the need for surgery [6]. There are multiple different burn first aid courses offered around the world, each tailored specifically for their local environment, but the basic tenets of burn first aid in any setting are:

1. Cool the burn with cool running water (preferably for 20 mins or more).
2. Remove all jewelry and clothing around the burned area.
3. Cover the burn with clean cloth or bandage.
4. Administer oral analgesia for pain control.
5. Seek immediate medical advice if the burn is large (>5% TBSA) or in a sensitive area of the body (face, hands, feet, genitalia, over major joints) [7].

Simply providing burn first aid training somewhere that previously had none can have a huge impact on the clinical outcome of burn patients. Additionally, burn first aid training has been shown to be long lasting. Even 5 years after attending a course, attendees' burn first aid knowledge was significantly better than those who did not attend [8].

Barriers to Care

Several barriers are likely to be encountered in providing high-quality, effective prehospital burn care. One common barrier consists of local beliefs and practices surrounding burn care. Whether you are in Boston, Massachusetts, or Lilongwe, Malawi, society at large often has preconceived notions, developed over many generations prior to the modern era of effective burn care, about how to care for burns. Oftentimes, these practices are not helpful (e.g., applying egg, milk, or butter to a burn wound) and sometimes can even be harmful (e.g., applying animal dung or hair as a dressing over a burn wound). These practices may be long standing, strongly believed in and practiced by local traditional healers in some LMICs. It is important to know what is the local practice and who in the community outside of the hospital is administering burn care. One is likely to be more successful with community outreach if the team collaborates with local leaders and traditional healers. Any community outreach about burn care should address prevention, first aid, and local wound practices. It must be culturally sensitive to the local practices while highlighting important principles of appropriate burn first aid and wound care.

Another barrier which is likely to be encountered in the prehospital setting is delays in seeking appropriate burn care. The Lancet Commission estimates that more than 5 billion people worldwide do not have access to needed safe, affordable surgical and anesthesia care [9]. This number is likely equal, if not larger when considering access to safe, affordable *burn care*. This lack of access is multidimensional, not simply bound by geographic proximity to a burn center. Someone may only live 10 km away from a health center but not have the money to pay for transportation, or they might even live close by but not have the funds to pay upfront for their treatment. Using the "Three Delays Framework" – delay in seeking care, delay in reaching care, and delay in receiving care – you can imagine how each delay can affect and exacerbate the other. One can also use this framework as a tool to better categorize barriers specific to any one area that delay care and then address them accordingly. Many international organizations concentrate on the third delay – delay in receiving care – by providing a certain specialty (such as burn surgery) that may not be present in the community. This model highlights the importance of having a plan in place to overcome all three forms of delay in order to be truly effective and successful. Many well-intentioned humanitarian projects have failed because they focused on one barrier to care only to uncover another barrier that was neither foreseen nor budgeted for.

Preoperative Management

Preoperative management of the burn injured patient begins as soon as they arrive at the health center and progresses in a stepwise fashion. The first step is stabilization of the burn injury and identification of any other traumatic injuries that could be life-threatening. Developing a regimented approach, such as the one in advanced trauma life support (ATLS) courses in the United States (primary survey, secondary survey, then adjuncts/imaging and tertiary survey), helps the team to avoid being distracted by the burn injury when the patient may have other traumatic injuries that are more acute. Once the patient is stabilized, then the burn injury can be properly addressed.

Unfortunately, most patients in LMICs present days or even weeks after the burn injury occurred, sometimes even with large burns and therefore are unable to be immediately resuscitated. Oftentimes, patients present chronically dehydrated and only after they have developed a complication related to their burn injury. They may exhibit signs of local infection of their burn wound or be frankly septic. They may also have other underlying ***undiagnosed*** medical comorbidities that require acute management before the burn wound can properly heal or be addressed surgically.

Fluid Resuscitation

If the patient suffers a burn >15% TBSA and presents to the health center within hours of the burn injury, then one can properly resuscitate the patient using one of several available burn fluid resuscitation formulas. The best known is the Parkland formula. There are several resuscitation formulas that have been developed for burn resuscitation (Table 31.2) [10]. The common endpoint for all of these formulas is an hourly urine output of 30–50 ml/hr. or 0.5 ml/kg/hr. for adults and 1 ml/kg/h for children (<5 years old). The fluid of choice in burn resuscitation is Lactated Ringers (LR) as it is an isotonic solution with physiologic electrolytes and does not cause metabolic acidosis like normal saline in large quantities. If LR is unavailable, however, any iso-

Table 31.2 Fluid resuscitation formulas during the first 24 h for major burns (>20% TBSA)

Formula	24-hour fluid requirement	Endpoint
Parkland	4 ml/kg/TBSA, first half given in 8 hours, second half in 16 hours	Urine output 30-50 ml/hr for adults, 1 ml/kg/hr for children less than 5 years old
Modified Brooke	2 ml/kg/TBSA, first half given in 8 hours, second half in 16 hours	
"Rule of ten"	TBSA x 10 = fluid rate per hour for first 24 hours For every 10 kg above 80 kg increase rate by 100 ml	
American Burn Association ABLS	Adult: 2 ml/kg/TBSA Children: 3 ml/kg/TBSA Electrical: 4 ml/kg/TBSA	

ABLS Advanced Burn Life Support

tonic solution will suffice to maintain intravascular volume during burn shock. It is important to note that these formulas help determine ***initial*** volume resuscitation for the first 24 h, i.e., they are meant as a guide to begin resuscitation at an appropriate volume rate. Frequent re-evaluation of the patient's urine output during the first 24–48 h is important to confirm that resuscitation is proceeding according to plan.

Once the patients are ~24–48 h post-injury and they no longer require large volumes of fluid, they can be transitioned to maintenance fluids such as 0.45% normal saline with or without dextrose. If the patient is not intubated, then oral intake should be encouraged with the addition of oral rehydration salts to maintain appropriate electrolyte balance. If available, a nasogastric tube should be placed for enteral access in any burn patient with a TBSA >20% (in children, >15% TBSA) both for administering enteral fluids and for nutrition.

Wound Evaluation

Determining overall burn size and depth is essential to burn resuscitation and all subsequent surgical planning and medical management. The most common way to estimate burn size is to use the "Rule of Nines" or a Lund and Browder chart (Fig. 31.4) [11]. It is essential to stress that *only second and third degree burns are included in TBSA estimates, not first degree burns.* Alternatively, you can use the Palmar method to measure burn size (where the *patient's* palm and fingers are equal to 1% TBSA). This is a useful method for patients with scattered burns on multiple parts of the body, such as scald burns. Burn depth is much more difficult to assess because the true extent of injury is often not visible on the surface for several days. Table 31.3 lists common characteristics of each burn depth from first to fourth degree. In general, most second degree burns will heal with just good wound care, early

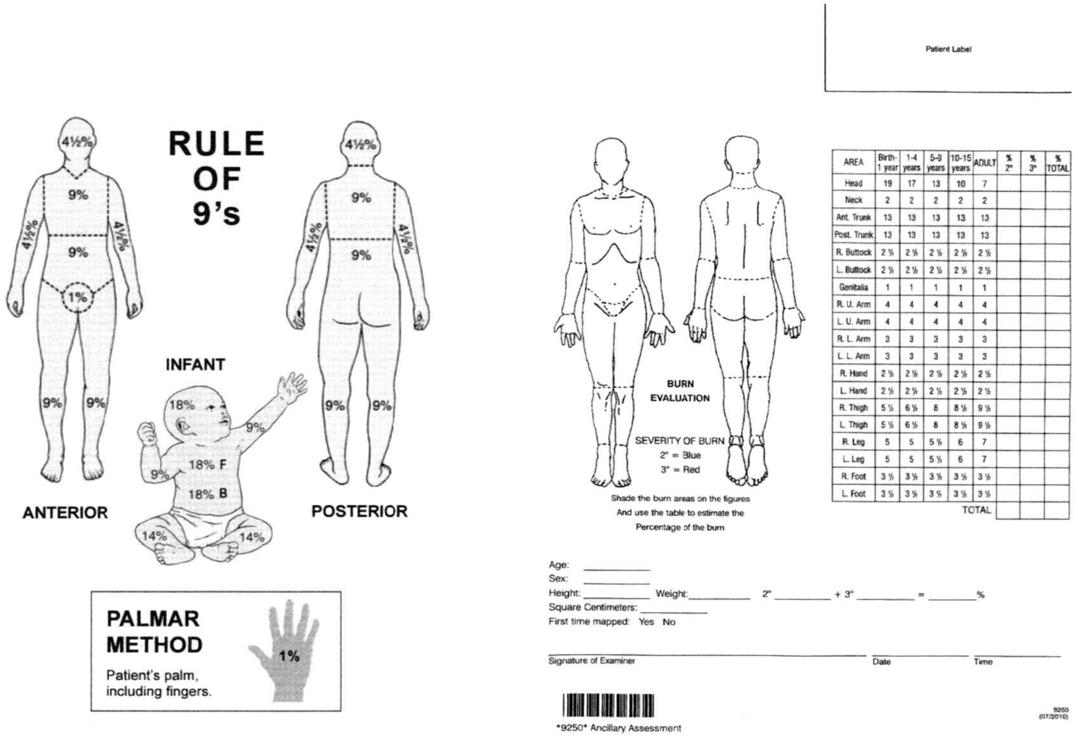

AREA	Birth-1 year	1-4 years	5-9 years	10-15 years	ADULT	% 2°	% 3°	% TOTAL
Head	19	17	13	10	7			
Neck	2	2	2	2	2			
Ant. Trunk	13	13	13	13	13			
Post. Trunk	13	13	13	13	13			
R. Buttock	2 ½	2 ½	2 ½	2 ½	2 ½			
L. Buttock	2 ½	2 ½	2 ½	2 ½	2 ½			
Genitalia	1	1	1	1	1			
R. U. Arm	4	4	4	4	4			
L. U. Arm	4	4	4	4	4			
R. L. Arm	3	3	3	3	3			
L. L. Arm	3	3	3	3	3			
R. Hand	2 ½	2 ½	2 ½	2 ½	2 ½			
L. Hand	2 ½	2 ½	2 ½	2 ½	2 ½			
R. Thigh	5 ½	6 ½	8	8 ½	9 ½			
L. Thigh	5 ½	6 ½	8	8 ½	9 ½			
R. Leg	5	5	5 ½	6	7			
L. Leg	5	5	5 ½	6	7			
R. Foot	3 ½	3 ½	3 ½	3 ½	3 ½			
L. Foot	3 ½	3 ½	3 ½	3 ½	3 ½			
					TOTAL			

Fig. 31.4 "Rule of Nines," Palmar method, and Lund and Browder chart for burn estimation

Table 31.3 Evaluation of burn size and depth

Burn degree	Depth of injury	Characteristics	Typical mechanisms
1st	Epidermis	Red, non-blistered skin, painful	Sunburns, contact, scald
Superficial 2nd	Dermis	Blisters, pinkish-red dermis, wet, painful	Scald and contact burns
Deep 2nd	Dermis	White, hemorrhagic petechiae, dry, painful	Multiple
3rd	Subcutaneous fat	Tannish-black, dry, insensate	Flame and chemical burns
4th	Soft tissue, bone	Exposed muscle or bone, deep concave wound	Electrical injuries

physiotherapy, and time, whereas third degree burns of any significant size (>1% TBSA) will require skin grafting surgery; otherwise, the wound will take weeks to months to fully heal and likely develop scar contractures. For burns of indeterminate depth (i.e., deep second degree with possible third degree injury), you often have to wait for them to "declare" themselves, which generally occurs by post-burn day 5. Once the true extent of the injury is determined, then you can begin operative planning if deemed necessary.

Wound Care

All burn wounds should be appropriately cleaned with either saline or chlorhexidine and dressed with a topical antimicrobial to prevent infection of the wound. There are a plethora of topical agents available, but likely there are only a few options available at the local pharmacies near your health center. Once the burn wound is covered with a topical antimicrobial, then you must decide what type of dressing to use. These can be separated into two broad categories: the exposure or "open" method and the occlusive dressing or "closed" method. The "open" method consists of leaving the burn wound open to air and not letting anything except for a topical antimicrobial or possibly vaseline gauze come in contact with the wound. The wound will weep and a dry eschar will form over top, acting as an occlusive dressing until new skin grows underneath (if it is second degree). The patient may have a metal cage placed over them that is then covered with clean cloth in order to maintain an ambient temperature for the patient. This method is still commonly used in LMICs because it is simple, is low-cost, and takes significantly less time and personnel to manage. The trade-off is that patients remain on bedrest until their wounds fully heal and therefore cannot participate in physiotherapy. There also is a theoretical increased infection risk (although not proven in studies) because the eschar that develops can just as easily trap bacteria underneath rather than keeping them out.

The occlusive dressing or "closed" method is what is practiced almost exclusively in HIC burn centers. It comprises a primary non-adherent dressing that is placed over the wound after the topical antimicrobial is applied, followed by a secondary absorbent layer of coarse mesh gauze +/− cotton. This dressing can be left in place for 2–3 days unless it becomes saturated with wound exudate, then it must be changed more frequently. If done well, this method is preferable since patients are not confined to their bed and can participate in physiotherapy. The downside to the "closed" method is that it is more expensive, more labor intensive, and if done improperly can lead to infection and possibly convert a partial thickness burn into a full thickness one. Whatever wound care method is chosen, one must always keep in mind the local practices and capabilities.

Since many patients present in a delayed fashion, their burn wounds often have the appearance of being infected. They may present with a crusty wound that is draining "pus." If the wound is large, the patient may exhibit systemic signs and symptoms that mirror sepsis (e.g., tachycardia, fever, leukocytosis). Additionally, it can be difficult to discern between burn wound erythema, which is a normal physiologic response versus early cellulitis. In general, if the burn occurred within the past 24 hours, then it is highly unlikely to be infected and only requires topical antimicrobials. If it has been longer than 24 hours, then the probability of infection increases significantly and a short course of IV antibiotics would be prudent. If after several days of proper cleaning and wound care the appearance of the burn wound improves, then IV antibiotics can be discontinued.

Nutrition

Equally as important as good wound care is proper nutrition support. Without adequate nutritional intake, a partial thickness burn wound can convert to full thickness and wound healing will be stunted. An initial nutritional assessment should be done when the patient is admitted; they should be weighed at least weekly. For patients with burns <10% TBSA no significant changes need to be made to their diet, unless they were malnourished before the injury. Patients with large burns (>15% TBSA) have a hypermetabolic response to the injury that increases their resting energy expenditure 1.5–2 times above normal [10]. There are multiple formulas that have been developed to estimate caloric requirements for burn patients, ranging from complex to nearly impossible to use without a calculator. The following simple formulas can be used to estimate your patient's daily caloric need:

Adults: 20 kcal/kg + 70 kcal/% TBSA burn; protein 1.5–2 g/kg.
Children: 60 kcal/kg + 35 kcal/% TBSA burn; protein 2.5–4 g/kg [12, 13].

The overall composition of macronutrients should be approximately 50–60% carbohydrates, 30% protein, and 10% fats. Patients should be encouraged to eat calorie-rich foods, such as eggs, milk, legumes, and groundnuts. Oftentimes the family has to provide the patient's food so educating the family on appropriate foodstuffs is critical. If their caloric needs are greater than they can consume, it can be supplemented with tube feeds (if tubes are available) that the kitchen prepares with a blender. If a blender is not available, then you can give liquid calories such as milk, eggs, oil, and dissolved sugar.

Operative Planning and Management

Timing of Surgery

The vast majority of burn patients will heal without the need for surgery if they receive good wound care and proper resuscitation. For those patients who do require surgery, an essential question is when to proceed with skin grafting. Early (i.e., <7 days) excision and grafting is the general practice in HICs; however in LMICs surgery will often be delayed for weeks until any partial thickness burns heal spontaneously and the patient has developed a healthy bed of granulation tissue. A recent meta-analysis comparing early vs. late excision and grafting failed to show a mortality benefit *in either HICs or LMICs* but did show decreased sepsis and length of stay in the early excision group [14]. These results directly challenge the dogma that early excision and grafting is the superior choice. The truth, as always, is more nuanced and requires sharp clinical acumen to know when a patient is physiologically ready for surgery given the resources available in a particular setting.

Type of Surgery

Once it is determined that a patient requires surgery for their burns, it is necessary to decide on the type and extent of surgery, as well as the timing. The mainstay treatment for an acute burn is split-thickness skin grafting. Many factors must be considered in preparation for surgery – such as availability of blood, anesthesia, surgical equipment, personnel, etc. – that surgeons in HICs generally take for granted. Practically speaking, without the availability of a blood bank or skin bank, it is not advised to excise more than 10% TBSA in a single operation. If donor sites are scarce, then priority should be given to grafting sensitive areas such as the face, hands, genitalia, and joints. This will hopefully lead to less hypertrophic scar and contracture in the long run (see Chap. 32).

Availability of anesthesia will dictate how extensive an operation can be. Most minor skin grafting procedures can be performed under conscious sedation with just ketamine and will not require a ventilator or an anesthesiologist. Lower extremity burns can be grafted under spinal anesthesia which provides approximately 2–3 hours of paresthesia. Any skin grafting of significant size (>5% TBSA) will require general anesthesia and knowledge of the options will help with safe operative planning.

Acute burn surgery, i.e., burn wound excision and split-thickness skin grafting, is inherently bloody. All attempts should be made to limit blood loss during surgery since blood replacement is difficult in most centers in LMICs. Some techniques can be used routinely, such as injecting dilute epinephrine under burn wounds and donor sites prior to excision or harvesting. Tourniquets should be used liberally for extremity burns. Since a tourniquet machine is not likely available in LMICs, one can fashion a tourniquet from two Foley catheters placed proximally on the extremity. By taking a few extra precautions, blood loss can be easily reduced by a third or more.

Escharotomy and Sloughectomy

Two surgical situations deserve special attention: escharotomy and sloughectomy. When a patient has a circumferential third degree burn on the trunk, neck, or an extremity, they can quickly develop compartment syndrome which can lead to muscle necrosis, respiratory failure, and even death. If a patient starts to exhibit the 5 P's of compartment syndrome (*pain, pallor, paresthesia, pulselessness, and paralysis*), then one should immediately perform an escharotomy of the involved body part. The goal of an escharotomy is to release the eschar along the sides thereby relieving the pressure and allowing the underlying tissue to swell. Circumferential second degree burns generally do not cause compartment syndrome since part of the dermis is intact and can stretch.

A sloughectomy is an operation that one will only see practiced in LMICs [13]. Essentially, it entails removing the slough – dead, moist tissue overlying the burned area – by excisional debridement. A sloughectomy is required if there is concern for infection of the burn wound or if the necrotic tissue is not spontaneously lifting after an appropriate period of time. Sloughectomy can be performed at the bedside. If extensive or if there is concern for bleeding, then the sloughectomy should be done in the operating theater. Once the wound has been adequately debrided you can either proceed with skin grafting if the wound bed appears ready or continue with wound care until healthy granulation tissue forms.

Postoperative Care

Postoperative care after burn surgery, whether sloughectomy, skin grafting, or scar contracture release, should follow the same principles whether in HICs or in LMICs. This includes appropriate wound care to protect both the surgical burn site and the donor site; appropriate splinting, positioning, and immobilization of any involved limbs; and daily evaluation for infection. Certain patients (i.e., children) may require placement of a cast to ensure appropriate splinting is maintained throughout the early postoperative period. If there is a physiotherapist available, their expertise should be enlisted to help with postoperative splinting and position monitoring. However, it would be useful for the care giver to be familiar with some basic splinting positions in case a physiotherapist is not available (Fig. 31.5). Since family members are often directly involved in a patient's medical treatment, they should also be educated on splinting and encouraged to participate in the

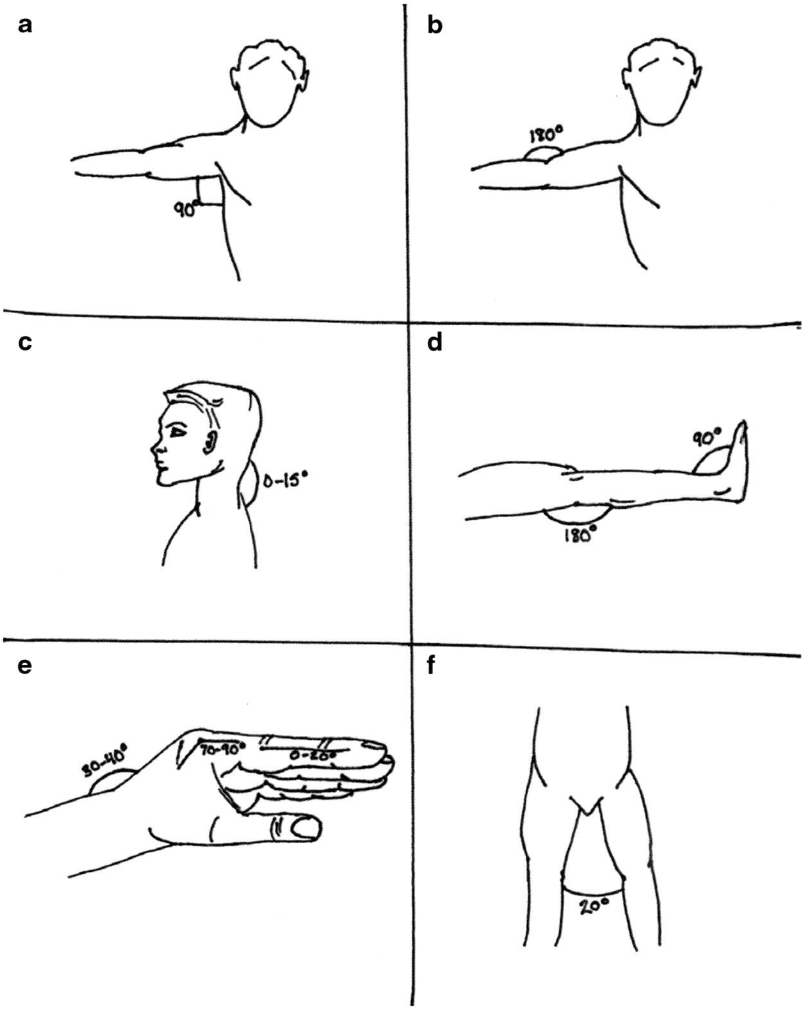

Fig. 31.5 Appropriate splinting and positioning after skin graft surgery. (**a**) Shoulder positioning at 90° of abduction, and slight horizontal adduction to prevent brachial plexus stretch. (**b**) Positioning of the elbow in neutral. (**c**) Positioning of the neck in neutral or slight cervical extension. (**d**) Positioning of the knee in neutral, positioning of the ankle in neutral. (**e**) Positioning of the wrist in the intrinsic plus position; 30°–40° of wrist extension, 70°–90° MCP flexion, 0–20° of IP flexion. (**f**) 20° of hip abduction, torso in neutral, lower extremities in neutral avoiding external rotation

patient's postoperative care. Until the local team is comfortable with managing burn patients postoperatively, we recommend visiting teams remain at the healthcare facility during the immediate postoperative period until it is clear that the surgery was successful. In general, this implies 5–7 days after skin grafting and 3–5 days after simple scar contracture releases. Even if the surgery was minor (e.g., <3% TBSA split-thickness skin graft or a simple z-plasty), it is important to ensure a successful outcome, especially if burn surgery is a new treatment modality in the region.

Postoperative care of the burn patient is unique compared to many other surgical specialties. For most, 4–6 weeks of healing time, whether for surgical incisions, hernias, or broken bones, is sufficient to say that the patient has "fully recovered" from surgery. For burn patients, however, remodeling of burn scar and skin graft sites is an ongoing process for *at least* a year. In order to guarantee the best aesthetic and functional outcome, they will require ongoing physiotherapy to prevent postoperative contractures, active scar management (i.e., scar massage therapy, compression dressings, possible serial splinting, physiotherapy exercises, etc.), and surveillance for hypertrophic scar formation and scar contractures. While this is common practice for multidisciplinary burn teams in HICs, it is often an overlooked but vital part of a patient's care towards full recovery from their burn injury. It is not uncommon for a patient to recover from their burn injuries while an inpatient, only to return 6 months later with a severe scar contracture at their prior burn site or even at an unburned site (see Chap. 32)! Patients and their family should be educated on appropriate postoperative physiotherapy exercises and encouraged to continue splinting affected joints at night. Regularly scheduled postoperative visits should be established for surveillance, either at the health center or possibly through outreach programs if patients cannot afford travel costs. As the patient gets farther out from their burn injury, visits can be extended out to longer periods of time until the patient develops a "mature" burn scar that is satisfactory to both patient and the practitioner (approximately 1–1.5 years from burn injury). By investing time and resources into helping develop a local structured postoperative protocol, one will achieve a higher degree of success and meaningful recovery for the burn patients in the region.

Role of Antibiotics Postoperatively

In general, systemic antibiotics are not required postoperatively unless the patient shows local or systemic signs of infection preoperatively (e.g., erythema, purulent drainage, fever, leukocytosis). Surgical removal of the infected eschar followed by dressing the area with local antimicrobials may be sufficient to control the infection if it is limited only to the wound. We recommend using systemic antibiotics sparingly in order to avoid development of multi-drug-resistant strains of bacteria. If available, culture swabs of the wound are important to determine the infectious pathogen. This will guide the antibiotic regimen. For *Pseudomonas* we recommend using acetic acid, sodium hypochlorite, and/or gentamicin topically as this is readily available in most LMICs. The use of antibiotics for burn patients is a common practice among local practitioners and may become a point of conflict between the visiting team and the local providers; a healthy level of deference goes a long way to building bridges.

Conclusion

Burn patients are arguably some of the most complex patients in a healthcare system. Often, when resources and personnel are not readily available, their care will suffer and they can languish for weeks or months on the ward with painful open wounds. The results of this neglect are visible to the world as severe contractures and hypertrophic scars (see Chap. 32). In HICs, over a quarter of burn patients never return to any form of employment [15] because of their burn injuries. This number is likely even higher in LMICs and represents a significant social and economic burden on families and communities. However, with a dedicated team to provide appropriate wound care, physiotherapy, and skin grafting when necessary, many of the complications and disabilities associated with burns can be avoided.

References

1. Peck MD. Epidemiology of burns throughout the world. Part I: distribution and risk factors. Burns. 2011;37(7):1087–100. https://doi.org/10.1016/j.burns.2011.06.005.
2. Burns. World Health Organization. https://www.who.int/news-room/fact-sheets/detail/burns. Accessed 2 Apr 2022.
3. Gibson C, Bessey PQ, Gallagher JJ. The global burn registry: a work in Progress. J Burn Care Res. 2020;41(5):929–34. https://doi.org/10.1093/jbcr/iraa078.
4. Allorto NL, Clarke DL. Merits and challenges in the development of a dedicated burn service at a regional Hospital in South Africa. Burns. 2015;41(3):454–61. https://doi.org/10.1016/j.burns.2014.07.021.
5. Borrelli MR. What is the role of plastic surgery in global health? A review. World J Plast Surg. 2018;7(3):275–82. https://doi.org/10.29252/wjps.7.3.275.
6. Harish V, Tiwari N, Fisher OM, Li Z, et al. First aid improves clinical outcomes in burn injuries: evidence from a cohort study of 4918 patients. Burns. 2019;45(2):433–9. https://doi.org/10.1016/j.burns.2018.09.024.
7. American Burn Association. Initial first aid treatment for minor burns. http://ameriburn.org/wp-content/uploads/2017/05/burnfirstaid.pdf. Accessed 2 Apr 2022.
8. Wallace HJ, O'Neill TB, Wood FM, Edgar DW, Rea SM. Determinants of burn first aid knowledge: cross-sectional study. Burns. 2013;39(6):1162–9. https://doi.org/10.1016/j.burns.2013.02.007.
9. Meara JG, Leather AJ, Hagander L, Alkire BC, et al. Global surgery 2030: evidence and solutions for achieving health, welfare, and economic development. Lancet. 2015;386(9993):569–624. https://doi.org/10.1016/s0140-6736(15)60160-x.
10. Alvarado R, Chung KK, Cancio LC, Wolf SE. Burn resuscitation. Burns. 2009;35(1):4–14. https://doi.org/10.1016/j.burns.2008.03.008.
11. Eastridge B, Putz B, Ward A, editors. Burn Clinical Practice Guideline. Austin, TX: Texas EMS Trauma and Acute Care Foundation Trauma Division; 2016. p. 1–20.
12. Carson JS, Khosrozadeh H, Norbury WB, Herndon DN. Nutritional needs and support for the burned patient. In: Total burn care. 5th ed. Elsevier; 2018. p. 287–300.
13. King M, Bewes P. Burns. In: Primary surgery: trauma, vol. 2. Oxford: Oxford University Press; 2013. p. 65–91.
14. Wong L, Rajandram R, Allorto N. Systematic review of excision and grafting in burns: comparing outcomes of early and late surgery in low and high-income countries. Burns. 2021;47(8):1705–13. https://doi.org/10.1016/j.burns.2021.07.001.
15. Mason ST, Esselman P, Fraser R, Schomer K. Return to work after burn injury. J Burn Care Res. 2012;33(1):101–9. https://doi.org/10.1097/bcr.0b013e3182374439.

32 How to Surgically Reconstruct Acute and Chronic Burn Wounds in Low- and Middle-Income Countries

Einar Eriksen

A great pleasure in life is doing what people say you cannot do.

– Walter Bagehot

Abbreviations

FTSG	Full-thickness skin graft
LMICs	Low- and middle-income countries
STSG	Split-thickness skin graft
TBSA	Total body surface area

Introduction

Burn casualties seem to be one of the most common mechanisms of injury in the third world. The majority of burns worldwide occur in low- and middle-income countries (LMICs). Burn injuries and poverty are quite often closely associated, where children and females are the main victims. These casualties seem to be linked to unprotected fireplaces and ground level cooking.

E. Eriksen (✉)
Children's Burn & Wound Care Foundation, Addis Ababa, Ethiopia

MCM Comprehensive Specialised Hospital, Addis Ababa, Ethiopia

Burn survivors frequently develop various degrees of handicaps and deformities which impose a heavy burden on the families and the society. The main reasons for the tragic post burn outcome are lack of designated hospital facilities, shortage of supplies and surgical equipment like dermatomes (manual or electric), skin meshers, skin staples as well as inadequate number of trained and motivated staff.

Aspects of Acute Burn Treatment

Diagnosis of Acute Burns

A basic knowledge of how to determine the **DEPTH** and **EXTENT** (Total Body Surface Area, TBSA) of thermal injuries will guide the health professional in providing the best possible treatment scheme for his patient.

The risk of future scarring and contracture development is closely associated with the depth as well as the location of the wound. The deeper the wound appears to be, the greater the risk of scar formation and contracture development if wounds are left without proper surgical care, like a skin graft.

M. A. Hardy, B. R. Hochman (eds.), *Global Surgery*, https://doi.org/10.1007/978-3-031-28127-3_32

The depth of a burn injury is traditionally classified into three different levels:

First degree burn: When the superficial part of the skin, the epidermis, has received too much of sunshine, it reacts with mild erythema and various degrees of pain.

Signs and symptoms: Mild erythema, pain, and discomfort. No blister formation. Will subside in a couple of days.

Second degree burn: Classified as superficial partial thickness or deep partial thickness, depending on how deep the injury penetrates into the dermis of the skin.

Signs and symptoms: Blister formation, Pain, Wet, Pink wound surface

Third degree burn: Both epidermis and dermis are destroyed, often described as a full-thickness burn. In special areas where the skin is normally thin, like the dorsum of the hand and foot, structures like tendons, fascia, and even bony structures may be exposed.

Sign and symptoms: Dry leather looking skin, no pain on touching the affected area

Clinical importance:

First degree burn (sunburn) has little clinical importance.

Second degree burn: Superficial wounds tend to heal quicker and will seldom leave any significant scar. The more superficial the wound is, the more pain the patient will experience. It heals usually within 2–3 weeks.

Third degree burn: If a wound has not healed properly within 3 weeks, the wound is classified as a third degree or full-thickness burn wound. This wound will eventually heal in most instances with scar formation.

Reference is made to other textbooks for more details about diagnosis of acute burns with assessment of depth and extent of burn wounds.

Principles for Improved Burn Care

A successful outcome for a burn victim starts with showing interest, concern and motivation about how best to provide care for the burn patient. The sooner the burn victim gets in contact with experienced health professionals, the better for the outcome. Even though a specialized multidisciplinary burn center is the preferred place for referral, such centers may not be easily available in LMICs. Motivated trained health professionals in any health facility can attend the acute injured patient with required emergency care, like IV fluids, observation of vital signs, measuring urinary output, assessment and dressing of the wounds until a planned referral has been organized.

It may sometimes be difficult to decide the depth of the wounds during the first 24–48 h. The signs and symptoms of second and of third degree burns should be applied when making a proper assessment of the burn victim.

Keeping the wounds clean, removing and peeling all loose blisters and changing the dressings on a daily/regular basis, is of paramount importance in order to prevent a second degree burn from getting infected and turning into a deeper wound.

Topical antibiotics, like Flamazine (silver sulfadiazine cream), are very helpful in preventing patients from ending up septic in deep burns.

Frequently, burns show up with a mixture of second and third degree burn. It is advisable to continue daily/regular dressing changes until all the second degree wounds have healed (2–3 weeks), before planning skin grafts on the remaining wounds.

Surgical Intervention in the Acute Stage

Surgical intervention is an emergency under the following conditions:

Escharotomy Circumferential deep (third degree) burns on the limbs, as well as the trunk, are regarded an emergency situation. The surgeon should without delay bring the patient to the operating room to perform two longitudinal escharotomy incisions of the limb to prevent compromised circulation. Likewise, two longitudinal and horizontal escharotomy incisions on the trunk need to be performed to make sure breathing is not compromised. In both instances, longitudinal incisions should run from just proximal to the circumferential burn until just below the distal margin of the burn.

Escahrectomy Surgical excision of dead tissue (escharectomy) needs to be performed whenever there is a clear demarcated deep infected third degree burn in order to remove necrotic tissue that otherwise may be a focus for septicemia. Tourniquet should always be used when operating on limbs.

Skin Graft Procedures during the Early/Acute Stage

The only way to prevent burn victims from ending up with severe handicap, is to treat the wounds as early as possible. Nothing will benefit the patient more than having the wounds covered with skin graft within 3–4 weeks post burn.

There are different approaches to deal with acute burns. The choices should be made based on the availability of experienced staff and how the facilities are equipped.

Early skin graft procedures within the first 2 weeks are regarded state-of-the-art treatment in standard burn centers. This requires optimal facilities with regard to experienced staff, ICUs, blood products, and laboratory support that often may not be available in many LMICs.

In general, there are many advantages of focusing on daily wound care until all second degree wounds have healed and then address the remaining deeper wounds that need skin grafts.

From our experience, wounds that have been dressed by dedicated and trained staff on a daily and regular basis for about 3–4 weeks appear clean and ready for skin grafts.

When there is an isolated deep partial thickness or full thickness burn, an experienced burn surgeon should consider early excision and grafting within the first 2 weeks. Early excisions significantly reduce the risk of infection.

Excision of necrotic tissue on extremities should be performed using tourniquet. This reduces blood loss. Furthermore, the surgeon will be able to determine the adequate depth of the excision when tourniquet is applied. Most often, early tangential excisions are followed by another 2–3 days to make sure no necrosis is left behind before applying skin grafts. Preventing graft loss should be of greatest concern, and most of the time it becomes a matter of whether or not the wound is clean and ready to receive a skin graft.

Experienced burn surgeons will also excise larger areas of third degree burns in the acute stage in order to reduce the load of necrotic tissue. From our experience, we usually cover the excised wounds with topical antibiotics. We do repeated surgical debridements, daily dressing changes and wound inspections until we feel sure the wounds appear free of necrotic tissue before applying the skin grafts (Figs. 32.1, 32.2, 32.3, and 32.4).

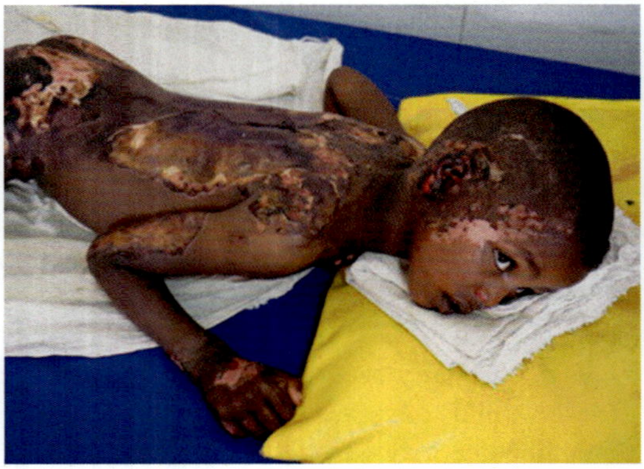

Fig. 32.1 6 years old boy with ext. flame burn injury. Admitted 5th day post burn

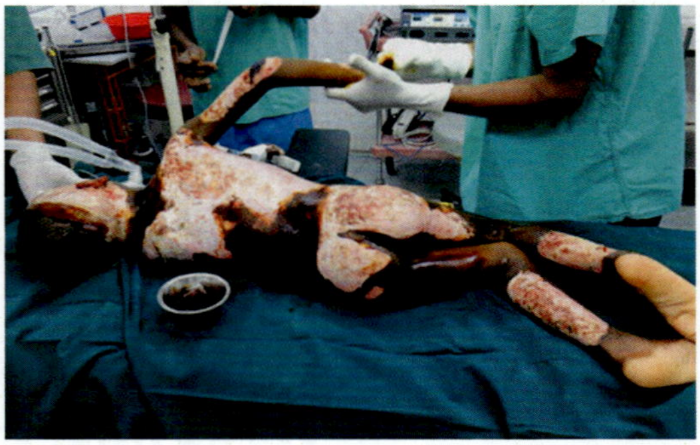

Fig. 32.2 Tangential excision of necrotic tissue as soon as patient is stabilized

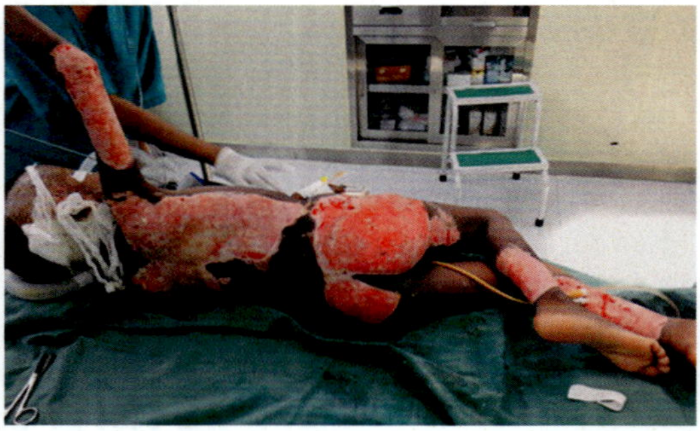

Fig. 32.3 Repeated surgical debridements until all necrosis are excised

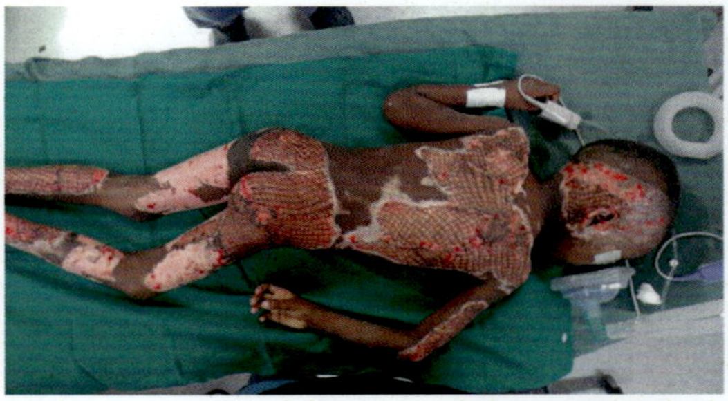

Fig. 32.4 Fully grafted before 2 weeks of injury

Basic Surgical Equipment

Proper treatment of acute and chronic burns, burn contractures require a standardized set of equipment.

The following equipment is recommended:

Skin graft Meshers are mandatory, whatever kind of surgical wounds are to be treated.

Graft take is enhanced markedly; larger areas can be covered using a Mesher (Figs. 32.5 and 32.6).

Although an electric dermatome is a great tool when dealing with extensive burns, the authors advise burn surgeons to get familiar of manual dermatomes. There are several reasons why that is important.

- **Humby knives** (Fig. 32.7) are inexpensive and may last for years when taken great care of.
- Blades are relatively inexpensive.
- Blades can be re-sterilized several times providing the edge is handled with utmost care.
- Humby knives can harvest wider grafts than electric dermatomes – an important point when dealing with reconstructive surgery.
- Electric dermatomes are expensive and difficult to obtain and to maintain.

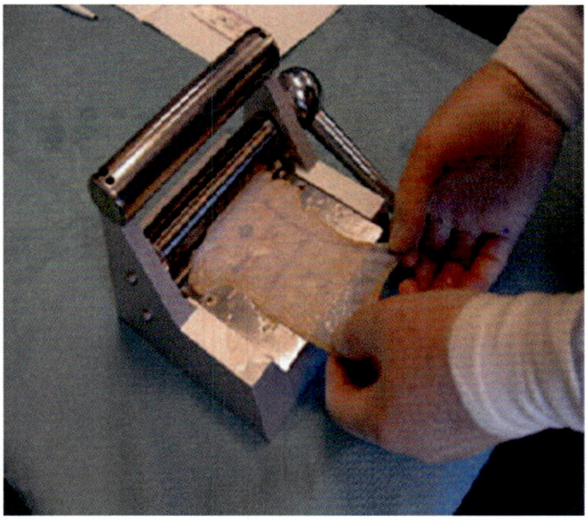

Fig. 32.5 STSG Mesher

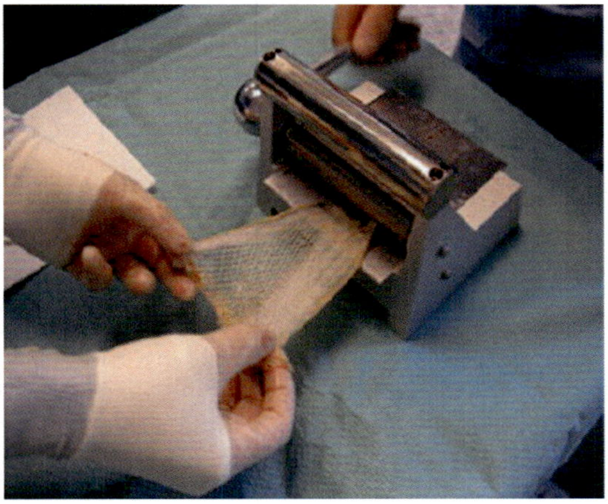

Fig. 32.6 STSG mesher without dermacarrier

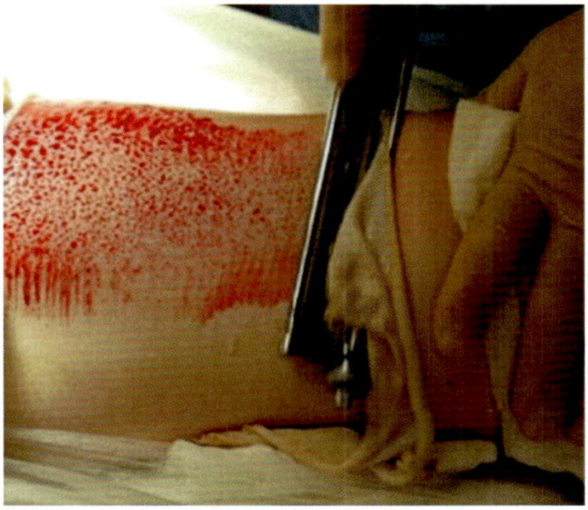

Fig. 32.7 Humby Knife

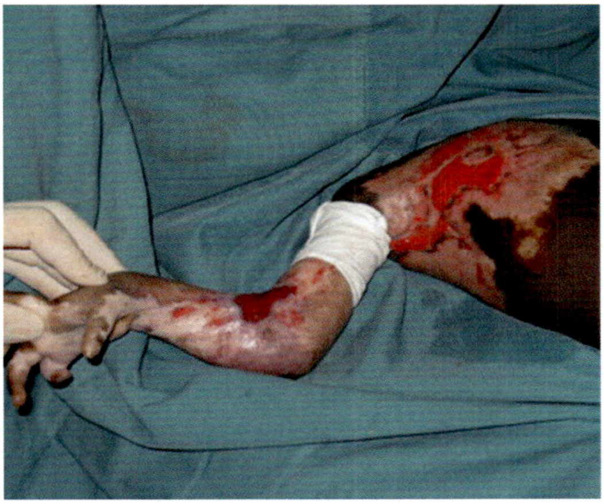

Fig. 32.8 Rubber Band Turniquet

Tourniquets (rubber bands) (Fig. 32.8) are highly recommended whenever surgery on the limbs is undertaken. Blood loss is significantly reduced. This helps the surgeon to distinguish necrotic from healthy issue. Surgery time is also shortened. There is lack of blood supply in LMICs so transfusions are limited.

Skin staples (Fig. 32.9) make burn surgery easier to perform. The equipment makes acute burn surgery as well as post burn reconstructive surgery far more efficient. Proper use of staples shortens the theatre time considerably.

Diathermy machine/electrocautery machine is needed to obtain meticulous hemostasis before applying a skin graft to the recipient

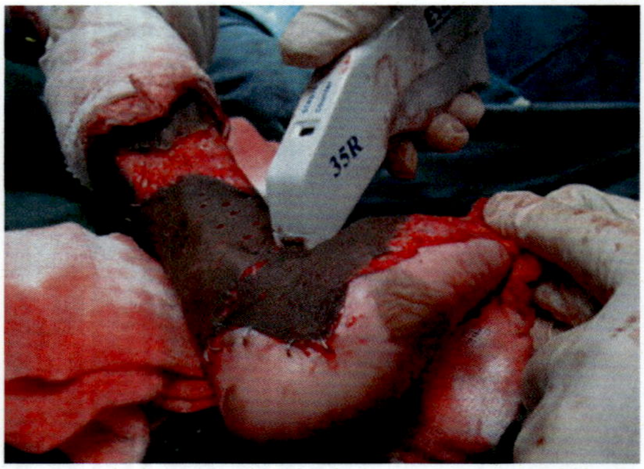

Fig. 32.9 Skin staple

wound area and this cannot be overemphasized. This is of particular importance in dealing with sheet grafts, FTSG and STSG. Adrenaline 1:1000 can be diluted and used topically to control bleeding. Usually 2 ml is added to 100–200 mL of saline.

Surgical Technique in Acute and Chronic Burns

The surgeon will have different options at hand for wound cover when planning closing an existing wound or releasing a contracture.

The Main Options Are

1. **Z-plasty:** The main indication is to correct post burn linear scars crossing joint related areas. Proper results depend on normal skin tissue located adjacent to the linear scar (see Figs. 32.75 and 32.76).
2. **Transposition flap:** Ideal when joints, tendons, and bony structures are exposed.

   These flaps are also very useful in post burn joint reconstruction, often in combination with STSG or FTSG.
3. **Distant flap:** Useful flaps in special challenging cases to be discussed under section "Post Burn Contractures."
4. **Skin grafts:** Skin grafts are differentiated in Split Thickness Skin Grafts (STSGs) and Full Thickness Skin Grafts (FTSG).

   Skin grafts give good results and are easier to deal with compared to flaps, and should always be considered when planning the closure of a wound or reconstruction of a contracture.

   In our experience, at least 80% of all burn patients, acute as well as chronic, can be treated very professionally using skin grafts alone.

Split Thickness Skin Grafts (STSG)

- Common donor sites are the thighs, legs, flanks, and gluteal areas. Avoid harvesting from forearms due to poor aesthetics.
- STSGs may vary in thickness, from superficial thin grafts to thicker grafts (~8 to 201000ths/inch).
- The degree of the dermal component of the graft determines the result of the surgery. The thicker the dermal component, the better appearance and functional result.
- On the other hand, the thinner the dermal component of the STSG, the sooner the donor wound will heal, but the graft at the recipient site may be subject for scarring (see Figs. 32.10 and 32.11).
- The donor wound from a medium, "standard" STSG will heal within 14 days and typically does not leave a noticeable scar.
- Thick STSG donor wound may take 3 weeks or more to heal.
- STSGs are frequently meshed in order to cover larger areas (Fig. 32.10).
- Sheet grafts are more functionally and cosmetically appealing compared to mesh grafts (Fig. 32.12).

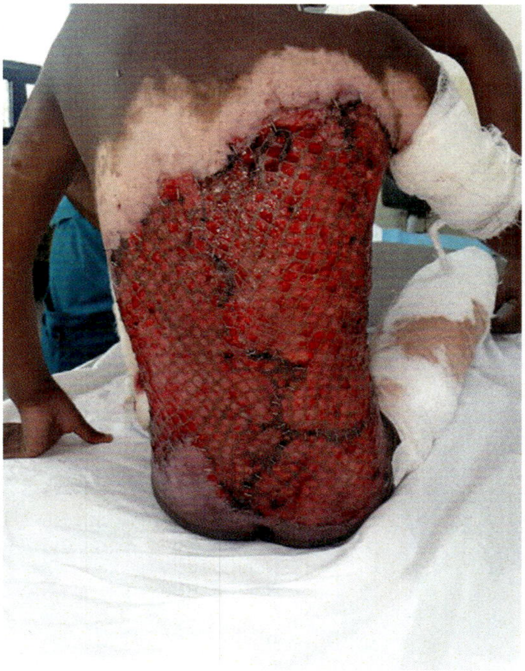

Fig. 32.10 STSG meshed 4:1, skin staples applied

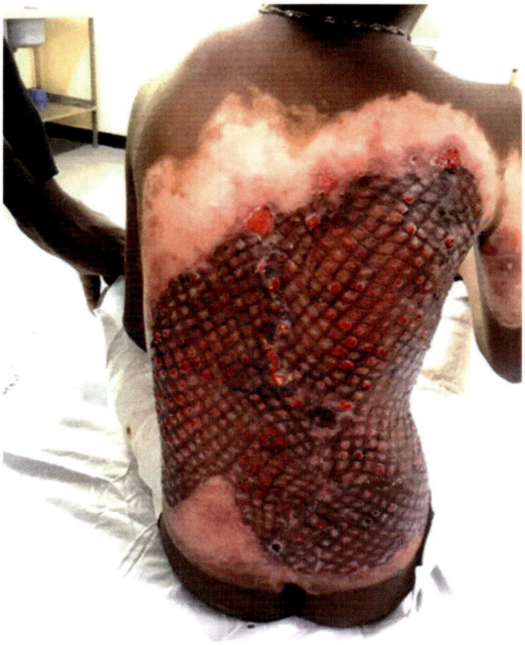

Fig. 32.11 Skin graft healed

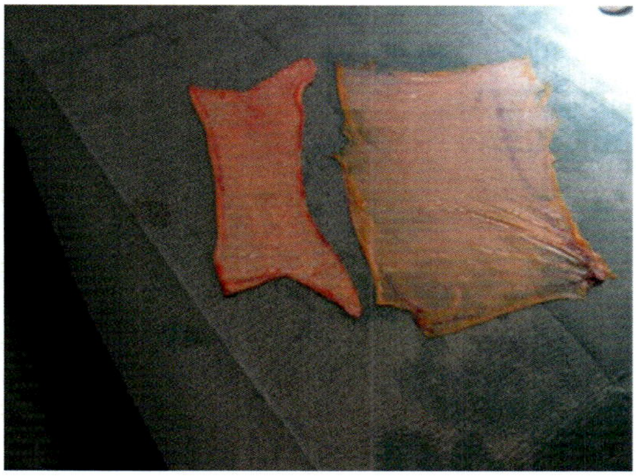

Fig. 32.12 FTSG & STSG

Full Thickness Skin Grafts (FTSG)

- A FTSG consists of the whole layer of skin – epidermis plus the whole dermal layer.
- Full thickness grafts are technically more difficult to harvest and to apply on the wound. Full thickness skin grafts require defatting of the undersurface of the dermis to enhance graft take (Fig. 32.13). Full thickness grafts are not meshed by a machine, but are often meshed by hand with a scalpel ("pie crusting") to allow blood and serous fluid to escape into the overlying dressing (Fig. 32.14).
- Meticulous hemostasis of the recipient wound is mandatory. Hematoma formation underneath the graft will inhibit graft take.
- FTSGs are preferred to STSGs when reconstructing facial defects and special joint areas:
  - Eyelids, lips, and cheek.
  - Anterior neck/axilla/elbow.
  - Volar aspect of the wrist and hand/fingers.
  - Groin/fossa poplitea/ankle.
- Smaller grafts may be harvested from the posterior aspect of the ear, supraclavicular area, and medial side of the upper arm. These donor wounds are usually easily closed.
- Hair follicles in grafts harvested from the groin will lead to hair growth at the recipient site and should be given concern. Harvesting from alternative places should be considered.
- When large FTSGs are required, the grafts may be harvested from the medial side of the

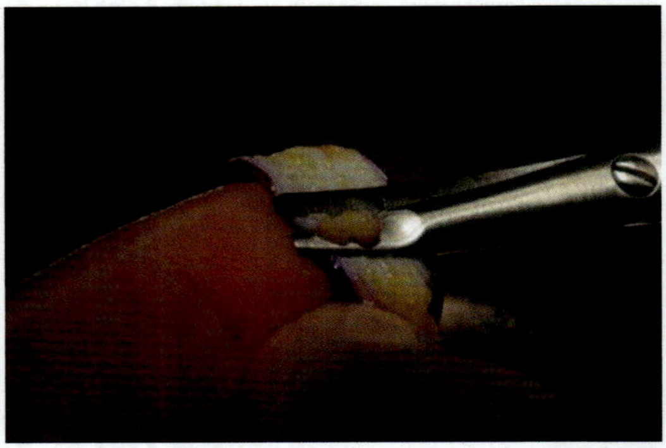

Fig. 32.13 Fat trimming of FTSG

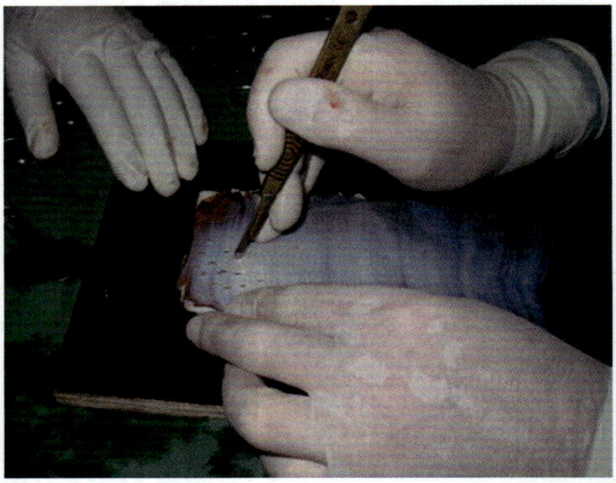

Fig. 32.14 Hand meshing of FTSG

upper arm, flank, abdomen, or from the thigh.

- FTSGs from medial aspect of upper arm or thigh will likely need to be closed with a meshed STSG (see Figs. 32.15 and 32.16).
- When harvesting FTSG from the thigh, the manual dermatome (Humby knife) can provide a wide graft.

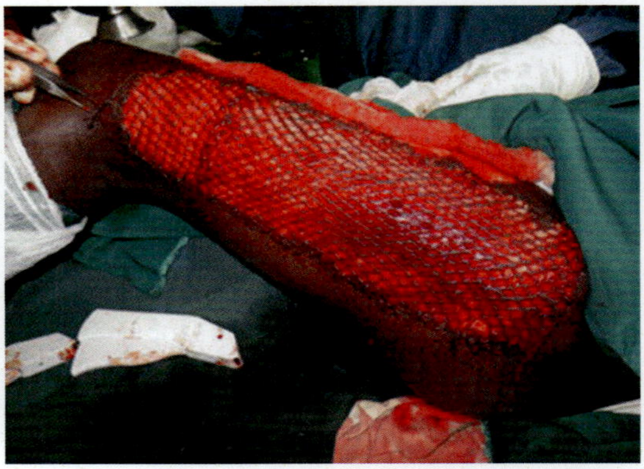

Fig. 32.15 Harvest of FTSG from lateral side of left thigh with application of STSG to donor site

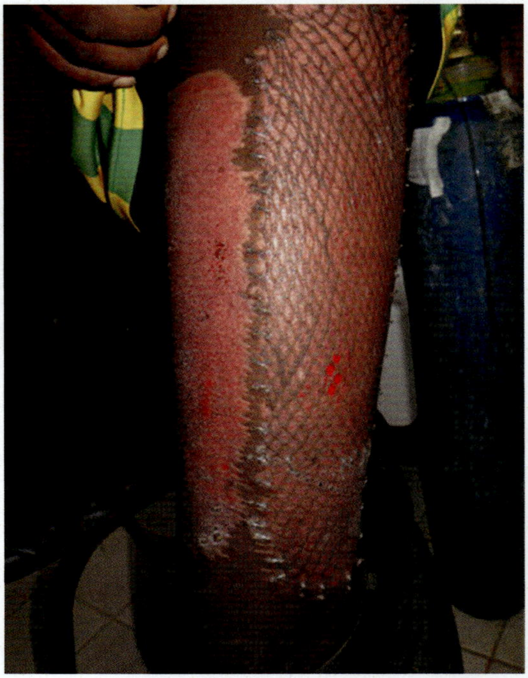

Fig. 32.16 Deep cut covered with 4:1 meshed STSG from medial side of same thigh

Harvesting and Application of Skin Grafts

As mentioned above, surgeons should be familiar with the use of a manual dermatome, the Humby knife (Fig. 32.7).

The thickness of the graft is determined by observing the gap between the roller of the dermatome and the blade. When the gap permits a scalpel or razor blade to gently slide in between the roller and the blade of the dermatome, a medium thickness STSG will be harvested – approximately 0.015 inch in thickness. The gap needs to be adjusted a bit to widen the space between the roller and dermatome blade to get a thicker FTSG graft. The thickness of the graft may also depend on several factors such as: The way the handle is used. Angle to the skin, force applied to the skin, whether the blade is new or used, from where on the body you harvest and whether the patient is a child or an adult.

It appears obvious that this procedure needs experience and practice.

Again, the following points all determine the thickness of the graft:

- The patients age – child or older adult?
- Consider that thickness of the skin varies from one place of the body to another.
- The angle between the dermatome and the skin surface.
- The pressure applied on the dermatome.

With experience, the surgeon will adjust their cut to obtain the desired thickness. Practice on pig skin is appropriate.

The thicker the graft, the deeper the donor wound, and the more likely the surgeon should consider re-grafting the donor area with mesh graft for quick healing. Joint areas should preferably be covered with thick STSG sheet grafts or FTSGs after hand meshing the graft in a few areas to permit serous fluid and blood to escape into the overlying dressing.

If a mesh machine is not available, split thickness grafts may still be meshed by hand through a number of small cuts thereby allowing expansion of the graft.

The application of proper bandage and dressing material is of greatest importance. Properly applied dressings will prevent hematoma formation and make sure the graft is not moving. This principle is applied to grafts wherever they are applied. A shear injury to the graft from sliding around is one of the leading causes of graft failure. The surgeon is responsible for the follow-up of all patients. The author advises the surgeon to do the first dressing change together with the nursing staff, and leave for the burn nurses to do the follow-up dressings. However, the surgeon should regularly inspect the wound in order to determine the appropriate timing for the skin graft procedure.

The right timing for post-op dressing changes may vary:

- Elective surgery with skin graft: First dressing change after 5 days.
- Unclean wounds/chronic hyper-trophic granulation wounds with skin graft: first dressing change first or second post-op day.

Care for Donor Wounds

Neglecting care for donor wounds may prolong hospital stay considerably!

Make all efforts to prevent donor wounds from becoming infected. Infected split thickness donor wounds may sometimes require a meshed skin graft for the donor wound to heal properly.

- If possible, avoid harvesting skin grafts from the posterior aspect of the lower limbs and trunk. Donor wounds from these areas may easily become secondarily infected.
- A simple and inexpensive dressing for donor wounds is Vaseline gauze (non-adherent gauze) covered with several layers of dry surgical gauze followed with a crepe bandage/roll gauze bandage.
- Make sure bed clothes and blankets do not touch the dressing. This is important in order

to keep the donor wound dressing dry and the best way of preventing donor site infection.

- Check the donor site dressing every day. If the dressing becomes wet – a sign of possible infection – the wet part of the dressing needs to be changed without delay.
- To prevent donor wound infection, it is advisable to change the outer bandage of the donor area the first post-op day. This may be repeated if dressing again gets soaked. Keep changing regularly until dressing stays dry.

Chronic Burn Wounds: A Challenge

Many patients present with chronic wounds with or without a contracture or deformity. Patients may have waited for months or sometimes even years before seeking help. Many of these patients, children as well as adults, show evidence of malnutrition.

This group of patients are difficult to treat. Before even considering surgical excision and grafting procedures, patients may need nutritional support for weeks to come. Measures need to be taken to address chronic anemia. Blood transfusions may be necessary but difficult to obtain in LMICs, unless the family members are willing to donate.

Sooner or later though, surgery has to be planned. In the meantime, various routines will be adhered to, like:

- 24 h nutritional support through a NG tube as necessary
- Routine work-up and treatment (scabies, parasites, HIV, etc.)
- Daily wound care with topical antibiotics.
- Physiotherapy training.

Chronic wounds always consist of a thick fibrous tissue that needs to be excised before any graft is applied. Skin grafts will be rejected in most instances, partly or in total, if applied to a fibrotic tissue floor.

The thickness of this fibrous tissue may exceed 1 cm or more. The only way to secure graft take is to undertake a complete excision of the fibrotic wound. Limb surgery must be performed under tourniquet control.

Chronic wounds are heavily infected. It is recommended to repeat surgical debridements at least a few times and obtaining a negative culture of the base of the wound before performing the final skin graft procedure.

Daily post-operative dressing changes should start from day 1, and continue every day until grafts are healing.

Sub-Acute to Chronic Wounds

Many patients present with wounds that are 6–8 weeks old. They are referred when the wounds do not heal properly. Small blisters may be a sign of an unstable scar.

When burn wounds do not heal within 3 weeks, they are categorized as third degree. Some of them may still heal given a little more time, which often is the right thing to do.

However, when wounds do not heal by 5–6 weeks, one should consider surgery, as the following cases underline (Figs. 32.17, 32.18, 32.19, 32.20, 32.21, 32.22, 32.23, 32.24, 32.25, 32.26, and 32.33):

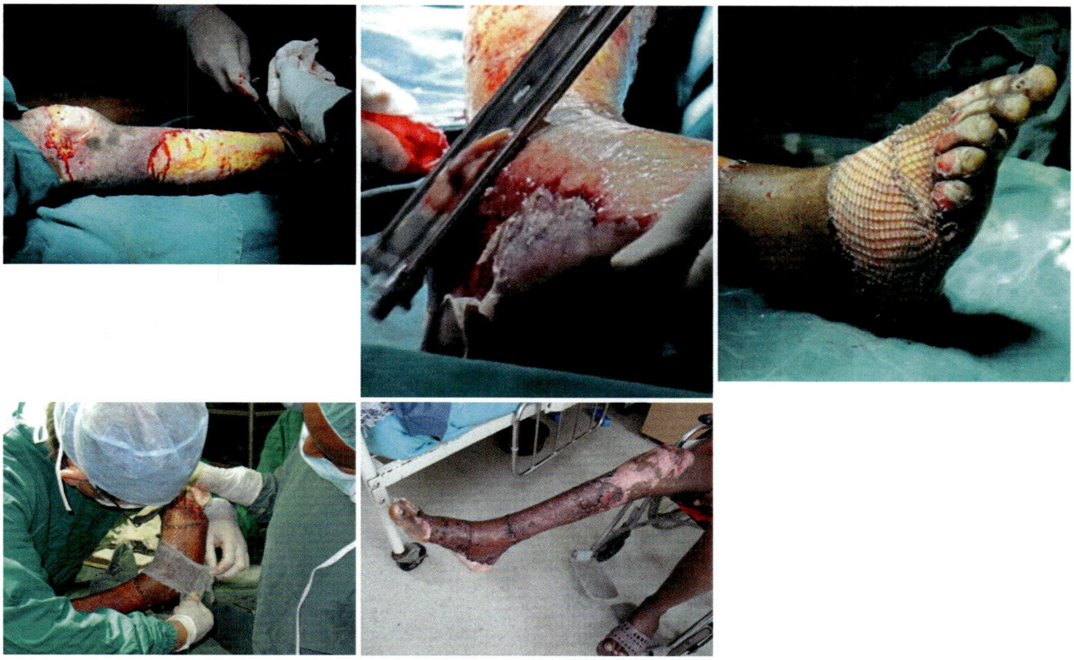

Figs. 32.17–32.21 Flame burn injury with unstable scar 7 weeks post injury. Tangential excision with Humby knife, FTSG across ankle area, meshed STSG on remaining wounds. Total procedure includes application of grafts under tourniquet

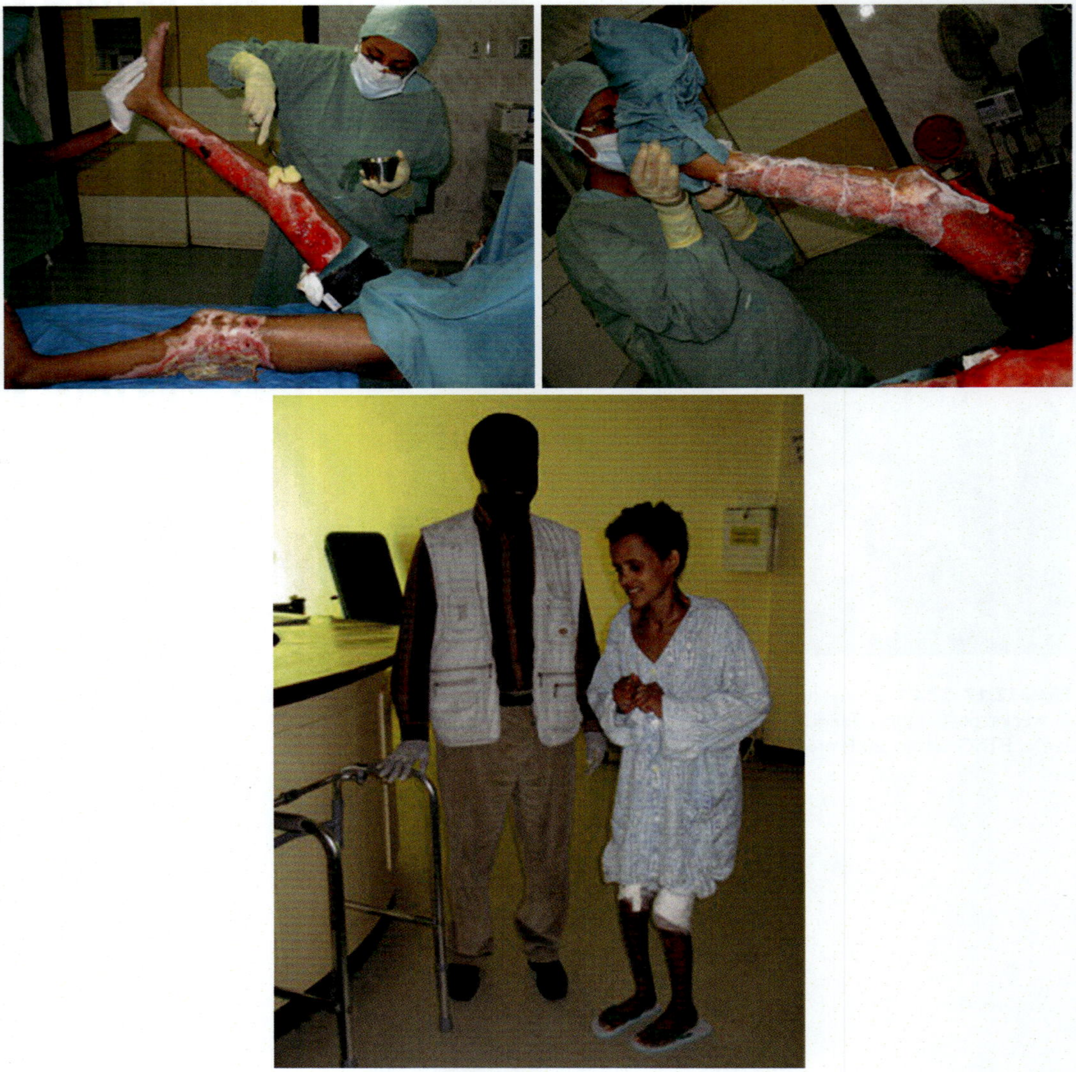

Figs. 32.22–32.24 12 months bedridden due to neglected flame burn injury. Severely malnourished. 24/7 NG tube feeding. Daily dressing change. Topical antibiotics. Surgical excisions of infected granulation tissue. Once debrided wounds appeared clean, meshed STSG was applied, (Figs. 22 and 23). After 4 weeks in hospital, patient was able to stand on 2 legs with good support from the physio-therapist, (Fig. 24). Discharged after 6 weeks in hospital

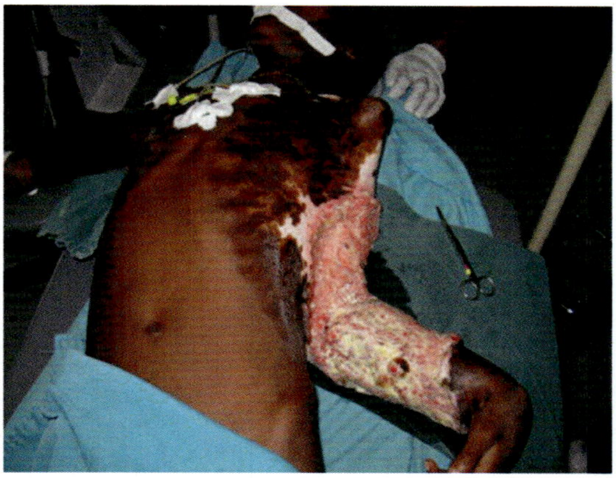

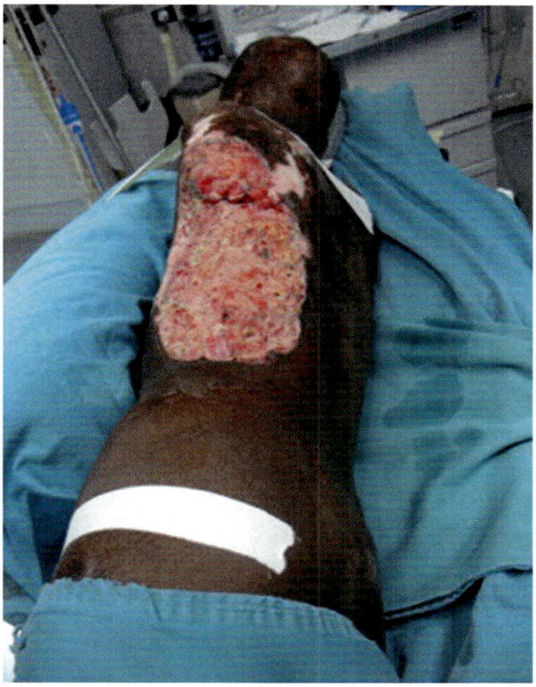

Figs. 32.25 and 32.26 Keep in mind that chronic burn wounds may degenerate into a Spinocellular Carcinoma (Squamous Cell Carcinoma) if left untreated for many years

Post Burn Contractures

Scar formation in neglected burns is the main reason for the subsequent development of deformities and handicap among burn victims.

Even though burn contractures may affect any neglected burn victim, the consequences among children are particularly of great concern. By nature, scar tissue will contract in order to minimize and close any wound. Contractures and deformities around joint areas in children will appear more pronounced as times goes by as a child is growing. The need for close follow-up after surgery is therefore of greatest importance among many pediatric burn victims.

Basic principles in post burn reconstructive surgery:

- Release of all contracting scar tissue contributing to the deformity.
- Z-plasty.
- Skin graft procedures.
- Transposition/pedicle flaps.

All scar tissue which contributes to the deformity needs to be released. The best cleavage line for dissection is the level between the scar and the underlying healthy subcutaneous tissue, which becomes an excellent recipient bed for a skin graft. The size of the wound following a complete release often appears to be much larger than the one that would be projected. Harvest of skin graft should always wait until the size of the wound has been revealed and accurately measured at its maximum size (e.g., in extension).

Z-plasty is an excellent way of releasing a linear scar in joint areas. The technique is very useful when the adjacent skin structure is normal without scar formation (see Figs. 32.75 and 32.76).

Sheet grafts, whether STSG or FTSG, are the main solution for the coverage in the majority of all post burn contractures (Fig. 32.12).

In joint related areas, a FTSG is usually the preferred choice. The functional and cosmetic result using FTSG in head and neck, elbow, hand, wrist, and fingers is far better than using STSG.

Meticulous hemostasis is of paramount importance when FTSG are applied in order to avoid "tenting" and graft loss.

Transposition flaps are very useful in joint areas. The donor defect may as well be closed directly, but often though a skin graft may be needed.

Distant/pedicle flaps are useful under conditions when a skin graft or local transposition flap may not solve the problem.

Application of the various reconstructive methods mentioned above will be described using specific case examples and accompanying photos throughout the remainder of this chapter (Figs. 32.27, 32.28, 32.29, 32.30, 32.31, 32.32, 32.33, 32.34, 32.35, 32.36, 32.37, 32.38, 32.39, 32.40, 32.41, 32.42, 32.43, 32.44, 32.45, 32.46, 32.47, 32.48, 32.49, 32.50, 32.51, 32.52, 32.53, 32.54, 32.55, 32.56, 32.57, 32.58, 32.59, 32.60, 32.61, 32.62, 32.63, 32.64, 32.65, 32.66, 32.67, 32.68, 32.69, 32.70, 32.71, 32.72, 32.73, 32.74, 32.75, 32.76, 32.77, 32.78, 32.79, 32.80, 32.81, 32.82, 32.83, 32.84, 32.85, 32.86, 32.87, 32.88, 32.89, 32.90, 32.91, 32.92, 32.93, 32.94, 32.95, 32.96, 32.97, 32.98, 32.99, 32.100, 32.101, 32.102, 32.103, 32.104, 32.105, 32.106, 32.107, 32.108, 32.109, 32.110, 32.111, 32.12, 32.113, 32.114, 32.115, 32.116, 32.117, and 32.118).

Facial Injuries

Eyelids

1. Thermal injuries to the upper part of the face/forehead will frequently affect the eyelids.
2. Second degree facial burns usually heal completely within about 2 weeks.
3. Wounds of the eyelids that have not healed properly within 3 weeks may easily contract and retract the eyelids.
4. Early reconstruction of retracted eyelids is of paramount importance in order to protect the cornea and restore normal eyelid function.
5. Technique:
   (a) General anesthesia is preferred.
   Inject lidocaine with adrenaline in the scar tissue/incision area to minimize bleeding. Allow 5–7 minutes before cutting.
   (b) Make an incision about 2–3 mm from the lid margin. Gently dissect the scar tissue from the underlying normal eyelid tissue. Bleeding points controlled by cautery. Make sure a complete release is done. If both eyelids are involved, release both together.
   (c) FTSG is harvested from behind the auricle, supraclavicular or medial side of upper arm. Fat tissue needs to be trimmed off, (Fig. 32.13), and the graft needs to be hand meshed (Fig. 32.14). Secure complete hemostasis. Use 4-0 or 5-0 nylon stitches.
   (d) Tarsorrhaphy is advised before applying the dressing. Apply ophthalmic ointment. The dressing should consist of Vaseline gauze, wet and dry gauze, gentle elastic bandage.
   Remove tarsorrhaphy and stitches within 2–3 weeks. Continue to apply dressing support to both eyelids for another 2–3 weeks (Figs. 32.27, 32.28, 32.29, 32.30, 32.31, 32.32, and 32.33).

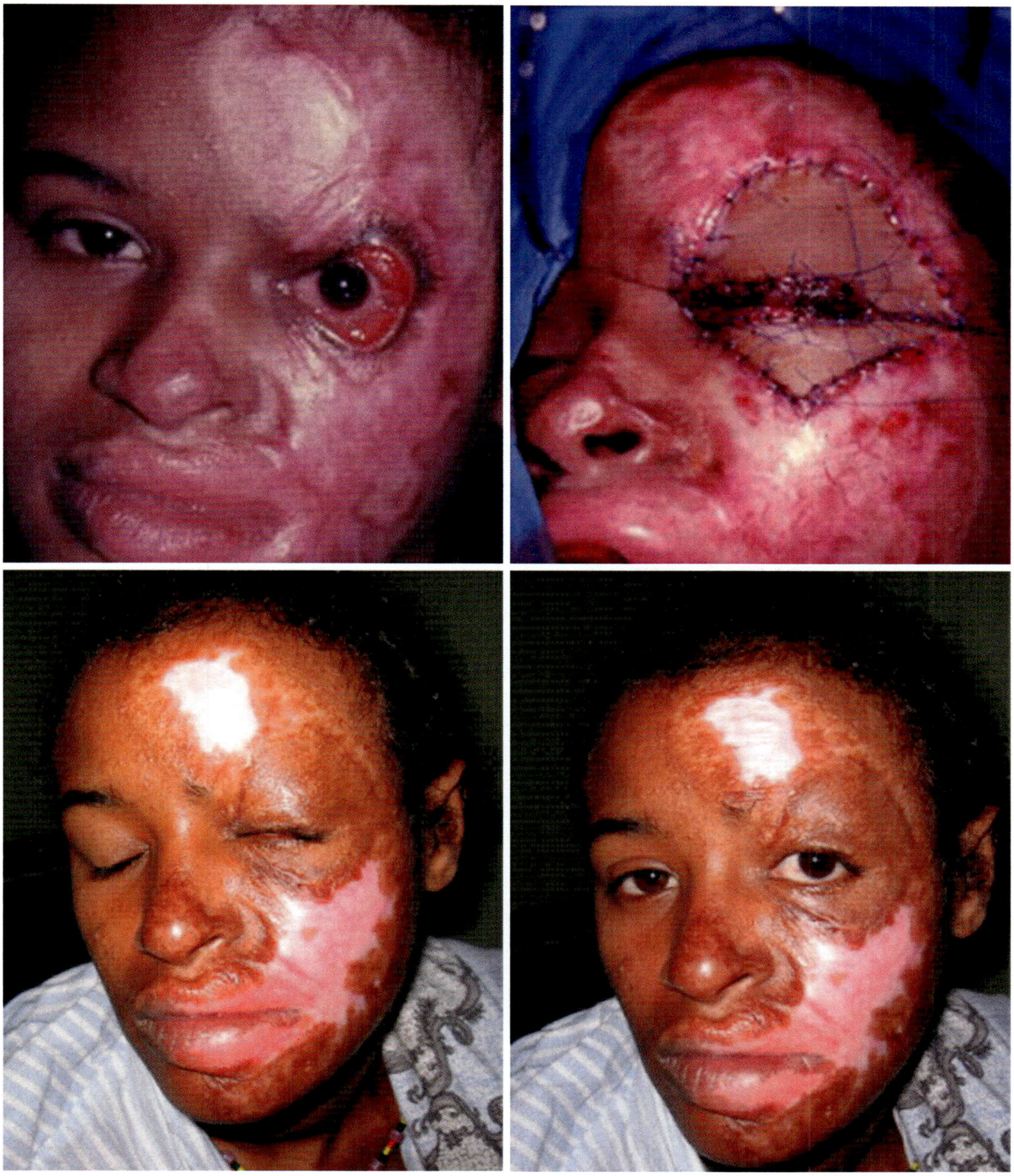

Figs. 32.27–32.30 Eyelid reconstruction with FTSG harvested from the supraclavicular region

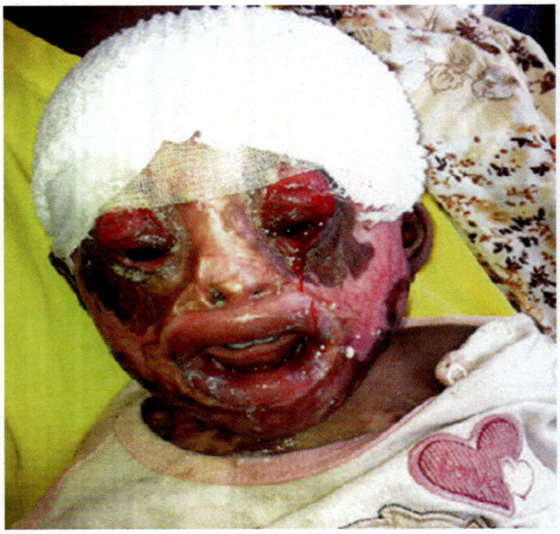

Fig. 32.31 8 month old girl who fell into the ground level cooking area with severe facial injury, all 4 eyelids retracted

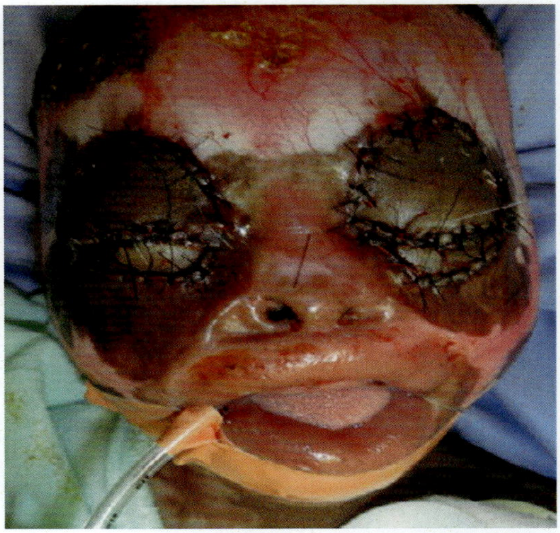

Fig. 32.32 Contracture release of all 4 eyelids. Reconstructed with FTSG harvested from medial side of upper arm. Tarsorraphy. Bandage support for 3 weeks before stitch removal

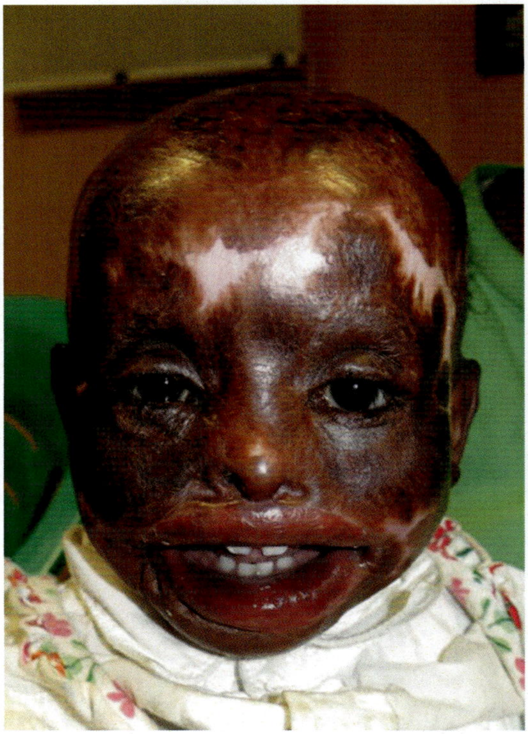

Fig. 32.33 12 month follow-up

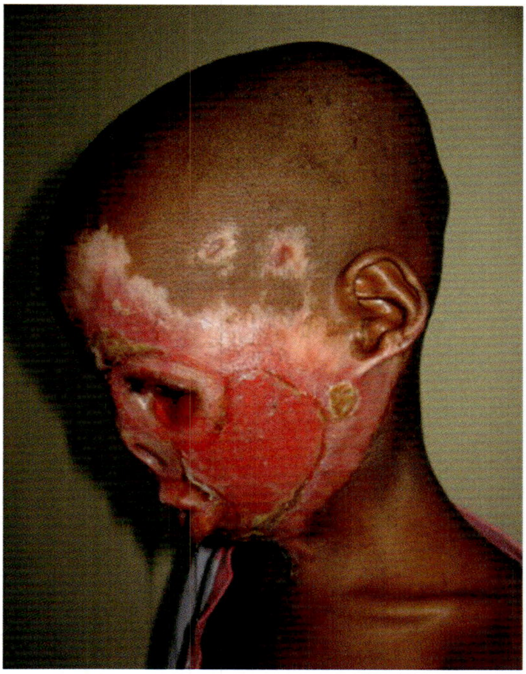

Fig. 32.34 Epileptic seizure 4 months before admission

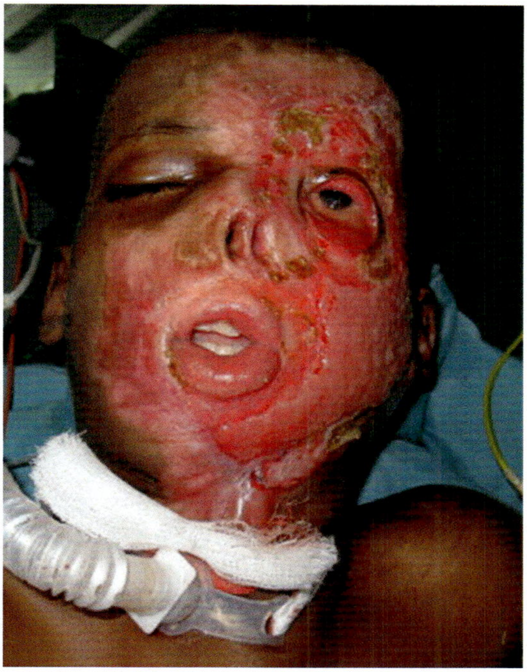

Fig. 32.35 Tracheostomy due to microstomia

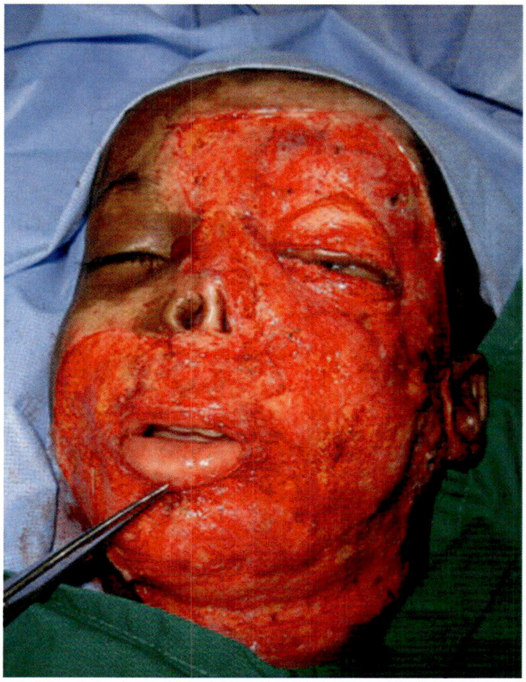

Fig. 32.36 Excision of all scar tissue

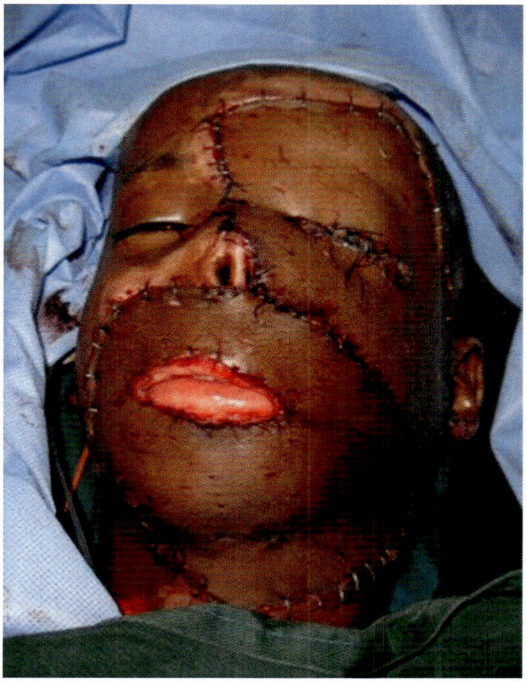

Fig. 32.37 2 large FTSG harvested from left flank and medial side of right upper arm

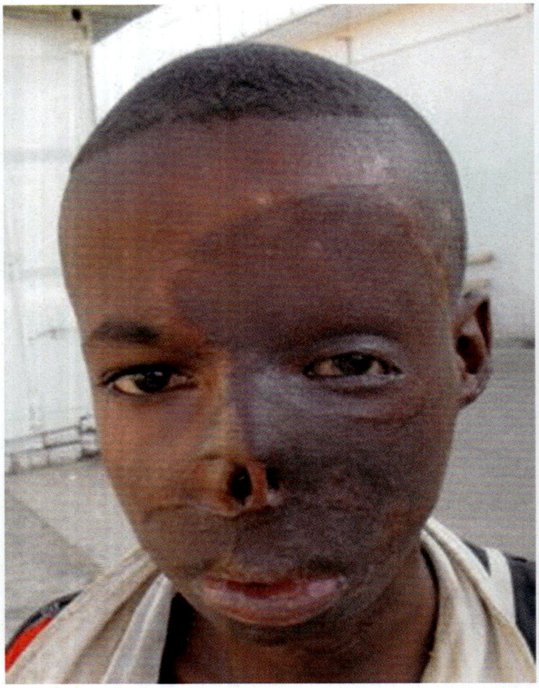

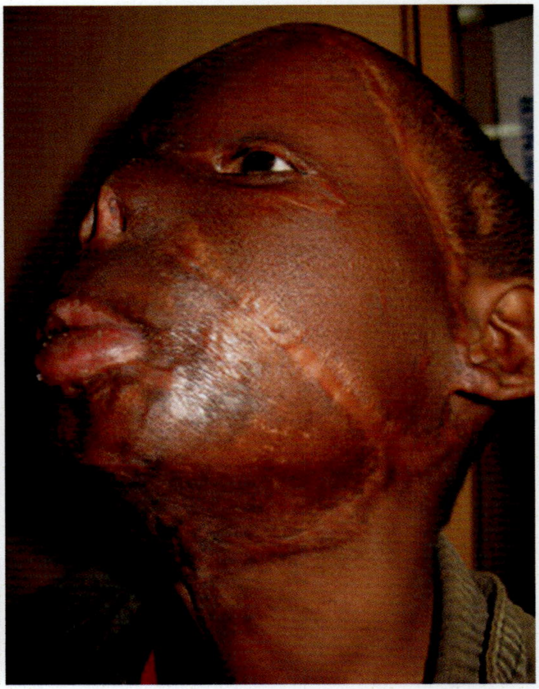

Figs. 32.38 and 32.39 15 month follow-up, Left lower eyelid reconstructed 3 months later. Bilateral oral commisurotomy due to secondary microstomia was later required

Radial Forearm Pedicle Flap

The pedicle version of the Radial Forearm Flap is a very good tool to solve highly challenging and critical conditions in burns as well as other trauma, particularly to the face and scalp area.

The fasciocutaneous flap is vascularized by a pedicle consisting of the radial artery and its 2 vena comitantes that are ligated distal to the bifurcation of the brachial artery in the elbow region. When the flap is raised, flow will enter the flap in a retrograde fashion, based on a normal functioning ulnar artery that needs to be tested prior to surgery with a positive Allen test.

This flap can be designed to fit the exact size of the defect.

As the flap leaves behind a donor defect of the forearm, donor morbidity is a concern.

The defect may be covered with a STSG, either a sheet graft or a meshed graft.

As microsurgery may not be readily available, the pedicle radial forearm flap is indeed a great tool to solve challenging problems.

The following two clinical conditions will demonstrate good indications for using this flap.

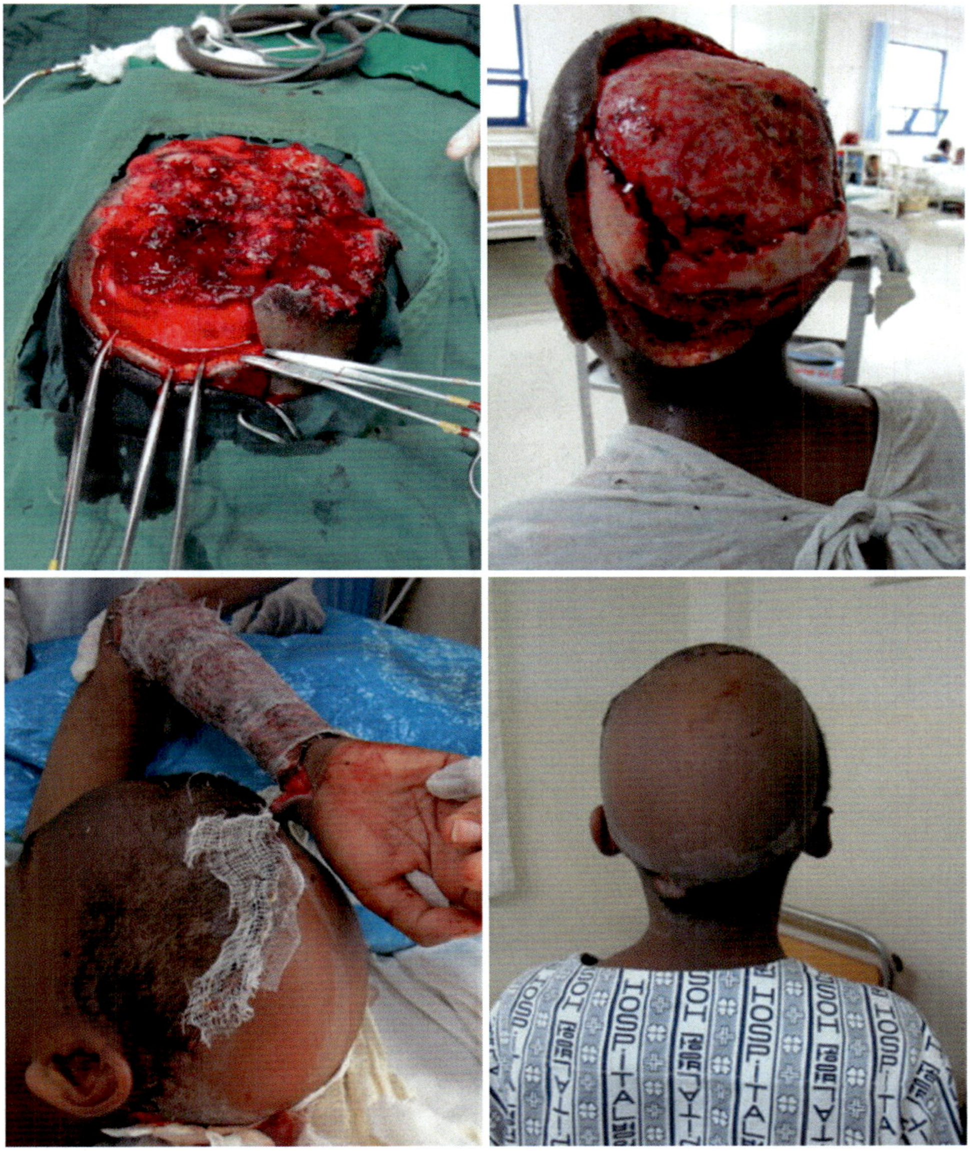

Figs. 32.40–32.43 A 13-year-old boy with a neglected flame burn to the scalp of 11 years duration. The chronic wound subsequently developed into a squamous cell carcinoma. During excision, it turned out a large part of the skull bone was eroded by the tumor, exposing the dura. Following 3–4 days with dressing change, the entire forearm skin was raised as a fasciocutaneous flap based on retrograde flow through the radial artery. The forearm was covered with meshed STSGSplit thickness skin grafts (STSG). Pedicle release on day 16. Good nursing care made it unnecessary to apply any kind of splint to keep the position of the hand. This case demonstrates that the entire scalp may be covered with this flap

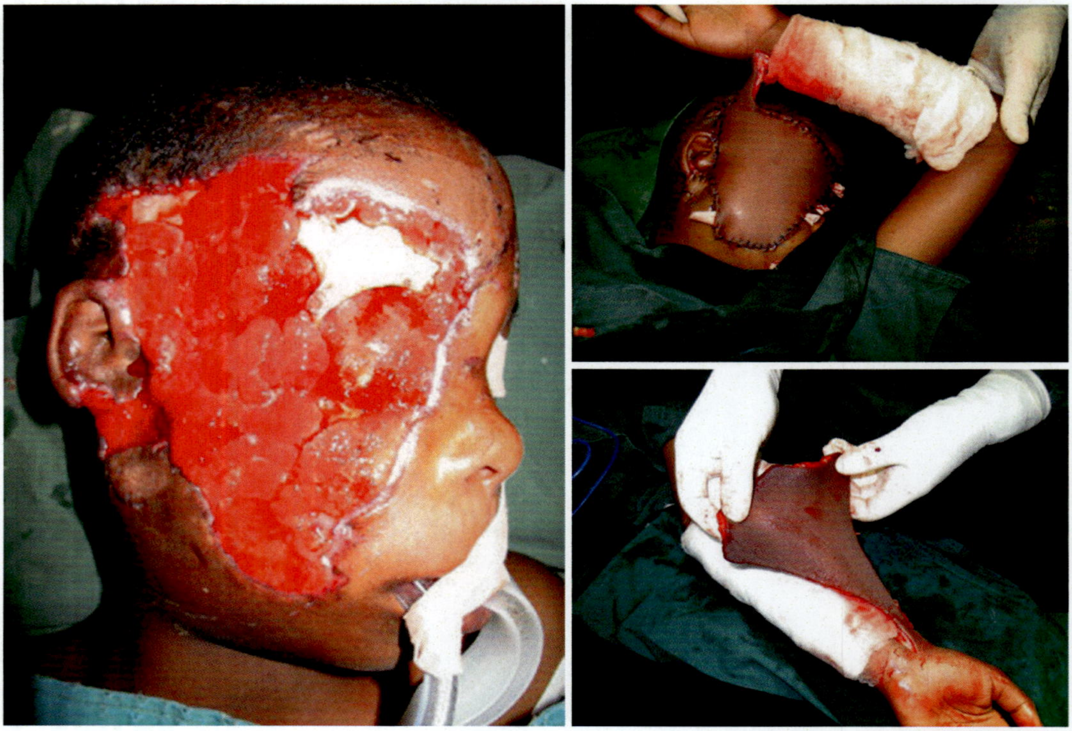

Figs. 32.44–32.46 A 16-year-old girl with a hyena bite. A huge defect exposing right side of forehead, upper rim of orbital with the eyeball missing. Repeated theatre visits for debridements. A pedicle radial forearm flap was designed to fit the defect and raised on the left forearm for better support and position of the arm. No splinting

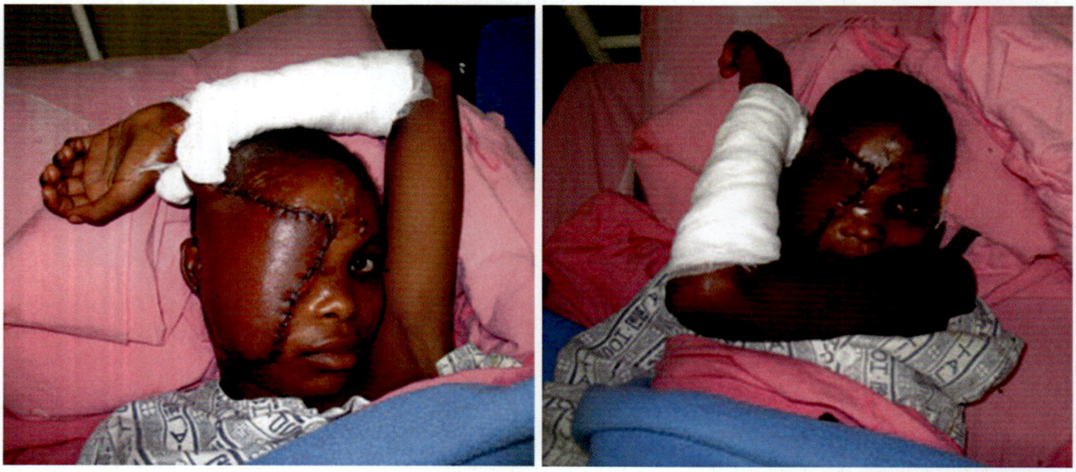

Figs. 32.47 and 32.48 Patient was encouraged to move shoulder joint while in bed to prevent shoulder pain and stiffness. Was up walking second post-op day

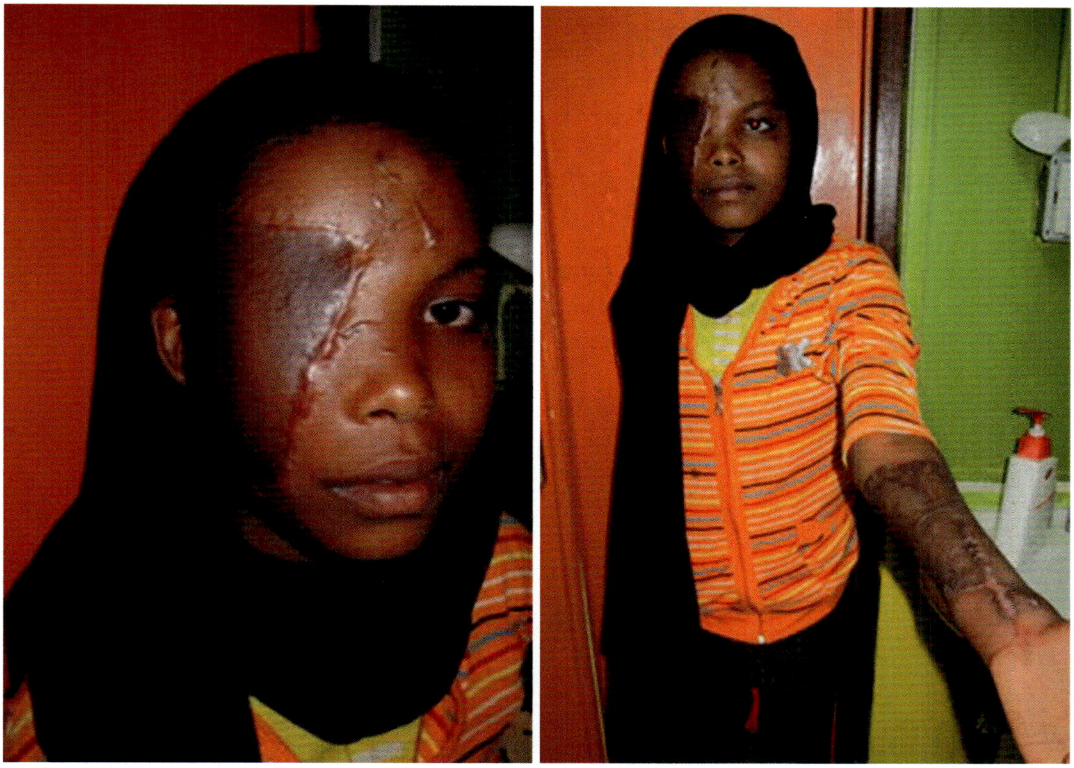

Figs. 32.49 and 32.50 Pedicle released on day 20

Neck Contractures

Anterior and lateral neck contractures are posing a real challenge to the reconstructive surgeon.

The scar tissue may involve a huge area of the neck. The chin may be pulled inferiorly towards the sternum making intubation a real challenge for the anesthetist. Most hospitals may not have access to fiberoptic intubation equipment. If intubation seems difficult, a preliminary release/incision of the scar under local anesthesia must be performed in order to have the patient intubated.

After intubation, the patient should be positioned with full neck extension in order to have proper access to the neck. All scar tissue contributing to the contracture needs to be excised. In severe anterior neck contractures, the resulting wound defect usually appears to be larger than one would think prior to surgery. The surgeon will frequently have to extend incisions into healthy skin tissue to obtain the best result.

Many surgical techniques have been described to reconstruct neck contractures:

- Skin graft procedures, STSG and FTSG.
- Local flaps and pedicle flaps.
- Expander techniques.
- Free flaps.

The author recommends reconstructing the wound defect using FTSG and STSG, frequently in combination with local advancement flaps. There are good reasons to stick to this method:

- The surgeon will not be sure about the size of the wound defect until scar release has been completed.
- Advancement of local cutaneous flaps from the lateral side of the neck will assist the sur-

geon to make sure to create a V- or Z-shaped junctions with normal skin, avoiding vertical scars.

- Once local flaps have been advanced and the actual wound size has been determined, it is time to plan harvesting the required skin grafts for resurfacing.
- FTSG is the main choice when resurfacing the anterior neck. During scar release, the cleavage plane will expose healthy subcutaneous tissue or platysma, a nice recipient tissue for FTSG. Once FTSG has been applied to recreate the neck contour, thick STSG may be used to resurface remaining part of the anterior neck (submental and sternal areas) in case there is shortage of FTSG for harvest.
- *Meticulous hemostasis* is of greatest importance before applying FTSG.
- FTSG may be harvested from the lateral aspect of the thigh using the Humby knife. Large FTSG may also be harvested from medial side of the upper arm or from the abdomen/flank, using the scalpel, followed by trimming of fat tissue. The donor areas need to be resurfaced with 4:1/3:1 meshed STSG (Fig. 32.15).
- A FTSG is elastic due to the dermis (Fig. 32.51). When applyinginserting the FTSG Full thickness skin grafts (FTSG) to the recipient site, make sure to gently stretch the graft across the wound surface to somehow match its original size at the donor site. OverstretchingNeck contractures should be avoided
- Keep the patient positioned with the neck extended post-op for 4–5 days with a thick dressing to support the grafts. A neck collar should be custom made for the patient to wear for 5–6 weeks post-op.

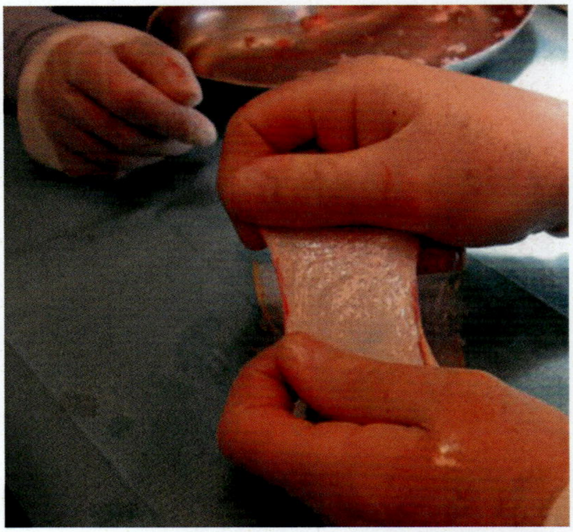

Fig. 32.51 The FTSG is elastic

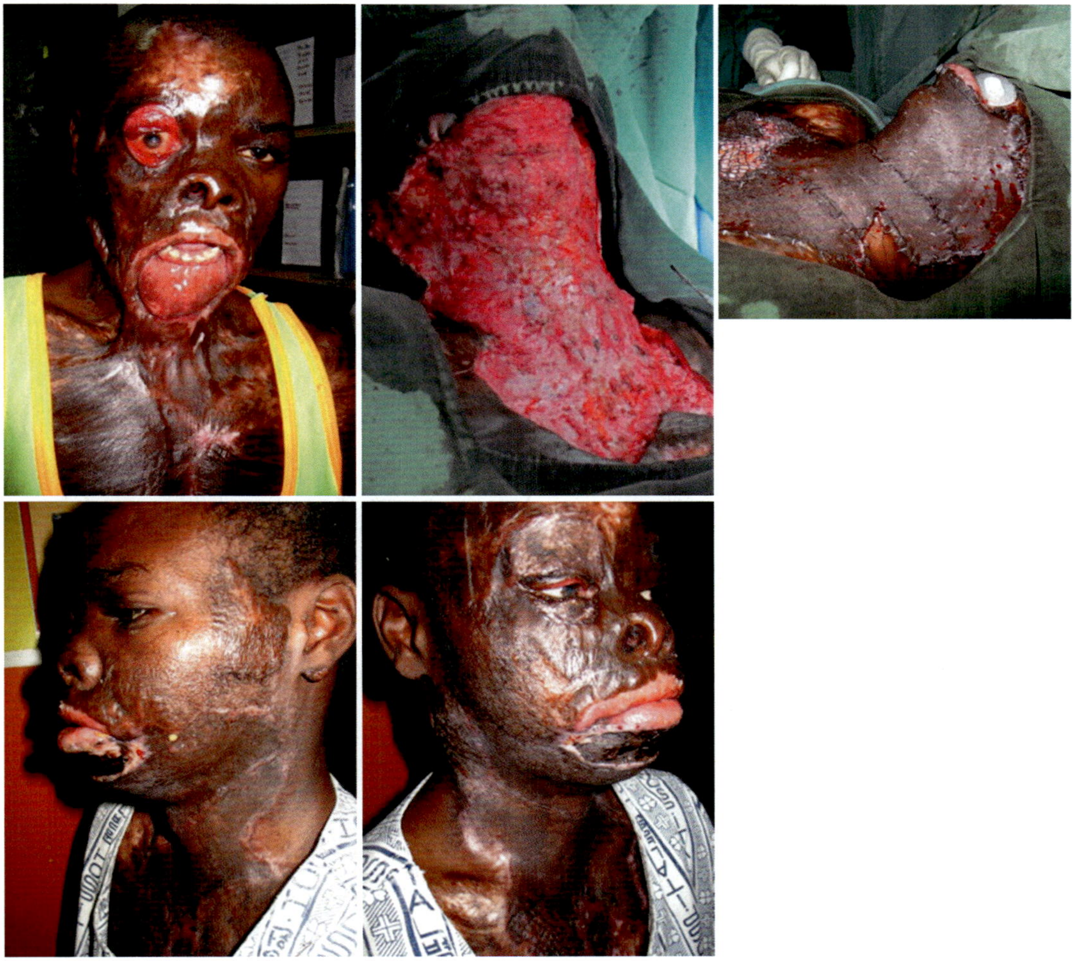

Figs. 32.52–32.56 A 22 years old man with a 5 years history of flame burn injury to the upper chest, ant neck, chin and large part of the face incl both eyelids on right side. A complete scar release was excised, revealing a huge wound. Reconstruction aimed at bringing the neck contour back to normal, extending the incisions beyond the middle of the neck. FTSG on anterior neck, STSG on upper chest, eyelids, and lower lip

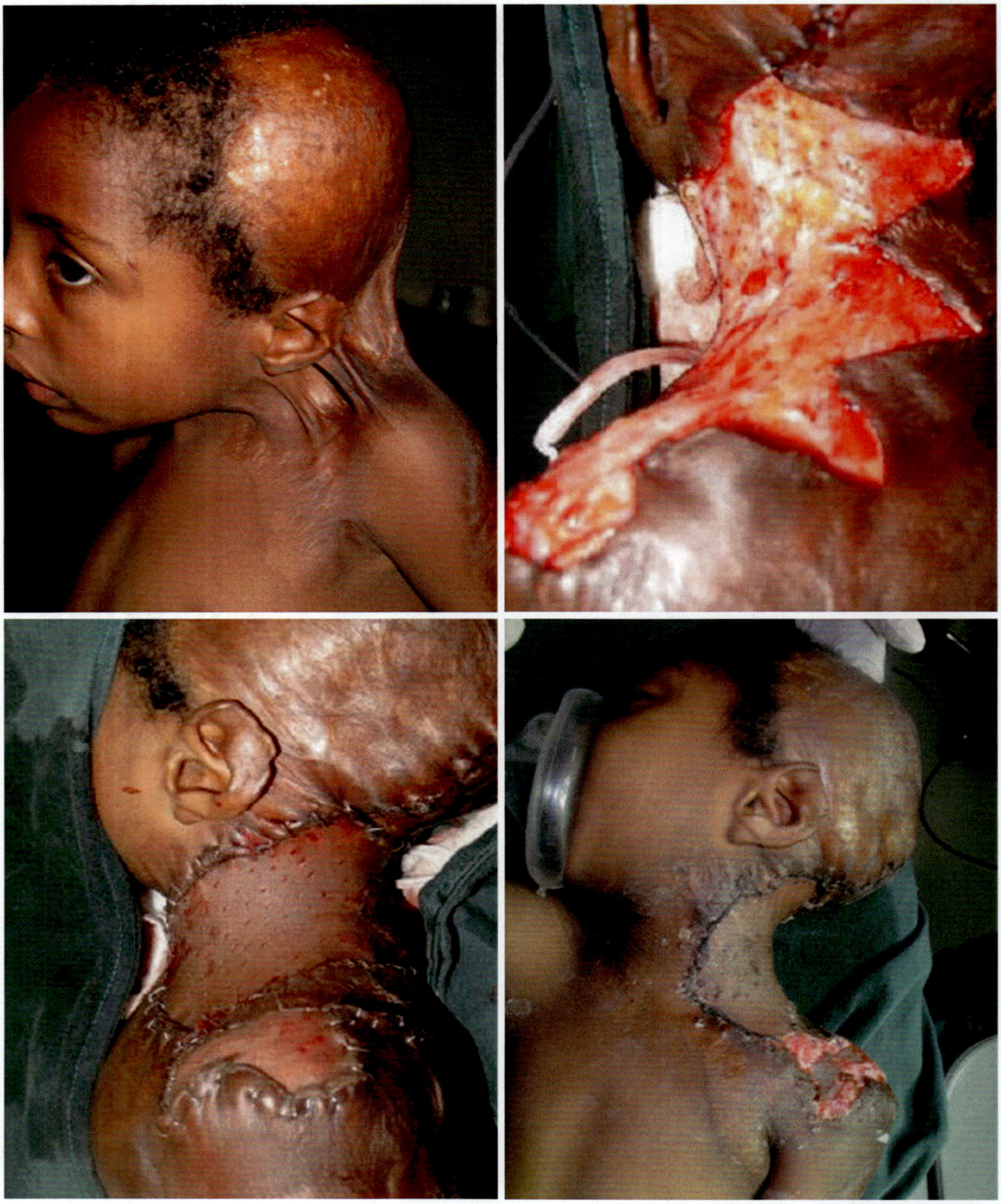

Figs. 32.57–32.60 A postero-lateral neck contracture in a small boy lasting from early childhood. The contracture stretches from the acromion area of left shoulder to the occipital region. Complete release of the deformity with scar excision. A FTSG was applied to the concave area of the neck. The remaining wounds were covered with hand meshed sheets of STSG

Upper Limb

Post burn contractures frequently affect anterior neck, shoulders, axilla, upper arms, and chest. A common mechanism is clothes catching fire during cooking on ground level kitchen facilities.

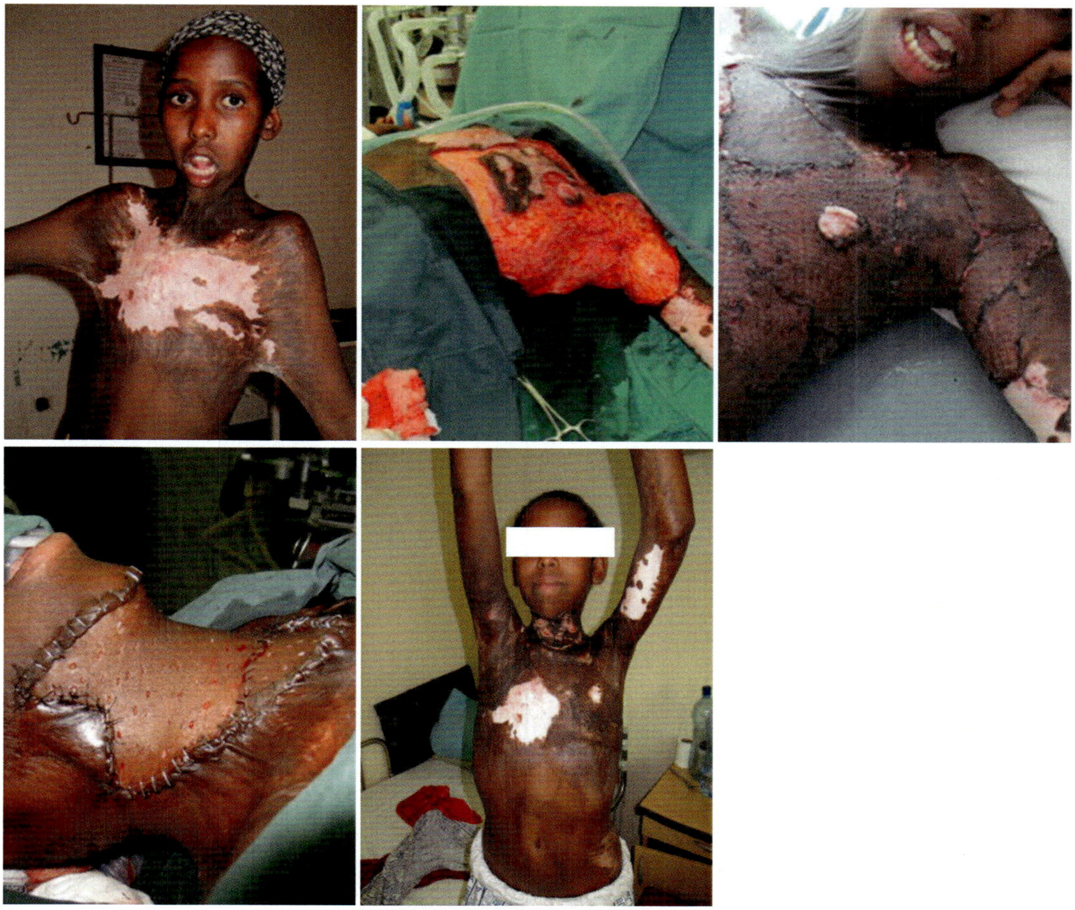

Figs. 32.61–32.65 A 15 year-old-girl with broad, thick scar affecting both axillae and the anterior neck, including scar adhesions between proximal upper arms and the chest. Three separate surgical procedures. Excision of scar. FTSG applied to both arm pits and anterior neck. STSG, meshed and sheets, applied to remaining wounds

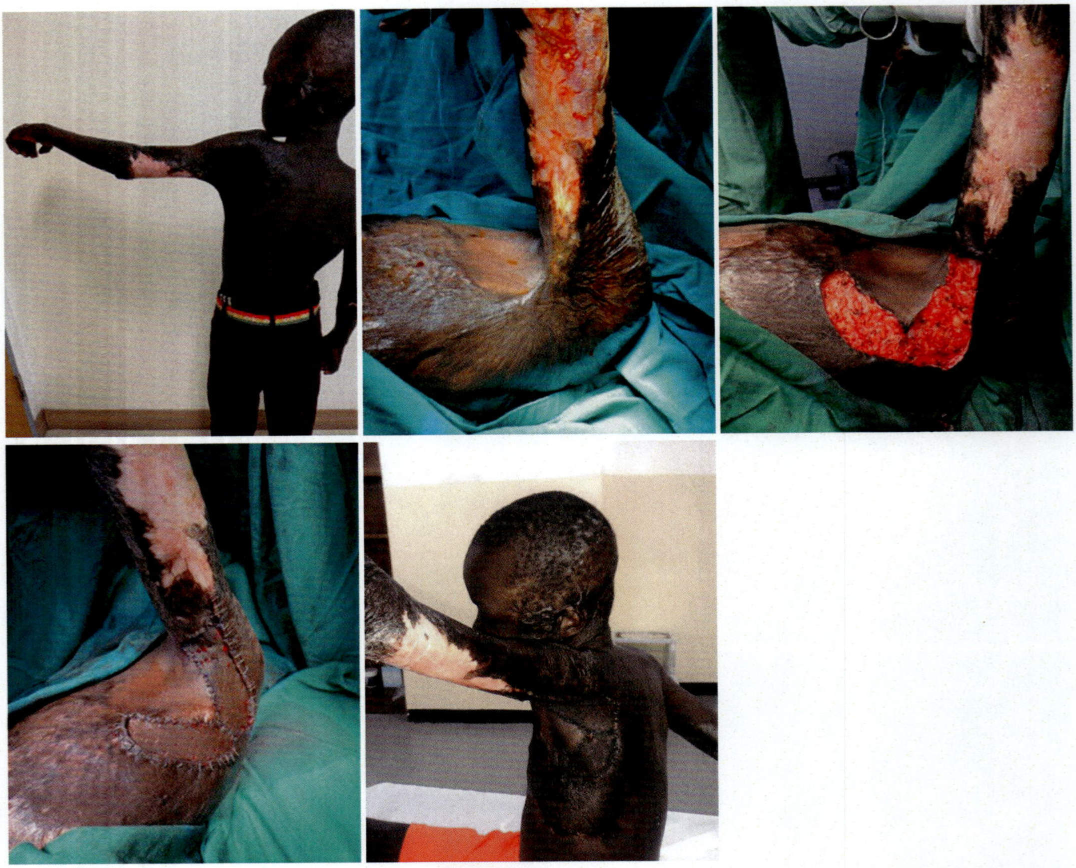

Figs. 32.66–32.70 A 14 year-old-boy with broad, thick scar from flame burn injury during early childhood, not able to elevate his arm above the horizontal line. The best option was to excise the thick fleshy scar to prepare a U-shaped area for a FTSG as a continuation of the normal armpit. A 90-degree splint was used for 6 weeks post-op. The U-shaped FTSG enabled the patient to raise the arm above the horizontal line without any problem. In due time, the boy should be able to raise the arm into a vertical position

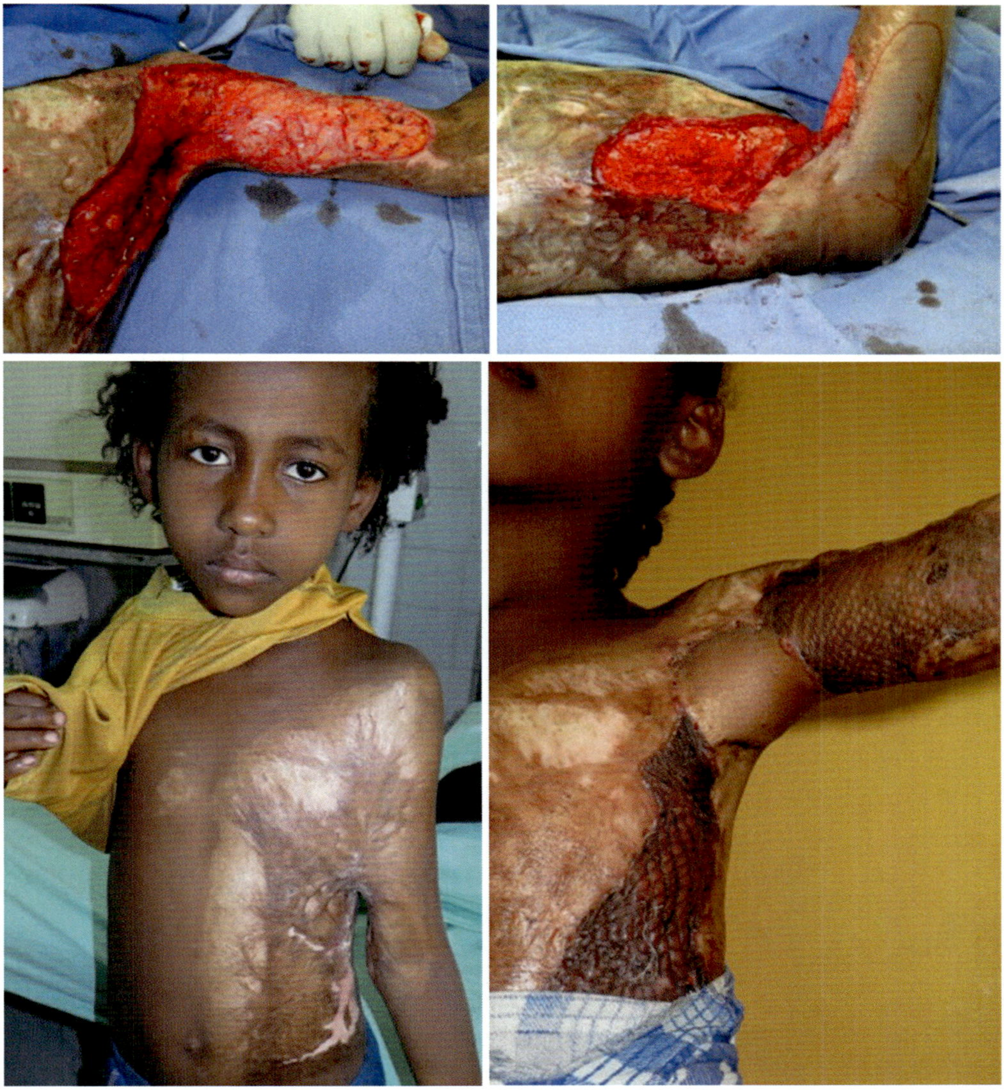

Figs. 32.71–32.74 Release of upper arm / chest contracture. Arm pit reconstruction with fasciocutaneous transposition flap from upper arm. Wounds covered with meshed STSG. Before/after shown here

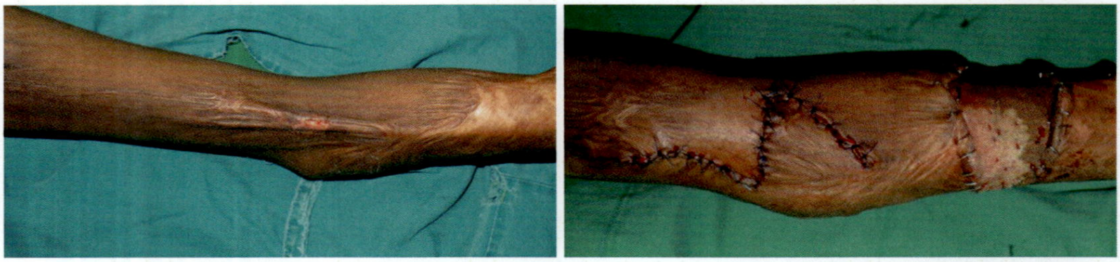

Figs. 32.75 and 32.76 Linear scar crossing the elbow joint. Thick scar proximal of upper forearm. Release of linear scar with Z-plasty. Thick scar release, covered with STSG

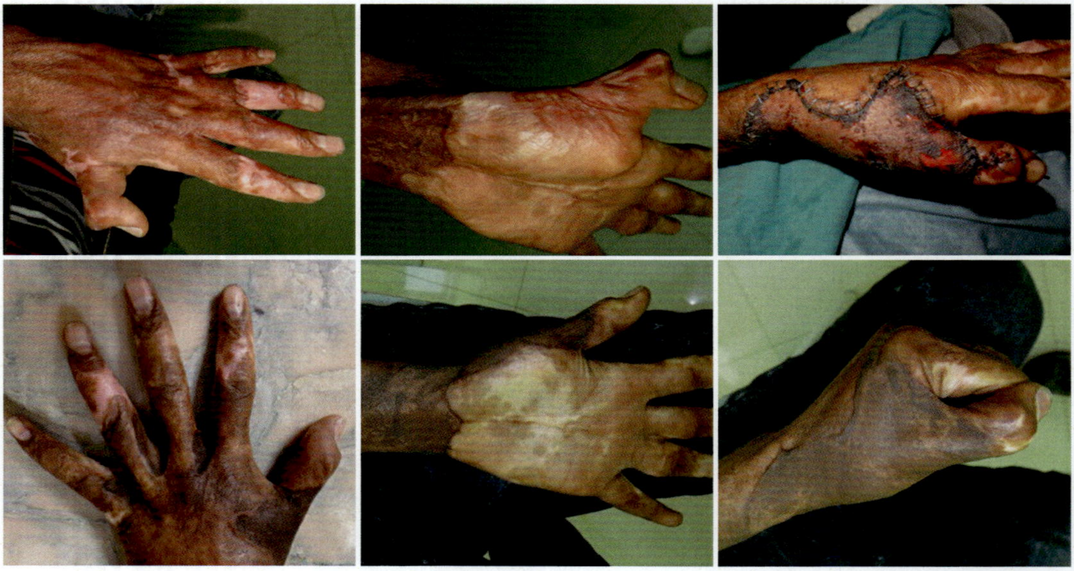

Figs. 32.77–32.82 A 24-year-old student with history of flame burn injury 5 years back. Post burn contracture of right hand with luxation of the IP joint of the thumb, wrist contracture, and moderate syndactyly between the ulnar fingers. Contracture release/excision of scar tissue of wrist and thumb. IP joint of thumb reduced and transfixed with a K-wire. FTSG applied to the wrist, thumb, and radial part of the dorsum of the hand, and release of ulnar syndactyly with FTSG

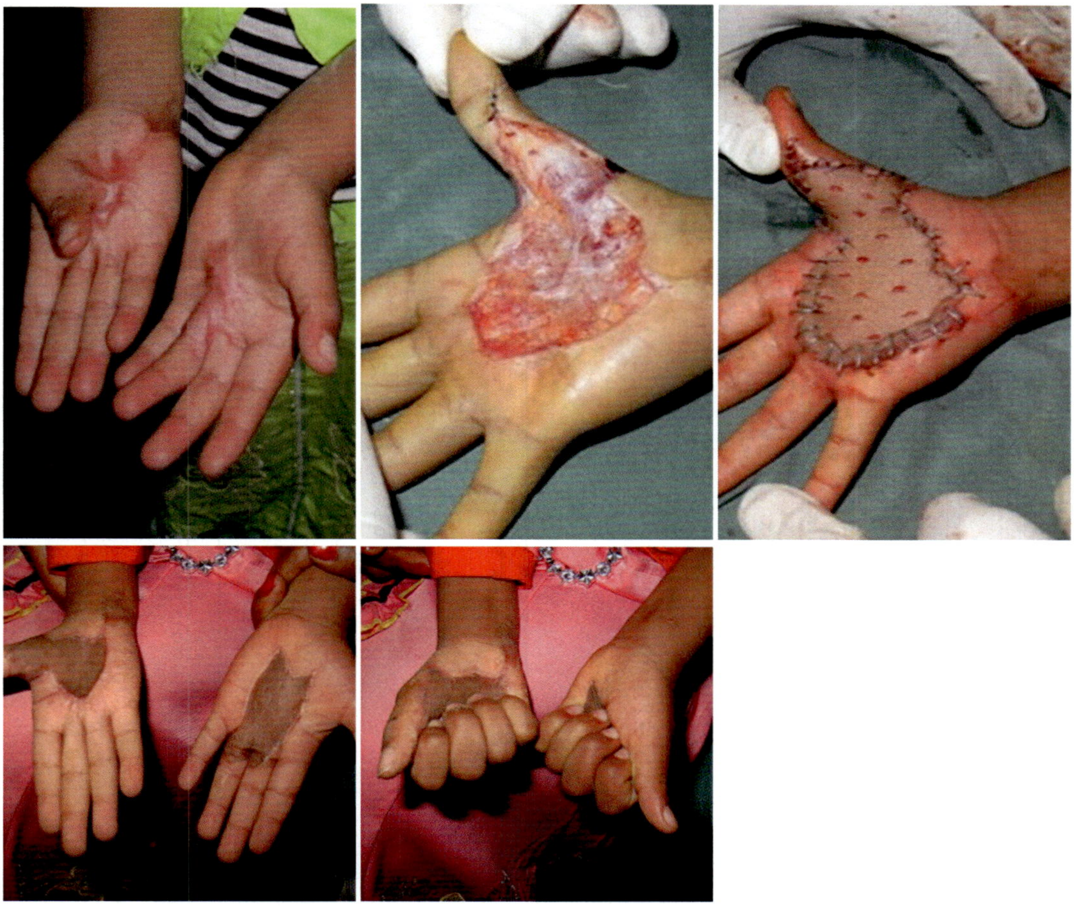

Figs. 32.83–32.87 *Case Presentation*: The patient had a third degree contact burn both palms from hot oven. Contracture release with FTSG

Groin and Lower Limb

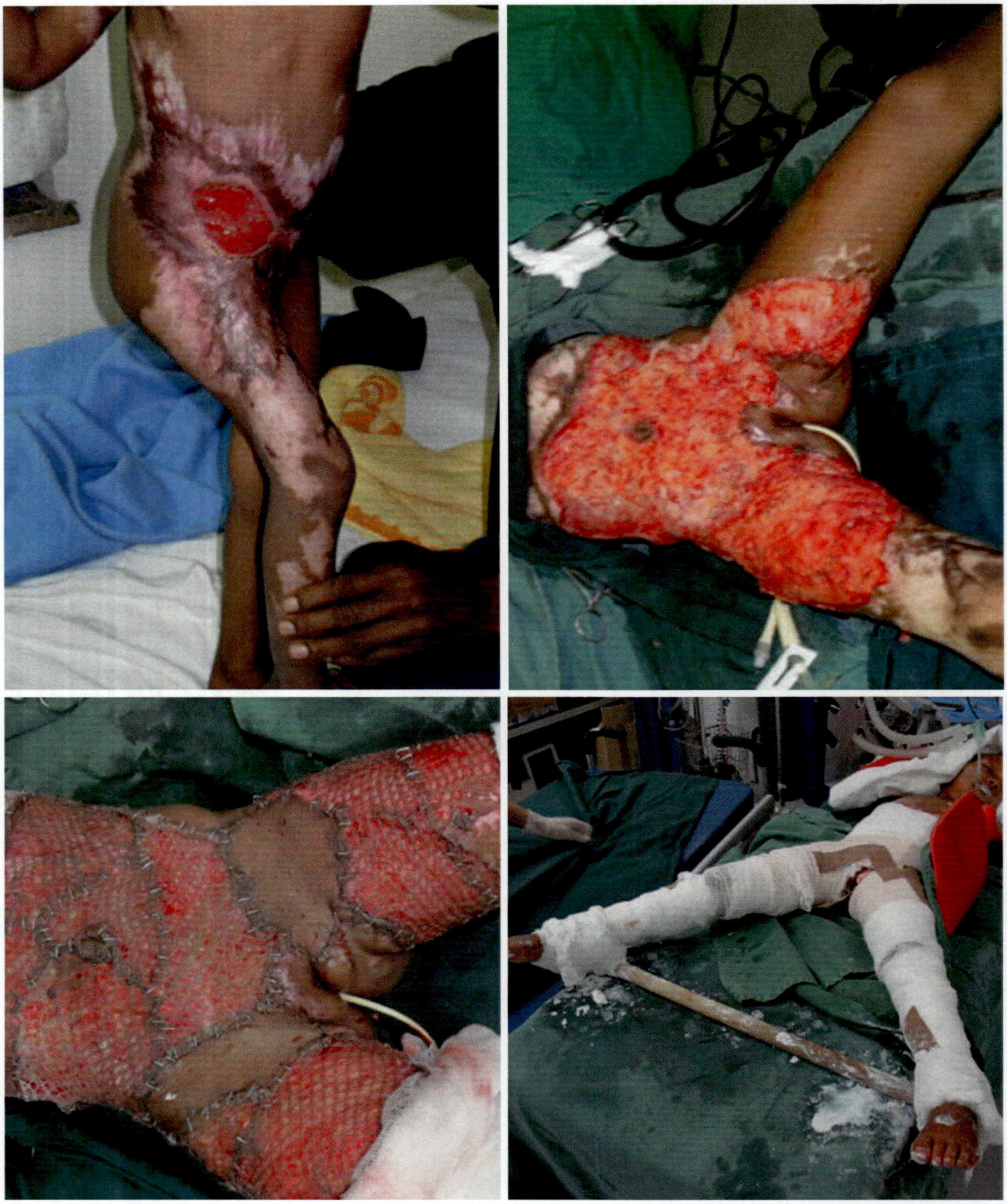

Figs. 32.88–32.91 A patient with a chronic abdominal and groin wound requiring wide excision. FTSG applied to both groins. Remaining wound covered with meshed STSG. The splint is practical in keeping the legs far apart, also helpful during dressing change

Knee Joint

1. Burn contractures of the knee joints are common and disabling. There are several important points to remember when planning knee joint contracture release.
2. The common peroneal nerve may easily be overstretched during the release procedure as it winds around the neck of the fibula.
3. The posterior joint capsule has most likely become tight.
4. The first step is to excise all scar tissue. This will certainly enable the joint to be carefully extended. No force should be applied to extend the joint. The joint should be stabilized either with an external fixator, or wooden bars. Continue with daily dressing.
5. Further extension of the joint may be done 2–3 times per week under sedation. No force to be applied. The joint will often reach full extension in a couple of weeks.
6. Once the joint is fully extended, the popliteal area should be covered with a FTSG. Remaining wounds with meshed STSG. Keep the external fixator until grafts have healed well. POP splints may be used for another 4–6 weeks, depending on the initial severity of the contracture.
7. In longstanding cases, the cartilage might have disintegrated, making the extended joint painful. The only solution would be arthrodesis to avoid a painful unstable joint.
8. One might argue that fasciocutaneous flaps may give a better solution to the popliteal joint compared to FTSG. This may certainly be the case, under favorable conditions, slim individuals, limited burns with ample healthy skin for a transposition flap. One must be sure the flap would reach the opposite side. In case of a bulky flap due to the amount of subcutaneous tissue, the situation is different.
9. The main advantages of using a FTSG are avoiding bulky flaps besides the advantage of harvesting the required size for the defect. The recipient wound bed must be very well prepared with no scar tissue for the FTSG to be successful (Figs. 32.92, 32.93, and 32.94).

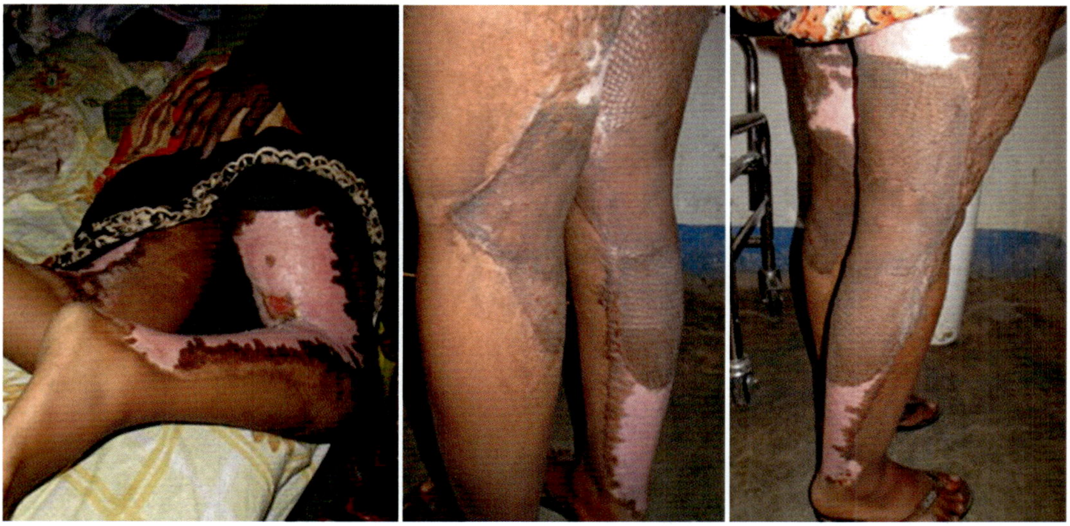

Figs. 32.92–32.94 An18-year-old girl (3 months pregnant) with post burn bilateral knee contractures of 3 months duration. Notice incisions reach mid-lateral line of knee joints to prevent post-op contracture lines. FTSG should always cover the popliteal areas as seen here. Remaining wounds covered with meshed STSG. Post-op POP splints were applied for 4–6 weeks

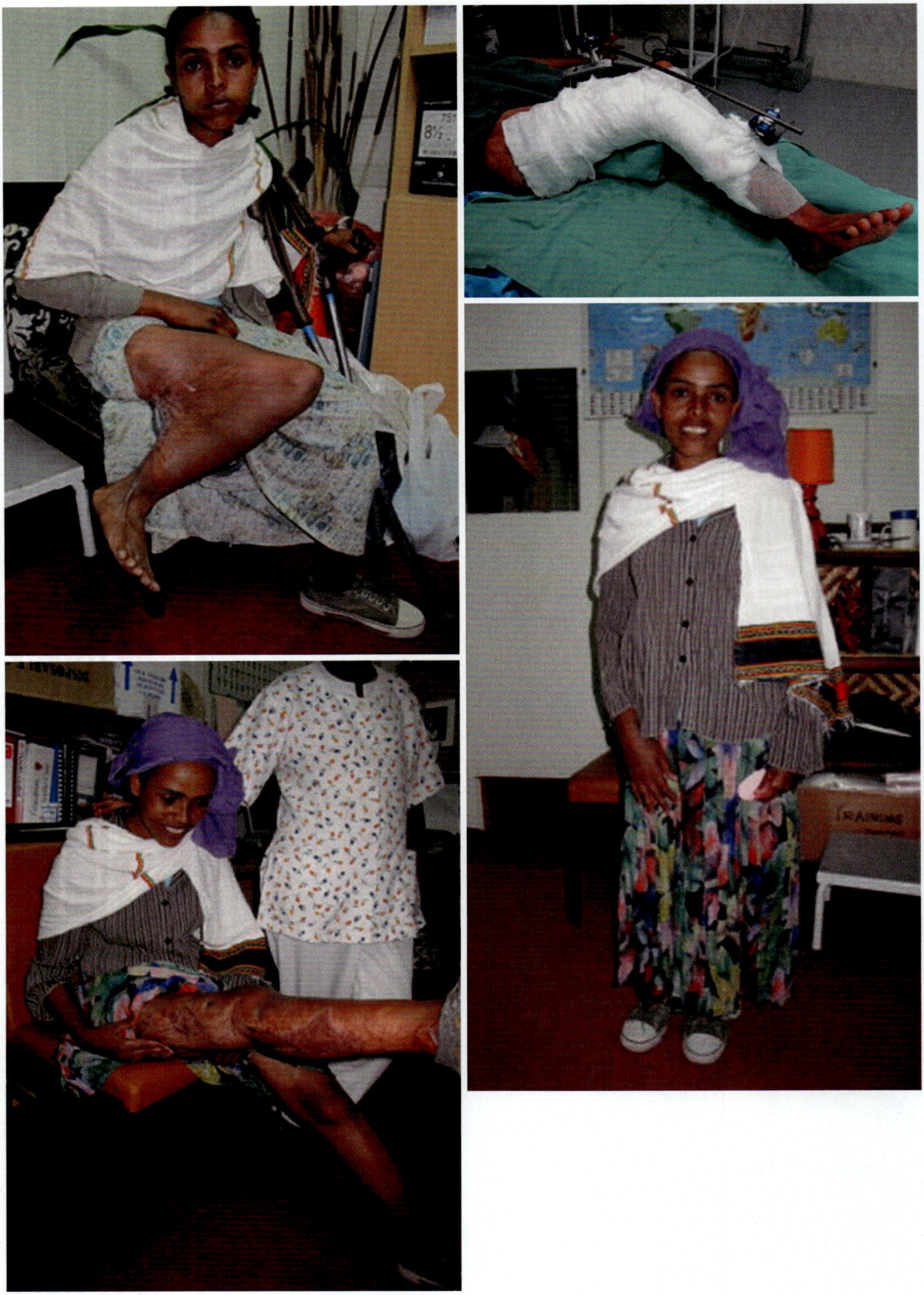

Figs. 32.95–32.98 A 21-year-old woman sustained a burn at the age of 6 months. She had never walked on two legs until she was admitted and underwent reconstruction in 2011. Contracture released, external fixation applied, wounds covered with meshed STSG. Arthrodesis of knee joint due to destroyed cartilage

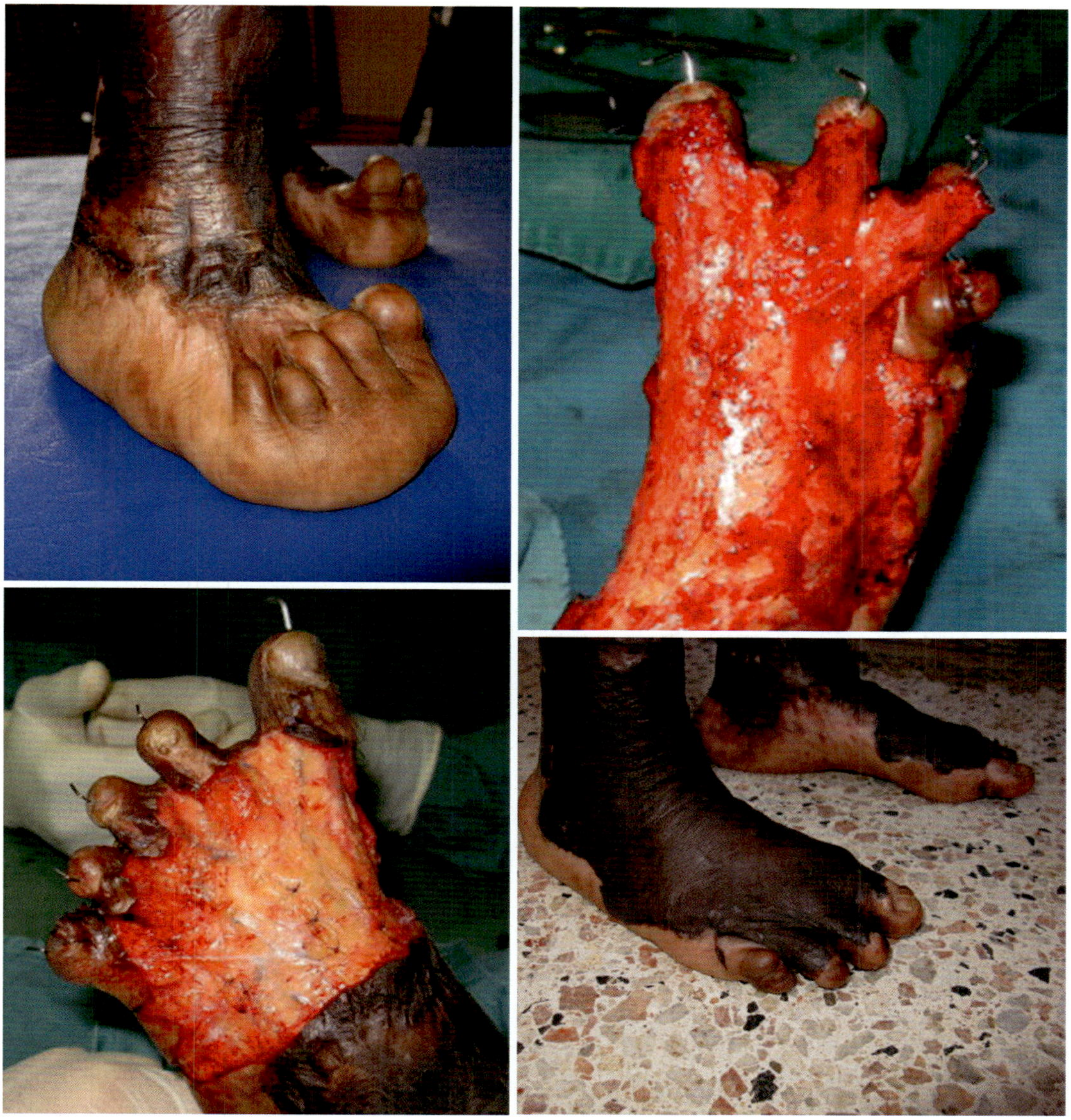

Figs. 32.99–32.102 A 14-year-old burned when stepping into burning trash while playing football 7 years previously. Note 90 degrees hyperextension of toes. Contraction release and pinning with K-wires, coverage with thick STSGs, 7 weeks in hospital

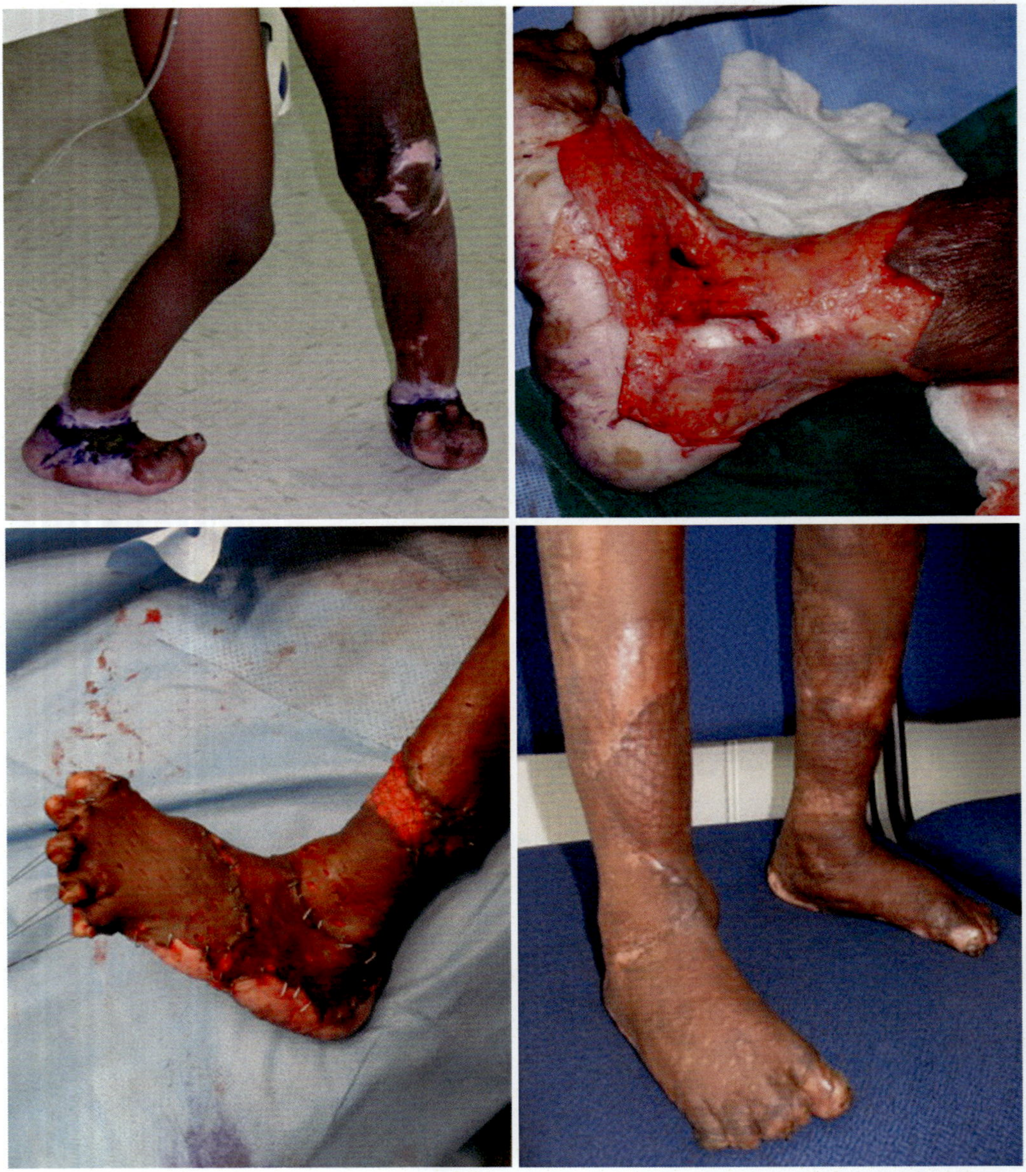

Figs. 32.103–32.106 Severely twisted/contracted ankle joints in a 4-year-old boy following stepping into burning trash. Ankle joints completely locked with no movement at all due to contracting scar tissue. Both knees flexed slightly so that heels would touch ground while walking. Even then, keeping balance was nearly impossible. Careful dissection under tourniquet to avoid exposure of tendon sheets, nerves, and joints. Toes dissected free and transfixed with K-wires. FTSG applied across the anterior ankle joint. The other areas covered with sheets of STSG. 1 year post-op visit, ankle close to normal range of movement

Heel Reconstruction

Heel reconstruction is a rather rare procedure. Surgeons will come across cases where heel reconstruction is necessary, either from traffic accidents, burns, or other casualties and tumors (Fig. 32.107).

Once the heel pad is missing, a skin graft – STSG or FTSG – may not yield a satisfactory result in the long run as pain will inevitably become a headache for the patient.

The sural reverse fasciocutaneous flap is frequently used in reconstruction of heel defects.

In this section, another reliable and easy to perform pedicle flap will be described through specific case examples: the tensor fascia lata (TFL) cross-leg flap. The distal part of the TFL muscle consists of a thick fascia that is included in the flap. Figure 32.108 shows the flap as it is raised from the lateral distal part of the right thigh. This flap produces predictably good results (Figs. 32.109 and 32.110).

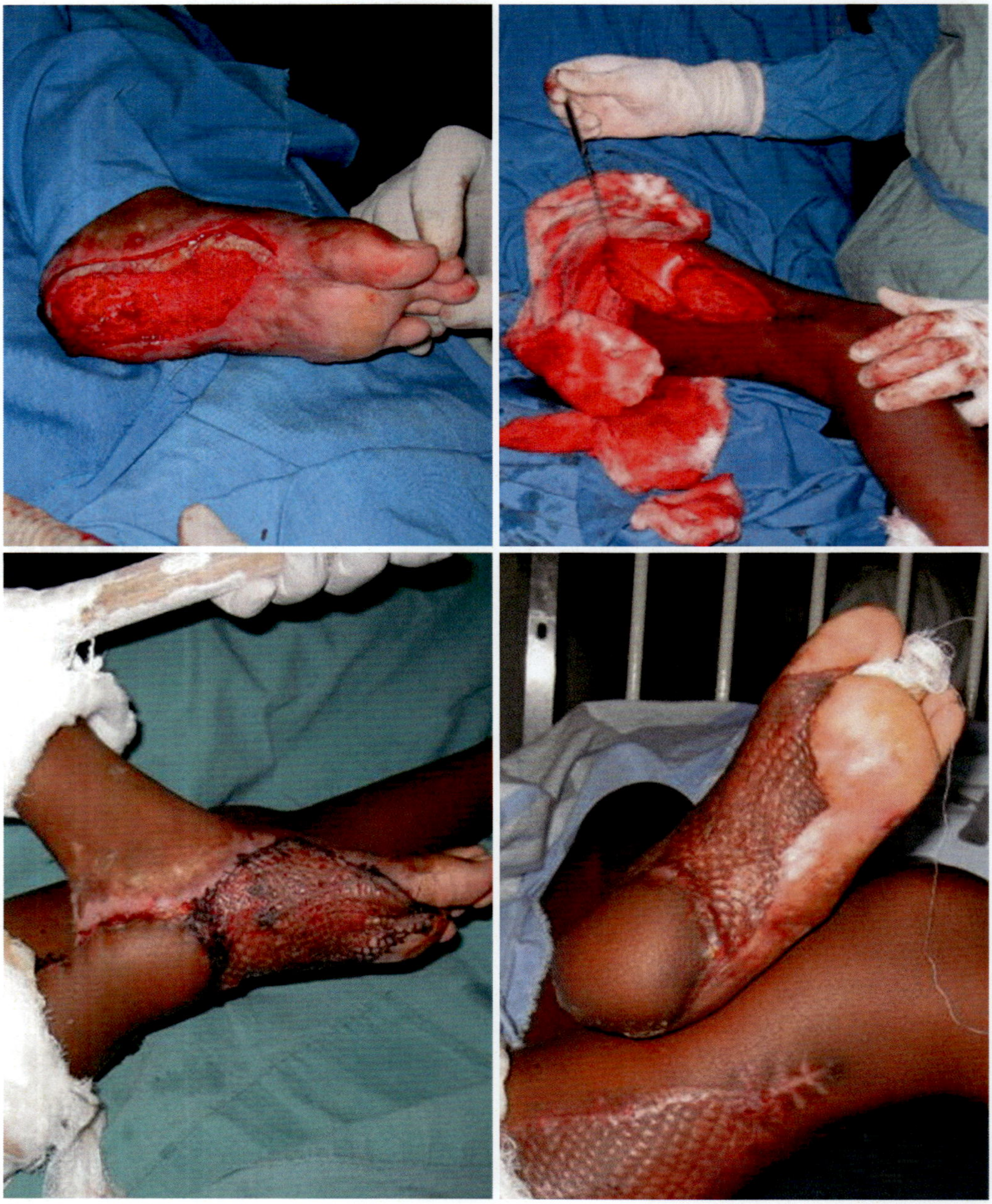

Figs. 32.107–32.110 Deep burn to left sole and heel on a 16-year-old boy. Excision of the necrosis reveals a huge defect. Left foot is brought across to the contralateral thigh where the TFL flap has been raised to be applied to the defect of the left heel. The remaining wound on the sole as well as the donor area on right thigh are covered with meshed STSG. Pedicle released 3 weeks post-op. No complaint of pain on follow-up

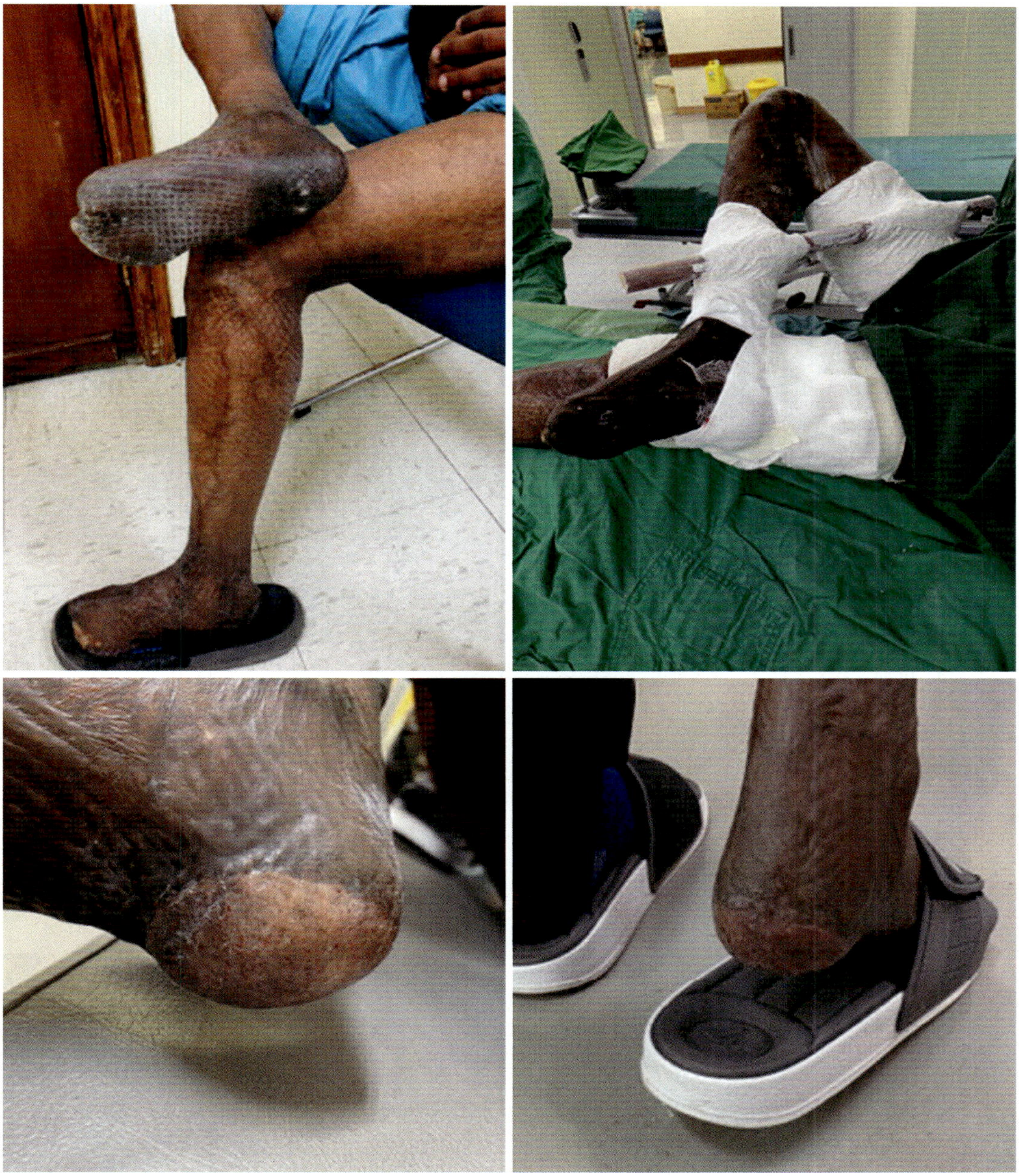

Figs. 32.111–32.114 A 20-year-old man with history of flame burn to both legs and feet at the age of 6. Right heel pad burned, was covered with STSG. Chronic pain from right heel during walking had been a big problem ever since. Heel reconstruction with cross-leg TFL flap 15 years after the incident. No discomfort as he gradually started walking during the next 3–4 weeks

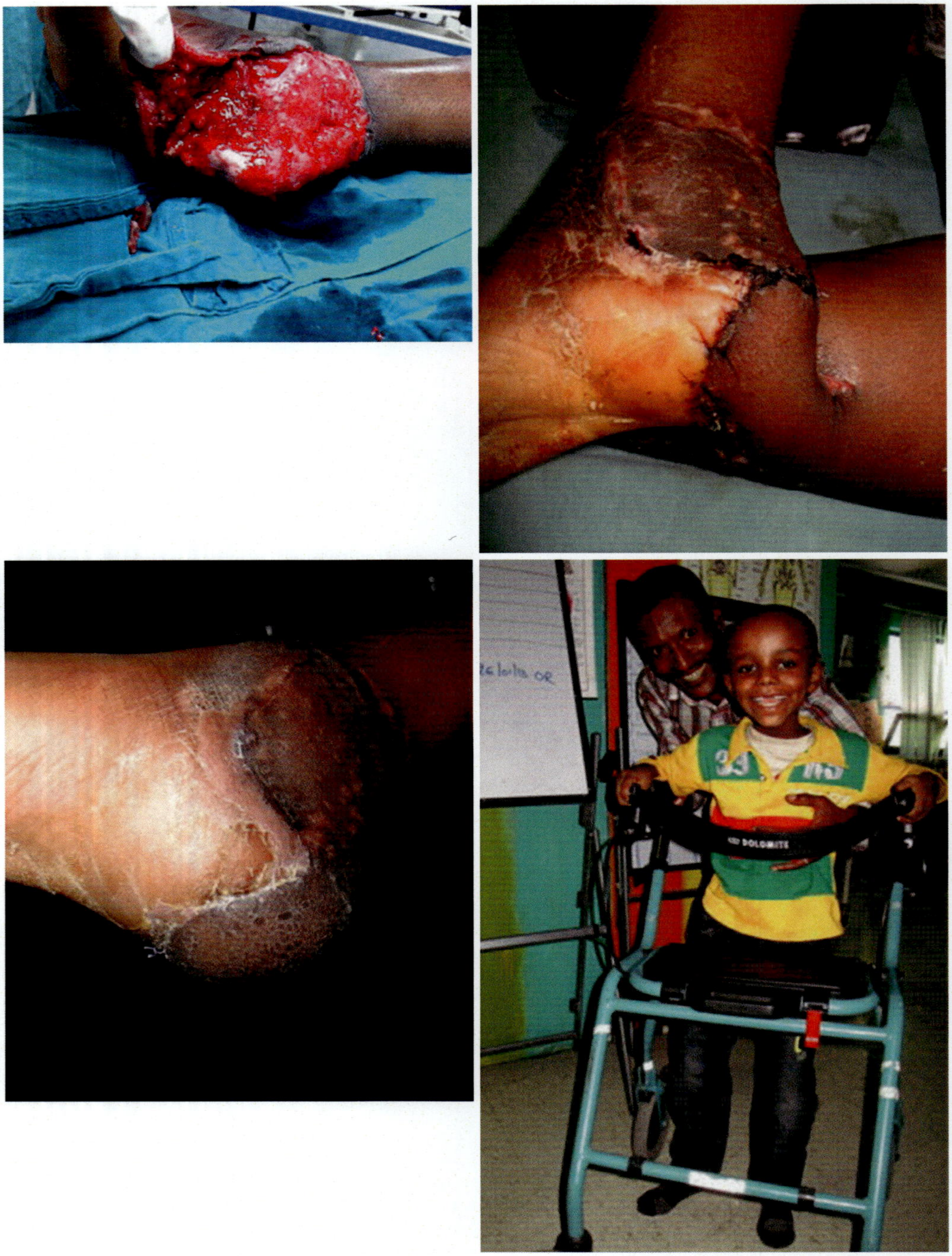

Figs. 32.115–32.118 A 5-year-old boy involved in a traffic accident resulting in a degloving injury with skin loss at the Achilles and ankle region. The heel pad was completely ripped off. Sheets of STSG were used to cover the Achilles and ankle area in advance of the TFL flap procedure. Child recovered well

Conclusion

Burns are the forgotten global public health crisis (WHO 2013). In LMICs it injures more patients than HIV and tuberculosis combined. We do hope this chapter will encourage surgeons who have sincere interest to help the many burn victims in their communities. The techniques needed for burn surgery depend only on a small set of basic instruments; they are inexpensive. Most of them will last for years once you have got them.

Even though burns can happen to any part of the body – from the scalp to the toes – the actual surgical technique is rather simple. There are some basic principles outlined in detail in this chapter. The principles are applied the same way in each procedure.

We hope that the reader of this chapter will join the many individuals currently involved in treating the unfortunate burn victims with modern burn care. The author has emphasized that every burn patient will receive best professional care by correctly applying the main building material – the skin grafts – to the painful wounds. The skin graft harvested from the patient himself is the solution to the misery that burn patients face after their injuries. Although a skin graft appears easy and simple, it is a phenomenal product for those that search for help.

Provision of better early care in the acute/early stage after burn injury will prevent subsequent disabilities that may be life-long and irreparable. Minimizing burn injuries is still the ultimate goal of all modern societies.

33 How to Manage Soft Tissue Infections and Injuries in Low- and Middle-Income Countries

Shailvi Gupta and Jaclyn Clark

So often in life things that you regard as an impediment turn out to be great, good fortune.
– Ruth Bader Ginsburg

Abbreviations

LMICs	Low- and middle-income countries
LRINEC	Laboratory Risk Indicator for Necrotizing Fasciitis
NSTI	Necrotizing soft tissue infections

Introduction

Necrotizing soft tissue infections (NSTI) are characterized by the presence of toxin-producing bacteria, widespread tissue necrosis, and fulminant inflammatory progression, leading to sepsis, multiorgan failure, and, if untreated, death. The mortality of this disease is high, estimated between 20 and 30% even in the best of care. Rapid identification and prompt surgical debridement of necrotic tissue are critical, and delays to surgical intervention are associated with increased mortality [1–3]. Necrotizing infections can occur after major traumatic injuries, as well as after minor breaches of the skin or mucosa (insect bites and abrasions), non-penetrating soft tissue injuries (contusions), or routine surgical procedures such as obstetrical and gynecological procedures [1].

S. Gupta (✉)
University of Maryland School of Medicine, Capital Region Health, Baltimore, MD, USA
e-mail: shailvi.gupta@som.umaryland.edu

J. Clark
University of Maryland School of Medicine, R Adams Cowley Shock Trauma Center, Baltimore, MD, USA

Diagnosis of NSTI

Diagnosing NSTI versus other more common clinical entities such as cellulites can be difficult. Clinicians often rely upon physical examination, diagnostic imaging, and clinical decision instruments to aid in diagnosing NSTIs. Classic physical examination signs described for NSTI include erythema, soft tissue edema, severe pain (pain out of proportion), fever, and hemorrhagic bullae. Hypotension and shock can be indicators of patients with NSTIs [4]. Various imaging modalities, if available, have also been utilized to help aid in the diagnosis. Plain radiography may demonstrate gas within the soft tissue [3].

If available, laboratory values can be utilized to aid in the diagnosis of NSTI. The Laboratory Risk Indicator for Necrotizing Fasciitis (LRINEC) score is a diagnostic clinical decision instrument validated for differentiating NSTI

M. A. Hardy, B. R. Hochman (eds.), *Global Surgery*, https://doi.org/10.1007/978-3-031-28127-3_33

from other soft tissue infections. LRINEC utilizes six laboratory values including white blood cell count, hemoglobin, sodium, glucose, creatinine, and C-reactive protein. A score greater than or equal to six indicates a "moderate" risk of NSTI (50–75% probability), whereas a score greater than or equal to 8 indicates a "high" risk (greater than 75%) probability [3].

Necrotizing soft tissue infections are deadly if left untreated and can be caused by a variety of organisms. Necrotizing infection types I and II are distinguished largely by whether the cause is polymicrobial (type I) or monomicrobial (type II) [1]. The polymicrobial Type I infections involve aerobic and anaerobic organisms and are usually seen in the elderly or in those with underlying illnesses; predisposing factors can include diabetes, decubitus ulcers, rectal fissures, and colonic or urologic or gynecologic procedures. Bacterial penetration into the fascial compartments of the head and neck may result in Ludwig's angina (infection of the submandibular fascial spaces), which may be life-threatening by compressing the trachea. The monomicrobial type II infection is most commonly caused by gram-positive organisms, with group A streptococcus being the most common pathogen followed by methicillin-resistant *Staphylococcus aureus* (MRSA). Type II infections may occur in any age group and in persons without any underlying illness [1] as may type I infections.

Clostridial gas gangrene (clostridial myonecrosis) is caused by anaerobic, spore-forming *Clostridium* subspecies, with *Clostridium perfringens* being the most common. It may occur spontaneously, often with the background of abdominal pathology or malignancy, or as a result of traumatic injury [5]. *Clostridium* infection is synonymous with myonecrosis and is characterized by rapidly progressive gangrene of the injured tissue along with the production of foul-smelling gas (like dead mouse). Historically clostridial gas gangrene was observed as a complication of battlefield injuries. More recently, trauma is responsible for the majority of cases; other predisposing conditions are bowel and biliary tract surgery, intramuscular injection, retained placenta, and intrauterine fetal death [1]. An anaerobic environment is necessary for progression of clostridial infections, and therefore, deeply penetrating injuries are more likely to develop an infection than more superficial wounds [6]. The potent bacterial exotoxins mediate the fulminant clinical features of the infection, and therefore clostridial myonecrosis is the most rapidly spreading lethal infection in humans. An immediate diagnosis and surgical debridement is the only way to save the patient's life.

Invasive fungal wound infections are devastating infections due to the presence of angioinvasive molds (such as *Mucorales*, *Aspergillus* species, and *Fusarium* species) [7]. The most common mechanistic and clinical factors associated with these infections include dismounted blast injury, above-knee traumatic amputations, extensive perineal/pelvic injury, immunocompetence, and massive blood transfusions. Almost all patients suffering from invasive fungal infections have a suspicious wound, defined as recurrent tissue necrosis following at least two surgical debridements. The hallmark of the diagnosis is continued necrosis in well-debrided wounds, and the mainstay of therapy is frequent aggressive surgical debridement, with topical and parenteral antifungal therapy [7].

Animal Bites

Animal bites are common worldwide. Based on recent data, the most important factor in treating animal bites is timely presentation to a medical facility and/or physician, as patients presenting 1–2 days post bite carry a 3.5 and 7 times increased relative risk of hospitalization or surgery respectively, compared to a patient who is able to be medically treated the same day of the bite [8]. Given that access to care may pose difficulties in low- and middle-income countries (LMICs) because of lack of roads and/or transportation, utilization of basic supportive care can be implemented and is a powerful tool in LMICs. Initial copious irrigation with saline or boiled water, debridement, and wound culture are often inexpensive and are within the algorithms of care in nearly all animal bites. Irrigating the wound with saline is an effective and readily accessible initial treatment for bite wounds. This should be followed by clinical assessment of the wound to determine its depth and extent. Radiology studies may be required if there is clinical concern for fractures. Supportive treatment options should be prioritized for animal bites as these are cost-effective and can be provided in resource-limited settings [9].

Given that various types of bites have different risks, it is critical that the offending animal be accurately identified to make sure that it is not a bearer of any infectious disease, such as rabies, to help guide medical and surgical algorithms.

Snakebites

Factors associated with increased snakebite prevalence include field labor, male gender, and residence in rural areas; environmental factors include monsoon seasons and evening hours. If the animal cannot be identified, a patient's presenting symptoms may prove useful in determining appropriate treatment interventions. Isolated fang marks can indicate the presence of a venomous bite with a demonstrated sensitivity of 100% and positive predictive value of 89%. The presence of multiple scratches, on the other hand, has demonstrated a positive predictive value of 100% of nonvenomous bites [9]. Symptoms largely include pain and swelling with accompanying erythema, ecchymosis, and paresthesia. Other symptoms may include hemotoxicity, syncope, neurotoxicity, ptosis, altered sensorium, and breathlessness.

Antivenom is recognized as the first-line treatment and is successful in the treatment of most bites, though antivenom is expensive and may not be accessible in LMICs. If antivenom is not available, ciprofloxacin may be used to cover gram-negative *Enterobacteriaceae* and enterococci [9]. Additional maneuvers should include the removal of clothing that may constrict the affected limb, maintenance of a patent airway, systemic support, and immobilization of the bitten limb at a level below the heart to prevent systemic spread. Despite appropriate treatment, systemic complications may arise within the pulmonary, neurological, and renal organ systems as well as local wound manifestations. Symptoms commonly include hemorrhagic blisters, pulmonary edema, compartment syndrome, cranial nerve paralysis, stroke, and shock. Sequelae including respiratory failure, dyspnea, systemic bleeding, sepsis, and shock have been shown to be strongly associated with fatal outcomes. Supportive care is critical in the setting of snakebites [9].

Crocodile Bites

Crocodile bites are a relatively common injury among people who live near rivers, estuaries, and even lakes. Worldwide, there are 23 crocodile species, but only one, *Crocodylus niloticus* (Nile crocodile), is found in the 43 countries of tropical Africa [10]. These areas of water where crocodiles inhabit are sources of fish and drinking water and are used for washing and other domestic activities within surrounding communities.

Crocodile bites commonly present as a result of penetrating, blunt, and shear forces, ranging from minor scratches and punctures to amputations and death, with deep punctures being the initial and most common presentation. The severity of presentation is often linked to crocodile or alligator size [9]. Despite a possibly small wound externally, crocodile wounds are usually deep, with severe tissue damage, and are frequently contaminated with unusual organisms, making them very difficult to treat (Figs. 33.1 and 33.2, reference 11].

The management of severe crocodile bites of the limbs is a challenge to the surgeon for two main reasons. Firstly, the bite injury is generally of a crushing and degloving nature with multiple wounds caused by the long rows of teeth. Small superficial puncture wounds can mask significant muscle damage with or without an associated fracture. Secondly, the wounds are contaminated with the normal oral flora of a crocodile, which consists of an unusual combination of bacteria. These can cause aggressive local tissue damage, as well as hemolysis. Thirdly, delay in referral often occurs and can contribute independently to the rate of complications [10].

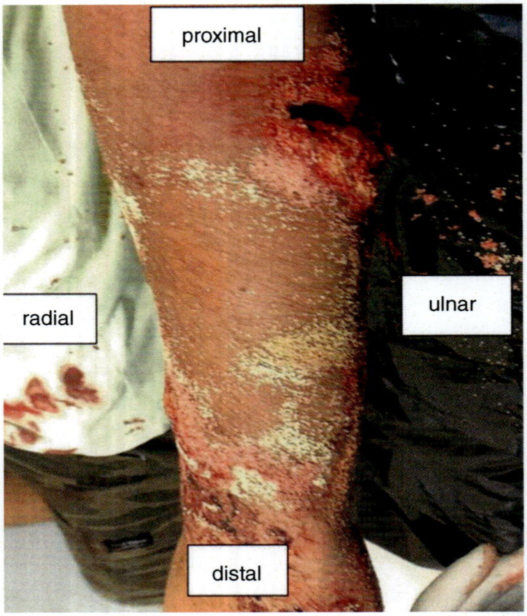

Fig. 33.1 Pre-operative patient photograph of the left forearm showing a deep puncture wound in the proximal part of the extensor compartment. Sand from the river bank is noted as the wound had not been cleaned

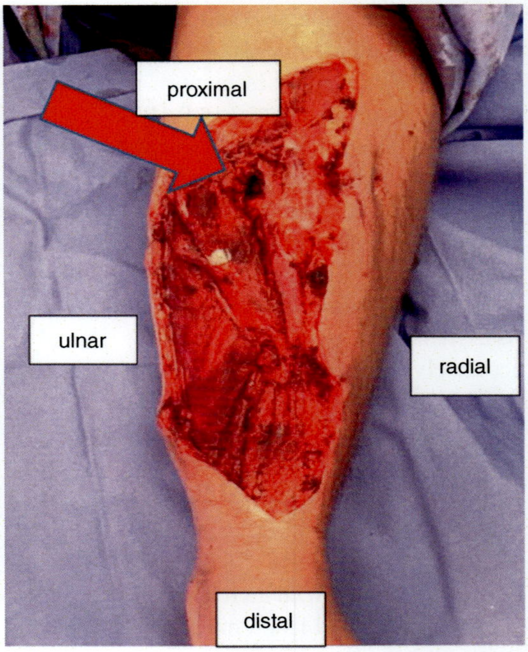

Fig 33.2 Intra-operative photograph of the patients left forearm post debridement demonstrating the extensive muscle damage in the flexor compartment and the depth of the puncture which had transversed the interosseous membrane and was visible within the flexor compartment (red arrow)

Initial management includes resuscitation, tetanus prophylaxis, empirical broad-spectrum antibiotics, and extensive surgical wound debridement under general anesthesia. Significant hemorrhage should be controlled with direct pressure and wound packing. If an associated fracture is present, the use of an external fixator can greatly assist with ongoing wound care. Repeated wound debridements are often necessary to control infection. Devitalized tissue should be debrided, and the remaining wound site should be left to heal by secondary intention or delayed primary closure. Most complications are related to serious deformities, reported in 40% of patients [9, 10].

Unusual gram-negative rods and anaerobes, including *Clostridia*, are found as part of the normal flora of the crocodile's mouth or are part of marine flora and therefore may infect crocodile bite wounds. Rhabdomyolysis can be seen in patients, which may be due to toxic products and enzymes released by microorganisms [10].

Some common pathogens include *Actinobacillus lignieresii* treated with a combination of tetracycline or streptomycin and potassium iodide, *Streptococcus anginosus* treated with vancomycin, *Streptococcus mutans* treated with ampicillin, *Campylobacter ureolyticus* treated with azithromycin, *Prevotella melaninogenica* treated with metronidazole, and *Bacteroides fragilis* treated with metronidazole [9].

Infections are usually polymicrobial bacteria, however, and may be difficult to culture and resistant to common antibiotics. Hemolysis can be associated with ongoing infection, and the hemoglobin should be monitored and the patient transfused as required. Amputation should be considered in view of the aggressive nature of the infections involved and the frequently present severe degree of tissue necrosis; amputation may be a life-saving procedure [10].

Spider Bites

Spider bites rarely cause medically relevant harm to humans. Ones that do are typically isolated to regions of Australia, except for the widow spider, *Latrodectus*. The venom produced by these spiders has been shown to cause long-lasting systemic and regional pain, patchy paralysis, agitation, and hypertension, among other symptoms. Calcium derivates were used historically to help relax the muscle, though they have not been shown to be effective. Antivenom has not been proven to be efficacious in the treatment of spider bites. Analgesics are typically used and have demonstrated effectiveness toward limiting pain and should be the primary method of treatment [9].

Rodent Bites

Rodent bites often occur during the summer months at night and typically present on the patient's face and hands. The most common pathogens include *Pasteurella multocida*, which is treated with beta-lactams, beta-lactamase inhibitors, and aggressive broad-spectrum antibiotics; *Bacillus subtilis* are treated with clindamycin and alpha-hemolytic *Streptococcus* treated with beta-lactams and vancomycin [9].

Landmines

Civilian injury from land mines is a consequence of modern warfare that unfortunately creates long-lasting effects among its victims. Anti-personnel landmines are an effective defensive weapon used to slow the enemy or deny certain areas of land to opposing personnel [12]. Their use, however, indiscriminately kills both military personnel and civilians alike. In addition to this, land mines leave a significant amount of land inaccessible to its communities for decades following a conflict [12]. It is estimated that at least 84 countries are infested with land mines, with about 80 million land mines buried worldwide [12, 13]. Most land mine victims, 80–90%, are noncombatants, mostly women and children carrying on with activities of daily living, and most living in LMICs, where access to healthcare and other rehabilitation services can be limited [14]. Land mine injuries often result in loss of limb, disability, psychological disorders, and loss of economic autonomy – affecting the victim and his or her community for years following the injury [12].

The severity of injury caused by antipersonnel landmines depends on the type of land mine, the proximity of the victim to the explosion, and the relationship of the victim's body to the mine at the time of its detonation [12]. The International Committee of the Red Cross (ICRC) has defined three injury patterns caused by land mines. Victims in Pattern I trigger an explosion by standing on a buried landmine. This usually causes a traumatic amputation of a part of the lower limb and less severe injury elsewhere. Such mines consist of an explosive and may include fragments of metal or plastic. Pattern II injuries are a random collection of penetrating injury caused by multiple fragments from an exploding land mine – injuries to the head, neck, or abdomen are common. Pattern III injuries result from handling a land mine, and victims tend to sustain severe upper limb and facial injuries [15].

Common with other war wounds, land mine injuries are frequently complicated by soft tissue maceration and gross contamination with vegetation, clothing, and soil. The degree of contamination is usually much greater than is initially apparent. Often, the wounds present late with necrosis, perhaps sepsis, and possibly systemic involvement [15]. The basic principle in treating these wounds is to first stop the hemorrhage and then debride the wound extensively until healthy tissue is present.

References

1. Stevens DL, Bryant AE. Necrotizing soft tissue infections. N Engl J Med. 2017;377:2253–65.
2. Bonne SL, Kadri SS. Evaluation and management of necrotizing soft tissue infections. Infect Dis Clin N Am. 2017;31:497–511.

3. Fernando SM, Tran A, Cheng W, Rochwerg B, Kyeremanteng K, Seely AJE, Inaba K, Perry JJ. Necrotizing soft tissue infection: diagnostic accuracy of physical examination, imaging and LRINEC score. Ann Surg. 2019;269(1):58–65.
4. Elliott DC, Kufera JA, Myers RA. Necrotizing soft tissue infections. Risk factors for mortality and strategies for management. Ann Surg. 1996;224:262–83.
5. Yang Z, Hu J, Qu Y, et al. Interventions for treating gas gangrene. Cochrane Database Syst Rev. 2015;10(12):CD010577.
6. Buboltz JB, Murphy-Lavoie HM. Gas gangrene. StatPearls Publishing; 2020.
7. Rodriguez CJ, et al. Treatment of suspected invasive fungal infection in war wounds. Mil Med. 2018;183:142–6.
8. Speirs J, Showery J, Abdou M, et al. Dog bites to the upper extremity in children. J Paediatr Child Health. 2015;51:1172–4.
9. Savu AN, Schoenbrunner AR, Politi R, Janis JE. Practical review of the Management of Animal Bites. Plast Reconstr Surg Glob Open. 2021;9(9):e3778.
10. Wamisho BL, Bates J, Tompkins M, Islam R, Nyamulani N, Ngulube C, Mkandawire NC. Ward round – crocodile bites in Malawi: microbiology and surgical management. Malawi Med J. 2009;21(1):29–31.
11. Venter M, Kelly A, Boffard K, Pretorius R, Younus A. African Nile crocodile bite of the forearm: a case report. East Afr Orthopaed J. 2020;14(2)
12. Ryken KO, Hogue M, March JL, Schweizer M. Long term consequences of landmine injury: a survey of civilian survivors in Bosnia-Herzegovina 20 years after the war. Injury Int J Care Inj. 2017;48:2688–92.
13. Walsh NE, Walsh WS. Rehabilitation of landmine victims, the ultimate challenge. Bull World Health Organ. 2003;81:665–70.
14. Mannion M, Chaloner E. Chapter 1. landmines and landmine injuries: an overview. Pain Med. 2006;7:S199–200.
15. Coupland RM, Korver A. Injuries from antipersonnel mines: the experience of the International Committee of the Red Cross. Br Med J. 1991;303:1509–12.

34 How to Approach NOMA and Facial Infections, Trauma, and Tumours Through Charity Missions: The Origins of Facing Africa and Lessons Learned

Chris Lawrence and Terry Lawrence

We are here to add what we can to life, not to get what we can from life.

– William Osler

Abbreviations

CL	Chris Lawrence
DNF	Dutch Noma Foundation
FA	Face Africa
MCM	Myung Sung Christian Medical Center
MdS	Marathon des Sables
TL	Terry Lawrence

Introduction

In 1998, one of the authors (CL) watched a WHO video about a disease called noma. It was so shocking for him to see that such a disease, related mainly by extreme poverty and malnutrition, should exist in the twentieth century and that so few know anything about it. He learned that noma was a bacterial infection that started in the gums of children under the age of 6 and spread very rapidly, and within 3–4 weeks, it ate away the lips and cheeks of small children. Noma exists predominantly in sub-Saharan Africa, but cases also appear in parts of SE Asia and South America. The WHO estimated at that time that 250,000 cases of noma occurred globally every year and that 90% of the victims would die within weeks unless it was diagnosed and cured with an antibiotic in the very early stages. Noma remains a disease still officially unrecognized by WHO and by most professionals. A large number of NGOs are still trying desperately to persuade the WHO to include noma in its listings of diseases.

Those who survive the ravages of this flesh-eating disease are left with gaping holes in their cheeks, nose and lips, thus causing terrible discomfort, pain, difficulty in drinking and eating and of course social rejection. Noma is usually considered a curse or a punishment from God, and as a result, the parents keep their affected children in the shadows out of shame. Since most Africans living in rural areas are often illiterate and know little of anything about doctors and hospitals, most of the parents' first port of call is to a "traditional healer" (witch doctors in our language), since the parents cannot afford the bus fare to a regional clinic or hospital.

One of the authors (CL) along with his wife, despite no medical background, were inspired and compelled to find a solution to this chilling disorder. The Dutch Noma Foundation (DNF) and Dr. Klaas Marck, an eminent Dutch surgeon who had been doing reconstructive surgery on

C. Lawrence (✉) · T. Lawrence
West Stowell House, Wiltshire, UK
e-mail: chris@facingafrica.org

M. A. Hardy, B. R. Hochman (eds.), *Global Surgery*, https://doi.org/10.1007/978-3-031-28127-3_34

noma sufferers in Nigeria four times a year, were contacted, which sparked the founding and registration as a charity of Facing Africa (FA) in the UK in 1998 by CL and his wife, Terry Lawrence (TL). This in turn resulted in a productive collaboration of CL and the teams of health professionals led by Dr. Marck from the DNF, together with a German charitable organization called AWD Kinderhilfe. The effort clearly needed assistance with fundraising to stabilize and broaden its activities. CL, with his extensive business and fundraising experience in the travel and fashion industries, along with his knowledge necessary to deal with potential difficulties or dangers in different countries and cultures, was an ideal administrative leader of this team of expert physicians and nurses. To overcome the many obstacles and challenges presented to each team on each mission, CL used some of his talent as a "hustler." Through his popularity as a recruiter for Marathon des Sables (MdS), an annual 245 km foot race across the Sahara in Morocco, CL was able to raise £ 250,000 each year, which were used to help fund the noma missions to Nigeria. As CL sold his travel company in 2005, he dedicated with his wife their organizational skills to develop an outstanding and innovative surgical care system for victims of noma.

Country and Site Selection

When the situation in Nigeria deteriorated because of wars and corruption, FA looked elsewhere in Africa for a country that was able to provide (a) direct flight connections to major European cities; (b) where corruption by bribing was not always required to innovate; (c) where government was relatively stable; and (d) where English was spoken. Another requirement was to (e) have access to a government hospital that was welcoming, well equipped for complex surgeries and affordable to FA. After exploring several West Africa countries, it was decided that Ethiopia was a suitable place to bring regular teams of surgeons, anaesthetists and wound care nurses to carry out reconstructive surgery on the victims of noma. Initially, a government hospital appeared suitable. The team was assured by the hospital director that specific drugs, consumables, disposables. and almost everything were available in abundance but that it would be wise to bring certain items that were unavailable in Ethiopia. In order to avoid excess customs duties and taxes on the suggested items, it was decided to address them to the hospital. This led to any unused medical items, such as very expensive sutures, to be used by the hospital rather than being kept for future use by the team. They had to be bought again for each mission. This lesson was followed by another, in that equipment and disposables of which FA was assured were on site were really unavailable and had to be sought elsewhere. With such experience, the staff was instructed to take all precautions against misunderstandings or devious interpretations of rules and regulations. They were also asked not to agree to or make any kind of promises regarding medical or surgical items. The FA continued to work at this hospital despite its difficulties with the hospital's management, facilities, staffing problems and insoluble negotiation issues.

This then led FA in 2009 to change site for future missions. CL along with a hired Ethiopian "fixer," experienced in public relations and communication (necessary hire to deal with local organizations and the public), focused now on a variety of privately owned and managed hospitals in and around Addis Ababa. After visiting a variety of private hospitals with attention to (a) location, (b) facilities, (c) cleanliness and (d) the cost to FA, six hospitals were screened by phone and e-mail in order to establish the level of fees, what would be provided by the hospital and what was expected of FA to bring. Five were eliminated: two for extravagant fees, two for inadequate facilities and equipment and one that insisted on their own surgeons participating actively in the operations beyond their skill sets. Finally, an American Christian foundation was selected to serve as the base for FA activities. Although satisfactory for one mission, on renewal of the contract, the hospital unflinchingly doubled the fees that had been charged for the previous trip. This resulted in another change of site in 2010 to another private hospital in Addis Ababa, South Korean MCM (Myung Sung Christian Medical) Hospital. It had four ORs, was well equipped and staffed and welcomed the team. As time progressed, however, the hospital continued to increase their charges for uncertain reasons, and FA had to find another site, primarily for financial reasons.

After 14 missions, the relationships between MCM and FA deteriorated on the basis of many financial and administrative reasons. Most importantly, the hospital neglected to obtain legal licenses for the staff and for FA during 14 missions as required by law, and for which, FA was charged. When it had become obvious that it was time to find an alternative hospital, FA moved briefly (two missions) to another new and well-equipped private Ethiopian hospital, before landing at a small, spotlessly clean and extremely well-maintained hospital (Nordic Medical Centre) built by a Norwegian friend of CL. This Scandinavian establishment was used for three surgical missions, and then came the pandemic. The missions had to stop not only because of COVID but also because of an ongoing civil war (tribal), which broke out in 2020.

As can be seen from this abbreviated story, an NGO focused on a rare surgical condition must choose its major site of operation carefully, and negotiate even more carefully, with the motto of "Trust and Verify" (President Reagan), on every occasion. Mission leaders must remain flexible in their activities and demand fair and just treatment from their hosts.

Facing Africa House and Rehabilitation Facility

Even cheap hotels would not accommodate people with open wounds on their faces for fear of alienating other guests who would automatically assume that these diseases were contagious. The original 35 patients who had agreed to have reconstructive surgery who were brought to Addis Ababa were accommodated in a most appalling, filthy hostel, which was totally unsuitable for people who were about to undergo complex surgery. This became an important factor in that 70% of the patients developed wound infections. The error that was never repeated was to check the site where patients would stay prior to scheduling their arrivals. A solution was required to accommodate these patients arriving from remote rural villages, many of whom had never owned a pair of shoes, been in a car, seen a building higher than one storey, or is some cases had never seen a white person. Accommodating these gentle but uneducated people in a suitable alternative site had to be found for pre-operative workup and for post-operative follow-up and rehabilitation.

The search for a site ended when CL and his wife found a delightful rehabilitation centre for children with polio located in a countryside setting about 20 miles outside Addis Ababa. The facility had several dormitories with showers, kitchen and dining room, a basic physiotherapy room, playroom and acres of lawn and gardens. The management of the facility was willing to accommodate up to 50 FA patients twice a year for up to 8 weeks on each mission. The new patients could stay there for 2 weeks prior to the arrival of the surgical team. During that time, a Western doctor and two wound care nurses along with six Ethiopian trainee nurses would be based at the facility throughout the 8 weeks. The trainees would be taught how to use many of the different dressings used in Western hospitals, pain management and general nursing and more intimate contact with the patients. This gathering of 30–40 people with severe facial deformities quickly realized on meeting each other that they were not the only people with such disfigurements and previously considered freaks in their villages. After meeting others, they gained immediate confidence and were seen to make new friendships. From being outcasts in their own village societies, they made friends. Children under the age of 14 were encouraged to come with a parent or guardian.

This beautiful facility was where FA patients would be fed, accommodated and clothed for 2 weeks prior to their operations, for 2 weeks while being hospitalized, and a further 2–4 weeks for recovery time and intense rehabilitation.

In 2011, the trustees of FA accepted the offer by the management of the facility to loan a part of their land for FA to build their own facility. The buildings designed by an architect would include four dormitories with ten beds in each for male and female patients, showers with hot water, toilets, dining room, recreation room, laundry room, doctor's office, storage room and a play area surrounding the buildings, for football and volleyball. The new facility, called "Facing Africa House", was officially opened by the British Ambassador to Ethiopia in 2012 after a cost overrun from £ 50,000 to £ 350,000. It became, and remains, a critical site for future patient intake through their rehabilitation.

Public Relations

FA was becoming noted for the amazing reconstructions, and soon, FA was being contacted by surgeons, anaesthetists and medical organizations wanting to offer their time, skills and help. Volunteers from different countries wanted to join FA teams; one trip included nine different nationalities among the team members. Few local surgeons, anaesthetists and nurses participated as assistants to learn new techniques and apply them to their own work.

Word of mouth and local newspaper articles helped generate interest and some contributions to the FA charity.

Once the BBC decided to make a documentary about the work being done by FA teams, which was first screened in the UK in 2010, more than US$ 500,000 was donated within a few weeks. Despite international interest, public interest in Ethiopia and WHO interest globally for these poor children with noma did not improve their preventive healthcare and antibiotic distribution as needed.

Meeting Legal Requirements and Licensing

An official charity licence issued by the Charity Commission in Addis Ababa was both desirable and necessary for FA's optimal function. Very little progress was made despite many meetings at the commission's offices. The Charity Commission put up obstacles until one was issued with conditions that were not only extremely cumbersome but would also entail maintenance an expensive army of local accountants, auditors, bookkeepers and lawyers. The promised tax-free concessions to FA were so convoluted that they were unattainable. Another obstacle that finally resulted in returning the license to the commission was the demand that the foreign charity/NGO must have an Ethiopian partner with the right to sign checks to open a bank account. In these unfortunate circumstances, FA appealed to the Federal Ministry of Health and was granted a special licence to carry out clinical work under their auspices. Similar obstacles are frequently encountered in many LMICs and need to be legally circumvented to continue the health work beneficial to the local population.

Direct appeal to the Ministers of Health will facilitate function as long as their priorities are included in the NGO's agenda. In the case of noma, the greater interest of the federal authorities as expressed by one famous Minister of Health (subsequent head of WHO) was in missions dedicated to the treatment of heart and kidney problems, diabetes, orthopaedics, cancer, strokes, bone fractures, etc. rather than to a disease like noma, which was almost unknown in Ethiopia in spite of the fact that there are probably thousands of children who die quietly in rural areas, disfigured and tortured by their infirmities.

The other issue is timely applications for individual permits to practice surgery in the host country. This process may be done through the hospital where one will practice. The problem with that may be that after all the fees are collected by the hospital for submission of applications and the fees for the applications themselves, nothing gets done until it is too late. It is important to check, verify and obtain the personal permits before embarking on the mission. Alternative processes may be to do this directly with the Ministry of Health or occasionally through the local consulate or embassy of the host country (more difficult).

Although laborious and sometimes costly, personal license must be secured, if required, to avoid practicing illegally, which could have disastrous consequences and must be avoided at all costs. Maintaining or obtaining malpractice insurance is also strongly advised.

Negotiations

The negotiations with the hospital and the Ministry of Health aimed to establish the rules and regulations governing foreign healthcare staff coming to Ethiopia as clinicians were the first order of business. In parallel, one must investigate and negotiate with the hospital about the availability of drugs, antibiotics, surgical instruments, consumables and disposables. Before proceeding further, it was advisable to find a local "fixer" bureaucrat who can help process the various licences and permits, as well as to identify and refer noma patients from rural areas and to negotiate with hotels for the team to base themselves and with the Ethiopian Airlines for any group concessions. All activities require some form of negotiations. These require patience, diplomacy, mutual understanding of limits and conditions and, most importantly, trust. Unfortunately, the latter can sometimes be questioned. All agreements must be checked and verified as well, especially regarding dedicated personnel and their compensation, as well as availability of equipment, drugs and space for recovery room, for hospitalization and for storage.

A walk through the designated hospital may be very helpful – preferably with a local witness.

Recruiting the Team of Professionals

FA initially reached out for volunteer surgeons or anaesthetists in the UK. CL sought qualified and experienced volunteers who might be interested in joining an FA surgical mission to Ethiopia for a few weeks. With little understanding of the different types of surgical specialities and no knowledge or understanding of anything other than noma being a flesh-eating disease, it was very challenging to find qualified individuals to work in LMICs in relatively basic hospital facilities with meagre resources. Once an experienced consultant plastic surgeon was identified in UK and was willing to join the FA team going to Addis Ababa, other healthcare workers began to volunteer. This included a prominent maxillofacial surgeon and a university professor who was also curious and interested in participating in the new FA undertaking. The original Dutch mentor agreed to lead the team to Ethiopia as the rotations to Nigeria ended. This small group was then able to recruit a very experienced anaesthetist, who in turn brought his friends, an anaesthetic ODP and his wife, a very experienced ward nurse. The FA program was ready to begin its work in Ethiopia in October 2007.

Recruiting the Patients with Noma

Once a team was prepared to work, it needed to identify appropriate patients, prepare them for difficult and lengthy operations, optimize them nutritionally and otherwise and obtain consents (with translators and with guardians as necessary). An Ethiopian native ("a fixer") was hired, who worked previously for TV news channels, and although he had no health contacts, he was familiar with officials in the ministries of immigration, media/PR and communications. He spent the coming months sourcing children and adults who had unsightly facial disfigurements caused by noma or injuries. Finding noma victims in the poorest areas of Ethiopia was expected, but identifying them was very difficult. Parents of noma children considered the disease as a curse; out of shame, therefore, they hid them at home and denied knowing anyone, child or adult, with severely damaged faces.

Despite these obstacles, there were 35 patients treated by FA in 2007, among which were 18 with noma and 17 with various trauma, animal bites, tumours and nose reconstructions. They understood from FA surgeons explanations that their original good looks may be only partially restored following surgery. Other people with noma declined the offer, believing in some cases that they would never wake up after an anaesthetic, while others preferred to take treatment from a traditional healer using herbs, prayers and lies.

Motivation and Maintenance of the Team

The members of the team are all volunteers who are motivated primarily by wanting to contribute to the treatment of the most unfortunate, disabled, disfigured, poor young individuals imaginable. The team members are all very talented, distinguished members of various medical and nursing specialists. They include plastic, maxillofacial and oral surgeons, anaesthesiologists, wound nurse specialists and ward and recovery room nurses and other specialists as needed. It is not unusual for some of these individuals to recruit others to participate in these 2-week missions where they all operate as a unit every day and care for the patients after their operations.

FA pays for all its volunteers' flights, hotels and meals on each trip and encourages social cohesion among the volunteers. During the 2-week mission, FA sponsors nightly joint dinners for the staff at one of the many excellent restaurants in Addis Ababa, which encourages relaxation and potentiates close interactions among members of the team. As a result, strong friendships have emerged from the trips, and there is always a strong feeling of bond and mutual assistance and appreciation for everyone's part in the mission. Teamwork is the fundamental quality needed for the mission's success. Fortunately, FA is well funded enough, to make this group, however large or small, work as a team by providing all the essentials and comforts that people did not expect. Providing and caring for each individual while in a strange country with very different cultures maintained the team spirit and a sense of gratitude for the organization. CL and his wife, based on a 35-year business experience in travel and fashion industry, focus on transferring the finest hospitality and appreciation to their hardworking team. FA missions have become the envy of most NGOs. They provide not only personal comforts but also the use of an excellent hospital with Western standards of nursing, equipment and facilities that people do not expect.

Lessons from Initial Missions

Besides the lessons described above on how to deal with the site that the mission will use where there has to be mutual trust and collaboration, there were many other lessons that had to be learned from FA's initial experience with the first 35 patients and subsequent missions.

1. Hospital and rehabilitation/recovery site. This needed to be addressed for pre- and post-operative care not only for patient comfort but also to test patients pre-operatively for endemic diseases, train in hygiene and wound care and train student nurses to eventually avoid the unacceptable high rate of post-operative wound infections and problems.
2. After each operation, the patients were sent to a surgical recovery ward staffed by young nurses who had limited training and were very restricted with basic essentials, including pain management drugs and bandages. Their form of wound care required total re-education, which was provided by the visiting nurses (see Chap. 40, under wound care) both at Facing Africa House for nursing students and following operations both at the hospital and at FA House.
3. Negotiations with the hospital authorities must be clearly defined on both sides. One must check everything regarding any verbal commitments by the facilities. With experience such as that of FA, all precautions for misunderstandings or devious interpretations of rules and regulations must be observed and all team members instructed not to agree privately to or make any kind of personal promises regarding medical or surgical items. Inspection of the facilities, "a walk-through", may be very valuable to avoid any misunderstandings.

4. Appropriate licenses to practice in LMICs must be obtained prior to the visit, relying primarily on the organizer of the mission or preferably on personal initiative if possible.
5. To continue and maintain high standards of each mission, there is an obvious need for a highly motivated, experienced and gifted administrator with a dedicated associate. They raise funds, recruit volunteer professionals and arrange and support flights, living quarters and living expenses. To maintain the team's cohesiveness, close clinical collaboration and patient selection and care, FA provides all the essentials and comforts. It helps maintain a high level of collaboration and individual satisfaction so that team members are eager to return and to train new cadre of individuals to continue this critical service not only to save lives but also to help their patients gain dignity and function within their communities.

Summary and Plans

There are a number of issues that needed to be addressed for future FA trips, many of which have been or are being addressed:

1. FA needs to take more of its own consumables, disposables and drugs because of the inadequacies and unreliability shown by the host on FA's first trip. All medical supplies should be taken as personal baggage on the flight so as to avoid having to argue with hospital management about ownership of any products at the end of the mission.
2. FA would need to find more suitable accommodation close to the hospital for patients coming from rural parts of Ethiopia. A small but clean and habitable hotel to provide all the rooms may be the best solution. FA solved this by building its own facility within a pre-existing rehabilitation centre.
3. It is essential to accommodate the patients for at least a week prior to their complex surgeries to carry out all essential pre-op medical tests for malaria, HIV, etc. as well as teaching them the basics of hygiene with showers and dental care. This was done following construction and opening of FA House.
4. All team members in the future had to agree never to make any offers of donations of equipment, consumables and disposables. Even using the word "maybe" is inappropriate since "maybe" could be considered a firm promise.
5. FA decided that future trips should include at least four, if not five consultant surgeons as well as having two consultant anaesthetists who specialized in difficult airways not to overtax a smaller group while instructing local health providers.
6. It would be agreed in writing on all future missions what was being provided by FA by way of medical and surgical equipment, drugs, consumables and disposables and what would be provided free of charge by the hospital. This includes overtime pay to some needed ancillary staff to have their allegiance (such as floor sweepers).
7. FA would, in the future, bring two experienced British ward nurses to cover the many nursing inadequacies and to train local staff in maintaining clean facilities (day and night), dressing changes and pain management. The training will begin at FA House prior to surgery (as is already being done). This is necessary to prevent infections and pain.
8. Once it is known that that very complex reconstructive surgery is being done, space is needed in the OR for medical students and local medical personnel to assist, observe and learn new surgical and anaesthesia techniques.
9. Evaluation following each mission visit will lead to improvement. It is never too late to make necessary changes. FA changed hospitals from one that was ill-equipped and insufficient to an alternative better managed with more ORs and more services and finally to another hospital more amenable to reasonable contracts, to develop and be able to use the world-class skills of volunteer surgeons, anaesthetists and nurses to capacity.

10. Once established, FA needed to decide how many missions it should carry out per year, how to staff them and how to fund them. Having gained experience of working in Ethiopia for three annual missions, it was decided that from 2010 onwards, Facing Africa would be confident enough and would be able to source two teams every year to take to Ethiopia instead of one.

This summary enumerates many details, both favourable and unfavourable, of the many FA missions as an example for other similar volunteer surgical missions. The presentation is extracted from the history of the many FA missions. It focuses on pertinent facts to illustrate the many problems that the missions have faced over the years and to present the many solutions that FA provided in full or in part to make the surgical visits very effective and successful. The public relations campaign has remained limited to raising the necessary funds to continue the mission in only one country so far. No plans have been made yet to expand the effort to other countries.

35 How to Approach NOMA and Facial Infections, Trauma and Tumours Through Charity Missions: Facing Africa Non-operating Mission

Hiroshi Nishikawa

Introduction

Much is known about the ideal proportions of the Western face. The horizontal thirds and the vertical fifths that make the proportions of the Western face (e.g. the correct proportions between the width of the eyes and the width of the nose or the distance the eyes are apart) were well known in the Renaissance. Leonardo drew cephalometric diagrams to help him paint and to understand the basis of human proportion (Fig. 35.1).

I find it fascinating that Leonardo's painting of the Duke of Milan's Mistress, the Lady with an Ermine drawn 500 years ago, still resonates to European minds as a girl of beauty (Fig. 35.2). We are conditioned, taught, educated or maybe genetically wired to appreciate her.

Yet when African art (face) influenced Picasso (see Desmoiselles d'Avignon, Figs. 35.3 and 35.4), then the frame of reference was thrown. This was partly because of the huge conceptual differences between the depiction of the African face and Western art and maybe because the known benchmarks of the Western face were invalid for the African one. Picasso (hence Western aesthetic appreciation) tried to explore this during his African phase of paintings, and he eventually produced quite outrageous art based upon African images and, at the time, its primitive and alien nature.

Western cephalometric proportions guide reconstructive and cosmetic surgery of the face, if one has been trained in Europe. The relative gross facial reconstructions we carried out in Addis Ababa for severe abnormalities will never achieve these ideals. The yardstick that we judge aesthetic results is based upon will never achieve these ideals. The yardstick that we judge aesthetic results is based upon our pre-conceptions, education, genes and exposure to a world that is distinctly *not* African. So when I look at the African face, I realize that I am not trained to fully analyse it. I am therefore curious to understand whether my concept of a normal or a beautiful African face will be the same as that of an indigenous person. This has inspired me to try and construct a study on the differences between my European-based perceptions of facial aesthetics and that of the African ones.

This study would take the form of a field trip involving two surgeons, an anaesthetist, the CEO of FA, and a translator, who ideally should be an anthropologist. The anthropologist should have a deep understanding of the indigenous people of Ethiopia and their languages, customs and social structures. The areas to be visited will be influenced by known previous referral patterns.

H. Nishikawa (✉)
Craniofacial/Plastic Multidisciplinary Department, Welbourne Center and Birmingham Children Hospital, Birmingham, UK

M. A. Hardy, B. R. Hochman (eds.), *Global Surgery*, https://doi.org/10.1007/978-3-031-28127-3_35

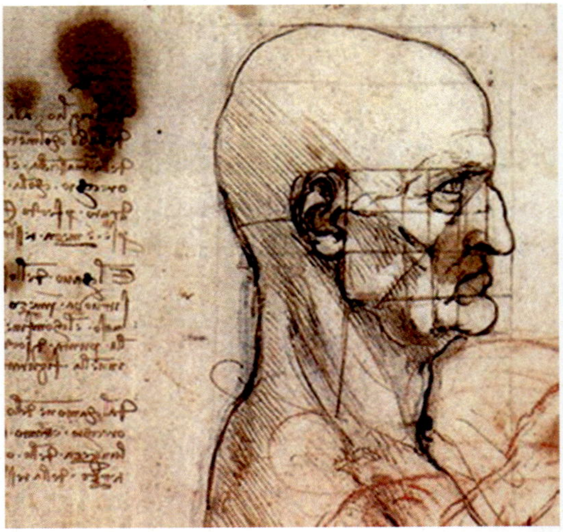

Fig. 35.1 Cephalometrics of the human face

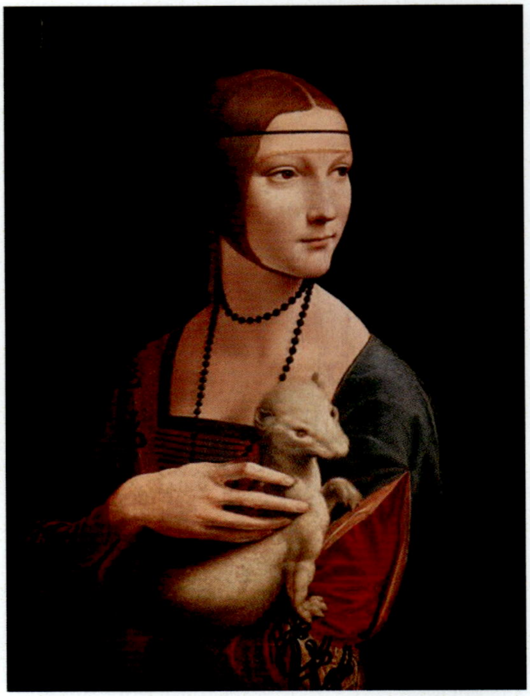

Fig. 35.2 The Lady with an Ermine. Leonardo Da Vinci

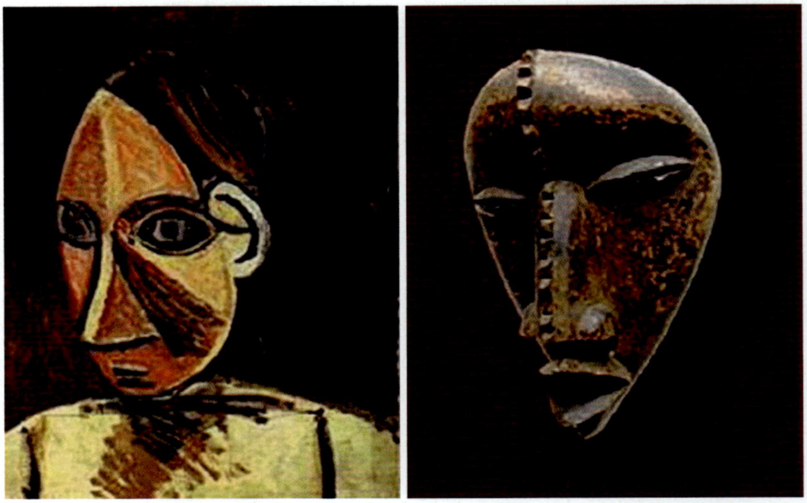

Fig. 35.3 Self Portrait. Piccasso

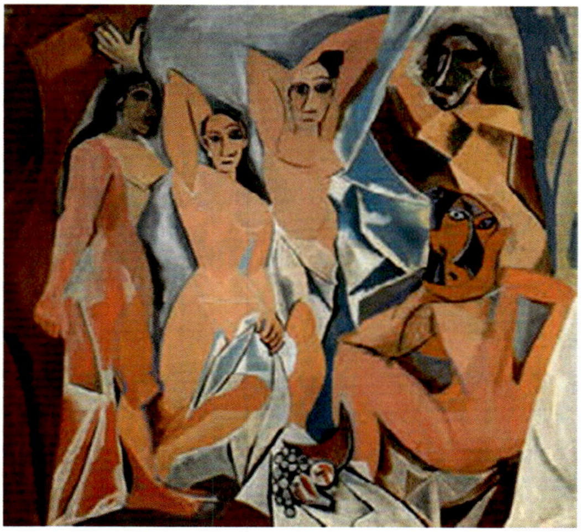

Fig. 35.4 Les Desmoiselles d'Avignon

Aims

There are several aims to the non-operating mission:

1. Improve our understanding of surgical outcome of patients treated for noma.
2. Pilot future potential studies for benchmarking the perception of normal and facially deformed patients in remote areas of Ethiopia.
3. Improve pre-assessment methods for noma patients.
4. Enhance the understanding of cultural and sociological differences that have a bearing on improving FA healthcare delivery.
5. Disseminate these findings in scientific publication and meetings.

Discussion

The primary purpose of this mission is for clinicians and the CEO to have a much clearer idea of the patient's true perception of the outcome of surgery carried out for complex facial deformity in Addis Ababa. This may in turn help improve FA healthcare delivery.

It is often unclear as to the real feelings of indigenous people from remote areas of Ethiopia, concerning the outcome of their facial surgery. The reasons for this are complex. Western surgeons usually cannot communicate effectively with these patients (there are over 90 languages in Ethiopia). Translation is often unreliable. It is also difficult for Westerners to understand behavioural and cultural cues (a nod may mean a no, a smile may indicate anger or disdain, yes may mean "go away"). There are also intrinsic difficulties of validated outcome measures for all facial surgeries.

Outcome measures have traditionally centred on functional changes (e.g. improved breathing and mouth opening) and noting measurable changes of appearance such as simple linear alterations (changes in the length of the nose or eyelids). For increasingly complex parameters involving volume, symmetry and shape changes, analysis is much harder. The mathematical comparison of these changes compared to the norm is the basis of complicated research involving digital mapping of thousands of coordinates topographically [1]. This is clearly still experimental, but simpler validated research based on the response of trained, unbiased observers to photographic appearances of pre- and post-operative patients have been used to assess cosmetic outcome [2–4]. This kind analysis is based on the assumption that the observer has a firm grasp of what a normal appearance is. However, probably the most important parameter is the patient's own perception of outcome. Patient-reported outcome measures (PROMS) have been used quite widely in the UK and the USA for the analysis of patient perceptions of surgical result. In Ethiopia and other developing countries, there are probably significant problems in a PROMS approach to outcome analysis because we have no idea what the benchmark of "normal" or "acceptable" is. There will almost certainly be problems for indigenous people to understand the concept of the questionnaire or looking at photographs comparatively for the purposes of assessment. However, unless we start to make some approaches along these lines, then the benchmark will never be understood, and FA will never grasp the true nature and ramifications of the complex surgery it carries.

Methodology of Study on Facial Norms in Ethiopia

One aspect of this mission is to pilot potential field studies on individuals we meet in the areas visited. The aim is to try and discover what their frame of reference is regarding normal and abnormal facial appearance. What do they consider attractive or less attractive? Are such concepts totally different compared to Western perceptions? The null hypothesis of a PROMS study in Ethiopia would be that both Western and Ethiopian aesthetic appreciation are based on similar parameters of facial proportions and structure (i.e. what we fancy so do they). However, the appearance of mature women of the Mursi tribe would tend to highlight how our aesthetic values are probably different (Fig. 35.5).

A possible method would be to show photographs of ethnic faces to age-matched cohorts to European and Ethiopian subjects and compare their responses statistically. Kappa analysis can be used to analyse subjective variables. There would be two sets of grouped responses permitted.

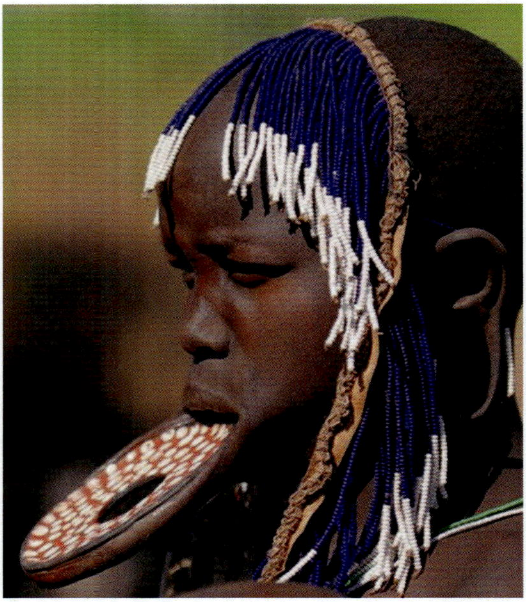

Fig. 35.5 Woman from the Mursi tribe

Normal or Abnormal Ordinary, Attractive, Beautiful, Ugly

First the responder will decide if the photograph of the face is normal or abnormal. Then a second question will be asked. Is the face, in terms of cosmetic appearance, ordinary, ugly, attractive or beautiful? We have to inform the informer that an immediate impression is all that we want. The methodology would not be valid if it transpires that communicating these requests is impossible or their responses are totally unreliable. It is also on the supposition that the words normal, beautiful, ugly, attractive and abnormal exist in their language.

It may also transpire that simple contact between our culture and theirs would instantly alter all natural behavioural responses. This is analogous to Heisenberg's "uncertainty principle"; we can never study anything accurately because as soon as we attempt to measure a phenomenon, it will instantly alter its natural steady-state characteristics. Therefore, it is important to have the services of an accurate translator if we ever attempt to carry out such a study. If the translator is an anthropologist, then further insight may be gained as to the nature of their aesthetic preferences rooted in culture and tradition.

The Effect of Facial Deformity in Ethiopia

I was very much personally moved on witnessing several very deformed noma patients breastfeeding (Fig. 35.6). Apparently, devoted spouses also usually attended them. It would be interesting to understand the sociological weight of the facial appearance in an individual's integration into African society. Maybe the anthropologist may inform us the width of the hips or the size of the breasts and buttocks or height is a far more valued aspect of beauty in their culture and for mate selection. I am not trying to be facetious but expressing my total ignorance of their cultural values. If, for example, we discovered that facial deformity has little sociological impact in their

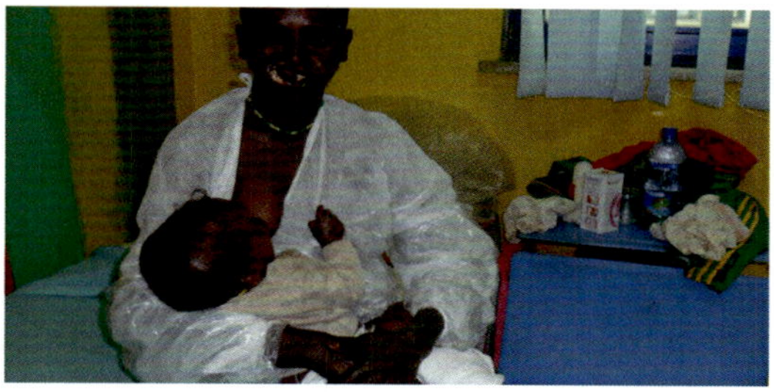

Fig. 35.6 Breastfeeding woman with facial deformity caused by noma

world, then it could be argued that the only purpose of treating a facial abnormality would be for functional reasons only. A searching analysis of motivation could have fundamental implications on patient selection by the FA. It is therefore desirable to meet potential patients with facial deformity during this mission to try and determine their status and condition in society. We should determine whether they are isolated or fully integrated.

Should any of these individuals we encounter wish for surgery, we should try and understand whether their motives are the same as our surgical aims and whether it is possible to make them understand how we intend to carry this out. It would be important to ascertain whether their motive is just financial or their expectations are in fact totally mismatched with what FA can technically offer.

Lastly, we need to try and find a patient that we have already treated for facial deformity and determine whether we have in fact improved the quality of life. An Ethiopian PROMS would undoubtedly be hard, and again a reliable translator/anthropologist will be required. The following questions may be asked:

- Are you better?
- Are you happier?
- Are you pleased?
- Are you less self-conscious?
- Are you more accepted by your friends and family?

These questions may have no meaning to them, or the answers may also be invalidated by a desire to please us. Perhaps the anthropologist could give us some insight as to how to ask such personal and blunt questions. We have no idea if such questions are culturally acceptable or understandable in their society. However, if it can be shown that surgery has been beneficial not only functionally but also sociologically, then this would be circumstantial evidence that many of our concerns about motivation and outcome are not valid and that aesthetic and social benchmarks are perhaps similar or comparable to ours.

Conclusions

1. A non-operating mission to remote areas of Ethiopia will allow us to initiate pilot studies on the indigenous perceptions of facial deformity and normality.
2. A benchmark of what is normal, abnormal, ordinary, beautiful or ugly (unacceptable) could be established.
3. It is an opportunity to educate operating clinicians as to the true outcome of complex surgery undertaken to correct facial deformity in the long-term setting of the patient's natural environment.
4. A more accurate picture of outcome (functional and psychosocial) may be achieved if analysis of potential pre-operative and definitive post-operative patients undertake a modified or simplified form of Ethiopian PROMS.
5. The data and impressions acquired may allow FA to improve pre-operative assessments for the future and could alter the type of cases that FA target.
6. There is likely to be some academic mileage if these pilot studies are undertaken.

References

1. de Jong M, Boehringer S, Kayser M, Wollstein A, Ruff C, Dunaway D, Hysi P, Spector T, Liu F, Niessen W, Koudstaal M, Wolvius E. An automatic 3D facial landmarking algorithm using 2D Gabor Wavelets. IEEE Trans Image Processing. 25(2):580–8.

2. Anand A, Campion NJ, Cheshire J, Haigh T, Leckenby J, Nishikawa H, White N. Analysis of cosmetic results of metopic synostosis: concordance and interobserver variability. Author information. J Craniofac Surg. 2013;24(1):304–8. https://doi.org/10.1097/SCS.0b013e318272dacb.
3. Ward J, Mc Alistair W, Drinivasan D, Rodrigues D, Solanki G, White N, Nishikawa H. A subjective evaluation of pre- and postoperative cosmesis following calvarial remodeling for non-syndromic sagittal synostosis. University of Birmingham, and The Healing Foundation.
4. Edler RJ. Considerations to facial aesthetics. J Orthod. 2001;28(2):159.

36 How to Approach Noma and Facial Infections, Trauma and Tumours Through Charity Missions: Ethics of Surgical Charity for Complex Patients

Hiroshi Nishikawa

Introduction

Medical ethics describes the moral principles by which doctors must conduct themselves. There are four pillars of medical ethics [1]:

1. ***Beneficence***: Doing good.
2. ***Non-malfeasance***: Do no harm.
3. ***Autonomy***: In medical practice, autonomy is usually expressed as the right of competent adults to make informed decisions about their own medical care. The principle is perhaps seen at its most forcible when patients exercise their autonomy by refusing life-sustaining treatment.
4. ***Justice*** (in the context of medical ethics): is the principle that when weighing up if something is ethical or not, we have to think about whether it's compatible with the law and the patient's rights and if it's fair and balanced. However, with regard to the principle of justice for healthcare delivery as a whole, it refers to a fair and equitable distribution of health resources.

H. Nishikawa (✉)
Craniofacial/Plastic Multidisciplinary Department, Welbourne Center and Birmingham Children Hospital, Birmingham, UK

The Meaning of Four Pillars

1. The four pillars of medical ethics imply that there must be a universality of medical standards [2]. In reality, this is primarily a theoretical foundation that frequently does coincide with practical reality. In practice, these ethical pillars have variable effects on the doctor working a long way from his native country, in a medically underdeveloped country, which may be very far removed culturally, socially and politically, from everyday practice. Such conditions certainly confront many foreign doctors working in Africa, Asia and South America. As an example, the charity Facing Africa was set up to help patients in Ethiopia suffering from a debilitating condition called noma. This disease usually affects children who are malnourished. It starts as an infection in the mouth that eventually destroys soft tissue and skeletal structures of the face. The mortality rate is 90%, and among the children who survive, many are left with severe facial deformity and functional problems such as ankylosis (the inability to open the jaw). The treatment is not possible without experienced reconstructive plastic and maxillofacial surgeons, anaesthetists, nurses, administrators as well as the brave scouts who explore the countryside for suitable patients. Management of these patients requires a system of pre-assessment and aftercare along

M. A. Hardy, B. R. Hochman (eds.), *Global Surgery*, https://doi.org/10.1007/978-3-031-28127-3_36

with means to deliver complex surgery. To perform the major reconstructive operations, specialised equipment is needed along with hospital facilities.
2. The strategy of collaborating institutions or specialist groups is to bring their expertise to the underserved countries without conditions but with certain prerequisites in order to be able to fulfil all the functions effectively and safely. The prerequisites include the services of a hospital with appropriate facilities and services to fulfil the goals of the mission and ensure that there is continuity of care once the visiting providers leave. The advantages of this paradigm is that usually the surgical and anaesthetic specialists have a range of skills which permit broader functions, which include a variety of operations other than noma and general anaesthesia for all procedures. The Facing Africa group, for example, has helped patients who had facial deformities as a result of trauma and large benign tumours and medical conditions such as vascular malformations, leprosy and neurofibromatosis. This group, by not restricting its contributions to treatment of patients only with Noma, has saved many lives, improved function and restored appearance in many patients over the years. The mission, such as Facing Africa, encounters many ethical problems illustrated by Samaya's case. She is a little girl who was found begging on the streets of Addis Ababa and brought for care by the group.

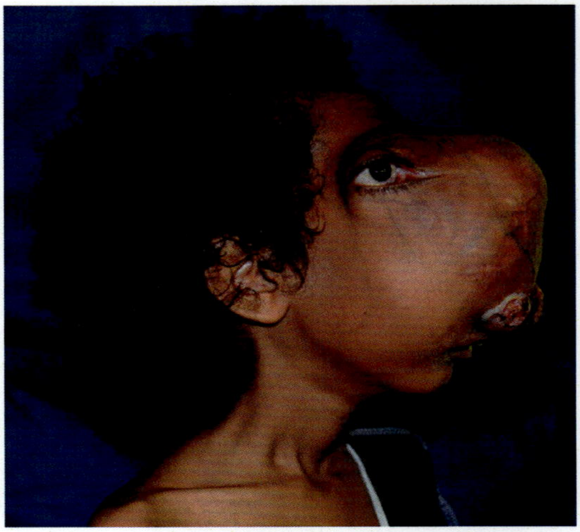

Fig. 36.1 Samaya. Preoperative lateral view

Illustrative Case of a Real Problem and its Solution

1. Samaya was an eight-year old girl who had a 6-month history of a rapidly growing facial tumour. The lesion was benign but aggressively expansile osteofibroma located within her midface. The tumour had obliterated her nose and stretched outwards (Fig 36.1). At the same time, her eye sockets were propelled forwards and sideways, causing visual problems (Fig. 36.1). She was still able to eat, but the tumour had filled and stretched her entire nasal cavity so she was no longer able to breathe through her nose. Clearly, it was only a matter of time before the tumour would start pushing her palate downwards and obliterate her mouth. This would mean certain death from starvation and as a terminal event asphyxiation. CT scans demonstrated that the tumour had not yet eroded through the skull base and into the brain.
2. At a pre-operative meeting, the entire team discussed whether it was right to treat Sumaya, given the risks of the operation. There were significant surgical and anaesthetic uncertainties about surviving the operative removal of such a gigantic facial mass. No one on the team had ever encountered such pathology. Based on close inspection of the scans, the tumour appeared resectable. However, it was uncertain whether resection would result in a cure or only in palliation. It was also clear that the operation would still leave the patient very disfigured. As a group, the team decided on the basis of the skill mix available that surgery was justifiable as it was the only chance which Samaya had of a prolonged life. The ethical issue of acceptance of the decreased quality of life was explained but unlikely well understood by the patient.

3. A consent was obtained from her father. Via a translator, we informed him that there was a good chance that Samaya may succumb from surgery, but without it, she would certainly die. He agreed, and he signed the consent with an X since he was illiterate.
4. The surgery involved the whole team and took all day. The tumour was removed. Limited facial and nasal reconstruction was possible. Samaya made a surprisingly uneventful post-operative recovery. After a few days, haemostatic packs were removed from a large residual midfacial dead space, and patient was rehabilitated sufficiently to be discharged 1 month later.
5. Evaluating Samaya's treatment from the ethical point of view alone, we need to look at it as sequential to the pillar of ethics. The first pillar leads us to the question: Did the treatment benefit the patient? In medicine, benefit can be measured in several ways. The outcome of either life or death is a straightforward binary analysis and certainly operative in this case. A more complex variable is to measure the functional change provided by the procedure, and again this was beneficial for Samaya; she could now eat and breathe better. The most difficult outcomes of all to analyse objectively are aesthetic improvements and the change in the quality of life after surgery as evaluated not only by society but especially by the patient. All these elements must be understood by the patient or their surrogate when signing the consent for the operation.

   For Samaya, there was clearly a good outcome on several levels. Her life was saved. Functionally, she was better regarding her airways and feeding ability, and even her vision improved as her tumour no longer obstructed her midface, nose or eyes.

   She remained facially deformed (Figs. 36.2 and 36.3). She had been converted from extreme to just major hypertelorism. Her nose was released from the depths of her tumour and was just recognised as a nose. She will still need some major surgical interventions to improve her features cosmetically. Did the team improve the quality of her life? Arguably yes. We saved her so that she could go back to her life of begging, and at the age of 8, she could continue to support her family.

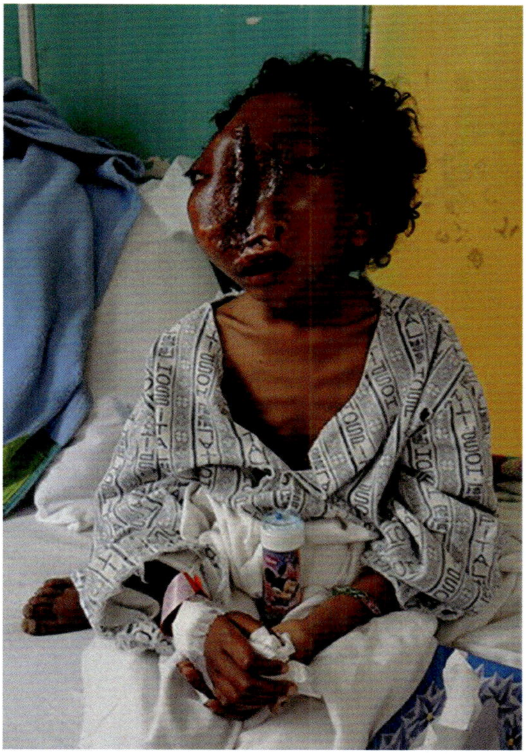

Fig. 36.2 Early postoperative view

6. The team's satisfaction with the outcome of this case emphasises the cultural and economic chasm between the wealthy, mostly Western, world that the team came from and the reality found in the underserved low- and middle-income countries (LMICs) that the team and others are trying to help. The benchmarks and the frame of reference of doing good become less certain.

   A specific lesson drawn from the previous case is that the concept of a good aesthetic outcome for most of the treated patients from LMIC's rural areas wish and espect to have a fully normal appearance is unrealistic. This would be appreciated and understood to be an impossibility in the extraordinarily

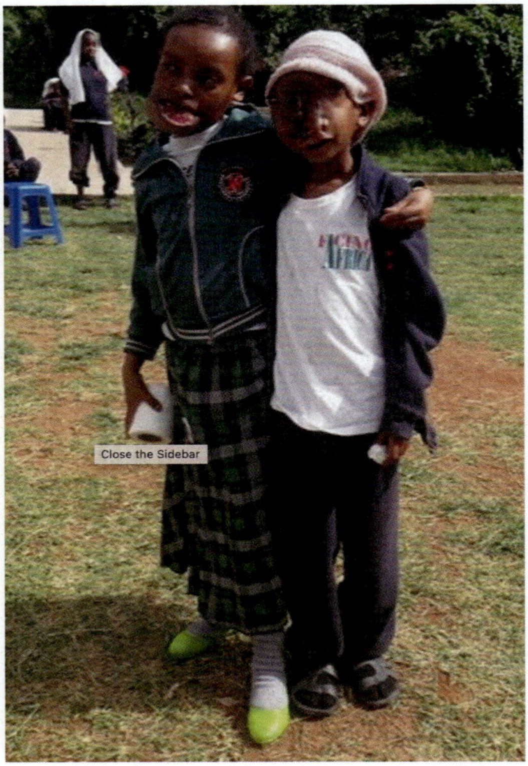

Fig. 36.3 Samaya 1 month after her operation with her friend with a large tumour of the jaw waiting for surgery

difficult cases like noma or the case described here of a huge facial tumour by most patients from a wealthy country. Unfortunately, from the perspective of the rural Ethiopian or other LMICs' patients, it is likely that the aesthetic outcome was disappointing for many of the major noma and other facial or contracture release operations carried out over the years despite some definitive functional improvements. For these patients, the concept of reconstructive surgery generally remains alien as they frequently don't appreciate the advanced treatments that many receive.

7. The importance and the complexities presented by the third pillar of medical ethics encountered in LMICs, which revolve around the right of the patient to make informed decision about whether to go ahead with their treatment, are especially challenging when majority of patients are uneducated and frequently illiterate and have no access to the Internet. Angell has written: "There must be a core of human rights that we would wish to see honoured universally, despite variations in their superficial aspects ...The forces of local custom or local law cannot justify abuses of certain fundamental rights, and the right of self-determination on which the doctrine of informed consent is based, is one of them" [3].

   Ethical treatment must of course be universal. *Doctor knows best* is a mantra rightly questioned. In Ethiopia and in other LMICs, trust in the infallibility of the surgeon still prevails as probably also extends to the local "traditional" doctors who treat illnesses based upon non-Western and often non-scientific, traditional techniques. In Ethiopia, there are over 100 different tribal languages; the high number of tribal languages is true in many other African countries. No single translator will be able to communicate clearly with all the patients that visiting teams or individuals propose to treat. Often, the consent is conveyed by a chain of interpreters. It is certainly not ethical to decide what is best for an adult without their informed consent or to carry out treatment in good faith alone, except for emergent, life/death situations. However, this inevitably and unknowingly occurs as a result of "something lost in translation" during the intense and time-restricted urgency of an operation.

8. Samaya's case raises some issues concerning the fourth pillar of ethics, i.e., justice. Was her treatment compatible with her legal rights? Was it fair to treat her ahead of other patients waiting to be treated by the team? Was it justified for the team to use all the team's resource for the whole day for one case when several other deserving patients could have benefited from the available time, personnel and resources? There are some parallels between the delivery of national healthcare in the UK and the strategy Facing Africa employs. The system of pre-assessment and follow-up is an acknowledgement that for many of these difficult,

chronic conditions, single fix solutions are often not possible. However, for surgical specialty teams, the presence of expertise is never continuous. Even though videoconferencing and instant communications are used, in reality, specialty teams can only deliver intense missions a few times per year. It is for this reason that training of local personnel must remain a priority for the visiting specialty teams, and this is almost an ethical obligation that is difficult, and sometimes impossible, to fulfil by all NGOs.

9. Utilitarianism principles *for the greater good* with the delivery of justice for as many deserving patients as possible is just not applicable to specialty teams. National healthcare systems ideally have the capability of treating all the medical conditions that confront a population. The system with fewer resources must resort to greater rationing. For specialty missions, the rationing, by necessity, has to be quite stark and in many ways brutal. This is because the constraints were created by the principles of the specialty team's aims and the target pathology that it funds. The constraints are partially justified in some cases by providing adequate training to qualified personnel, if such personnel exists. Most of the large number of patients that the Facing Africa encounter on the first day of its mission do not achieve "justice". Many have journeyed hundreds of miles to gain access for a few fleeting minutes to gain access to expertise. The *lucky* few are treated. The doctors of the visiting team have to employ the "bully" principle of treatment, which selects only those patients who are winners. The surgery must be successful, and there should be complete recovery within the time span available to the mission. If these aims are not achieved, harm is done, unless local teams are taught sufficiently to take over the care. The initial process is often heartbreaking.

   The other arm of justice related to healthcare is that it must have a system of self-perpetuation in order to treat future patients. This involves training surgeons, anaesthetists and nurses. Facing Africa only recruit experienced and dedicated experts. Trainees that come are sponsored separately by the regional or central government health system with support from the hospital. Replacement of expertise should ideally be aimed at local doctors. In many cases, such as Facing Africa, very few Ethiopian surgeons have benefited in terms of application to their own practices from what could have been learnt from these missions, and there has been a relative lack of long-term engagement of national surgeons. In reality, the participation of local surgeons in super-specialty training and participation such as Facing Africa is not the fault of the local doctors but is a reflection of a critical lack of resources. The treatment of complex conditions is probably unattainable for most healthcare systems in LMICs except for the rich minority, which usually seeks care abroad. Therefore because there is no resource to manage some of these really difficult problems, the incentive to do so for local clinicians is severely tested. It can only be achieved by close collaboration of the specialty teams and local healthcare providers and the support and active involvement of the federal government, with support and pressure from the public and interested international funding foundations and agencies.

10. The aim of all the ethical pillars discussed so far is to prevent harm. The second pillar of "Do no harm" is not frequently discussed because it is so self-evident in most circumstances. It is sometimes not quite so clear when specialty missions or even well-meaning individual assistance is provided. If doctors take on patients, however deserving, who are beyond their capability to treat, harm will inevitably be done. Unfortunately, distant shores can make some immature and arrogant visiting clinicians braver and more adventurous because subconsciously they feel that it is better to do something, than to do nothing, and they may feel that they are beyond the reach of local clinical governance. Any mission, individual or team, that

becomes a surgical playground is destructive and potentially lethal. It behoves individual volunteers to be, and the teams to select, the most experienced and compassionate clinicians who understand their own limitations and the aims of their participation in this volunteerism. In this way, individual volunteers and specialty teams can provide fleeting episodes of excellence and at best influence and inspire local doctors and governments to make appropriate changes to improve their own healthcare systems.

Conclusion

These ethical pillars are guidelines. They should be non-negotiable, but in reality, the. intrinsic stresses of specialty missions may lead to some inevitable ethical distortions. However, individual volunteers and members of surgical specialty teams must aim to provide the same quality of planning and care as they would in their countries of origin. All patients, no matter where they are on the planet, deserve this.

References

1. Gillon R. Medical ethics: four principles plus attention to scope. BMJ. 1994;309:184.
2. Beauchamp TL, Childress JF. Principles of bioethics. 7th ed. Oxford University Press; 2013.
3. Angell M. Ethical imperialism? Ethics in international collaborative clinical research. N Engl J Med. 1988;19(16):1081–3.

How to Approach Noma and Facial Infections, Trauma and Tumours Through Charity Missions: Noma – A Neglected Disease

37

Alexander J. Rickart and Graham Merrick

Abbreviations

FA	Facing Africa
NTDs	Neglected tropical diseases
WHO	World Health Organization

Aetiology and Epidemiology

Aptly described as the face of poverty, noma rapidly progresses from oral ulceration to oro-facial gangrene (Fig. 37.1) [1, 2]. An opportunistic infection with a name derived from the Greek term meaning 'to devour', the disease aggressively spreads through the hard and soft tissues. With a mortality rate thought to be as high as 90% and with so few able to access treatment in its active phase, very little is understood about the disease. Most commonly affecting children under the age of 6, the World Health Organization (WHO) estimates a worldwide incidence of 140,000 new cases a year [3, 4]. Predominantly reported in sub-Saharan countries in a belt run-

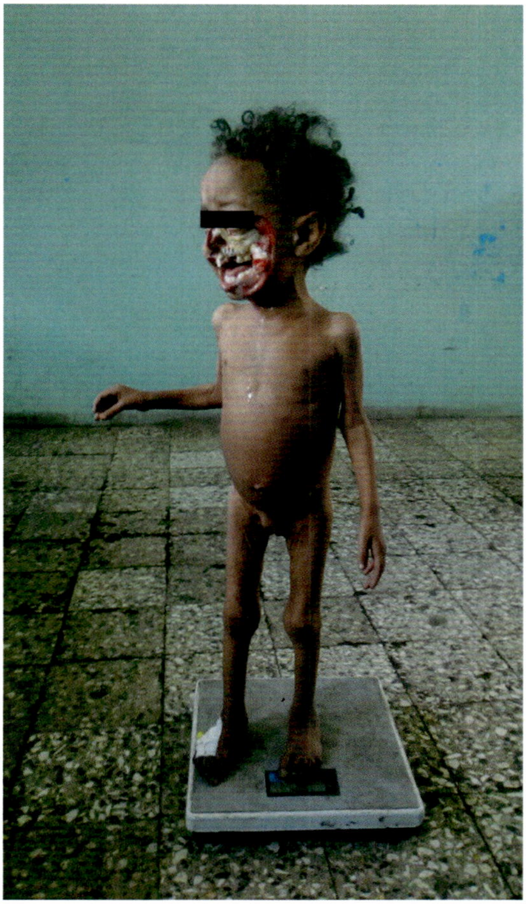

Fig. 37.1 A three-year old girl with acute noma; this image encapsulates why the term 'the face of poverty' is so fitting. The destructive and aggressive nature of the disease is clearly seen alongside the hallmarks of protein energy malnutrition

A. J. Rickart (✉)
Department of Oral and Maxillofacial Surgery, Great Ormond Street NHS Foundation Trust, London, UK
e-mail: alexander.rickart@nhs.net

G. Merrick
Department of Oral and Maxillofacial Surgery, Taunton and Somerset NHS Foundation Trust, Taunton, UK

M. A. Hardy, B. R. Hochman (eds.), *Global Surgery*, https://doi.org/10.1007/978-3-031-28127-3_37

ning from Mauritania to Ethiopia, the incidence is highest in West Africa [3]. In spite of this, there is a consensus that noma is prevalent in marginalized communities internationally but is chronically under-reported.

Risk factors can broadly be held under the umbrella of poverty. However, specific factors identified from affected populations highlight viral co-infection, poor oral hygiene, the low coverage of immunizations, malnutrition, poor sanitation and lack of access to clean water alongside an increasing incidence in those affected by the HIV and AIDS pandemic [2, 5, 6].

What turns the preceding oral ulceration or necrotizing ulcerative gingivitis into noma is as yet undefined, though it is probably due to a combined pathological oral flora in the presence of a child with limited physiological resources and impaired immunity secondary to poor nutrition and concurrent disease. *Fusobacterium necrophorum* and *Prevotella intermedia* are purported microbiological isolates, although an unfavourable shift in oral microbiota is more likely than a singular causative organism [7–9]. Sub-Saharan Africa, in keeping with the rest of the world, sees faltering growth most frequently noted before the third year of life, with some infants predisposed following intrauterine growth restriction [10]. As a result, it is unlikely to be a coincidence that the average age of onset of noma is analogous with the timing of the linear phase of growth retardation and often affects those most profoundly stunted [10].

Facing Africa: Our Experience in Ethiopia

Facing Africa (FA), described in detail previously in Chap. 34, is an NGO that has focused on the rehabilitation of patients suffering from the late complications of noma in Ethiopia since 2007. With an estimated incidence in Eastern Ethiopia between 1.6 and 13.4 per 100,000 children aged 0–9 years, the need to provide resources and care to those at the Eastern edge of the 'noma belt' is clear [11].

Treatment for the acute phase of the disease includes addressing the underlying malnutrition, provision of oral antibiotics and good oral hygiene. However, timely access to care alongside accurate diagnosis and management is missing from local settings. Regardless, vertical programs to address noma will always be less effective when compared to wider efforts addressing the root cause of the disease: poverty [12].

For those who survive, predicted to be numbering 770,000 people worldwide, the functional, psychological and aesthetic sequalae are significant [2]. In an effort to determine the global burden of the disease, it was calculated that there are between 1 and ten million disability-adjusted life years lost due to noma, which is analogous to other neglected tropical diseases [12]. A retrospective review of patients treated by FA for deformity and functional impairment secondary to noma between 2015 and 2019 provided insight into each patient's quality of life [13]. It is clear that it is not just the aesthetic and functional side of disease that reconstructive surgery aims to address but mental wellbeing and a feeling of belonging being of upmost importance.

Defects secondary to noma frequently cause trismus, nasal fistulae, loss of teeth and incompetent lips, which makes eating, drinking and talking a significant challenge. Several studies have also reported that the physical appearance carries a stigma, which can lead to social isolation, bullying and an inability to integrate into society, be this through work, education or finding a partner [14].

Pattern of Disease

Classification of the defects of noma patients treated by FA enables us to describe the pattern of disease [13]. Montandon's classification of noma defects has been adopted by the WHO, and the distribution of our cases is demonstrated in Fig. 37.2 [4, 15]. The distribution of defects seen by our group is similar to that described in a

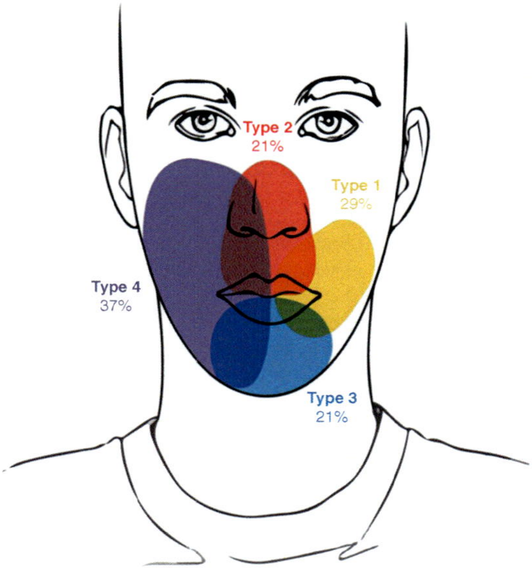

Fig. 37.2 Pattern of disease distribution, as classified by Montandon, of cases seen by *Facing Africa* between May 2015 and May 2019 [13]

series by Pittet et al. [16] Most commonly, they are laterally based, with the majority being classified as Type I or IV. These cases can be surgically challenging to manage, often with significant ankylosis, and the required scar excision leaving an even larger defect than initially appears.

Over time, treatment has evolved considerably as initial management predominantly focused on local or pedicled delto-pectoral, latissiumus dorsi or supraclavicular island flaps [17]. It still remains true that local flaps are generally used where possible, conferring excellent tissue match, reliability and reduced morbidity. Certainly, FA has also found the submental island flap particularly useful in the reconstruction of noma. In spite of this, large pedicled flaps are now generally discarded in favour of free tissue transfer, which has been shown to be safe and reliable even in resource-poor, developing countries [18, 19]. Although there are challenges in obtaining long-term follow-up, a validated, noma-specific tool for recording patient-reported outcome measures is a potential focus for future collaborative work [20].

Summary

For nearly 25 years, extreme poverty has been steadily declining. However, as the disruption of the COVID-19 pandemic is compounded by conflict and climate change, global poverty is currently increasing. Previous progress in health, education and living standards are at risk of becoming undone, and consumption distributions show that the poorest are becoming even poorer. It is this small subset where noma is most prevalent, and the inequality is not easily overcome.

Noma will continue to affect those with the least, representing a preventable loss of life and devastating those who survive. A commitment to the United Nation's Sustainable Development Goals, with particular relevance to addressing poverty and hunger alongside improvements in immunization coverage, water, sanitation and hygiene, would go a long way to eradicating noma.

In the interim, there has been a drive to include noma in the WHO list of neglected tropical diseases (NTDs). This diverse list of 20 diseases, all borne out of poverty, includes analogous conditions such as leprosy and buruli ulcers. This would provide the benefits of being swept along with the WHO NTD 2021–2030 road map, facilitating integrated approaches, multisectoral coordination and improved access to funding and research. It seems that the 'noma paradox' holds true in that by the time a country has developed the resources to manage the disease effectively, the associated economic developments have caused it to disappear [19, 21]. Until progress is made, the need to help those devastated by noma will continue, and our approach to the surgical management of these complex patients will be the focus of this chapter.

Ethical Approval Consent for publications of photographs was kindly provided by the patients or their guardians.

References

1. Ashok N, Tarakji B, Darwish S, Rodrigues JC, Altamimi MA. A review on Noma: a recent update. Global J Health Sci. 2016;8(4):53.
2. Enwonwu C, Falkler W Jr, Idigbe E. Oro-facial gangrene (Noma/cancrum oris): pathogenetic mechanisms. Crit Rev Oral Biol Med. 2000;11(2):159–71.
3. World Health Organization, Regional Office for Africa. Evaluation of the WHO Africa Regional Programme on Noma Control (2013–2017). Available from: https://www.afro.who.int/publications/evaluation-who-africa-regional-programme-noma-control-2013-2017. Accessed 30 Mar 2022
4. World Health Organization, Regional Office of Arica. Information brochure for early detection and management of noma. Available from: https://www.afro.who.int/publications/information-brochure-early-detection-and-management-noma. Accessed 30 Mar 2022
5. Galli A, Brugger C, Fürst T, Monnier N, Winkler MS, Steinmann P. Prevalence, incidence, and reported global distribution of Noma: a systematic literature review. Lancet Infect Dis. 2022;22:e221.
6. Chidzonga MM, Mahomva L. Noma (Cancrum oris) in human immunodeficiency virus infection and acquired immunodeficiency syndrome (HIV and AIDS): clinical experience in Zimbabwe. J Oral Maxillofac Surg. 2008;66(3):475–85.
7. Farley E, Mehta U, Srour ML, Lenglet A. Noma (Cancrum oris): a scoping literature review of a neglected disease (1843 to 2021). PLoS Negl Trop Dis. 2021;15(12):e0009844.
8. Falkler W, Enwonwu C, Ewell A, Idigbe E. Isolation of fusobacteria from the oral cavities of malnourished Nigerian children living in agricultural and herding villages. Oral Dis. 2000;6(2):103–5.
9. Marck KW. Noma: a neglected enigma. Lancet Glob Health. 2013;1(2):e58–9.
10. De Onis M, Blössner M. The World Health Organization global database on child growth and malnutrition: methodology and applications. Int J Epidemiol. 2003;32(4):518–26.
11. Lafferty N. Changing the face of Africa. In: Estimating the burden of noma in rural Ethiopia and identifying options for prevention and improvement in its diagnosis and management Liverpool School of Tropical Medicine; 2012.
12. Srour ML, Baratti-Mayer D. Why is Noma a neglected-neglected tropical disease? PLoS Negl Trop Dis. 2020;14(8):e0008435.
13. Rickart AJ, Rodgers W, Mizen K, et al. Facing Africa: describing Noma in Ethiopia. Am J Trop Med Hygiene. 2020;103(2):613.
14. Wali IM, Regmi K. People living with facial disfigurement after having had Noma disease: a systematic review of the literature. J Health Psychol. 2017;22(10):1243–55.
15. Montandon D, Lehmann C, Chami N. The surgical treatment of Noma. Plast Reconstr Surg. 1991;87(1):76–86.
16. Pittet B, Jaquinet A, Montandon D. Clinical experience in the treatment of Noma sequelae. J Craniofac Surg. 2001;12(3):273–83.
17. Rüegg E, Baratti-Mayer D, Jaquinet A, Montandon D, Pittet-Cuénod B. The surgical management of extra-articular ankylosis in Noma patients. Int J Oral Maxillofac Surg. 2018;47(12):1527–33.
18. Giessler GA, Schmidt AB. Noma: experiences with a microvascular approach under west African conditions. Plast Reconstr Surg. 2003;112(4):947–54.
19. Rodgers W, Lloyd T, Mizen K, et al. Microvascular reconstruction of facial defects in settings where resources are limited. Br J Oral Maxillofac Surg. 2016;54(1):51–6.
20. Speiser S, Langridge B, Birkl MM, Kubiena H, Rodgers W. Update on Noma: systematic review on classification, outcomes and follow-up of patients undergoing reconstructive surgery after Noma disease. BMJ Open. 2021;11(8):e046303.
21. Marck KW. A history of noma, the "Face of Poverty". Plastic and Reconstructive Surgery. 2003;111(5):1702–1707.

38 How to Approach Noma and Facial Infections, Trauma, and Tumours Through Charity Missions: The Management of Trismus and Ankylosis in Noma

Will Rodgers and David Dunaway

Introduction

Trismus is defined as a restriction in the range of motion of the jaws from any cause. Trismus may cause difficulties in feeding, speech and maintaining oral health and may compromise protection of the upper airway. The differential diagnosis for trismus is large, in this chapter, we will focus on trismus as a sequela of noma. Trismus is common in noma, and it is estimated that up to half of all noma patients have a degree of trismus. Trismus forms part of the NOITULP noma classification (see Table 38.1) ranging from normal mouth opening to absolute trismus or ankylosis [1]. Ankylosis is defined as a fusion of the mandible to the skull base and may be articular (involving the temporomandibular joint) or extra-articular.

Trismus occurs as a late sequela of noma and is dependent on the site and severity of the acute phase of the disease and subsequent scar formation and tissue contraction. The pathogenesis of trismus in noma is often multifactorial and may result from:

Table 38.1 NOITULP noma classification

Degree of trismus	Mouth opening
T-0	≥40 mm
T-1	>20–40 mm
T-2	>0–20 mm
T-3	Ankylosis

- Extra-articular ankylosis.
  - Fibrous extra-articular ankylosis.
  - Bony extra-articular ankylosis.
- Intra-articular ankylosis.
- Myostatic contracture.

Myostatic contracture, where the muscles are not directly affected by the disease but contract due to a lack of full passive range of motion, is secondary to scarring and wound contracture in local tissues, leading to a reduced soft tissue envelope which is insufficient to allow full opening. Where the muscles of mastication are involved in the acute phase, the resulting myositis commonly leads to fibrotic extra-articular ankylosis. As a rule of thumb, when scarring is seen distal to the anterior border of the masseter, at the level of the first molar tooth, trismus is likely. Where there is prolonged fibrous ankylosis, or in cases where the acute phase of noma involved the bone, a bony extra-articular ankylosis may be seen. If the temporomandibular joint is affected in the acute phase, a true intra-articular ankylosis arises. In any prolonged trismus, it is common to find hypertrophy of the coronoid pro-

W. Rodgers (✉)
Craniofacial Unit, Great Ormond Street Hospital for Children NHS Foundation Trust, London, UK

D. Dunaway
Great Ormond Street Hospital for Children NHS Foundation Trust, London University Hospital, London, UK

M. A. Hardy, B. R. Hochman (eds.), *Global Surgery*, https://doi.org/10.1007/978-3-031-28127-3_38

cess, which mechanically obstructs normal mouth opening both on the ipsilateral and contralateral sides [2].

In this chapter, we report our experience of 49 cases of trismus secondary to noma infections.

Assessment

Assessment of trismus in people with noma should include an assessment of the functional effects caused by limitation of mouth opening. Difficulty with feeding may lead to malnutrition and a low BMI. Speech may be affected, and it is likely that there will be poor oral health due to obstructed access to the oral cavity. Although patients may be severely affected by the condition, there is a significant subgroup that manages to function effectively even with severe trismus.

Clinical examination should document the range of movement at both TMJs. The surrounding soft tissue should be assessed and any obvious extracapsular restrictions noted.

A careful intraoral and full dental exam should be performed. Extensive intraoral scarring is often found. Caries and periodontal disease are common, and frequently multiple teeth will require extraction.

Patients with trismus are often underweight and may require pre-surgical optimisation prior to intervention. In our experience, patients often present several weeks prior to possible intervention, whereupon they receive nutritional assistance and anthelmintics as required.

Radiological assessment is essential for accurate diagnosis and treatment planning. An orthopantomogram aids in dental assessment and can give an indication of the site of bony ankylosis. Computed tomography is ideal for radiographic assessment in those with severe trismus (T-2) and ankylosis (T-3) for adequate pre-surgical planning (see Fig. 38.1). Contrast enhancement may be of use if there is concern with regard to the relation of bony ankylosis to vasculature.

Anaesthetic assessment is essential prior to surgery. An anaesthetist experienced in the

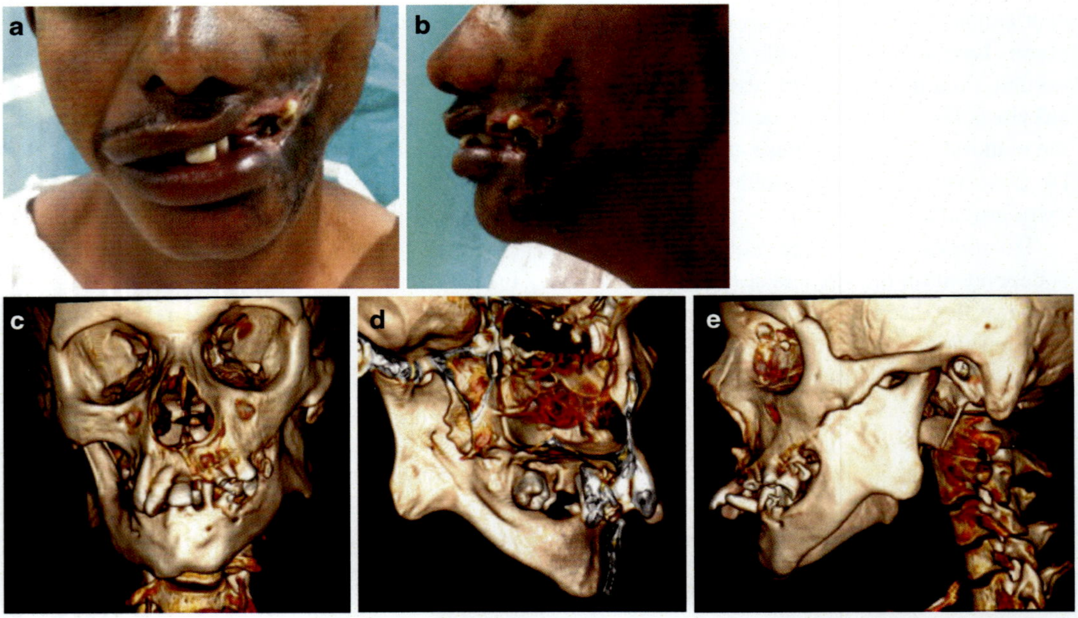

Fig. 38.1 Patient with complete ankylosis (NOITULP stage T3) as a late sequela to noma showing significant post-infection scarring. Note the 'anarchie dentaire'. (**a**) frontal view, (**b**) lateral view, (**c**) CT lateral view showing bony ankylosis from mandible to zygoma (**e**) showing lingual surface of mandible with bony ankylosis from pterygoid plates to mandible

management of difficult airways is a key member of the noma surgical team. Typically severely affected patients require an awake fibreoptic intubation. Tracheostomy is occasionally necessary, and it is important to have a well-prepared theatre team experienced in airway emergencies.

Management

Our experience of 49 noma patients treated over 2 missions in 2011 and 2012 found 16 to have trismus of grade T2 or higher. Of the 16, 8 were male and 8 female. Patients were aged between 6 and 40 years with a mean age of 17. Mean BMI was 16 compared to the mean BMI for all patients seen during the missions of 17.3. Over the 2 missions, 12 patients had procedures to improve trismus, of whom 5 had true ankylosis requiring ankylosis release with bilateral coronoidectomies. Post-operative in-hospital stay ranged from 1 to 7 days with a mean stay of 4 days. Of the nine patients who were treated for trismus release in the first mission, three required further procedures for trismus release on the following mission.

Patients with mild trismus and opening of ≥20 mm usually function normally and consideration should be given to the merit of release of trismus, which may paradoxically worsen function due to post-operative scarring in settings where close follow-up is unavailable. Those with trismus of grade T-2/3 (opening of <20 mm) often benefit from treatment.

The key to the management of trismus is post-operative physiotherapy, therefore intervention should only be considered in those who are able to tolerate this, careful judgement is necessary to avoid an unnecessary procedure.

Surgical Management

In those unable to tolerate significant intervention or the required post-operative physiotherapy, dental extractions of affected teeth alone may provide a sufficient aperture to increase oral intake and improve nutrition.

Definitive surgical management is directed at the cause of the trismus. In noma, trismus is often multifactorial [3].

Fibrous Extra-Articular Ankylosis

Noma causes extensive soft tissue necrosis, and healing is usually accompanied by extensive fibrosis and wound contracture. Post-noma fibrosis is a particularly difficult condition to treat and has a great tendency to recur after treatment.

Limited areas of fibrosis can be treated by fibrous band release followed up with intralesional steroid injections to discourage re-fibrosis of the area. This treatment should be accompanied by regular physiotherapy.

It is usually necessary to excise areas of fibrosis in order to mobilise the temporomandibular joint. Excision of fibrotic areas should be accompanied by soft tissue reconstruction with local or distant flaps.

Extra- and Intra-Articular Bony Ankylosis

Treatment requires release of the bony bridges, which extend between the mandible and skull base. In noma, bony bridges often exist at sites quite distant from the temporomandibular joint. It's not uncommon for the coronoid process or body of the mandible to be fused to the skull base or maxilla.

If there is a significant risk of recurrence of ankylosis. Surgical techniques to reduce the risk of ankylosis include:

Gap arthroplasty with or without interpositional flap or graft.
Costochondral graft.
Distraction osteogenesis.
TMJ replacement.

The additional complexities of temporomandibular joint replacement and distraction osteogenesis along with their associated complications and follow up requirements make these treatments inadvisable where long-term regular local specialist follow-up is unavailable.

Coronoid Process Hyperplasia

Hyperplasia of the coronoid process of the mandible frequently occurs in trismus associated with noma. The elongated coronoid process may impinge on the medial surface of the zygomatic arch and act as a further cause of trismus. The treatment of this condition is coronoidectomy. Coronoidectomy has a lower relapse rate than simple coronoidectomy.

For those with severe trismus, examination under anaesthesia is indicated, followed by a stepwise approach to releasing the ankylosis. Our preference is to measure the mouth opening on-table following intubation; we then proceed to the release of intraoral scarring and relevant dental extractions followed by re-assessment of mouth opening. If adequate opening is not achieved, then ipsilateral coronoidectomy via an intraoral approach combined with release of the masseter is undertaken. Contralateral coronoidectomy and release is often required if adequate mouth opening is not achieved.

In those cases of true ankylosis (T-3), an extraoral Al-Kayat approach may be required to release the mandible from fibrous and bony bridges to the facial skeleton and skull base. Following release, it may be appropriate to insert an interpositional dermal fat graft, temporoparietal flap or vascularised tissue graft (Fig. 38.2) to reduce the risk of re-ankylosis.

In noma, patients will frequently require soft tissue reconstruction concurrently, and it may be possible to design the reconstruction to provide an interpositional graft.

Procedure: Coronoidectomy

The coronoid process can usually be removed via a transoral approach though an extra-oral approach as described below may be used. Following local anaesthetic infiltration, a vestibular incision is made in the free gingiva extending up the external oblique ridge. A subperiosteal dissection should expose the ramus to the sigmoid notch laterally. The attaching fibres of the temporalis muscle to the coronoid should be sharply dissected to facilitate access, and care should be taken medially with subperiosteal dissection to avoid injury to the inferior alveolar neurovascular bundle. When the coronoid is adequately dissected, an osteotomy is made from anterior to posterior in the Frankfurt plane at the level of the sigmoid notch. Prior to completing the osteotomy, it is recommended to gain control of the coronoid with Kocher's forceps to avoid displacement of the coronoid fragment superiorly when the osteotomy is completed. Releasing temporalis muscle attachment to the coronoid allows delivery.

Procedure: Ankylosis Release

An extraoral Al-Kayat approach is extended temporally to ensure adequate access with exposure of the temporalis fascia, temporalis muscle, zygomatic arch and the full extent of the ankylosis. Noma causes significant fibrosis to local tissues, and tissue planes may not be readily distinguishable. To protect the temporal branch

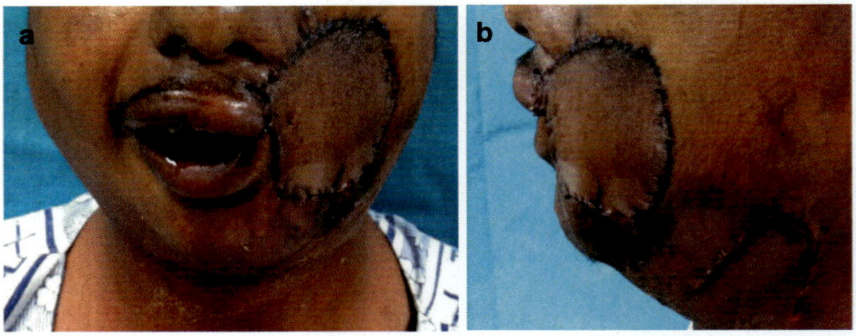

Fig. 38.2 Patient following ankylosis release with bilateral coronoidectomy, dental extractions and radial forearm free tissue transfer. (**a**) Frontal view showing improved mouth opening; (**b**) lateral views

of the facial nerve, it is therefore advisable to incise the temporalis fascia to the temporalis muscle above the zygomatic arch generously at a 45° angle continuous with a periosteal incision at the base of the zygoma with subperiosteal dissection continued anteriorly and inferiorly over the ankylotic mass until the unaffected ramus is identified. Stripping the masseter muscle from the zygomatic arch facilitates access. Excision of the entire ankylotic portion, including medial extent, is crucial to reduce recurrence, leaving a gap of at least 15 mm and ensuring a full range of passive opening. In noma, it may be the case that the temporomandibular joint is preserved though there is bony ankylosis more anteriorly. Function of the joint in this case will need to be assessed on table following ankylosis release. A coronoidectomy may also be performed through the same access, and an interpositional flap or graft can then be placed [4].

Post-Operative Management

Relapse following trismus release is common. Regular physiotherapy is key to maintaining adequate mouth opening and can be achieved with stacked wooden spatulas or bespoke devices. Physiotherapy should start as soon as possible post-operatively and may require analgesia initially. Seven exercises seven times per day, ideally supervised, for at least 3 months followed by ongoing three times daily exercise is a typical routine to maintain mouth opening. Maintaining compliance with these arduous and uncomfortable physiotherapy regimes is difficult. In spite of good physiotherapy, our experience is that at least a third of patients suffer relapse to a degree such that further intervention is warranted. Careful patient selection and education is therefore essential prior to any trismus or ankylosis release.

Complications

Complications related to trismus and ankylosis release include:

- Infection. Antibiotic prophylaxis should be given according to local protocols.
- Haemorrhage. The maxillary artery may be abnormally situated and close to the site of bony ankylosis. The abnormal anatomy combined with challenging access increases the risk of significant haemorrhage. If available, pre-operative CT angiography will help define the anatomy.
- Facial nerve injury. The position of the facial nerve may be distorted by scar contracture, and the dense fibrous tissue can make the nerve difficult to identify.
- Injury to the parotid gland or its duct may result in a sialocoele or parotid fistula.
- Injury to the external auditory meatus can result in canal stenosis and hearing impairment.

Conclusion

Trismus and ankylosis release in noma is challenging with a high risk of recurrence. Long-term follow-up and physiotherapy are essential, and further surgical intervention is often required. Patient motivation and support with arduous post-operative physiotherapy regimes can be challenging. The chance of success is greatest at the first operation, and complication rates are higher for subsequent interventions. In situations where close follow-up is not possible, operative trismus release may not achieve long-term success, and alternative strategies to ensure adequate nutrition and oral health should be considered [5].

References

1. Speiser S, Langridge B, Rodgers, et al. Update on Noma: systematic review on classification, outcomes and follow-up of patients undergoing reconstructive surgery after Noma disease. BMJ Open. 2021;11:e046303. https://doi.org/10.1136/bmjopen-2020-046303.
2. Kaban LB, Bouchard C, Troulis MJ. A protocol for Management of Temporomandibular Joint Ankylosis. Children. 2009;67(9):1966–78. https://doi.org/10.1016/j.joms.2009.03.071.

3. Rüegg EM, Baratti-Mayer D, Jaquinet A, Montandon D, Pittet-Cuénod B. The surgical management of extra-articular ankylosis in Noma patients. Int J Oral Maxillofac Surg. 2018;47:1527. https://doi.org/10.1016/j.ijom.2018.07.012.
4. Rodgers W, Lloyd T, Dunaway D, et al. Microvascular reconstruction of facial defects in settings where resources are limited. BJOMS. 2016;10:11.115. https://doi.org/10.1016/j.bjoms.2016.11.115.
5. Bos KE, Marck KW. The surgical treatment of Noma. Uitgeverij Belvédère/Medidact; 2006.

39 How to Approach Noma and Facial Infections, Trauma, and Tumours Through Charity Missions: Anaesthesia Considerations in Noma

Peter Lee and Patrick Seigne

Abbreviations

FOB Fibre-optic intubation
HIV Human immunodeficiency virus

Pre-Operative Status

Most patients are young and healthy, but it is critically important that a full pre-operative evaluation is carried out looking for any evidence of cardiac, respiratory or other medical conditions that might be optimised before embarking on such major surgery in locations where the management of post-operative complications may be challenging. Conditions such as tuberculosis and infection with human immunodeficiency virus (HIV) are not uncommon in this patient population. In a minority of the severe cases, patients may have absolute trismus due to extraarticular ankylosis bridging the gap between the mandible and the maxilla. Apart from the obvious airway issues this causes for intubation, it may have led to poor nutritional intake and poor dental hygiene with their attendant sequelae. Dental review plus admission for nutritional supplementation a month in advance of planned major surgery has proved beneficial in improving post-operative recovery. Pre-operative assessment is best carried out in multidisciplinary clinics consisting of maxillofacial surgeons, plastic surgeons, dentists, operating theatre nurses, ward nurses, wound care specialists, local doctors and translators. The experience of all involved health professionals is vital at this stage to allow a balanced assessment of risk and potential benefit to each patient. Our practise is to have the patients and all healthcare workers in the same room together at the time to facilitate open and immediate communication and dialogue between the patient and the team. Careful note taking and medical record maintenance are also critically important – the conduct of airway management and anaesthesia provision during previous surgery is very useful in the planning process, many of these patients having had multiple surgical procedures for this condition. The availability of laboratory testing is somewhat limited in resource-poor situations such as this, but a full blood count and HIV test are useful in all but the most minor of procedures. Electrocardiography and cardiac echo are useful in select cases. Pre-operative radiography of the upper airway is useful for both surgical planning and airway assessment. Chest radiography is indicated in patients with unexplained respiratory symptoms or a history of tuberculosis.

P. Lee (✉)
Bon Secours Hospital, Cork, Ireland
e-mail: plee@bonsecours.ie

P. Seigne
Department of Anaesthesiology and Intensive Care Medicine, Cork University Hospital, University College Cork, Cork, Ireland

M. A. Hardy, B. R. Hochman (eds.), *Global Surgery*, https://doi.org/10.1007/978-3-031-28127-3_39

Airway Management

An airway management plan is made for each patient following pre-operative assessment. A key part of that plan is the experience of the anaesthesiologists involved. It has always been our practice that two consultant anaesthesiologists would be present for the induction and intubation of any patient having surgery for facial deformity subsequent to noma infection. In general, one of these anaesthesiologists would have a lot of experience with airway management of these patients, and one may be gaining experience. This structure provides the safest possible conditions for the patient and allows knowledge transfer and the accumulation of experience for the clinicians. A nurse experienced in complex airway management is a crucial part of this team. Regardless of the airway management plan, a wide range of airway management equipment must be checked and immediately available. Conventional laryngoscopes, video laryngoscopes, fibre-optic bronchoscopes and screens, supraglottic airway devices such as laryngeal mask airways, front of neck access equipment, airway topicalisation devices and a full range of sizes of endotracheal tubes, including reinforced tubes and Rae tubes, must all be at hand. A minority of patients with noma have severe trismus or bony ankylosis, reducing the inter-incisor distance and preventing subluxation of the mandible. Oral intubation in such cases would be extremely difficult or impossible. Hence it is critical that anaesthesiologists working with victims of noma must have a detailed knowledge and experience with fibre-optic intubation (FOB). It is our experience that noma is a disease of the anterior facial and oral structures and the lower airway in survivors is unaffected [1]. Awake FOB with application of topical local anaesthesia of the airway and maintenance of spontaneous ventilation, until intubation has been achieved, is indicated in a select few cases where induction of general anaesthesia may compromise airway patency and the ability of the anaesthesiologist to successfully perform bag-mask ventilation. The use of awake FOB in this setting may be additionally complicated by the fact that patients may never have attended a hospital before and where language barriers may hinder communication and reassurance of the anxious patient. We have found asleep nasal intubation to be safe for the majority of noma patients. Regardless of the airway management plan, following induction of general anaesthesia bag-mask ventilation can be facilitated by a number of techniques: two-handed application of the face mask, use of smaller-size oropharyngeal airways, use of paediatric face masks to ventilate via the nose with occlusion of the mouth and use of adhesive dressings to temporarily close cheek defects. In patients with trismus and bony ankylosis, nasal intubation is necessary using either oral video laryngoscopy or nasal fiber-optic bronchoscopy. Nasal blood vessels should be vasoconstricted using topical phenylephrine to reduce the risk of bleeding and consequent obstruction of the view. We would recommend against elective tracheostomy for these patients (except in emergent "can't intubate, can't ventilate" scenarios, because of the lack of local experience in their short- and long-term post-operative management).

The airway management plan should also cover extubation. In general, extubation is straightforward in these patients although clearly additional care has to be taken where flaps have been used to cover orofacial defects. As excess pressure applied to the face via the face mask may damage the surgical repairs, a nasal airway is a useful adjunct to extubation and immediate recovery. In rare cases where soft tissue swelling or oedema of the airway is a possibility, an Aintree airway exchange catheter may be briefly left in situ over which the endotracheal tube can be removed.

Anaesthesia

Standard monitoring (electrocardiogram, pulse oximetry, capnography, end tidal anaesthetic gas analysis, non-invasive blood pressure monitoring) is recommended where available. In the few cases where excessive blood loss is a possibility, where surgery is likely to be prolonged or in those cases where the use of a free flap is necessary, invasive blood pressure monitoring may be required. Our experience is that this is rarely warranted particularly where blood gas analysis is not available. Central venous lines are generally not indicated – they could interfere with surgical access or damage critical vascular structures, and rapid infusion of blood products or vasoactive agents are rarely needed.

Induction is with routine agents. Maintenance is with oxygen and nitrous (available in large cylinders, as no central gas supply is usually available) plus halothane or isoflurane. An oxygen concentrator is usually available also and may supply oxygen concentrations up to 50%. Multimodal analgesia is the norm, but morphine remains the main agent, and supplementary regional blocks were used in selected cases.

Careful fluid management is important, particularly where flaps are used as part of the surgical repair. Urinary catheterisation should be performed for complex cases and output monitored to ensure adequate hydration. Blood products are rarely available in this environment and are reserved for only the most critical cases. Thankfully, with careful, experienced surgical technique, transfusion is seldom necessary.

Post-Operative Care

Recovery room and intensive care facilities are usually very limited. It is also unlikely that local nursing staff would have extensive experience in caring for the complex airways and surgical repairs seen in these patients. Post-operative care should be performed by nursing staff experienced in this area, generally members of the team. However, integration and education of local staff for effective post-operative care are important. For at least the first post-operative night and in some cases for longer, the patients should be nursed in a high dependency environment with regular observations. On-call cover must be immediately available in the early post-operative period and should consist of experienced senior surgeons, anaesthesiologists and nursing staff.

Reference

1. Coupe MH, Johnson D, Seigne PW, Hamlin B. Airway Management in Reconstructive Surgery for Noma (Cancrum Oris). Anesth Analg. 2013:117210–7.

How to Approach NOMA and Facial Infections, Trauma and Tumours Through Charity Missions: Wound Management and Nursing

40

Pat McCluskey

Key Messages

- Healthcare professionals (HCPs) who care for patients with wounds should have knowledge of wound healing physiology and recognise the physiological pathway across all wound healing processes.
- Healthcare professionals (HCPs) who intentionally create surgical wounds hold a responsibility to provide evidence-based care that minimises risk factors to ensure optimal wound healing.
- General wound management incorporates comprehensive assessment of both the patient and their wound including assessment of pain, nutrition and general health status.
- Aseptic technique is fundamental in wound care management to reduce the risk of infection.
- Dressings are adjunctive and provide protection and the ideal wound healing environment.
- Animal bites that are contaminated/dirty require dedicated wound hygiene.

Abbreviations

FA	Facing Africa
HCPs	Healthcare Professionals

Introduction

Although globally the underpinning principles remain the same, there are certain factors that need to be considered in the context of Facing Africa (FA) in Ethiopia. Nurses in Ethiopia have the same standard of nursing education and acquire a Bachelor of Science at qualification. However, exposure to wound care is minimal, and consequently the 'theory-practice' gap is very evident. Much of wound care practice is skill based, and the basic principles of aseptic technique and handwashing need to be explained rationally and repeatedly. Language used needs to be clear and concise whilst regularly checking that the concepts are fully understood.

Access to dressing products and cleansing agents are diminished, and greater emphasis needs to be concentrated on technique as opposed to 'dressing the wound'. Furthermore, due to

P. McCluskey (✉)
Advanced Nurse Practitioner in Wound Care, Wound Healing, and Tissue Viability, Cork University Hospital, Cork, Ireland

M. A. Hardy, B. R. Hochman (eds.), *Global Surgery*, https://doi.org/10.1007/978-3-031-28127-3_40

easy access of dressing products and diagnostics in the developed world, there is less reliance on the sensory aspects of wound care such as smell, touch, hearing and visual. Conversely, in Ethiopia, strengthening the sensory skills of nursing staff is paramount, thus enabling the nurses to listen to their patients; observe for signs of infection through smell, and observe for the presence of erythema, exudate and pain. Sensory skills generally impact their ability to learn when the signs and symptoms characterize how the patient is actually presenting and progressing.

Education

Education is therefore a key aspect of the 2-week surgical mission with FA, and the Ethiopian staff are eager and quick to learn and practice their skills. This aspect of the mission cannot be understated, and it may take a little longer to complete tasks such as dressing changes and medication rounds; however, during subsequent visits with FA to Ethiopia, the evidence that learning had been achieved was notable, and nurses had grown in confidence as their skills improved.

Irrespective of where nurses work, there are key elements in wound management practice that need to be embedded to achieve good outcomes, and these include understanding what wounds are, factors that affect wound healing, impact of nutrition, aseptic technique, management of specific wounds (skin grafts, donor sites, animal bites), the role of bacteria in wound healing and the ability to recognise when there is bacterial imbalance, which needs to be promptly treated [1].

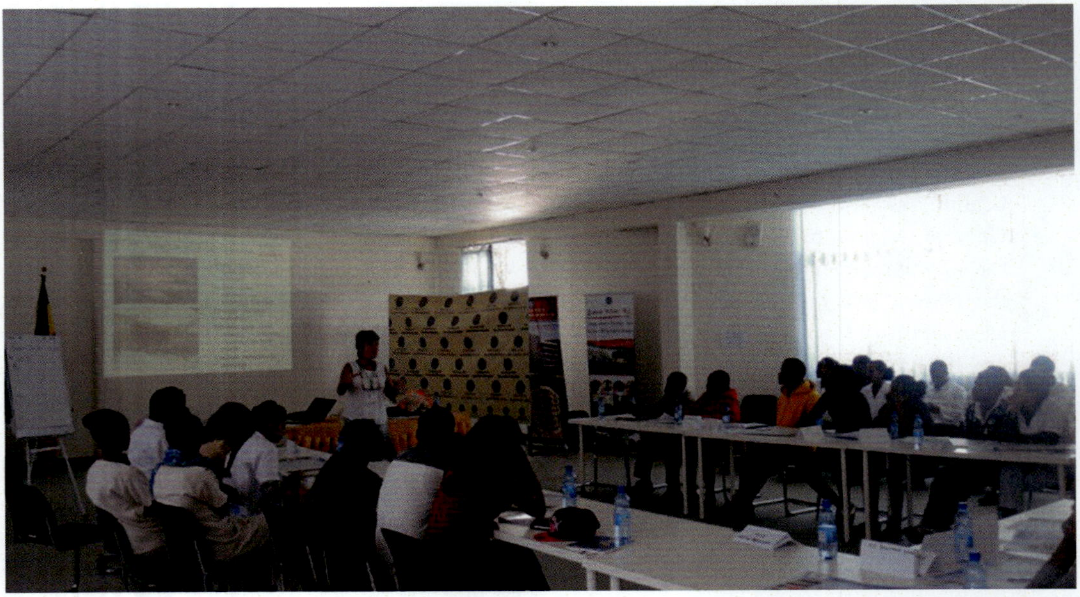

Definition and Classification of Wounds

A wound is defined as a cut or break in the continuity of the skin caused by injury or surgery [2]. There are two basic classifications of wounds: open, when there is a degree of tissue loss, and closed, when there is trauma with underlying tissue damage without a break in the continuity of the skin. Surgical wound classification is further subdivided into:

1. Clean: An incision where there is no inflammation encountered during the surgical procedure and there is integrity of the sterile technique.
2. Clean-contaminated: An incision where the respiratory, alimentary or genitourinary tract

is entered under controlled conditions and no contamination is incurred.

3. Contaminated: An incision where there is a major break in sterile technique or spillage from the gastrointestinal tract or an incision where acute, non-purulent inflammation is encountered. Open traumatic wounds present for greater than 12 hours are also considered contaminated wounds.
4. Dirty or infected: An incision created surgically in which the viscera are perforated or when acute inflammation with pus is encountered. Traumatic wounds where treatment has been delayed for a prolonged duration may also be included in this category.

Wounds encountered in FA are a mixture of all of the outlined. Many of the wounds reviewed during the assessment period are well-established wounds such as noma, wounds that have been previously reconstructed and not fully healed, tumours of the face and neck and some hyena or other animal bite wounds. Additionally, some of the more established wounds may be heavily contaminated, and it is not unusual to have maggots feasting on the wound debris. Prior to the arrival of the FA surgical team, the patients requiring or hopeful for treatment will already have been admitted to FA house for a minimum of 2 weeks.

Factors that Affect Healing

Acute wounds will generally proceed through an orderly and timely process to produce a healed wound that has anatomic and functional integrity. However, there are physiological factors that may impede wound healing such as aetiology, comorbidities, nutrition, pain, duration and size of the wound, inflammation and/or infection [3]. Additionally, patients who attend FA will have travelled for days or maybe weeks on foot on meagre resources. When they arrive, they are exhausted, nutritionally deplete and dehydrated. The factors that will have contributed to their delayed or obstructed healing will be attended to, and the factors that can be managed prior to assessment will be dealt with, such as nutritional deficits, infection and personal and wound hygiene.

Wound Healing in Children

Many of the patients attending Facing Africa are children who have been affected by noma. When they present, infection is often present, children are underweight and the impact of traveling to a new place and meeting other people with a variety of obvious wounds can cause anxiety and distress. Children who present with tumours of the face and neck are often outcasts in their own communities and have lived with ridicule and suspicion; the added stress of presenting to a new community in fear and anticipation can be an additional stress. However, having to live 2 weeks in a community prior to assessment and treatment, sharing meals and engaging in arts and crafts in the care of the nurses and doctors whilst having their needs addressed can greatly relieve the stress.

Wound healing in children generally follows the same process as adults; however, there is an increased production of collagen and elastin. Granulation tissue is created at a faster rate than in adults, resulting in a faster healing process [4]. Considerations for the child should therefore be included in all prevention, assessment and management strategies.

Pre- and Peri-Operative Care

Healthcare professionals (HCPs) who intentionally create surgical wounds hold a responsibility to provide evidence-based care that minimises risk factors to ensure optimal wound healing, and the Facing Africa surgical team is very attentive to this responsibility. Minimising risk requires attention to bacterial screening, excellent hand decontamination throughout all phases of surgical care, promotion of nutrition and hydration (protein and calorie requirements are increased in wound healing), pain management, minimising length of stay pre-operatively and provision of prophylactic antibiotics when required [5]. Personal hygiene is attended to, and patients are encouraged to participate in hand cleaning and changing soiled clothes and cloths that are used to cover their wounds and disfigurement.

Nutrition

Identifying patients who are malnourished and addressing their nutritional needs prior to surgery are necessary. Deficiency in protein and other nutrients may have an adverse effect on tissue/body structure, function and clinical outcomes [6]. Hydration is an integral component of nutritional assessment. Dehydrated tissue becomes inelastic, fragile and more susceptible to breakdown. Tissue perfusion at a wound site may also be impacted due to a decreased blood volume, limiting the supply of oxygen and nutrients [7]. Whilst 2 weeks would appear to be a short time to address many of these factors, children respond quickly to a balanced diet and increased protein and caloric intake and vitamins, which are provided by Facing Africa.

Post-Operative Care

Attention to hand decontamination and aseptic technique during dressing changes minimises cross contamination and reduces the risk of infection. Surgical wounds heal mostly by primary intention where the wound edges have been opposed and the method of closure will be either through sutures, clips, surgical glue or Steri-Strips. Appropriate surgical wound care is essential in preventing surgical-site infections, wound dehiscence and haematoma formation. HCPs must be able to identify the physical signs of infection such as redness, warmth, pain, swelling, increased exudate, odour and purulent discharge or systemic signs of infection such as raised C-reactive protein and white cell count. Patient education in the recognition of these symptoms is pivotal to assist in early detection [8].

Dressings

Surgical wounds epithelialise in approximately 48–72 h [9]. The new epithelial cells are fragile and need protecting. The Facing Africa surgical team provides very specific instructions on how the wounds are to be managed and usually recommend that the surgical wound is left undisturbed for at least 48–72 hours post-operatively.

The use of an aseptic, non-touch technique for dressing changes is encouraged after all procedures, using only sterile saline to clean the wound, and the application of an interactive, sterile, post-operative dressing. Dressings should maintain a moist wound environment to support epithelialisation, provide a protective barrier against bacteria or contamination, be atraumatic on removal and have the capacity to absorb the minimal exudate that is produced during the normal inflammatory period [10].

These procedures are initially performed by the FA nursing team and assisted by the Ethiopian nurses. The rationale for the techniques is explained at each stage, and the choices made are outlined. At each assessment of the wound, what is visually observed is discussed, and patients are listened to and heard. This practice works extremely well in the sharing of knowledge and skill and helps build confidence. When the surgical team departs, nurses are able to continue managing these wounds seamlessly.

Head and Neck Surgery

Surgical wounds in head and neck surgery can be extensive and include skin and muscle flaps and varying suture lines due to reconstruction. These constitute the majority of surgeries performed by the FA surgical team. There are many variables to consider in graft failure, and nursing staff need to be encouraged to gain an understanding of these variables to ensure that complications are observed quickly and communicated to the team to ensure that they can be treated in a timely fashion. It is important not to presume that staff will already be aware of the possible risks and that these risks are communicated to the nursing staff and reiterated at every opportunity so that the standard of care becomes more of a habit than act. To ensure this, nursing staff need to understand precisely what is being observed so the terminology does not become a barrier in itself. Close observation and consistent monitoring of these wounds is essential to identify early complications such as:

Poor Vascularity Vascular status is compromised; colour change, diminished capillary refill time, temperature change and oedema will be observed.

Haematoma or Seroma Formation On observation, a swelling will be detected, and exudate/blood can be aspirated under aseptic technique, by the surgeon, and sent for microbiological examination.

Infection Overt or subtle signs of infection may be observed, and if infection is confirmed from a culture of the aspirate with sensitivities to antibiotics attained, antibiotics will be prescribed by the surgeon. This is especially important at FA where infection with endemic viruses is prevalent. Many of the organisms are anaerobic, and infection can be rapid with dire consequences.

Mechanical Shearing Graft failure may occur as a result of excess or inappropriate movement, which may affect new blood vessel growth or encourage haematoma formation. Take steps to reduce swelling by elevation, and secure dressings adequately to optimise graft adherence.

Transparent, semi-permeable, sterile dressings are usually chosen to facilitate graft inspection [11]. However, the site and depth of the graft may require a foam dressing. It is important that the dressing should facilitate high moisture vapour transmissibility. Excess moisture underneath a dressing can cause maceration and interfere with graft adherence.

Head and neck wounds that are exposed after surgery should be cleaned twice daily under aseptic technique using sterile saline. An antibiotic ointment may be prescribed by the surgeon for a period of 5–7 days. Ointment should be applied in one direction (from cleanest aspect), using sterile gloves and using one fingertip for each new application. This reduces the possibility of cross-contamination.

Split-Skin Graft

A split-skin graft involves excision of the epidermis and part of the dermis. The most common donor site is the thigh [12].

Donor Site Management

Donor sites are invariably more painful than the graft site, and there is great variation in their management. However, re-epithelialisation usually occurs within 7–10 days. Appropriate analgesia for pain and elevation to reduce oedema is provided. Dressings that ensure haemostasis, absorb increased exudate in the acute inflammatory phase and have non-slip properties are chosen. Alginates (for their haemostatic properties) are often the dressings of choice with a secondary absorbent layer and secured with non-slip bandages. Dressings remain in situ for 7–10 days and removed only if contamination occurs. If the donor site has any evidence of an increased bacterial burden (increased pain, malodour), then an antimicrobial dressing regime is implemented. Other dressing regimes include silicones, hydrofibres, foams and hydrocolloids [13]. Techniques in bandaging are improved with practice and by observation, and the rationale underpinning choices is explained at each stage. This ensures that best practice based on evidence is applied at each stage.

Oral Care Pre- and Post Surgery

Oral cavity wounds heal in a saliva-filled environment that contains millions of microorganisms. Oral hygiene pre- and post-operatively is essential to reduce the risks of infection [14]. A soft toothbrush or mouth swab is provided to each patient when they are admitted to FA to clean the mouth from saliva, debris and blood post-operatively and the rationale clearly outlined. As it is necessary to implement a food regime as quickly as possible, this is a further challenge. In the immediate post-operative period, a soft suction cannula may be used to remove the excess saliva as required. Antiseptic mouthwash (according to local protocol) is also encouraged twice daily and after food ingestion to minimise bacterial growth.

Animal Bites and Wound Management

Animal bites are very common on the African continent, and injury can be inflicted from hyenas, dogs, snakes or crocodiles. Infection and hard-to-heal wounds are often a consequence if early intervention is not implemented. The general management of bites, irrespective of their origin, remains the same and consists of meticulous wound hygiene. Wound hygiene describes the cleansing, debridement, refashioning and dressing of wounds [15]. Nursing staff at FA are taught how to clean the wound with intent by irrigating the wound bed and surrounding tissue regularly and repeatedly based on clinical assessment. Debridement of any devitalised tissue, biofilm, debris and organic matter with gauze or curettes is recommended based on HCP's skill and knowledge base. However, these skills require training and practice, and Ethiopian nurses approach this practice tentatively after close observation and with experienced clinical supervision. Refashioning of the wound edge allows for the removal of senescent cells and helps agitate epithelial cell growth. Dressings should provide protection, absorption, moisture and warmth and be non-occlusive to prevent bacterial proliferation. Anti-microbial dressings that contain surfactants (loosen devitalised tissue) may be beneficial. However, wound irrigation and hygiene are essential components in early management until surgical intervention is appropriate. Nursing staff are advised on the necessity of urgent referral for appropriate management.

As there is a high risk of infection in these wounds from the flora in the animal's mouth, antibiotics are an early and necessary intervention [16].

References

1. Health Service Executive; National Wound Management Guidelines (2018) Office of the Nursing & midwifery services director. Health Service Executive.
2. Harman TF, Bordoni B. Wound classification (Updated, 2021, May 4). In: StarPearls (Internet). Treasure Island (FL): StarPearls Publishing; 2021.
3. Wounds International. International consensus, 'the role of proteases in wound diagnostics' an expert working group review. London: Wounds International; 2011.
4. Bryant R, Nix D. Acute and chronic wounds – E Book. Elsevier Health Sciences; 2016.
5. National Institute for Health and Care Excellence (2008) Prevention and Treatment of surgical-site infection. https://.org.uk//337;a1924. Accessed 9 Apr 2022.
6. Elia M (2000) The malnutrition advisory group consensus Guidelines for the detection and Management of Malnutrition in the community. Last Updated in 2020. www.researchgate.net. Accessed 15 Mar 2022.
7. Thorpe J. Nutritional assessment of people with wounds. Wound Essentials. 2014;9(1)
8. Verdon A. Ten top tips for patient management of surgical wounds. Wounds Essentials. 2014;9(1)
9. Winter GD. Formation of the scab and the rate of epithelisation of superficial wounds in the skin of the young domestic pig. Nature. 1962;193:293.
10. HSE National Wound Management Guidelines. Office of the Nursing & midwifery services director. Health service. Executive. 2018;
11. Mathes SJ. Plastic surgery. In: General Principles, vol. 1. 2nd ed. Philadelphia: Elsevier; 2006.
12. Coull A. Making sense of split-skin graft donor sites. Nurs Times. 1991;87(40):52–4.
13. Beldon P. What you need to know about skin grafts and donor site wounds. Wound Essentials. 2007;2:149–55.
14. Shah R, Domah F, Shah N, Domah J. Surgical wound healing in the oral cavity: a review. Oral Surg. 2020;47(2):135–40.
15. Murphy C, Atkin L, Swanson T, Tachi M, Tan YK, Vega de Senja M, et al. International consensus document: defying hard-to-heal wounds with an early anti-biofilm intervention strategy: wound hygiene. J Wound Care. 2020;29(Suppl. 3b):S1–28.
16. Stevens DL, Bisno AL, Chambers HF, et al. Practice Guidelines for the diagnosis and management of skin and soft tissue infections. Clin Infect Dis Soc. 2014;59:e10.

How to Manage Vascular Trauma and Emergencies in Low- and Middle-Income Countries

41

Adam Lee Goldstein, Jacob R. Krimbill, Alberto Saltiel, and Mark A. Hardy

Optimism is the faith that leads to achievement. Nothing can be done without hope and confidence.

– Helen Keller

Abbreviations

ABI/API	Ankle-brachial index or arterial pressure index
ALI	Acute limb ischemia
AT	Aspirating thrombus
ATLS	Advanced Trauma Life Support
BKA	Below-knee amputation
CDL	Catheter-directed lysis
CLTI	Chronic limb-threatening ischemia
CT	Computed tomography
DFS	Diabetic foot syndrome
DPL or DPA	Diagnostic peritoneal lavage or aspiration
FAST	Focused Assessment with Sonography in Trauma
GSV	Greater saphenous vein
HIC	High-income countries
IPC	Intermittent pneumatic compression
IV	Intravenous
LMICs	Low- and middle-income countries
NCDs	Non-communicable diseases
OR	Operating room
PAD	Peripheral arterial disease
PE	Pulmonary embolus
PTFE	Polytetrafluoroethylene
PVD	Peripheral vascular disease
REBOA	Resuscitative endovascular balloon occlusion of the aorta
TIA	Transient ischemic attack
TPA	Tissue plasminogen activation
US	Ultrasound
WHO	World Health Organization
WIfI	Wound, infection, and ischemia

A. L. Goldstein (✉)
Department of Surgery, Trauma Unit, Wolfson Medical Center, Holon, Israel
e-mail: adamleeg@wmc.gov.il

J. R. Krimbill
General Surgery, Columbia University Medical Center and NY Presbyterian Hospital, New York, NY, USA
e-mail: jk4226@cumc.columbia.edu

A. Saltiel
Vascular and Endovascular Surgery Department, Tel Aviv Sourasky Medical Center, Tel Aviv, Israel

M. A. Hardy
Department of Surgery, Columbia University Vagelos College of Physicians and Surgeons, New York, NY, USA
e-mail: mah1@cumc.columbia.edu

M. A. Hardy, B. R. Hochman (eds.), *Global Surgery*, https://doi.org/10.1007/978-3-031-28127-3_41

Introduction

Vascular surgery often needs to be performed by general surgeons in low- and middle-income countries (LMICs). This is especially true for emergent interventions due to traumatic injuries or acute pathologies, limb-saving procedures, and common necessary elective cases, since transfer to a major hospital may be delayed or untenable. Basic vascular surgical skills are essential for the rural/global surgeon and are life (and/or limb)-saving in many situations. With a strong understanding of vascular surgery principles and techniques, the general surgeon must be able to perform temporizing procedures that may give the patient critical time (hours to days) until transfer to a specialized center or arrival of an experienced vascular surgeon or necessary special supplies (i.e., grafts, anticoagulation medications).

While trauma remains a significant source of vascular disease, the etiology of vascular disease/injury is changing in LMICs as the prevalence of risk factors for peripheral vascular disease (PVD), including geriatric age, continues to rapidly grow in populations that were previously spared from these conditions [1, 2]. This has led to a growing need for vascular surgery competency, diagnostics and therapeutics, and infrastructural resources to support patient monitoring, access to anticoagulation therapy, and preventative health resources [1].

In managing vascular trauma, the treating physician must always follow the principles of trauma care and Advanced Trauma Life Support (ATLS), understand the source of injuries, prioritize what needs treatment first, and understand and treat the overall condition of the patient. To best decide what definitive or temporary vascular surgical care to provide, the surgeon must remember first of all to save the life over the limb. In this chapter, we aim to provide an outline of vascular trauma and non-traumatic emergencies, with a focus on essential diagnostics, surgical techniques, and follow-up that might be most helpful in limited-resource environments.

Mechanism/Epidemiology

Trauma remains the major cause of death worldwide, especially on the African continent, and often requires emergent vascular interventions. It is not surprising that vascular injuries are more commonly associated with hemorrhagic shock and death than other types of injuries [3], and reliable quantification of the burden of vascular injuries is hindered by death in the field prior to transport. More broad trauma metrics including the general ratio between blunt versus penetrating trauma, socioeconomic status of the population (i.e., rural or urban), and current armed conflicts are also often not well captured, making development of targeted solutions to improve care more challenging. The epidemiology of vascular trauma drastically differs in LMICs depending on the presence of armed conflict, a high percentage of remnant landmines, rural or urban settings, and the availability and quality of prehospital care [1].

In regard to prehospital care, the Stop the Bleed campaign was formed in the United States in 2015 in response to the persistently increasing volume of mass shootings. This campaign was born from evidence-based research showing the high number of potential preventable deaths in both combat and civilian settings by simple prehospital/bystander interventions to slow/stop hemorrhage [4]. Severe limb hemorrhage as a cause of preventable death has been reported as high as 14% in recent combat literature [4], with similar percentages in civilian trauma. Stop the Bleed campaigns have also shown success in LMICs [5] and remain an important public health tool worldwide.

Diagnosis

There is a drastic difference between LMICs and high-income countries (HICs) in available vascular interventions and diagnostic capabilities. The approach to vascular.

trauma regardless of environment is consistent: hard signs of injury (Table 41.1) require

Table 41.1 Hard and soft signs of vascular injury

Hard signs	Soft signs
Pulsatile bleeding	Non-pulsatile bleeding
Expanding hematoma	Non-expanding/non-pulsatile hematoma
Loss of distal pulses	Diminished pulses
Bruit/thrill	History of arterial bleeding/ hypotension
	Previously applied tourniquet
	Neurological deficit
	Wound proximity to named vessel

operative exploration, whereas soft signs of injury call for further evaluation or monitoring before vascular injury may be ruled out. Patients with neither hard nor soft signs of vascular injury and with no other indication for admission/operation may be safely discharged. The surgeon responsible for vascular trauma patients, especially a non-local surgeon, must be prepared for different methods within the capabilities and limits of the hospital to successfully diagnose and ultimately treat these patients.

A recent estimate showed that there is less than one computer tomography (CT) scanner per million people in LMICs, compared to almost forty per million people in HICs [6]. Therefore, the surgeon must be prepared to diagnose and treat vascular injury with a total reliance on physical exam, ankle-brachial index or arterial pressure index (ABI/API), ultrasound (US), and even surgical exploration when question remains. Due to the lack of interventional radiology in many LMICs, we will not discuss their use in this chapter despite its obvious value in vascular injury when available [7].

Apart from hard signs of vascular injury (Table1), physical examination may be a difficult and insensitive tool in diagnosis of traumatic vascular injury. In the multi-trauma patient, there might be a delay in diagnosis of peripheral vascular injury due to other distracting injuries, hypovolemia due to hemorrhage, and/or vasospasm, which temporarily may decrease active bleeding. The significance of vascular injury might not be completely appreciated until the patient is resuscitated. It is not uncommon for the surgical team to finish a damage control laparotomy only to discover a newly bleeding wound that was previously underestimated. Strict adherence to the principles of ATLS will help decrease these missed/underappreciated injuries.

A blast injury (locally from bullet trajectory or blast mechanism) may also cause occult injuries to vasculature that require intervention yet are not initially realized; unfortunately, they are often diagnosed only after there is critical limb or organ damage, as is discussed later. Concomitant orthopedic injuries such as displaced fractures or dislocations should be reduced as soon as possible so as to permit spontaneous return of peripheral blood flow to the extremity and change the definitive care plan for the patient.

Hard signs are an indication for immediate surgical intervention without further diagnostics or imaging necessary. A hard sign, however, does not indicate that the basic principle of ATLS may be shortened or compromised. After the primary/secondary survey and adjuvants of ATLS are completed, an unstable patient must be taken to the operating room (OR). A stable patient with multi-trauma or one who responds to resuscitation and has a hard sign of vascular trauma, with or without imaging (when available), might still be required to go to the OR to rule out other organ system injuries before vascular operative intervention. Bleeding must be temporarily controlled either by direct pressure or proximal tourniquet to consider imaging, and if unable to do so, then the patient will need an immediate operation.

The use, and possible complications, of tourniquet are discussed below. When a patient arrives from the field with a tourniquet already in place, it must be established that (1) the tourniquet is functioning as needed; (2) the time the tourniquet was placed is known and recorded; and (3) the tourniquet is actually indicated. In approaching trauma patients, the ATLS protocol starts with the evaluation of airway and respiratory status, followed by circulation. If a tourniquet is present, it will ultimately need to be removed to characterize the injury (if one ever existed). However, one must do so when prepared to handle the consequences; prior to taking down a tourniquet, it is important to have a second tourniquet placed proximally that is not tightened but ready to be engaged if needed. Evaluation of the true necessity of the tourniquet is important because of the high percentage of tourniquets placed that are not necessary, together with the potential iatrogenic damage caused to the limb by the tourniquet.

Ankle-brachial index (ABI) (or arterial pressure index, API) is an important test for the evaluation of all extremity trauma (penetrating and blunt) with proximity to vasculature and without hard signs of vascular injury. It is a readily available rapid test with high negative predictive value, and it is especially useful in resource-constrained settings where CT and angiography are not available, since the only necessary equipment is a blood pressure cuff. When no hard signs of vascular injury are present, and there is a normal ABI (>0.9), then arterial damage may be safely excluded without further imaging or monitoring [8]. Utilization of the ABI/API has significantly decreased unnecessary imaging, surgical exploration, and hospital admissions. Its efficacy has been shown for both blunt and penetrating trauma [9]. Therefore, we believe evaluating the ABI/API is a requirement in any suspected vascular trauma regardless of the setting.

Doppler ultrasound (US) has clear potential for identifying acute vascular trauma, especially where CT scans are not readily available. However, ultrasound is highly operator-dependent and has a high rate of false-positive results in populations with chronic vascular disease. Thus, it is more useful in helping diagnose vascular injury in children [10] and is also informative for post operative monitoring [1].

Despite the accuracy of the physical exam and the value of ABI/API, surgical exploration remains necessary to rule out vascular injury if the patient remains unstable or appears to have continual hemorrhage, especially when CT scans are not available.

Treatments

Arterial Trauma

When managing vascular trauma or any operation for ischemic injury or gangrene, it is important to consider general operative principles. Like in all vascular surgeries in any environment, the cornerstone of exposure is securing proximal and distal control of the vessel. Once this is obtained, treatment options will be considered depending on the overall condition of the trauma patient and the contamination of the surgical field. In non-trauma patients, planning of exposure and control of the vessels also applies. If the patient remains stable, then preferably, a definitive repair is to be performed. If the patient is unstable in a trauma patient, further debridement is necessary, or major orthopedic surgery is needed, then a temporary shunt may be used.

The first step in treating vascular trauma is hemostasis. This ideally will be obtained in the field or the emergency room by direct pressure, proximal arterial compression, or judicious temporary use of the tourniquet. With regard to direct pressure, it is important that the one maintaining pressure does not let go for any reason (to test if it is bleeding) to avoid losing the clot that may have formed. Pressure by the scrubbed hand (using knuckles/fist instead of extended fingers) is only released when the surgeons are ready to gain control of the bleeding vessel operatively. This avoids cramps and may be sustained for longer amounts of time.

Tourniquets have a clear role in saving lives, yet their adaptation from military to civilian use has been met with controversy. Despite the controversy, most recent studies continue to show a benefit in overall survival, blood product use, and limb outcome [11]. In LMICs, tourniquets may be anything that can be tightened and tied, be it a cloth, a belt, or a shirt. The principles of proper tourniquet use include the following:

1. Know when to apply a tourniquet.
   (a) Bright red pulsatile bleeding.
   (b) Large amounts of dark red bleeding.

    (c) Bleeding that cannot be stopped by direct pressure.
2. Place the tourniquet as close to the injury as possible in order to avoid damage to healthy/viable tissue.
3. If there were distal pulses before the tourniquet was placed, make sure that there are none after.
4. Make sure the bleeding has stopped (that the tourniquet is doing its job).
5. Lastly, record the time of placement – either on the tourniquet, on the leg, on the forehead of the victim – wherever it may be easily seen by any of the teams taking care of the patient. Junction tourniquets and prehospital endovascular exclusion have begun to gain popularity, yet this is still far from mainstream or relevant for LMICs.

The goal for surgery is to restore blood flow distally to the injured area to avoid gangrene. This should be done urgently. However, if the patient's hemodynamic status does not allow for revascularization, ligation of an injured vessel might be the most accurate option available. Especially when it comes down to choosing to save either life or the limb. When proximal ligation is performed, the distal extremity must be frequently assessed closely for signs of worsening ischemia, which will mandate urgent revascularization or amputation in case revascularization is not permitted due to the patient's status [12]. Endovascular surgery has risen in popularity in HIC and has allowed for minimally invasive treatment of low-flow arteriovenous fistulas, pseudoaneurysms, and active bleeding of nondominant arteries by transcatheter embolization, or by the placement of intravascular stents to exclude the injured areas of the vessel or to treat focal intimal injuries. These minimally invasive techniques are not generally available in other major centers in LMICs, and thus, open surgery remains the gold standard in the treatment of most vascular trauma, especially that of the extremities.

The multi-trauma patient requiring surgery in more than one compartment should be prepped and draped from the chin to the knee. In limb vascular injuries, the prep needed includes total length and circumference. To also ensure rapid access to vein graft harvesting, the contralateral uninjured limb should also be circumferentially prepped and draped. Venous harvesting may sometimes be done from the ipsilateral limb, but this is not advisable, especially in blast injuries.

If hemostasis has not been obtained (or adequately obtained) in the operating room, a Foley catheter may be used for temporary tamponade [13]. This may also be done in the emergency room or field. This is an important option to understand in LMICs with limited, or overwhelmed, resources. Once a bleeding vessel is identified intraoperatively, a proximal balloon occlusion with a Fogarty catheter (Edwards Lifesciences, Irvine CA), if available, may be considered. The balloon may be inserted blindly and should be accurately fitted to the vessel's diameter. We strongly discourage the use of blind clamping of vessels to avoid possible damage to the vessel intima and wall.

A longitudinal incision should be carried out above and below the injured area to allow for complete control of the vessel above and below the site of injury. In certain cases, a tourniquet may be applied (or reapplied) proximally, to allow for hemorrhage control until surgical access is gained and proximal control is achieved. Once control has been gained, the incision can be extended over the injured area, where the damaged vessel will be exposed. For trauma to the proximal lower extremity, a retroperitoneal incision may be required to gain proximal control of iliac vessels. Further proximal control would be at the bifurcation of the iliac artery and veins via an abdominal approach. In proximal upper extremity trauma, a supraclavicular or infraclavicular incision may be warranted to gain control of the vessel or even a sternotomy in rare cases. For excellent outline of various quick vascular exposures, we strongly recommend Henry's book, *Extensile Exposures*, for every surgeon's library [14].

Clamping with vascular clamps the artery proximally and distally is recommended under direct vision, and never blindly, prior to exposing the injured vessel. If specific vascular claps are unavailable, then it can be done be done with double-looped thin rubber drains as close to the injury as possible or with surgical Adsons dressed in rubber booties and closed with the minimal amount of tension needed for hemostasis. Anticoagulation can be achieved locally by injecting 1000 U heparin into each limb prior to clamping. If all other sources of bleeding have been controlled, systemic heparinization can be performed with 5000 U heparin and repeated every 4–6 h as needed. If the patient begins to become coagulopathic, then no systemic heparin is given. The proximal and distal areas of the vessel should be exposed, and surrounding area is debrided including edges of the vessel if injured by blunt or gunshot trauma or by explosion. It is necessary to assess inflow and backflow bleeding from the proximal and distal vessels prior to final vascular repair. If inflow or outflow are not thought to be appropriate after distal and proximal irrigation (or passage of a Fogarty balloon, if available), one must search other areas for flow-limiting injuries. If a basic c-arm x-ray is available, a single-shot intraoperative (on-table) angiography may be performed and to determine if there is any occlusion of flow. We use a 21 or 22G needle, with a mix of $\frac{1}{3}$ contrast to $\frac{2}{3}$ heparinized saline (1000 U heparin in 1 l of saline). If there is any question of indirect damage, we support immediate repair in order to avoid complications, possible limb loss, and/or the need to return to the operating room.

Wide debridement of all soft and boney injured tissue is mandatory prior to coverage of the vascular repair and closure, preferably with surrounding viable muscle and skin. This is needed to prevent vascular conduit/graft infection or disruption. Muscle and/or soft tissue flaps may become extensive originating from parts of the lower abdomen, flanks, and other parts of the ipsilateral extremity. Muscle flaps may need to be temporary if further debridement is necessary for large contaminated tissue defects.

Arteriotomies on damaged vessels should be carried out longitudinally, allowing for its extension if the damage to the vessel is greater than previously assessed. Longitudinal arteriotomy also permits easier exploration of the posterior vessel wall including presence of an arteriovenous fistulas and of intimal tears.

Following exploration, indications for a definitive (or temporary) repair can be checked. Repair (or bypass) is the goal for vessels that are vital for limb function and survival while remembering the mantra of "life over limb." In hemodynamically unstable patients, a more aggressive approach toward vessel ligation should be considered, especially when the vessel is not essential to distal tissue viability. Venous ligation is usually well tolerated in the extremities without significant sequelae. Ligation may even be utilized for large central and major veins such as the portal vein or the inferior vena cava (IVC) in extreme situations with unstable patients [15]. If necessary, arterial ligation may be done safely to the following vessels:

- Subclavian artery.
- Radial or ulnar arteries (if intact palmar arch is present and a normal backflow is perceived during surgery).
- Internal iliac artery.
- Superficial femoral artery (with a patent deep femoral artery).
- Single tibial artery (when other tibial arteries are intact).

Surgical repair may be done **with** *primary repair, patch repair, end-to-end anastomosis of the damaged artery, the creation of an interposition graft, or a bypass*. Primary repair may be considered for stab wounds when there is minimal damage to the arterial wall and there are no flow restrictions. It is done by using a non-absorbable single or running suture. We prefer Prolene (if unavailable, then silk) 6–0 or 7–0 depending on the size of the vessel (larger for the aorta). A vessel defect involving more than 1 cm but less than 3 cm, or a full transection of the artery in which both edges of the vessel are less than 3 cm apart after debridement of the edges, can be reapproximated by an end-to-end anastomosis once both ends of the vessel are sufficiently mobilized to avoid any tension. Figure 41.1

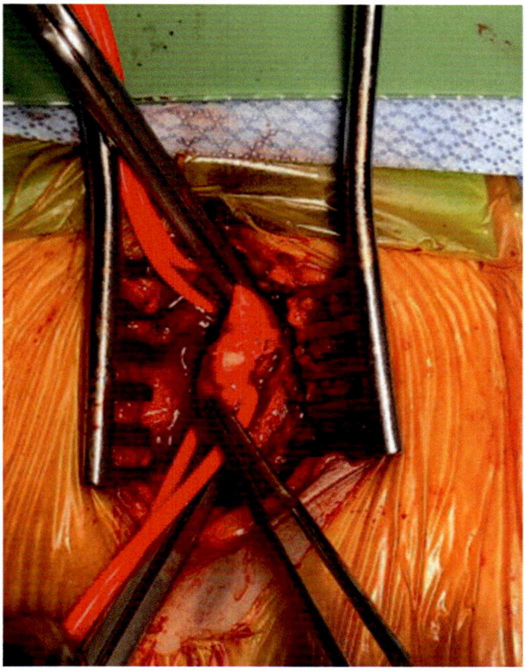

Fig. 41.1 Laceration to the common femoral artery that was repaired by primary closure *Source: Photos courtesy of authors A.G. and A.S*

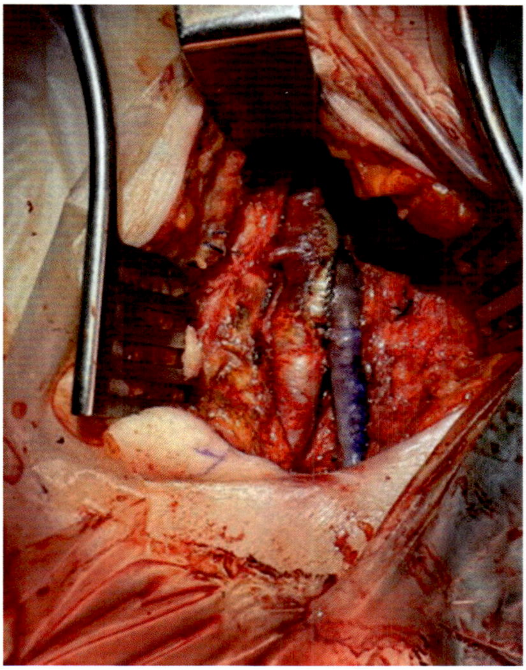

Fig. 41.2 A combination of a patch repair to the common femoral artery and an interposition reverse SVG replacing the deep femoral artery and proximately sewn to the patch repair (the vein graft is marked with purple and the patch more white) *Source: Photos courtesy of authors A.G. and A.S*

shows a laceration to the common femoral artery that was repaired by primary closure.

When a broader arteriotomy is required in order to debride the damaged vessel, a patch angioplasty is indicated, which may be obtained from the contralateral greater saphenous vein (GSV). If question remains regarding the viability of the vessel, then it might be safer to perform a formal resection and repair with an interposition graft. A patch repair is shown in Fig. 41.2 together with a GSV graft repair (Fig. 41.3).

When a tension-free primary anastomosis is not possible, then an interposition graft may be used. The conduit of choice should be an autogenous vein (especially for vessels <5 mm in diameter), obtained from the contralateral limb (the neck for large vessels). When a whole segment of an artery is involved and the inflow and outflow vessels are not the same, a bypass with a reversed (because of valves) GVS autogenous vein graft should be performed. To increase the diameter of the vein graft panel, reconstruction [16] or other methods may be used (Fig. 41.4). The GSV autologous conduit, when used for either patch angioplasty, interposition grafts, or bypasses, has been shown to have good short-, mid-, and long-term patency rates [17].

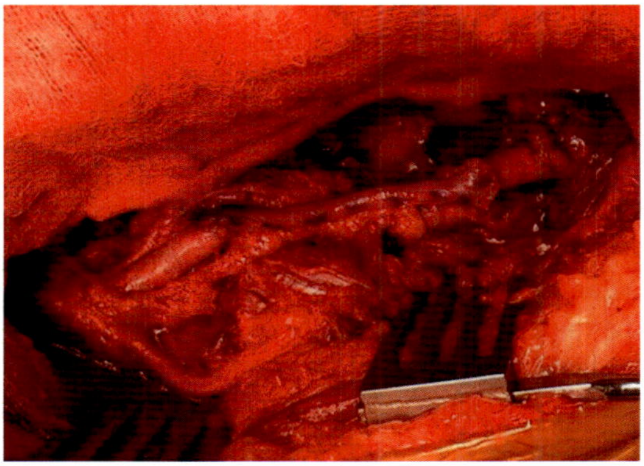

Fig. 41.3 Superficial femoral artery repaired with reverse SVG. *Source: Photos courtesy of authors A.G. and A.S*

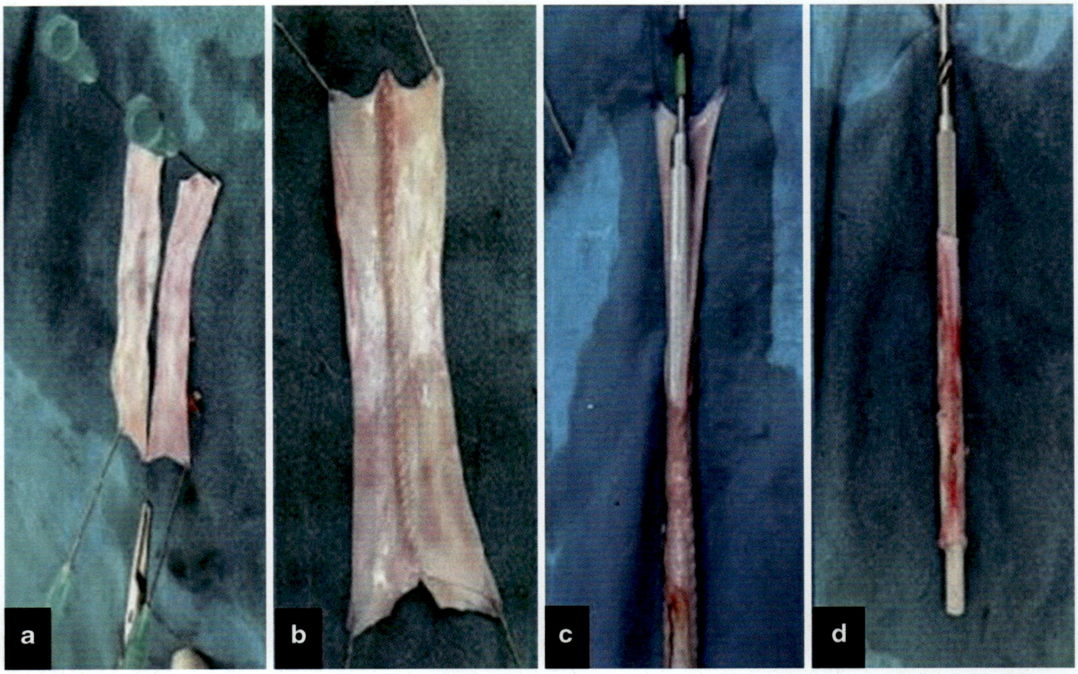

Fig. 41.4 GSV graft repair of the superficial femoral artery. *Source: Photo courtesy of author M.A.H.* (**a**) The saphenous-vein is longitudinally opened and divided. Two equal rectangular pieces are created. (**b**) First, the pieces of saphenous vein are sewn side by side. (**c**) Free borders of the saphenous veins are coiled up in a sterile cylindrical rod and sewn each other with a 6/0 Prolene monofilament suture. (**d**) The neo-vein conduit has been performed with a caliber twice the original vein's diameter. Source: Ketenciler S, et al. Annals of Vascular Surgery. 2018 Nov 1;53:117–22

For larger-vessel injuries, redo reconstructions, or if the GSV is not available or adequate, then the contralateral femoral vein or jugular vein for short segments is a good (and underutilized) option. These much larger vessels may be harvested with limited morbidity and good long-term results. Ideally, the femoral vein is harvested distal to the insertion of the profunda (deep) femoral branch, allowing for adequate limb drainage.

Occasionally, a synthetic graft is needed but is usually not readily available in LMICs. Preserved veins from cadavers may be used and should be obtained when possible and maintained sterilely in an antibiotic solution in the refrigerator. Synthetic grafts are undesirable for use in the nonsterile penetrating, blast, or open blunt trauma injuries. In civilian trauma, usually for knife and bullet wounds to vessels that are centralized or proximal enough that are too large for GSV grafts, synthetic grafts are commonly used in HICs, but the jugular vein may be employed in LMICs.

Once the repair is completed, an assessment of revascularization should be done before closure. The return of distal pulses, arterial Doppler signal distal to the repair, return of normal capillary filling time, and an increase in distal extremity temperature are all positive findings. Primary closure of the debrided wound may be considered for clean and clean/contaminated wounds. However, if a large soft-tissue defect is present, muscle coverage of the vessel is critical to prevent vascular infection, and a vacuum dressing (available or created) should be employed. Negative-pressure dressings may be readily formed using suction machines or drainage systems [18].

Temporary vascular shunting is a critical tool for any surgeon. This procedure has acquired widespread recognition as a temporary solution that allows for distal perfusion of the extremity when additional treatment is mandated prior to definitive vascular repair. The use of vascular shunts has been utilized since the early 1900s. Originally, the use of prosthetic tubbing was meant to be permanent. Utilization of temporary shuts are valuable when (1) the bleeding has been controlled yet the patient is too unstable to continue with definitive vascular surgery; (2) when significant orthopedic surgery must also be performed to the ipsilateral limb; or (3) if damage control surgery needs to be done before the patient can either be transferred to a higher level of care or when specialist surgical help can be obtained. When used for short periods of time (1–3 h), shunt patency rate reaches 100%, even when systemic anticoagulation is not utilized. Temporary shunts may remain open for more than 2 days without systemic anticoagulation [19]. The goal is to perform definitive surgical repair within 48 hours, with initiation of DVT prophylaxis anticoagulation if the bleeding has stopped. The diameter of the shunt should be similar to that of the artery. Sterile IV set tubing, nasogastric feeding tubes, or even chest tubes may be used as shunts with care not to damage the vascular intima using double-looped vessel loops or thin Penrose drains. The shunt may be also secured using either 2–0 or 1–0 silk ties. By placing a longer silk tie in the middle of the shunt, it can be easily identified and followed for any slippage out of place in one direction or the other. It must be inserted into the proximal vessel first while allowing for inflow bleeding assessment and elimination of air and then inserted distally into the target vessel. Distal perfusion must be assessed after placement of the shunt, ideally with Doppler signals.

Venous Trauma

There is no unanimous decision on whether or not to treat large venous injuries. Venous repairs acutely thrombose much more often than arterial repairs, although they are known to frequently spontaneously recanalize eventually. Peripheral edema following acute venous thrombosis or venous ligation may be avoided in 50% of patients with venous repair as compared with ligation, although in both scenarios, a complete resolution of edema usually happens with time [20]. If repair is feasible and safe, it may be done by simple lateral suture venorrhaphy, end-to-end anastomosis, patch venoplasty, or interposition graft, all depending on the anatomy and extent of the injury. With larger veins, especially the vena cava, it is important to perform a transverse repair in order to avoid narrowing of the lumen. Ligation should be done, and not postponed, if the patient may not be able to tolerate prolonged surgery. Whenever there is venous trauma, regardless of the approach taken to treat it, postoperative leg elevation and light compression of the extremity may help reduce edema.

Fasciotomy

With all vascular trauma, especially to the lower extremities, it is important to focus on the possible need for prophylactic distal fasciotomies. Although they have potential morbidity and complications (especially wound infection and length of hospital stay), a four-compartment fasciotomy of the distal lower limb may be needed with all combined arterial and venous injuries with blast or blunt injuries and, even sometimes, with sharp injuries of the vessels accompanied by soft tissue injuries. The use of prophylactic fasciotomy remains controversial, yet, especially in LMICs, it might be the safest option to prevent potential limb loss due to compartment syndrome. The risk factors and formal clinical grading scores are not yet accurate enough to predict with any certainty who might benefit from a prophylactic fasciotomy [21, 22].

A special understanding of blast injury with soft tissue damage is very relevant to vascular ends that appear normal but are microscopically damaged. Along with soft tissue damage and contamination, this creates the perfect storm for conduit/graft infection, potential breakdown, and local wound infections. Therefore, with blast injuries, it is important to perform multiple debridements, be liberal with the use of a temporary graft, and use synthetic

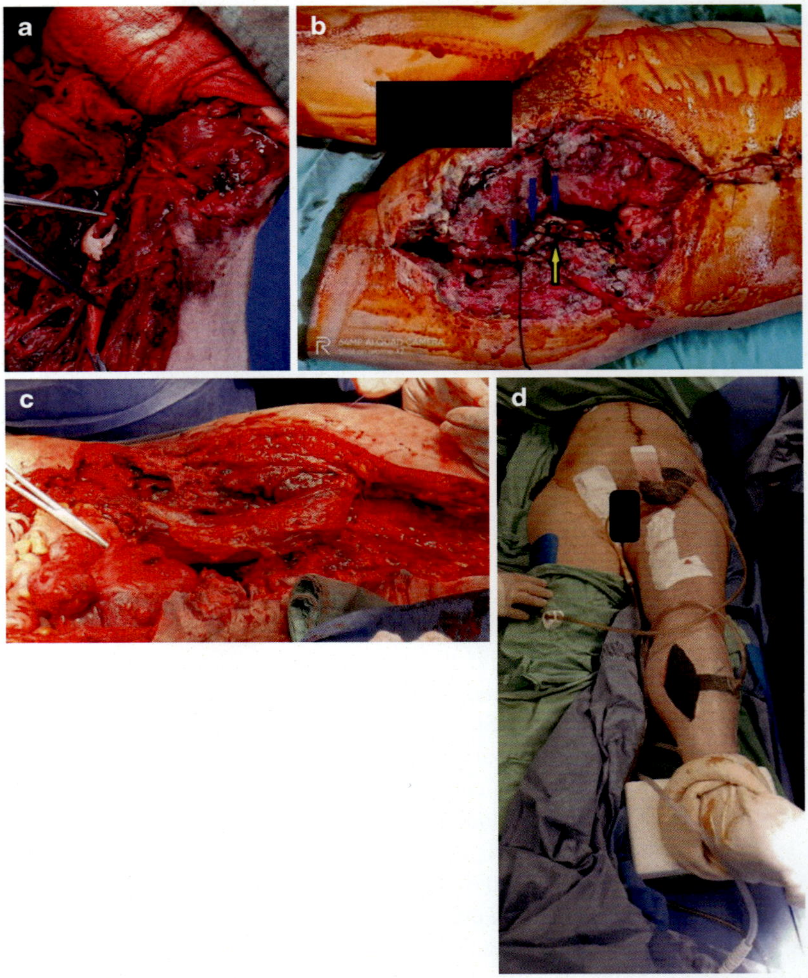

Fig. 41.5 Different stages of repair for a large inguinal blast defect. (**a**) Distal and proximal control of the vessel (femoral artery). (**b**) Temporary shunt with the silk ties – the yellow arrow showing the middle silk tie for placement reference. (**c**) Coverage of definitive repair with ipsilateral rotated sartorius muscle flap (**d**) Final bandaging with negative pressure dressings including prophylaxis fasciotomy

grafts only as a last resort. It is important to understand the challenges of these complex cases to save first the life and then the limb. Figure 41.5a–d illustrates the steps taken following a blast injury.

Nonoperative Management

Not all vascular trauma will require surgical intervention. Patients with low-velocity injuries, patients who have intact circulation or perfusion, patients who are not actively hemorrhaging and have no hard signs of bleeding, and those with minimal vessel defects or small (<2 cm) pseudoaneurysms detected on duplex ultrasound are candidates for initial observation and nonoperative management. Patients who do not present signs of distal ischemia and do not have a defect greater than 2 cm, nor have any extravasation on initial evaluation, also deserve to be observed. Out of these, only 9% required further surgical treatment [23]. In another report by the same authors about 309 patients with injuries in proximity to major vessels who were all observed clinically without any imaging study, only 4 progressed to requiring surgery. This concludes that physical examination alone is safe to evaluate occult vascular injuries, which results in excellent long-term outcomes. These results, along with many others, have proven that there is no need for initial invasive diagnostic evaluations that may be very difficult, if not impossible, in LMICs. As long as there are no hard signs of bleeding, suspected ischemia, or danger to the limb, nonoperative management is both indicated and feasible, especially in LMICs. The nonoperative approach, however, mandates close follow-up of the patient with a duplex ultrasound for at least 2 weeks (stay near the center) and a low threshold for surgical intervention in case of any change in the limb status.

Follow-up remains a critical component of vascular surgery. Anticoagulation use is strongly dependent on availability and resources. Trauma patients in LMICs (wars and road traffic accidents (RTAs) usually have the luxury of being young with healthy vessels or have few risk factors for atherosclerosis. For most vascular repairs (short conduits/grafts) in such patients, no anticoagulation is needed with the exception of those over 45 who might benefit from aspirin therapy.

Abdominal Vascular Trauma

Abdominal vascular trauma is a major challenge under any circumstances and worse in a station rural hospital in LMICs with likely shortage of necessary resources. The vast majority of such injuries are secondary to gunshot wounds and knife wounds along with blast wounds, usually secondary to armed conflicts. Blunt injuries can also cause vascular injuries, especially rapid deceleration, crushing injuries, or falls from heights, which all can result in avulsion of vessels or intimal tears, which then leads to thrombosis or to pseudoaneurysms.

Initial Assessment

Any patient who is hypovolemic and/or in shock should be considered as bleeding until proven otherwise. If there are no obvious signs of bleeding, intraabdominal vascular source of exsanguination is a high suspect if the abdomen has been injured. Abdominal distention and/or peritonitis may be initial physical signs, but the patient may initially present with minimal or no signs and respond adequately to fluid replacement. With retroperitoneal tamponade of a vascular injury, patient may become asymptomatic before crashing or may be asymptomatic initially with a thrombosis or intimal injury. Regardless of the patient's condition, large-bore access, preferably in the upper extremities, is the primary intervention along with an attempt to prepare matched blood for transfusion if it becomes necessary. Permissive hypotension technique, if possible, is an alternative until intraoperative control is obtained.

Radiologic assessment with an abdominal X-ray with wound markers may be helpful to trace the track of a penetrating injury with bullet or knife. A Focused Assessment with Sonography in Trauma (FAST) may be helpful to identify hemoperitoneum but is not useful for retroperitoneal bleed. CT scan with contrast is most useful to identify specific vascular injuries but generally is available only in major medical centers in LMICs. To ascertain that abdominal hemorrhage is the cause of blood loss, diagnostic peritoneal lavage or aspiration (DPL or DPA) is indicated in the emergency room, done with a little cutdown, under direct vision.

As stated previously, unstable patients should be immediately transferred to the operating room. If they appear terminal in the emergency room, the only way to stop the bleeding, besides thoracotomy and cross clamping of the aorta above the diaphragm, is the use of the resuscitative endovascular balloon occlusion of the aorta (REBOA) (Fig. 41.6). Visiting faculty may bring this with them since it may not be available in most areas in LMICs. REBOA insertion may be taught to non-physicians and is relatively simple and minimally invasive while offering an excellent temporizing control of intraabdominal bleeding on the way to the OR.

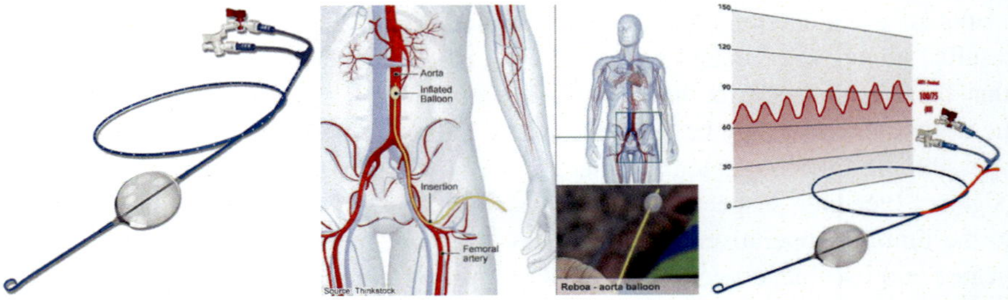

Fig. 41.6 Placement of catheter and ER-REBOA PLUS and pREBOA-PRO catheters. *Source: Copyright Prytime Medical Devices, Inc. All Rights Reserved. Reprinted with permission*

Operative Approaches to Intraabdominal Bleeding

Initial exploration is vital to rule out any other injuries. To avoid further clotting problems, the OR should be warm. There should be blood available and a cell saver, if possible. One can be created to be maintained on call [24]. Once inside the abdomen, all four quadrants are packed, and after removal of all free blood and clots, the three zones of the retroperitoneum are systematically explored. Here any bleeding vessels which should be temporarily clamped off with vascular clamps, vessel-loops, or Rummel tourniquets; with large vessels the intraluminal use of Foley catheters may be very useful. Zone 1 contains all middle vessels including the aorta and IVC with their branches. Zone 2 extends laterally from the renal vessels to the paracolic gutters, and Zone 3 does the same from the bifurcation of the aorta to the pelvis. In Zone 1, all hematomas should be explored, while in Zones 2 and 3, hematomas from penetrating trauma should be explored, while those from blunt injury should be left alone, unless they are expanding.

Initial control of any bleeding vessels is done with manual compression prior to proximal and distal direct control of the vessel. If control of bleeding cannot be obtained, then temporary compression or cross clamping of the aorta is done above the stomach or preferably the use of REBOA directed manually. As soon as control of the bleeding vessel(s) is obtained, aortic occlusion is released. Surrounding the vena cava is fraught with risk of tearing lumbar veins, and compression with sponge sticks should precede any manipulation of the large veins.

Management of Individual Abdominal Vessels

It is beyond this chapter to describe the various maneuvers to approach the front and back of the various large vessels, and the reader is guided to a standard text on vascular surgery. Suffice it to say that due to excellent collateral circulation, the celiac trunk and its branches may all be ligated if needed. Ligation of the common hepatic artery, if necessary, should be done proximal to the gastroduodenal artery takeoff to maximize collateral flow to the liver. Injury to the mesenteric artery may benefit by a bypass from the aorta to the distal segment of the transection with ligation of the proximal segment to avoid injury to the pancreas and its subsequent leak. As to injuries to the portal vein or the superior mesenteric vein, they can both be ligated with the proviso that that the subsequent bowel swelling will require vigorous postoperative fluid resuscitation to control peripheral hypovolemia. The left renal vein over the aorta can be divided and ligated to expose the ventral part of the aorta. Renal artery injuries may lead to sacrifice of one kidney if it is known that the other is well functioning, since renal artery reconstructions in emergency conditions may be very difficult and will usually require a bypass from the aorta or the ipsilateral iliac artery. Any injuries to the superior mesenteric artery should be repaired to avoid bowel ischemia; if it is ligated, second-look operation is required to evaluate small bowel viability. Hematomas over the duodenum should be explored even with blunt injury to confirm no duodenal injury. Injury to the infrahepatic vena cava repair may be difficult because of the lumbar veins. Compression with sponge sticks or use of an intravascular balloon for control of the vessel may be easiest. Approach to repair of the posterior wall is easiest through the anterior laceration if rotating by ligating the lumbar veins is difficult. Inferior vena cava may be ligated while the vena cava superior to the renal vein on the right needs to be repaired to preserve the right kidney. Portal vein may be ligated if the hepatic artery is preserved but will also require vigorous fluid resuscitation because of sudden intestinal edema.

Retroperitoneal Bleeding

Bleeding in the right upper quadrants, behind the liver is extremely difficult to control and packing this area for 24–48 hours is acceptable. If upon removal of the packs there is recurrent bleeding then the liver has to be elevated out of its fossa and there may be a need for passing a chest tube from the inferior vena cava to the right atrium to repair the back of the retrohepatic vena cava.

Injury to the right renal vein usually results in loss of that kidney (if the left is normal); if repair is needed, the easiest approach is to autotransplant it to the right iliac artery and vein after first cooling it with iced heparinized saline solution to prolong the tolerable 4–6-h ischemia time. Hematomas overlying the kidneys should be examined before making any decisions. Reconstruction of the arteries can be done with an interposition graft with saphenous or jugular vein (assuming that prosthetic graft is not available), from renal artery to hepatic on the right and to splenic artery on the left.

Injury to iliac vessels is exposed by extension of the midline incision, and after controlling the bleeding, internal iliac artery can be used to bypass an injury to the external iliac artery or be ligated and divided, which will better expose the iliac veins. The iliac veins may be ligated, preferably at the common iliac rather than external iliac to preserve better the pelvic collaterals. Their repair risks narrowing with thrombosis and possible pulmonary emboli. Distal injury to the internal iliac vein is best controlled by packing. In all these dissections, special care must be taken of the femoral nerve laterally next to the vein and the ureter medially as it crosses the common iliac artery.

Vessels smaller than 3 mm can be ligated, while those greater then 3 mm should be suture-ligated or if larger than 5 mm closed with a running suture for low-pressure vessels and two layers for high-pressure arteries. During repairs, it is important to touch the intima only very delicately, or not at all, and use stay sutures instead. Sizing of the patch is important to avoid oversize and aneurysmal dilatation and thrombus formation. With small vessels, both ends should be spatulated, and the use of a sterile angiocath or sterile feeding tube in both ends of the anastomoses will facilitate avoidance of suturing two walls together.

Repairs

The types of repairs are similar to those described previously for peripheral vessels and include primary repair or end-to-end anastomoses, patch repair with vein or prosthetic graft, or interposition graft with a vein or prosthetic graft. Sutures generally used are 3–0 or 4–0 polypropylene (Proline(R)) for large vessels like the aorta and IVC, 4–0 to 5–0 for smaller vessels (iliacs), and 5–0 or 6–0 for still smaller (mesenteric or renal); silk sutures may be substituted if Proline is not available. Prior to completing the repair, the proximal clamp should be released to flush out any clots or debris and heparin solution instilled into the vessel. Heparinization following repair of vessels in trauma is highly debatable and generally avoided as discussed previously in this chapter. All repair and suture lines should be separated from the intestine and other organs with soft tissue such as an omental pedicle to avoid fistula formation.

Postoperative Care

Patients who have their portal vein or superior mesenteric vein ligated will need.

intense fluid resuscitation, while some may have to return to the OR for a second look at bowel viability. Ligation of IVC or iliac veins requires leg elevation and elastic stockings or Ace bandage wrapping to avoid leg edema. Possible thromboses of small vessels, pseudoaneurysm formation, embolism, and vascular breakdown of the anastomoses with infection or without are problems that may be encountered and require patient proximity to hospital staff for about 3–4 weeks.

Nontraumatic Vascular Emergencies

Introduction

Nontraumatic vascular pathology represents a heterogeneous group of conditions and a growing concern worldwide. In 2010, a study from the Global Burden of Disease reported the incidence of peripheral vascular disease had doubled [25]. The very rapid rate of aging among the global population and rapid urbanization, sedentary lifestyles, tobacco use, and poor dietary habits have led to seven out of ten deaths in LMICs to be due to noncommunicable diseases (NCDs) Additionally, life expectancy is increasing in LMICs, resulting in a concomitant rise in chronic vascular diseases [25, 26]. The incidence of well-described risk factors for vascular complications including hypertension, cardiovascular disease, obesity, diabetes mellitus, and chronic kidney disease also continues to rise in LMICs, not only in the elderly but also in the younger age group. Despite that, many hospitals in LMICs still perform more vascular procedures for injury than for peripheral vascular disease (PVD). Many vascular conditions exist along a continuum of disease, which can make discerning acute changes from chronic problems challenging in resource-poor settings. Delays in recognition and timely triage of vascular emergencies portend increased morbidity and mortality in patients in LMICs and strain their underequipped, understaffed, and undertrained healthcare systems. Unfortunately, surgical assessments in LMICs have rarely focused on essential equipment, supplies, and personnel for provision of vascular care.

In 2016, multinational consensus recommendations were published in an effort to better characterize the services and resources needed to provide essential vascular care [26]. This assessment was designed to outline the resources and services needed to assess and triage common vascular conditions at various levels of a national healthcare system, regardless of national income. As the burden of vascular disease continues to increase, it is essential for providers to understand the assessment and treatment options available in LMICs in order to provide high-quality patient care in any environment. Existing data suggest that outside of tertiary centers, perioperative equipment and supplies were not reliably available, even such as basic airway equipment and electronic cardiac monitoring. At some tertiary hospitals, there was lack of mechanical ventilation support, electronic cardiac monitoring, or arterial blood gas and blood chemistry analysis [25].

The advances in endovascular treatment of arterial and venous pathology in the last decade have been widespread in HICs. Endovascular treatment of vascular diseases has now replaced open surgical interventions in 70–80% of cases in majority of HICs. These advanced techniques have reached only a few major medical centers in LMICs for various reasons. The two main ones are lack of specialist training and lack and high cost of needed equipment and instrumentation. We will therefore focus in this chapter only on the urgent open surgical techniques for vascular interventions that are practical and safe when done by trained general surgeons. While general surgeons in HICs are now trained less in vascular surgery, general surgeons in LMICs continue to be trained in most surgical disciplines prior to entering the field of specializations, making them more qualified to perform urgent vascular operations where specialists are not available. The gap between PVD burden and vascular care capacity in LMICs remains wide and needs to be corrected, both in the local and regional hospitals, and especially in university centers as previously well described in a study in Ghana by Gyedu et al. [26].

Chronic Limb-Threatening Ischemia

Peripheral arterial disease (PAD) is diagnosed by abnormal or absent pedal pulses on physical exam. An essential additional diagnostic exam, that can be performed at any setting, is to perform and interpret an ankle-brachial index (ABI). The result of <0.9 as well as toe pressures <70 mmHg indicates arterial insufficiency and can be useful in patients with diabetes mellitus or with significant vessel calcifications. In early stages, PAD may be asymptomatic or patients can experience exercise-induced leg pain (claudication). The presence of rest pain, tissue loss, or gangrene for more than 2 weeks in patients with PAD is considered diagnostic for chronic limb-threatening ischemia (CLTI).

The prevalence of CLTI worldwide is unknown and likely variable based on regional epidemiologic risk factors and different cultural and social practices. Large population-based studies tend to assess the prevalence of PAD, which can be extrapolated to estimate the prevalence of CLTI. In 2013, a systematic review published in *The Lancet* estimated that approximately 202 million people were living with PAD; however, they did note significant discrepancies across the six WHO-defined regions [27]. Survey-based data of the US population estimated the overall prevalence of PAD at 4.6% [28] as compared to two countries identified in sub-Saharan Africa where by observational studies, prevalence of PAD was higher at 14.8% [29] The lack of accurate prevalence data in LMIC, especially within healthcare systems where patients present with late-stage pathology, makes the estimation of the PAD burden in LMICs very difficult. In any context, patients with evidence of CLTI merit urgent referral to a vascular specialist at a tertiary center to minimize complications and improve outcomes.

In 2019, a committee comprised of members from three multinational vascular surgical societies published the Global Vascular Guidelines for the management of CLTI [30]. Within these recommendations, the authors advocate strongly for (1) accurate staging the extent of disease with CLTI, (2) appropriate recommendations for evidence-based revascularization, and, most importantly, (3) transfer to an adequately equipped tertiary center with well-trained staff. Classically, chronic limb ischemia was defined using the Fontaine or Rutherford classifications; however, in 2014, the Society for Vascular Surgery proposed a new classification for stratifying chronically threatened limbs based on three clinical parameters: wound, infection, and ischemia (WIfI) classification [31]. This new grading system offered several advantages but specifically accounted for the presence or absence of infection, which dramatically impacts the success of limb salvage. Although revascularization is the mainstay treatment of CLTI, patients should continue to receive appropriate medical therapy to minimize the damage from vascular disease including cardiac optimization, glycemic and lipid control, daily exercise, and, most importantly, insistence on tobacco cessation. Discussion of CLTI must include a wide variety of vascular insufficiencies with a variety of pathologies that are beyond the purpose of this chapter since the major chronic vascular problems, as compared to the acute events, need to be addressed in LMICs in tertiary (usually university) centers, which are adequately staffed by trained personnel and have adequate diagnostic and therapeutic equipment, as well as vascular instruments, sutures, and prosthetic grafts. These are usually lacking in primary local and even in many regional hospitals [25]. Aortoiliac atherosclerotic disease, often described as inflow disease, should be suspected in vasculopaths with nonpalpable femoral pulses. These patients should be promptly transferred to tertiary centers whenever possible, once stabilized. The approach to ruptured aortic aneurysm is similar to that described briefly to management of the traumatic injury of the aorta. Elective treatment of infrainguinal disease and tibioperoneal disease should also be promptly transferred to the care of specialists unless gangrene with sepsis has intervened, in which case an amputation may be required to save the patient's life. Even the presence of early gangrene should prompt transfer to a tertiary center for revascularization and to save as much of the leg as possible with adequate blood supply to the skin flap to allow good healing of the stump and fitting of a prosthesis.

Acute Limb and Cerebral Ischemia

As contrasted with chronic limb-threatening ischemia, acute limb ischemia (ALI) is the onset of new ischemic symptoms with duration of less than 2 weeks. Outside of the context of trauma, ALI is most commonly attributed to thromboembolic disease frequently associated with cardiac arrhythmias and/or plaques in the aorta and main.

vessels. Brain ischemia can also be acute and transient and must be promptly addressed to avoid a devastating neurologic complication. It also is frequently due to emboli but may be due to gradual narrowing of the internal carotid artery, which may need early intervention at a tertiary center.

Thromboemboli

Legs

The emboli to the legs, and rarely to the arms, should be clinically suspected in patients with new onset of sudden acute limb pain, paresthesia, and pallor of the extremity. Pulselessness and paralysis represent late findings. The Rutherford classification for acute limb ischemia is used to assess the severity of a threatened limb and is based on physical examination, which includes skin color, venous filing, and motor and sensory function. It also includes the presence of Doppler flow signals in pedal arteries. The differential diagnosis between an embolus coming from above, usually the heart or the aorta, and a thrombosis on the basis of progressive narrowing of the arteries secondary to atherosclerosis may be difficult without an arteriogram, which is generally not available in regional or local hospitals in LMICs. If the episode is acute, with an arrhythmia preceding it, and if there is no previous history of claudication, rest pain, or chronic skin changes, it is most likely due to an embolus. Therapeutic anticoagulation with intravenous (IV) heparin should be promptly instituted. If transfer to a tertiary center is impossible in the next 8–12 h and the leg is deteriorating, an attempt at removal of the clot may be attempted cautiously by a general surgeon. The pulse by palpation or Doppler will be strongest just above the clot and decreased or absent below it by palpation or preferably by Doppler. The clot usually stops at the bifurcation of the vessels (superficial/profunda femoral or at the division of the popliteal artery in the leg or the division of the radial/ulnar in the arm). The skin incision should be made over the suspected site of clot, and if a Fogarty balloon catheter is not available (which is likely in LMICs), an attempt at aspirating the thrombus (AT) should be made with a fine catheter and a 60 cc syringe by gently "milking" the clot out of the vessel by pressing on the leg and "rolling" a rolled towel upward, without breaking the clot. AT is typically reserved for a small *thrombus* that is discrete. It is generally not effective for long occlusions or large thrombus burden. AT is suited for an embolus lodged at the bifurcation of tibial vessels or within a stenotic segment of a vessel. The closer the diameter of the vessel size to the outer diameter of the guiding catheter tip, which should reach the clot, the more likely a good suction mechanism may be quickly generated, and the thrombus is aspirated. A 60 cc syringe is used, and a fast aspiration is created as shown in Fig. 41.7. Once the thrombus lodges itself in the catheter, aspiration stops. Keeping the negative pressure on the syringe and pulling the guiding catheter out will show the trapped thrombus in the catheter. 1.

Once the clot is extracted, the vessel should be irrigated with heparinized saline solution and closed with 5–0 Proline, if available, or silk. An alternative approach is to try to dissolve the clot by direct thrombolysis with a percutaneous catheter using tissue plasminogen activator (TPA) if it is available by slowly infusing it over 12 h into the vessel. This is a preferable method for acute venous thrombosis of the iliac veins. It may lead to bleeding from other sites and from the site of cannulation; it should be used, even by experts, only where close monitoring, adequate nursing, and radiologic support are available.

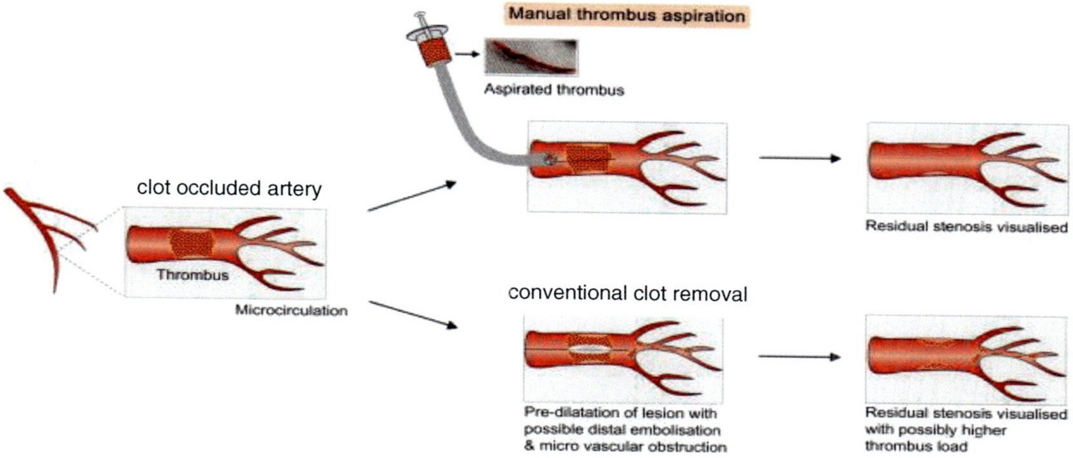

Fig. 41.7 Aspiration thrombectomy may be particularly effective for popliteal and tibial vessels. A large-lumen catheter (6 F–8 F) connected to a 60 mL syringe is advanced into the proximal aspect of the occlusion, vacuum is attached by aspirating the syringe, and the thrombus is aspirated into the catheter and removed from the artery [32]. *Source: Nicolas W.Shammas Chap. 32 - Thrombotic Lesions in the Lower Extremity Peripheral Arteries: Diagnosis and Management, Editor(s): On Topaz, Cardiovascular Thrombus, Academic Press, 2018, Pages 459–467) Academic Press*

Brain

The emboli can also go to the brain and lead to a stroke following transient ischemic attack (TIA). Diagnosis can be made by history of sudden weakness or paresis on one side (paresis), sudden transient monoclonal blindness (amaurosis fugax), and slurred speech. The symptoms generally resolve in 24–48 h. The patient should be anticoagulated if the diagnosis is confirmed by history (especially an arrhythmia), a bruit over the carotid artery on one side and decreased pulse, and, most importantly, an arterial Duplex ultrasound (USD), which may not be available and which requires a trained and experienced practitioner and/or technician. When such diagnosis is suspected, the patient should be transferred promptly to a tertiary center where diagnosis can be confirmed, therapeutic anticoagulation be undertaken, and operative intervention, if indicated, be carried out with appropriate anesthesia and recovery room support.

Acute Limb Ischemia

Similar to CLTI, data regarding the prevalence of ALI within LMIC is limited. Understanding the impact of acute limb ischemia is critically important as ALI confers significant morbidity and mortality. Healthcare systems in LMIC may have limited ability to urgently provide rapid care. Prolonged time to revascularization is associated with worse outcomes. In Ethiopia, a 2014 review of patients presenting with ALI reported an average time to intervention was 9 days and no patients presented within 24 h of symptom onset. ALI is a surgical emergency, and its best treatment is expeditious referral to a tertiary center.

Need Assessment

Many vascular care capacity assessments in LMICs have demonstrated marked deficiencies in items of diagnosis and perioperative and vascular surgical care. Deficiencies were most often due to absence of equipment, lack of training, and technology breakage. Imaging studies such as Doppler ultrasound in expert hands and contrast-enhanced cross-sectional imaging are important adjuncts in making the diagnosis and can provide additional information for operative planning. Unfortunately, they are almost never found in local or even regional hospitals in most LMICs and are even sometimes not available in major hospitals [25]. Assessing distal arterial signals with a handheld Doppler probe, which is more frequently available, is also an important part of the assessment of a patient with ALI. Therapeutic anticoagulation with heparin should be promptly initiated in the absence of strong contraindication. The surgical management of ALI centers upon assessing the viability of the afflicted extremity and then performing revascularization, almost always following transfer to a tertiary center, or a limb amputation as indicated by sepsis and/or by long delay following the onset of gangrene and of indicated transfer. Patients with prolonged ischemia, even without overt signs of tissue necrosis, may not be amenable to limb salvage due to the risk of reperfusion injury.

When the limb is considered salvageable, there are several techniques that can be used to reestablish flow. The feasibility of these different approaches is likely to be dictated by available resources. Providers in local hospitals in LMICs are often non-surgeons with little to no vascular training or experience. While these providers are valuable for patients with common risk conditions for PVD that require preventive instructions and prophylactic treatment with medications such as aspiring, statins, and beta-blockers, they have at best moderate skill to treat ALI effectively (e.g., amputation for lower-extremity gangrene or even toe amputations). They are relatively ineffective, except for diagnosis, for patients with complex surgical conditions, especially those who require advanced vascular surgery. Such patients must be promptly transferred to a tertiary center where an open surgical bypass of an occluded segment using an autologous vein graft or a PTFE (polytetrafluoroethylene) graft (if available) needs to be performed for thrombosis secondary to atherosclerosis. For embolism, clot extraction by Fogarty embolectomy, which revolutionized the ability to restore perfusion within the native vessel, or by an earlier basic aspiration technique with soft rubber catheters is indicated. Ready access to standard-sized #3, #4, and #6 Fogarty embolectomy catheters has been recognized by expert consensus as essential and is recommended [25]. Catheter-directed lysis (CDL) and percutaneous thrombectomy are newer treatment approaches and are typically performed in well-equipped tertiary centers for acute occlusions due to thrombotic etiologies. Both of these techniques require the expertise of an endovascular specialist and the ability to perform angiography. CDL/Percutaneous thrombectomy needs expensive medications, post-op monitoring, and higher rates of reintervention, all of which may not be feasible in most LMICs at this time. Training in these areas is badly needed, and dedication of appropriate resources should be guided by individual countries' need evaluations and action.

Diabetic Foot Syndrome

In 2019, the International Diabetes Federation estimated the global prevalence of diabetes to be 493 million people and is expected to increase by 25% by the year 2030 [33]. Diabetes mellitus is a well-described risk factor for multiple vascular conditions including coronary artery disease, cerebrovascular disease, and PAD. The microvascular sequelae of poorly controlled diabetes mellitus pose significant personal and social burdens including retinopathy, renal failure, and poor wound healing. The WHO has proposed the term diabetic foot syndrome (DFS) as an all-encompassing term to describe any ulceration distal to the ankle in a diabetic patient and any associated stigmata of infection or ischemia [34]. This ulceration is most commonly attributed to diabetic neuropathy and occurs along pressure points of the foot; however, it can also be secondary to chronically non-healing wounds or minor traumatic injuries. For inexperienced practitioners, diabetic foot syndrome can be challenging to manage as it may present with either a minimally symptomatic minor wound or a severe life- and limb-threatening infection.

The estimated prevalence of diabetic foot syndrome within LMIC is variable depending upon different risk factors, diet, and access to primary care. One cross-sectional study in Kenya estimated the prevalence of DFS at their tertiary referral center as 4.6% [35]. Other studies have reported that up to 15% of patients with diabetes will develop a foot ulcer during their lifetime. Improving glycemic control, appropriate footwear (not walking barefoot), and regular foot exams are important first steps in the prevention of diabetic foot syndrome.

Limb Salvage: Treating Ischemia and Infections

Once infection develops in the foot or toes in a diabetic patient, intravenous antibiotic treatment must be initiated and with the patient admitted, at any sign of progression and/or lymphangitis (red streaking), and drainage of pus from the web space between toes, amputation of the toes, or even a partial foot amputation must be considered. Prompt transfer to a tertiary hospital is indicated. If that cannot be done, amputation of the toe(s) should be performed as drainage procedure and should extend to the area of tissue bleeding of the cut surface. After careful homeostasis using fine absorbable sutures (*not silk or Proline*) and cutting the bone at least 1 cm back of the cut surface of muscles followed by copious irrigation with saline, the wound should be loosely packed and left open to granulate and drain. Daily moist dressing changes should follow during postoperative care along with intravenous antibiotics.

If the patient presents with neglected foot infection that has ascended beyond the ankle with physical findings of swelling, redness, pain, drainage of pus from the toe web space or any site, fever, and/or other signs of sepsis, below-the-knee leg amputation (BKA) must be considered. If there is no improvement or if there is progression in ascending infection or sepsis despite intravenous antibiotics and leg elevation, amputation is urgent to avoid septic death. Patient should be transferred to a tertiary center if possible. If a delay is unavoidable, a general surgeon should be capable to perform BKA by cutting the skin circumferentially a handbreadth (6 inches) below the distal patella and then in "cone"-like fashion cutting back the groups of muscles securing homeostasis with non-absorbable sutures, except for large vessels (tibial, peroneal, popliteal) with silk sutures; the nerve should be cut as high as possible and allowed to retract and not be tied to avoid a neuroma. The bones should be cut well above the level of the cut muscles (at least 1.5 inches) and beveled on their external surfaces to avoid sharp ends that may impinge on the skin. Closure following irrigation with saline should be in layers with fascia and subcutaneous layer closed loosely with interrupted non-absorbable sutures and the skin reapproximated without tension with interrupted nylon or silk sutures tied loosely (avoiding compressing the skin with forceps) (Fig. 41.8). We do not recommend drains as long as homeostasis is well secured. Carefully applied dressing with padding over the stump and wound, without any pressure to allow for swelling, is a critical part of this procedure with the concern of skin necrosis due to borderline vascular supply. The stump should be elevated, and dressing should be changed in 3–5 days, if there is no bleeding, fever, or pain, each of which would prompt earlier change. Steps in the amputation are outlined in Fig. 8 showing the incision (can be circumferential or "fish mouth with longer posterior flap"), amputation with bone cut back, and stump closed in three layers.

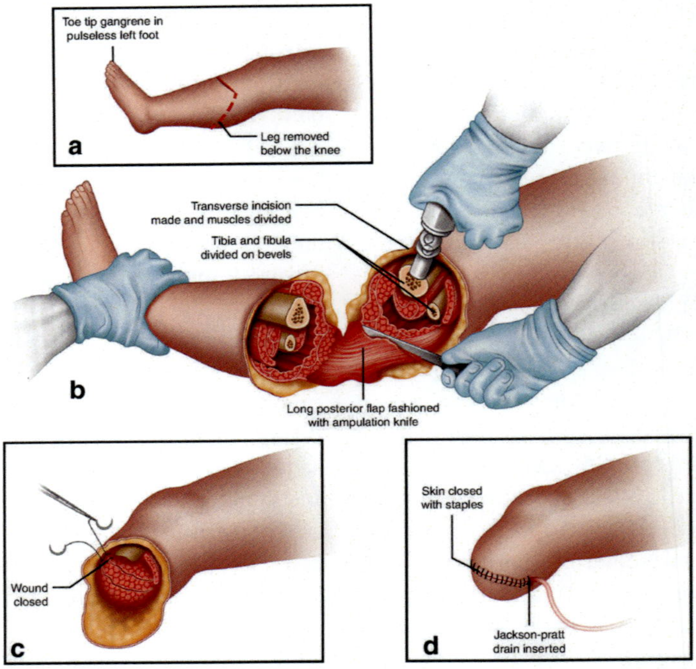

Fig. 41.8 The Stages of a Below Knee Amputation (BKA). (**a**) To mark location of incision & level of amputation, (**b**)Amputation with maintaining posterior muscle flap, (**c**) Wound closure, showing posterior skin flap, (**d**) Skin closure showing the posterior flap brought anterior, with drain placement. *Source: Ahmad, I. (2020). In: Karamanos, E. (eds) Common Surgeries Made Easy. 2020, Springer, Cham*

Deep Vein Thrombosis

A major effort needs to be directed to the prevention and early identification of patients at risk of deep vein thrombosis (e.g., hospitalized, injured, and postsurgical procedures). This requires few resources but may be life-saving in preventing pulmonary emboli, which may be fatal. This risk is especially high after orthopedic, or any major operative procedure, when the patient remains supine and immobile for a long time on the operating table and may not be adequately prophylaxed with heparin and/or intermittent pneumatic compression (IPC) device (not likely to be available).

Detection and treatment of deep vein thrombosis consist mainly of history of acute pain, swelling of the lower extremity, and appropriate history of prolonged sitting (as in an airplane) or being supine (as in hospital for a fracture). On physical examination, there is pain on squeezing the swollen calf and on dorsiflexion of the foot. This should be confirmed with a Doppler exam, if it is available to localize the clot. Treatment with therapeutic heparin should be promptly instituted on high suspicion alone, if Duplex confirmation is not available. Continuation of anticoagulation with warfarin should be initiated only by a center that has monitoring capability and where the patient should be transferred.

Conclusion

In conclusion, vascular emergencies in any economic setting are challenging and require a thorough understanding of the pathophysiology of trauma and fundamental competency of the practice of vascular surgery. If the treating surgeon remembers the basic principles—life over limb, to use temporary shunts, to perform aggressive/multiple debridements, and to perform fasciotomies if there is any doubt – outcomes will be favorable in any geographic location. There are desperate needs for adequate vascular surgical skills in much of the world, especially in LMICs, and therefore potential role for bidirectional partnerships is important. It permits and encourages local surgeons to share and exchange knowledge and skills – between different academic and clinical centers.

References

1. Stewart BT, Gyedu A, Giannou C, Mishra B, Rich N, Wren SM, Mock C, Kushner AL, Alexander P, Amponsah-Manu F, Dardik A. Consensus recommendations for essential vascular care in low-and middle-income countries. J Vasc Surg. 2016;64(6):1770–9.
2. Song P, Rudan D, Zhu Y, Fowkes FJ, Rahimi K, Fowkes FG, Rudan I. Global, regional, and national prevalence and risk factors for peripheral artery disease in 2015: an updated systematic review and analysis. Lancet Glob Health. 2019;7(8):e1020–30.
3. Gebregiorgis D, Nega B, Seyoum N. A perspective of extremity vascular trauma epidemiology and its management in a resource limited set up. Clinical Surgery Research Communications. 2021;5(3):27–34.
4. Eastridge BJ, Holcomb JB, Shackelford S. Outcomes of traumatic hemorrhagic shock and the epidemiology of preventable death from injury. Transfusion. 2019;59(S2):1423–8.
5. Parvin-Nejad FP, Padmanaban V, Jalloh S, Barrie U, Sifri ZC. Stop the bleed in rural Sierra Leone: one year of interventions and outcomes by nursing trainees. J Surg Res. 2022;273:79–84.
6. Frija G, Blažić I, Frush DP, Hierath M, Kawooya M, Donoso-Bach L, Brkljačić B. How to improve access to medical imaging in low-and middle-income countries? EClinicalMedicine. 2021;38:101034.
7. Jamil H, Tariq W, Ameer MA, Asghar MS, Mahmood H, Tahir MJ, Yousaf Z. Interventional radiology in low-and middle-income countries. Annals of Medicine and Surgery. 2022;77:103594.
8. Kobayashi L, Coimbra R, Goes Jr AM, Reva V, Santorelli J, Moore EE, Galante J, Abu-Zidan F, Peitzman AB, Ordonez C, Maier RV. American Association for the Surgery of Trauma–World Society of Emergency Surgery guidelines on diagnosis and management of peripheral vascular injuries. J Trauma Acute Care Surg 2020 89(6):1183–1196.
9. Hemingway J, Adjei E, Desikan S, Gross J, Tran N, Singh N, Starnes B, Quiroga E. Lowering the Ankle–Brachial Index Threshold in Blunt Lower Extremity Trauma May Prevent Unnecessary Imaging. Ann Vasc Surg 2020 62:106–113.
10. Rehman ZU, Riaz A, Nazir Z. Peripheral arterial injuries in children: an audit at a University Hospital in Developing Country. Ann Vasc Dis. 2020;13(2):158–62.
11. Kauvar DS, Dubick MA, Walters TJ, Kragh JF Jr. Systematic review of prehospital tourniquet use in civilian limb trauma. J Trauma Acute Care Surg. 2018;84(5):819–25.
12. Orcutt MB, Levine BA, Gaskill HV, Sirinek KR. Civilian vascular trauma of the upper extremity. J Trauma. 1986;26(1):63–7.
13. Navsaria P, Thoma M, Nicol A. Foley catheter balloon tamponade for life-threatening hemorrhage in penetrating neck trauma. World J Surg. 2006;30(7):1265–8.
14. Henry A. Extensile Exposures. New York, London: WB Saunders; 1973.
15. Kobayashi L, Coimbra R, Goes Jr AM, Reva V, Santorelli J, Moore EE, Galante JM, Abu-Zidan F, Peitzman AB, Ordonez CA, Maier RV. American Association for the Surgery of Trauma–World Society of Emergency Surgery guidelines on diagnosis and management of abdominal vascular injuries. J Trauma Acute Care Surg 2020 89(6):1197–1211.
16. Ketenciler S, Boyacıoğlu K, Akdemir İ, Kömürcü G, Polat A. Autologous saphenous vein panel graft for vascular reconstruction. Ann Vasc Surg. 2018;53:117–22.
17. Klocker J, Bertoldi A, Benda B, Pellegrini L, Gorny O, Fraedrich G. Outcome after interposition of vein grafts for arterial repair of extremity injuries in civilians. J Vasc Surg. 2014;59(6):1633–7.
18. Maduba CC, Nnadozie UU, Modekwe VI, Nwankwo EU. Comparing hospital stay and patient satisfaction in a resource poor setting using conventional and locally adapted negative pressure wound dressing methods in management of leg ulcers with split skin grafts: a comparative prospective study. Pan African Medical Journal. 2020;36(1)
19. Granchi T, Schmittling Z, Vasquez J Jr, Schreiber M, Wall M. Prolonged use of intraluminal arterial shunts without systemic anticoagulation. Am J Surg. 2000;180(6):493–7.
20. Timberlake GA, Kerstein MD. Venous injury: to repair or ligate, the dilemma revisited. Am Surg. 1995;61(2):139–45.
21. Kluckner M, Gratl A, Gruber L, Frech A, Gummerer M, Enzmann FK, Wipper S, Klocker J. Predictors for the need for fasciotomy after arterial vascular trauma of the lower extremity. Injury. 2021;52(8):2160–5.
22. Ratnayake A, Worlton TJ. Role of prophylactic fasciotomy in contemporary vascular trauma practices. Injury. 2022;53(2):811–2.
23. Dennis JW, Frykberg ER, Veldenz HC, Huffman S, Menawat SS. Validation of nonoperative management of occult vascular injuries and accuracy of physical examination alone in penetrating extremity trauma: 5-to 10-year follow-up. J Trauma Acute Care Surg. 1998;44(2):243–53.
24. How to Build a Cell Saver - YouTube https://www.youtube.com
25. Stewart BT, Gyedu A, Giannou C, Mishra B, Rich N, Wren SM, Mock C, Kushner AL. Essential vascular care guidelines study group. Consensus recommendations for essential vascular care in low- and middle-income countries. J Vasc Surg.

2016;64(6):1770–1779.e1. https://doi.org/10.1016/j.jvs.2016.05.046. Epub 2016 Jul 16. PMID: 27432199; PMCID: PMC5121001

26. Gyedu A, Stewart BT, Nakua E, Quansah R, Donkor P, Mock C, Hardy M, Yangni-Angate KH. Assessment of risk of peripheral vascular disease and vascular care capacity in low- and middle-income countries. Br J Surg. 2016;103(1):51–9. https://doi.org/10.1002/bjs.9956. Epub 2015 Nov 12. PMID: 26560502; PMCID: PMC4715606
27. Fowkes FG, Rudan D, Rudan I, Aboyans V, Denenberg JO, McDermott MM, Norman PE, Sampson UK, Williams LJ, Mensah GA, Criqui MH. Comparison of global estimates of prevalence and risk factors for peripheral artery disease in 2000 and 2010: a systematic review and analysis. Lancet. 2013;382(9901):1329–40. https://doi.org/10.1016/S0140-6736(13)61249-0. Epub 2013 Aug 1. PMID: 23915883.
28. Selvin E, Erlinger TP. Prevalence of and risk factors for peripheral arterial disease in the United States: results from the National Health and nutrition examination survey, 1999-2000. Circulation. 2004;110(6):738–43. https://doi.org/10.1161/01.CIR.0000137913.26087.F0. Epub 2004 Jul 19. PMID: 15262830.
29. Desormais I, Aboyans V, Guerchet M, Ndamba-Bandzouzi B, Mbelesso P, Dantoine T, Mohty D, Marin B, Preux PM, Lacroix P. EPIDEMCA investigators. Prevalence of peripheral artery disease in the elderly population in urban and rural areas of Central Africa: the EPIDEMCA study. Eur J Prev Cardiol. 2015;22(11):1462–72. https://doi.org/10.1177/2047487314557945. Epub 2014 Nov 6. PMID: 25376847
30. Conte MS, Bradbury AW, Kolh P, White JV, Dick F, Fitridge R, Mills JL, Ricco JB, Suresh KR, Murad MH, GVG Writing Group. Global vascular guidelines on the management of chronic limb-threatening ischemia. J Vasc Surg. 2019;69(6S):3S–125S.e40. https://doi.org/10.1016/j.jvs.2019.02.016. Epub 2019 May 28. Erratum in: J Vasc Surg. 2019 Aug;70(2):662. PMID: 31159978; PMCID: PMC8365864
31. Mills JL Sr, Conte MS, Armstrong DG, Pomposelli FB, Schanzer A, Sidawy AN, Andros G. Society for Vascular Surgery Lower Extremity Guidelines Committee. The Society for Vascular Surgery Lower Extremity Threatened Limb Classification System: risk stratification based on wound, ischemia, and foot infection (WIfI). J Vasc Surg. 2014;59(1):220–34.e1-2. https://doi.org/10.1016/j.jvs.2013.08.003. Epub 2013 Oct 12. PMID: 24126108
32. Shammas NW. Chapter 32 - thrombotic lesions in the lower extremity peripheral arteries: diagnosis and management. In: On topaz, cardiovascular thrombus. Academic Press; 2018. p. 459–67. https://doi.org/10.1016/B978-0-12-812615-8.00032-6.
33. Baril DT, Ghosh K, Rosen AB. Trends in the incidence, treatment, and outcomes of acute lower extremity ischemia in the United States Medicare population. J Vasc Surg. 2014;60(3):669–77.e2. https://doi.org/10.1016/j.jvs.2014.03.244. Epub 2014 Apr 24. PMID: 24768362; PMCID: PMC4492305
34. Saeedi P, Petersohn I, Salpea P, Malanda B, Karuranga S, Unwin N, Colagiuri S, Guariguata L, Motala AA, Ogurtsova K, Shaw JE, Bright D, Williams R. IDF diabetes atlas committee. Global and regional diabetes prevalence estimates for 2019 and projections for 2030 and 2045: results from the international diabetes federation diabetes atlas, 9th edition. Diabetes Res Clin Pract. 2019;157:107843. https://doi.org/10.1016/j.diabres.2019.107843. Epub 2019 Sep 10. PMID: 31518657
35. Jeffcoate WJ, Macfarlane RM, Fletcher EM. The description and classification of diabetic foot lesions. Diabet Med. 1993;10(7):676–9. https://doi.org/10.1111/j.1464-5491.1993.tb00144.x. PMID: 8403832

How to Manage Common Pediatric Surgical Conditions: Infant Emergencies, Hernias, Congenital Malformations in Low- and Middle-Income Countries

42

Rie Seu and Vincent Duron

It is easier to build strong children than to repair broken men.

– Frederick Douglass

Abbreviations

AFP	Alpha-fetoprotein
ARM	Anorectal malformation
BA	Biliary atresia
BWS	Beckwith-Wiedemann syndrome
CDH	Congenial diaphragmatic hernia
EA	Esophageal atresia
GER	Gastroesophageal reflux
HD	Hirschsprung's disease
HIC	High-income country
LHR	Lung-to-head ratio
LMIC	Low- and middle-income country
NICU	Neonatal intensive care unit
PN	Parenteral nutrition
PPV	Patent processus vaginalis
PS	Pyloric stenosis
TEF	Tracheoesophageal fistula
TFLV	Fetal lung volume measurement
TPN	Total parenteral nutrition
WHO	World Health Organization

R. Seu (✉)
Albert Einstein College of Medicine, Bronx, NY, USA
e-mail: rie.seu@einsteinmed.edu

V. Duron
Columbia University Vagelos College of Physician & Surgeons, NYP-Morgan Stanley Children's Hospital, New York, NY, USA
e-mail: vd2312@cumc.columbia.edu

Introduction: Pediatric Surgical Problems in Global Context

This text is not meant to be an exhaustive review of pediatric surgery or even pediatric surgery in developing countries. Rather, this chapter highlights several pediatric surgical conditions that the health practitioner caring for infants and children in a developing country should be able to recognize and diagnose. The chapter offers guidance to determine, depending on the skills and resources available, which conditions may be treated at the receiving facility and which need to be transferred to a higher level of care.

M. A. Hardy, B. R. Hochman (eds.), *Global Surgery*, https://doi.org/10.1007/978-3-031-28127-3_42

Stomach and Small Intestine

Pyloric Stenosis

Epidemiology

The prevalence of pyloric stenosis (PS) is 2 to 4 per 1000 live births [1]. The prevalence varies depending on the region, in which those of Caucasian descent have a higher prevalence of PS than Asian and Black populations [1]. The male-to-female ratio is 4:1 [2]. A study has also shown that PS is more common in less urban areas [2].

Etiology and Pathophysiology

The cause of the development of PS is unknown. It is thought that it is a combination of both genetic and environmental factors. With a hypertrophied pylorus, the gastric outlet is mechanically obstructed.

Due to excessive vomiting, there will be loss of gastric contents, leading to dehydration. As a result, the renin-angiotensin-aldosterone system (RAAS) will be activated. Aldosterone will stimulate the excretion of potassium and absorption of sodium. As potassium depletion worsens, sodium is resorbed in exchange for hydrogen ions, creating a paradoxical aciduria. This leads to *hypochloremic hypokalemic metabolic alkalosis.* Diagnostic delay can lead to hypoglycemia and hypoalbuminemia [1].

Risk Factors

Several risk factors have been associated with PS development. Maternal alcohol use and cigarette smoking are thought to be associated with PS [3]. Furthermore, prenatal and postnatal exposure to medications such as erythromycin has been associated with increased incidence of PS [4]. Other perinatal risk factors include being firstborn, prematurity, undergoing a cesarian delivery, young maternal age (less than 20 years old), and bottle-feeding [5]. Breastfeeding has been shown to be a protective factor [1].

Clinical Manifestations

Infants with PS are usually term infants who are otherwise healthy. They usually show up between 2 weeks and 3 months (median is 6 weeks) with *projectile, nonbilious emesis* after feeds [5]. The emesis resembles the feeds and should not be yellow/green, as the hypertrophied pylorus prevents bile reflux [4]. There may also be signs of dehydration and weight loss [4]. The infant may also display signs of jaundice. Hyperbilirubinemia occurs due to hepatic glucuronyl transferase activity deficiency from decreased PO intake [4].

Upon physical exam, one may be able to feel an olive-shaped mass in the right upper quadrant of the abdomen when the abdominal wall is completely relaxed [4]. If abdominal US is available, repeat palpation to feel the olive should be avoided, since it will only increase the irritation of an infant who is already fussy.

Management

If PS is suspected, an upper abdominal ultrasound is the image modality of choice. In the longitudinal view, muscle thickness greater than 3 mm and channel length greater than 15 mm is highly specific and sensitive for PS. In the transverse view, a target sign is seen [4] (Fig. 42.1). If US is not available, then transfer to higher level of care is advisable. If that is not possible, and an olive-shaped mass is palpated with the right clinical history, then surgical intervention should be considered.

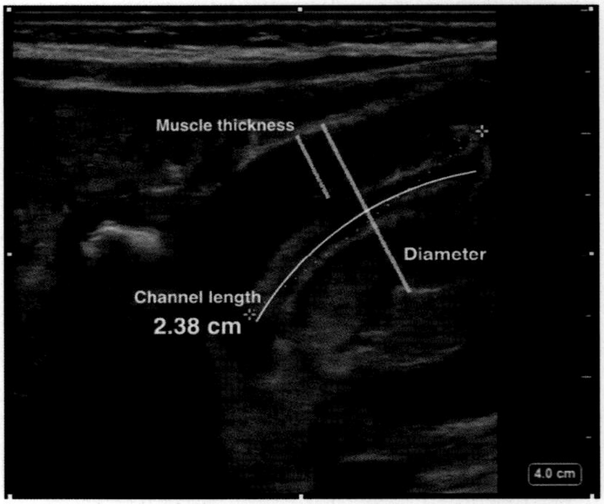

Fig. 42.1 Ultrasound images demonstrating pyloric stenosis. (https://med.emory.edu/departments/emergency-medicine/_images/ultrasound/image-week/channel-length.jpg)

Serum electrolytes should be measured prior to surgery, as electrolyte derangements are common with prolonged vomiting. Intravascular access should be promptly established. Preoperatively, electrolyte derangements and fluid depletion should be addressed. If the electrolyte disturbance is mild, it can be corrected with 0.45% normal saline (NS) with 5% dextrose (D5) solution. If there are severe disturbances, then 0.9% NS bolus of 10–20 mL/kg, followed with 0.9% NS with D5, should be used. Electrolyte disturbances, specifically severe hypochloremia and metabolic alkalosis, need to be corrected prior to surgery. For standard fluid management, 120 mL/kg using 0.45% NS and D5 with 10 mmol potassium chloride of 500 mL is advised only after the patient has urine output. If dehydration is severe, fluids can be increased to 150 mL/kg per 24 h [1]. Feeds should also be stopped when diagnosis is made. A nasogastric or orogastric tube can be used to empty gastric contents if there is persistent vomiting [4].

When the patient is stabilized and electrolyte levels are corrected, the infant can undergo surgical correction. A pyloromyotomy can be performed open, through a right upper quadrant or periumbilical incision, or laparascopically [4]. The steps elaborated here will be for the open approach [1] (Fig. 42.2):

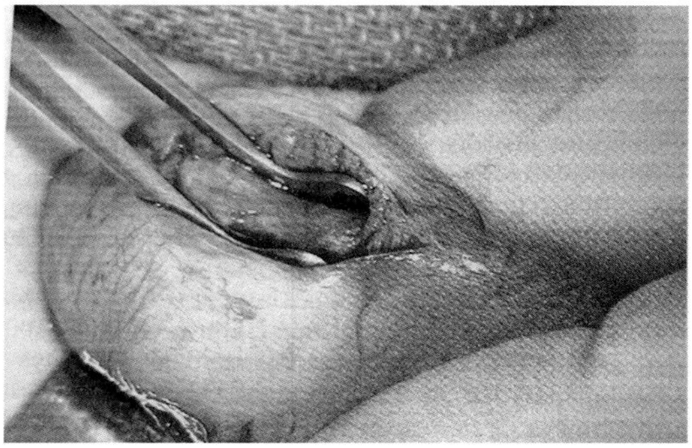

Fig. 42.2 Pyloromyotomy for hypertrophic pyloric stenosis. The thickened pyloric musculature has been cut and then spread apart to reveal the underlying mucosa. Source: Sabiston Textbook of Surgery, 17th Ed. Warren BW Chap. 70 p.2108, Fig70–8 (Elsevier)

1. A transverse incision is made in the right upper quadrant over the rectus muscle, 1 fingerbreadth below the costal margin.
2. The peritoneum is entered, and the omentum is brought into the wound to lift the transverse colon and identify the antrum of the stomach. The lower third of the stomach is elevated and mobilized to deliver the pylorus to through the incision.
3. At the mid-anterior surface of the pylorus, a longitudinal incision is made through the serosa and superficial muscularis. The incision is started 1–2 mm from the pyloroduodenal junction, marked by the vein of Mayo proximally to 0.5 cm into the lower antrum muscle layer.
4. Using a clamp or pyloric spreader, blunt dissection is performed to divide the firm fibers. Relief of obstruction is demonstrated by an upward protrusion of the gastric mucosa. Care is taken not to deepen the incision and injure the underlying mucosa.

Postoperatively, feeds can be started 3 h after returning from the recovery room. Maintenance fluids can also be continued postoperatively until the patient tolerates a diet [4].

Possible immediate surgical complications are mucosal perforation most frequently at the duodenal end. In this case, bilious fluid would be seen. This can be repaired using interrupted fine absorbable sutures. Other complications include bleeding, infection, and wound dehiscence [1]. Incomplete pyloromyotomy may occur if it is not of adequate length, most often because of a failure to extend the cut onto the stomach.

Neonatal Bowel Obstruction

Epidemiology

Neonatal intestinal obstructions arise from a variety of congenital anomalies of the gastrointestinal (GI) tract. More than 1 in 4000 births are affected by an obstruction of the duodenum, jejunum, ileum, and colon. Congenital atresia or stenosis of the duodenum is the most common intestinal atresia, which occurs in 1 in 5000–

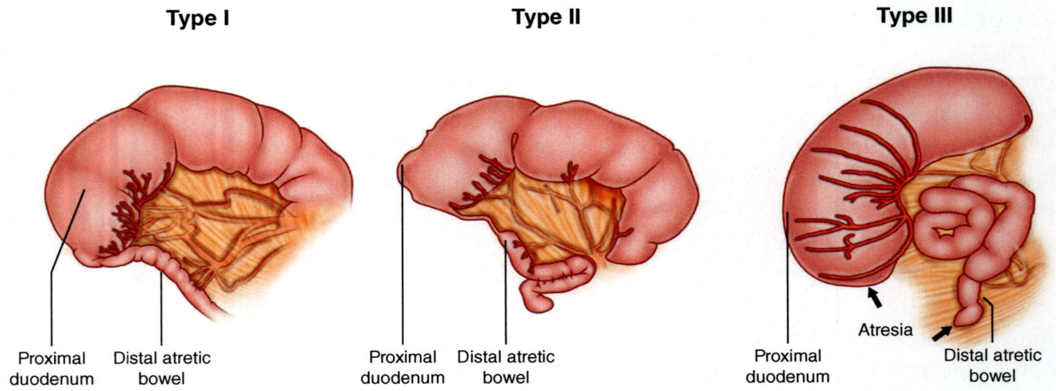

Fig. 42.3 Schematic of different types of duodenal atresia. Type 1, membrane or web causing duodenal obstruction; type 2, complete obliteration of duodenal segment with proximal and distal segments attached by fibrous cord; type 3, complete separation of proximal duodenum from distal duodenal segment (Reprint with permission, Artwork by Linda Li, MD, 2020)

10,000 live births [6]. Intestinal malrotation occurs in 1 in 6000 live births, although the true incidence is expected to be as high as 1% of the population [7].

Pathophysiology

Duodenal atresia is thought to occur because of failure of recanalization normally occurring by vacuolization of the duodenal lumen (Fig. 42.3) [8]. This mechanism differs from that which is thought to cause other types of intestinal atresias, which are thought to result from a vascular accident later on during gestation [9]. Intestinal rotation and fixation occur from the fifth to 12th weeks of gestation. During this time, the midgut naturally herniates through the umbilical ring as there is rapid intestinal growth. Any disruption of the steps of rotation and fixation will lead to rotational abnormalities or malrotation [10].

Risk Factors

The incidence of duodenal atresia is similar in males and females [11, 12]. Duodenal atresia is associated with other congenital anomalies in about half of patients, which include cardiac malformations, other intestinal atresias, biliary atresia, malrotation, gastroschisis, Hirschsprung's disease, anorectal malformations, renal defects, vertebral defects, and polysplenia. Duodenal atresia is associated with chromosomal and genetic syndromes. Approximately a third of patients with duodenal atresia have trisomy 21 [13–16].

In terms of jejunoileal atresias, one third of patients are premature. Maternal cigarette smoking and the use of vasoconstrictive medications in the first trimester of pregnancy have been shown to increase the risk of small bowel atresia [17]. Other congenital anomalies are seen in less than 10% of patients with jejunoileal atresia. Most common associations are gastroschisis, malrotation, and cystic fibrosis [18, 19].

Clinical Manifestations

In newborn infants, four signs raise the suspicion for and guide diagnosis and management of intestinal obstructions: [20].

1. Maternal polyhydramnios on prenatal ultrasound imaging.
2. Bilious vomiting, indicative of a proximal obstruction.
3. Failure to pass meconium in the first 48 h of life.
4. Abdominal distension, concerning for lower tract obstruction.

The presence of bilious vomiting in a newborn is a pathologic process and should raise the suspicion for malrotation with midgut volvulus until proven otherwise. Bilious vomiting occurs in infants when the obstruction is distal to the ampulla of Vater. A proximal obstruction will not usually be accompanied by abdominal distension (e.g., duodenal atresia, midgut volvulus). A more distal obstruction (e.g., ileal atresia, anorectal malformation) will usually be accompanied by abdominal distension.

The first step to diagnosis is a complete history and physical exam, including a prenatal history and any abnormal ultrasound findings if there was prenatal care. While 98% of women receive prenatal care and 94% give birth under the care of a skilled healthcare practitioner, the WHO estimates that less than 65% of women in LMICs do not receive adequate prenatal care [21, 22]. As such, there is a significant chance that a diagnosis of newborn intestinal obstruction will be made after birth in developing countries.

Management of these patients is as follows: (1) insertion of a nasogastric tube for decompression; (2) intravenous access to replenish GI losses and to hydrate for at least several days, most likely several weeks; and (3) parenteral nutrition, if available within 3 days if the infant is not feeding, and should include protein (many healthcare centers in LMICs will not have access to peripheral nutrition (PN), so crystalloid fluid will be administered).

Chest and abdominal x-rays should be obtained. If there is concern for malrotation, then an upper gastrointestinal intestinal contrast study should be obtained. In an infant with bilious vomiting and signs of distress – tense, red, or shiny abdomen, poor peripheral perfusion, lethargy, hemodynamic instability, electrolyte abnormalities – then an urgent exploratory laparotomy needs to be performed. In centers without access to radiologic studies or a pediatric surgeon, the patient should be stabilized and transferred to a higher level of care.

Infants with *duodenal atresia* will often also present with bilious vomiting. An abdominal x-ray will reveal a pathognomonic double bubble sign, delineating a dilated stomach and a dilated duodenum, most often without distal gas (Fig. 42.4). Unlike the management required of malrotation with midgut volvulus, duodenal atresia repair is not emergent and can be delayed until workup for associated anomalies has been completed. Until then, gastric decompression and IV fluid support are required.

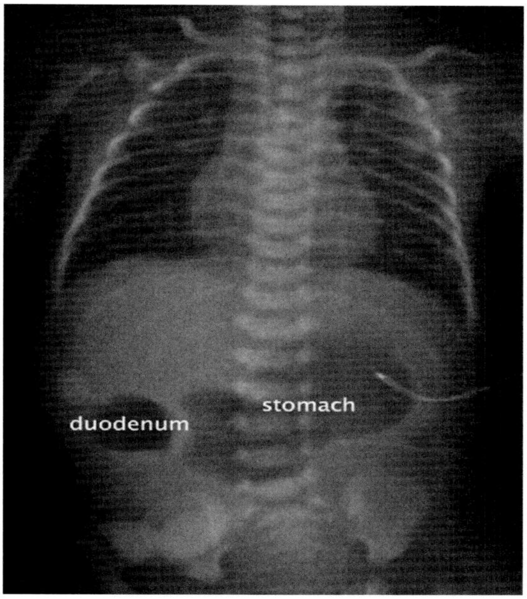

Fig. 42.4 Abdominal radiograph of neonate with double bubble sign with paucity of distal air, consistent with duodenal atresia

Jejunal and ileal atresia may be suspected on abdominal x-rays with dilated proximal loops of bowel and no distal air. A retrograde contrast enema will identify a microcolon which occurs from lack of passage of amniotic fluid during fetal life. As with duodenal atresia, repair may be planned after the patient has been rehydrated and prepared for surgery.

Short bowel syndrome may result from intestinal atresia if a there is insufficient length or inappropriate function of the small intestine. This is a chronic condition that may require long-term PN and specialized care for electrolyte, fluid, and bowel management. This condition is very difficult to treat in LMICs if resources are not available. Early transfer to centers with PN availability is necessary.

Management

Surgical repair of duodenal atresia is most often accomplished through a right upper quadrant incision. An exploration of the abdomen to examine organs and rotation of the intestines is first performed. The duodenum is mobilized using a Kocher maneuver. The anastomosis is classically performed with a diamond-shaped duodenoduodenostomy in which the proximal segment is opened through a transverse incision and the distal end through a longitudinal incision to connect the two ends in a diamond-shaped configuration. This is thought to maximize the lumen of the duodenum at the level of the anastomosis (Fig. 42.5). When this technique is difficult because of patient anatomy and in small or premature infants, a duodenojejunostomy is a good option. Prior to performing the anastomosis, a small-caliber Foley catheter should be passed proximally into the stomach and distally into the jejunum and pulled back with the balloon inflated, to ensure that there is no windsock deformity or additional web. A web may be resected or may be bypassed.

The classic procedure for malrotation with midgut volvulus is a Ladd procedure. The steps of a Ladd procedure are reproducible and include:

1. Evisceration of the bowel.
2. Counterclockwise detorsion of bowel until no longer torsed.
3. Division of Ladd's bands.
4. Broadening of the small bowel mesentery.
5. Appendectomy.
6. Placement of small bowel along the right abdomen and large colon along the left abdomen.

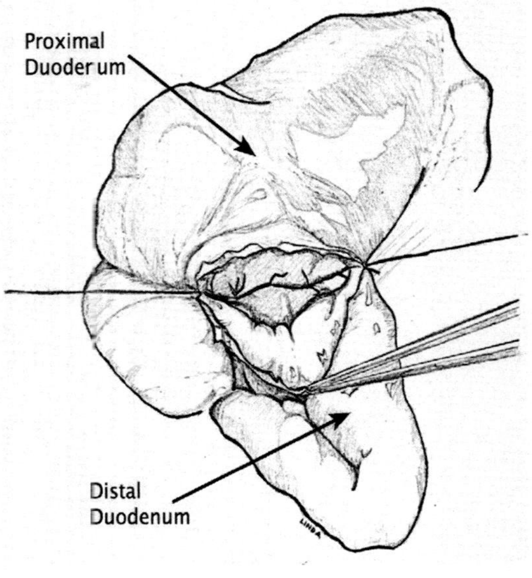

Fig. 42.5 Representation of diamond anastomosis technique (Reprint with permission, Artwork by Linda Li, MD, 2020)

During the Ladd's procedure, particularly if there is presence of midgut volvulus, temporary abdominal closure may be necessary if the abdomen is not able to be safely closed or if there is doubt about the viability of the remaining bowel. A temporary mesh may be sewed or a silo placed. A second look laparotomy within 24–48 h will allow the bowel to reperfuse, thus minimizing the length of resected bowel.

Biliary Atresia

Clinical Manifestations

The newborn will present to the healthcare facility with jaundice, acholic stools, dark urine, and hepatomegaly. If the condition continues for a few months, the infant may present with weight loss, irritability, and worsened jaundice. If presenting late, the infant will most likely have developed splenomegaly due to portal hypertension, ascites, and hemorrhage due to impaired vitamin K absorption. If biliary atresia (BA) is not treated, it will lead to cirrhosis and death [23].

Management

If an infant presents with jaundice for 2 weeks or more, they should be evaluated for biliary atresia. An evaluation can be done first via serologic tests, imaging, and biopsy. Liver function tests will show conjugated hyperbilirubinemia as well as elevated alkaline phosphatase and gamma-glutamyl transpeptidase [1]. An ultrasound can be done to differentiate different causes of infant cholestasis. After an infant fasts for 12 h, an infant with BA would show shrunken gallbladder, hyperechogenic liver hilum, or a cyst at the liver hilum and no bile duct dilation. A cholangiogram can also be done to assess the patency of the biliary tree. A percutaneous liver biopsy will show bile plugs, ductular proliferation, portal edema, and fibrosis [23].

Once diagnosis is made, treatment of BA is a Kasai hepatoportoenterostomy procedure. The failure to obtain bile drainage or the development of cirrhosis-related complications would be an indication of liver transplantation. Prior to the Kasai operation, the infant should be optimized with normal preoperative care, vitamin K provision several days prior to surgery, and monitoring of coagulation factors [1]. *The Kasai procedure is a technically challenging procedure that should be performed by a surgeon who has experience performing this surgery, in a hospital that has the resources to care for this complex patient.* Transfer to this type of setting should be done early during the diagnostic phase to optimize the patient's outcome.

Hernias

Inguinal Hernia

Epidemiology

The global incidence of inguinal hernias in children less than 18 years old ranges from 0.8 to 4% [24]. The most common type of inguinal hernia is on the right side (60%), although left-sided (25%) and bilateral hernias (15%) are found [25]. Indirect inguinal hernias make up more than 95% of inguinal hernias [25]. In infants and young children, incarceration of an unrepaired inguinal hernia could be as high as 31%, which could pose intestinal and testicular complications [26].

Pathophysiology

During fetal development, the testicle descends via the inguinal canal into the scrotum via the processus vaginalis, a sac-like protrusion of the peritoneum. Most of the time, this obliterates into a fibrous cord. If the processus vaginalis does not obliterate, it is called a patent processus vaginalis (PPV). This creates a canal for fluid or abdominal contents to pass. If only fluid passes, it is called a communicating hydrocele. If intestine, omentum, ovaries (in females), or other abdominal contents pass, it is an indirect inguinal hernia. It can be confined to either the inguinal region or in the scrotum. The cause of this is not completely understood [27].

Direct inguinal and femoral hernias are uncommon in young children. Direct inguinal hernias form medial to the inferior epigastric vessels in Hasselbach's triangle, due to weakness in the floor of the inguinal canal or after surgical repair of indirect inguinal hernias [1]. Femoral hernias form medial to the femoral vessels and are below the inguinal ligament [28].

Risk Factors

Inguinal hernias are more common in premature infants: a third of premature infants weighing less than 1000 g are predicted to develop a hernia [29]. Boys are six times more likely than girls to have inguinal hernias [27]. Other risk factors include family history of inguinal hernias, hypospadias, epispadias, exstrophy of bladder, and ambiguous genitalia [1].

Clinical Manifestations

Inguinal hernias can be apparent from the time of birth. They usually appear as an intermittent, painless bulge along the inguinal canal, in the scrotum, or in the labia [1]. An inguinal hernia may spontaneously reduce or be reduced manually. It may appear in situations of increased abdominal pressure, such as when the child is crying, coughing, or walking [1]. Upon physical exam, the physician can palpate the processus vaginalis over the pubic tubercle; a thick cord structure (silk glove sign) can signal the presence of a hernia sac [30].

Complicated inguinal hernias occur when hernia contents are not reducible. Symptoms can include tenderness and firmness of the bulge, vomiting, and refusal of feeds [29]. The hernia contents may be incarcerated, in which the mass is not tender [1]. An incarcerated hernia needs to be reduced and, if unable to be manually reduced, then needs to be surgically reduced and repaired. Incarcerated hernias can become strangulated or obstructed [1]. In the case of strangulation, the blood supply to the hernia contents is compromised, leading to infarction if not repaired. The child may have erythema at the site of the bulge, tachycardia, hypotension, and peritonitis [31]. This is a surgical emergency.

Management

Surgical herniotomy under general anesthesia within 2 weeks of diagnosis is advised for inguinal hernias, due to its possible complications such as incarceration, strangulation, and obstruction [29].

There are various methods to approach a herniotomy. The high ligation technique is most commonly performed in children. It is described below: [32].

1. An incision is made at the groin just superior and lateral to the pubis. The external oblique aponeurosis and external ring are exposed and incised in the direction of the muscle fibers.
2. The indirect hernia sac is identified and dissected; the cord structures are separated from the hernia sac, paying close attention not to injure the vas deferens, testicular artery, and testicular vein. Usually, the hernia sac is retracted anteromedially as this is its habitual anatomic location.
3. The hernia sac is opened, and the abdominal contents are reduced.
4. The sac is suture ligated at the preperitoneal level and transected distal to ties.
5. Hemostasis is ensured, and the external oblique aponeurosis is closed.
6. Scarpa's layer and the skin are closed, and a dressing is applied.

Complicated inguinal hernias are a surgical emergency. In addition to obstruction and strangulation, it can lead to bowel gangrene and perforation, peritonitis, septicemia, and intra-abdominal abscess formation [1]. Furthermore, there are concerns for not only the incarcerated bowel but also testicular vessels that are compressed in the hernia sac. If the child does not have signs of strangulation and if 24 h have not elapsed since the onset of symptoms, a manual hernia reduction can be attempted. If available, sedation and analgesia can be given to facilitate the reduction. While having the patient in as much Trendelenburg position as tolerated, the non-dominant hand should pull the hernia to make elongate it and make it more narrow. The dominant hand should gently compress the contents of the hernia in the direction of the inguinal canal to massage them into the abdominal cavity [31]. If manual reduction is not possible, surgical intervention is necessary.

Umbilical Hernia

Epidemiology and Risk Factors

The global incidence is 10–25%, although it seems to be more common in African countries for currently unknown reasons [33]. Umbilical hernias are more common in low-birth-weight and premature infants. There is also an increased risk of an umbilical hernia in children with Down and Beckwith-Wiedemann syndromes [1].

Pathophysiology

Umbilical hernias form due to the incomplete closure of the umbilical ring, where the umbilical vessels pass, during the first few weeks of infancy [30]. The full-thickness protrusion can include peritoneal fluid, preperitoneal fat, intestine, or omentum [1]. Small defects that are less than 1 cm are more likely to close, than larger defects that are greater than 2 cm [1].

Clinical Manifestations

Umbilical hernias manifest as a palpable protrusion at the umbilicus, which are reducible. They can be asymptomatic or tender upon pressure and palpation. Most umbilical hernias close by the second or third year of life, especially when small, although it can take until their teenage years.

Complications of concern are incarceration, strangulation, and rupture of umbilical hernias, although rare, about 1% [1]. The physical exam is essential to detect cases of these complications. Children will experience localized tenderness or pain, erythema of the skin or increased sensitivity at the umbilicus, and/or wound drainage [34].

Management

Non-operative management is advised during the first 4 years of life, especially if the defect is small and asymptomatic. In contrast, surgical repair is recommended for large hernias that become larger, for those that do not close by 4 years of age, and hernias with significant proboscoid components [1].

Treatment is advised if the child experiences signs or symptoms of incarceration or strangulation. If the defect is less than 0.5 cm, strangulation is less likely. However, studies have shown that both medium- and large-sized defects may be associated with incarceration and strangulation, although, again, the risk of this is low [35].

An open hernia repair under general anesthesia is advised, with an infraumbilical incision. The surgeon should remove the hernia sac, sew together the tissue along the muscle edge, and resecure the umbilicus to the underlying fascia. For complicated umbilical hernias or large defects, a mesh could be used to lessen the tension of the fascia and prevent the development of abdominal compartment syndrome. Although rare, patients can experience postoperative pain, seroma, hematoma, infection, and recurrence [36].

It is uncertain when surgery should be advised in LMICs. Earlier surgical treatment may also be considered for large hernias, as they are more likely to incarcerate and least likely to spontaneously close. Patients living more than 1 h away from surgical availability should also be considered for repair [1].

Abdominal Wall Defects

Gastroschisis

Epidemiology

The prevalence of gastroschisis ranges from 2.9 to 6.5 per 1000 infants [37]. It is more prevalent in the fetuses of younger mothers, particularly those less than 20 years old [37]. In HICs, survival rate exceeds 90%, due to improvements in neonatal care and nutrition [38, 39]. Nevertheless, in LMICs, mortality varies depending on the availability of NICU facilities and total parenteral nutrition (TPN) [40]. Some areas, such as in Zimbabwe and Uganda, report a mortality rate of more than 80% [41]. Gastroschisis is usually an isolated defect, although it has been associated with defects of other organ systems in 16–35% of cases, in particular gastrointestinal anomalies such as atresia [42].

Pathophysiology

The pathophysiology is not completely understood but is suspected to be due to a malformation during ventral wall closure in the embryonic period, possibly from an ischemic event, which leads to the herniation of bowel [42]. There may also be a gene-environment interaction, in which polymorphism and maternal smoking increase the risk for gastroschisis development in the fetus.

Clinical Manifestations

Gastroschisis is a ventral body wall defect, in which the intestines are freely floating in the amniotic fluid, *without an amnion covering* [42]. The fascial defect is usually at the right of the umbilicus. It is identified prenatally via ultrasound, most commonly during the second trimester [43] (Fig. 42.6). If laboratory tests are available, gastroschisis would show elevated maternal serum alpha fetoprotein when performed between 15 and 20 weeks' gestation [43].

Gastroschisis can be simple or complex. Complex gastroschisis describes a gastroschisis that is accompanied by intestinal complications, such as bowel atresia, stenosis, volvulus, perforation, or ischemia. These compounding factors can lead to greater morbidity and mortality of the infant. This occurs in 11–28% of gastroschisis cases [43].

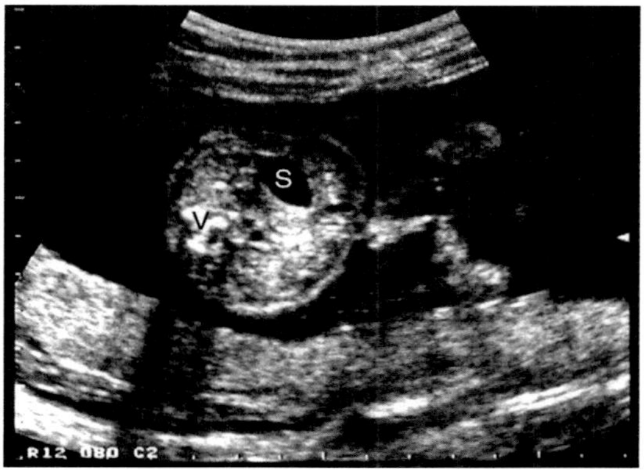

Fig. 42.6 Prenatal ultrasound image of gastroschisis

Management

If gastroschisis is diagnosed during prenatal care, it is recommended that the mother receives serial growth ultrasounds, due to the risk of intrauterine growth restriction, as well as twice-weekly antepartum fetal heart rate testing starting at 32–34 weeks [43]. It is important that delivery occurs in a tertiary pediatric surgery center, for surgical management post-delivery. Recent studies are attempting to determine the optimal time for delivery. A cost-effective analytical study showed that 38 weeks may balance the risks of respiratory distress syndrome and stillbirth [44]. It is recommended for the mother to undergo a vaginal delivery, unless indicated otherwise [43]. When the baby is born, *fluid resuscitation and minimization of insensible losses are the priority.* The patient must have large-bore IVs placed and be started on crystalloid fluid. The intestines must be placed in a bowel bag to prevent fluid loss from the exposed GI tract. A plastic bag may be placed over the lower half of the newborn. An NG tube will be placed. Surgical closure or silo placement may then be performed.

Surgical Management is Necessary The two most common methods are primary closure under general anesthesia or silo placement for several days followed by closure with or without a general anesthetic [1].

- **Primary closure**: the defect is slightly enlarged, and the abdomen is first explored to exclude other gastrointestinal anomalies. The bowel is then reduced into the abdomen. The fascial and skin layers are closed separately.
- **Silo closure**: A silo is used to encase the exposed bowel contents. If a silo is not available, IV solution bags or blood bags can be fashioned into silos. The infant should be in an incubator in supine position, with the silo hanging from the roof of the incubator. The bowel is gradually reduced into the abdominal cavity over several days, preferentially less in less than 7 days. The wound can be closed using a sutureless technique in which the preserved umbilical cord is used to cover the defect and covered by non-adherent dressing (Fig. 42.7). The advantage of this technique is that it may be performed at the bedside without anesthesia. Surgical closure may also be performed.

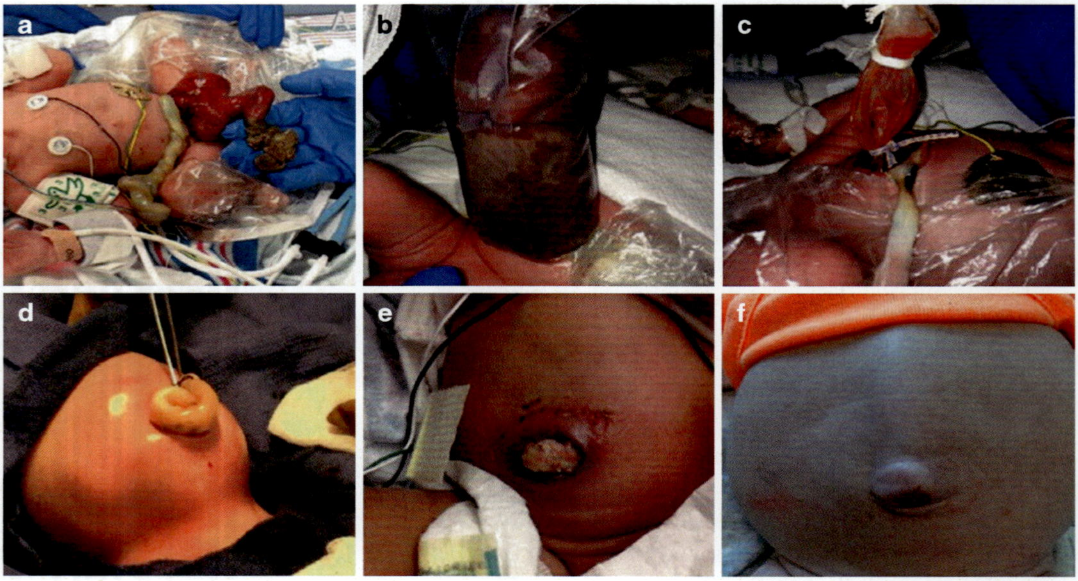

Fig. 42.7 Silo placement and sutureless closure of gastroschisis: (https://media.springernature.com/full/springer-static/image/art%3A10.1038%2Fs41372-019-0321-1/MediaObjects/41372_2019_321_Fig1_HTML.jpg)

Postoperatively, antibiotics are administered, and the patient is closely monitored. Possible complications of gastroschisis closure include abdominal compartment syndrome and respiratory distress due to splinting of the diaphragm. Reduced cardiac output and splanchnic perfusion pressure can cause oliguria and gut mucosal acidosis. Bowel ischemia can lead to necrotizing enterocolitis. Wound complications are also possible, which can lead to dehiscence, sepsis, and enterocutaneous fistula. Therefore, the infant should be closely monitored [45].

Previous studies have shown that silo closure may reduce need for respiratory support, reduce time to first feed, and lower infection rates without changes in outcomes, when compared to primary closure. In LMICs, silo closure may be advisable. NICUs are often not fully resourced or may be nonexistent in LMICs, which poses a problem as neonates recovering from the surgery and general anesthesia will need cardiorespiratory support after primary closure. Furthermore, neonates may often present to the hospital late with edematous and matted bowel, which increases the risk for abdominal compartment syndrome. Silo placement allows progressive reduction of the bowel as swelling decreases [46].

Parenteral nutrition is often needed for neonates with gastroschisis, as bowel function slowly improves. In cases of simple gastroschisis in high-income countries (HICs), TPN is given for 23 days and even longer in complex gastroschisis [46]. Early transfer to a higher level of care is recommended.

Omphalocele (Exomphalos)

Epidemiology

The incidence of omphalocele ranges from 1 in 4000 to 7000 live births [47]. Multiple anomalies are seen in 78–88% of cases of omphalocele [47]. Cardiac anomalies are seen in 50% of omphalocele births, gastrointestinal anomalies in 40% of the cases, and chromosomal anomalies in 30–40% of the cases [47].

Pathophysiology

Omphalocele is a midline abdominal wall defect that occurs between the sixth and 11th week of development. It occurs when bowel loops fail to rotate and return to the abdominal cavity after physiological herniation through the umbilical cord [45]. Although the bowel may be malrotated, it is functionally normal. The defect can include the small intestine and the liver and, in rare occasions, the spleen, stomach, bladder, uterus, and ovaries [48].

Risk Factors

Maternal risk factors include extremities in age, with increased incidence among those born to mothers with a BMI greater than 30 and aged less than 20 and more than 35 years old. Black infants were also more likely to have omphalocele than white infants. Patient risk factors included genetic and chromosomal anomalies, with trisomy 13, 18, and 21 as well as Beckwith-Wiedemann syndrome (BWS) being the most common [48]. 80–90% of newborns with trisomy 18 have omphalocele [48]. BWS is also associated with overgrowth, macroglossia, predisposition to embryonal tumors, and neonatal hypoglycemia [49].

Clinical Manifestations

Omphalocele is usually diagnosed prenatally via ultrasound, as early as 11–14 weeks' gestation. On the imaging, an anterior abdominal wall defect covered by a membrane is visualized (Fig. 42.8). A small omphalocele is less than

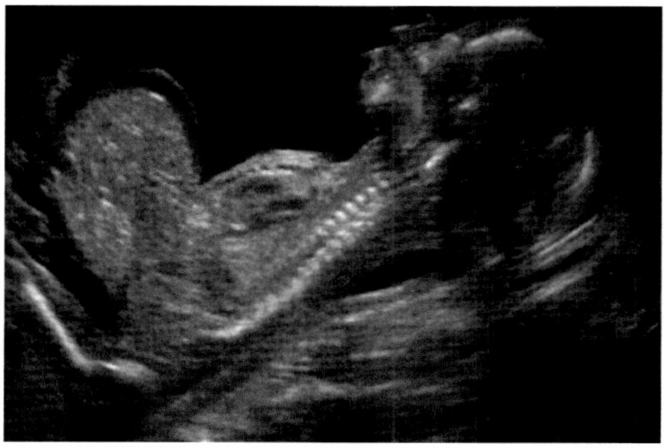

Fig. 42.8 Prenatal ultrasound showing giant omphalocele containing bowel and liver (https://www.chop.edu/sites/default/files/styles/gallery--main/public/ultrasound-fetal-ompha-canonical_0.jpg?itok=mkQ4KO5v)

5 cm and may contain parts of loops of small bowel. A large defect or "giant omphalocele" is usually defined as greater than 5 cm and containing liver [50].

Management

Herniated abdominal contents covered by a membrane are apparent on prenatal ultrasound (Fig. 42.6). Elevated maternal alpha-fetoprotein (AFP) levels are also associated with omphalocele. As omphaloceles are associated with other organ and genetic anomalies, comprehensive genetic testing should be done if possible. If resources are available, the mother should undergo chorionic villous sampling to detect for chromosomal abnormalities [50].

If the omphalocele is small, then a term vaginal delivery could be attempted. However, a cesarian section at term is usually indicated for large omphaloceles, to prevent sac rupture and organ damage [50]. If diagnosed prenatally, it is critical that the delivery takes place in a tertiary care center, where pediatric surgical care is available

After delivery, the pediatric team must assess cardiopulmonary function, due to concerns for cardiac anomalies. Giant omphaloceles are associated with pulmonary hypoplasia, which may require intubation and ventilation. If available, an echocardiogram and abdominal ultrasound should be done to assess for organ anomalies. Another concern is neonatal hypoglycemia, especially if the infant is suspected to have BWS. Intravenous access is necessary for fluid resuscitation, particularly if the sac has ruptured. A nasogastric or orogastric tube should be inserted and put on suction. A primary closure may be entertained for small- to medium-sized defects (2–4 cm) [45].

More commonly, a staged abdominal wall closure will be performed, as the fascial layer often cannot be closed without undue tension. If the sac is unruptured, the "paint and wait approach" can be undertaken (Fig. 42.9). In LMICs, this approach is recommended for all but the smallest omphaloceles. Topical agents, such as silver sulfadiazine, are used for eschar formation over the

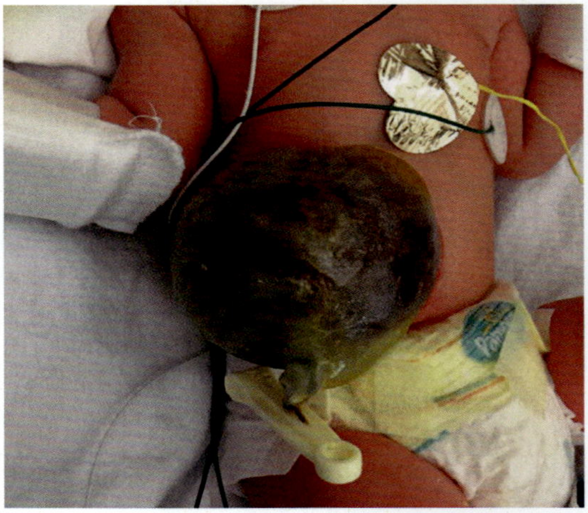

Fig. 42.9 Eschar formation over hernia sac during "paint and wait" treatment of giant omphalocele

amniotic sac, which promotes epithelialization over time. This will form a ventral hernia, which will be repaired later in life. Topical agents that have been used are mercurochrome solution, 70–90% alcohol, and silver sulfadiazine. Our preference is silver sulfadiazine. A crepe bandage is applied around the circumference of the abdomen, to maintain constant pressure to the omphalocele. The bandage and gauze can be changed every one to two days and should be checked for infection. With this method, the infant's hospital stay may be reduced to 7–10 days, with outpatient follow-up. Once the hernia sac is epithelialized, a compression dressing is fashioned to allow progressive reduction of abdominal contents, usually within a few months [1, 45].

Thoracic Congenital Malformations

Esophageal Atresia

Epidemiology

The global prevalence of esophageal atresia (EA) and tracheoesophageal fistula (TEF) is approximately 1 in 3000 births [51]. In more than 50% of infants, EA/TEF is associated with other clinical defects, particularly VACTERL (vertebral, anorectal, cardiac, tracheoesophageal, renal, and limb defects) and CHARGE (coloboma, heart defects, atresia choanae, retarded development, genital hypoplasia, ear abnormalities) associations. It is also associated with chromosomal anomalies, such as trisomy 18 and 21 and DiGeorge syndrome [51].

Pathophysiology

Esophagotracheal anomalies develop around 3–4 weeks of gestation, as both the trachea and esophagus develop from the common primitive foregut. The respiratory and digestive tubes are separated by lateral ingrowth of the epithelial ridges. Defects in mesenchymal proliferation during this process have been associated with EA or TEF formation [51]. There are five types of EA and TEF: (a) EA without fistula (7%), (b) EA with proximal TEF (2%), (c) EA with distal TEF (86%), (d) EA with proximal and distal TEF (<1%), (e) H-type TEF (4%) (Fig. 42.10).

Risk Factors

The most recent classification method of risks regarding EA was created by Spitz et al. in 1994. According to the study, the two major factors of survival of newborns with EA are birth weight and the presence of cardiac anomalies. If the newborn's birth weight is greater than 1500 g and without any cardiac anomalies, survival could be as high as 97%. However, if the newborn's birth weight is less than 1500 g or has cardiac anomalies, the survival is around 59%. If the newborn has both factors, the survival is 22% [52]. This classification system may be used early when deciding what intervention to offer the patient and whether to transfer the patient to a facility with more resources.

Clinical Malformations

Prenatal diagnosis is challenging – it occurs in 24–32% of the cases. A prenatal scan is known to be approximately 42% sensitive and a positive predictive value of 56% [1]. The main signs are maternal polyhydramnios, a small or absent stomach bubble at the 20-week anomaly scan, or blind-ending dilated upper esophageal pouch (also known as the "pouch sign") at 32 weeks.

Diagnosis of EA is usually made during the first 24 h of life. An orogastric catheter is not able to be passed more than 11 or 12 centimeters. Furthermore, in the nursery, the newborn could have symptoms of excess salivation, cyanotic episodes, and suffocation during breastfeeding [53].

The most common anomalies are of the cardiovascular system (23%), musculoskeletal system (18%), anorectal and intestinal organs (16%), urogenital system (15%), head and neck anomalies (10%), mediastinum (8%), and chromosomal anomalies (5.5%). The most common cardiac anomalies are ventricular septal defects and tetralogy of Fallot [53].

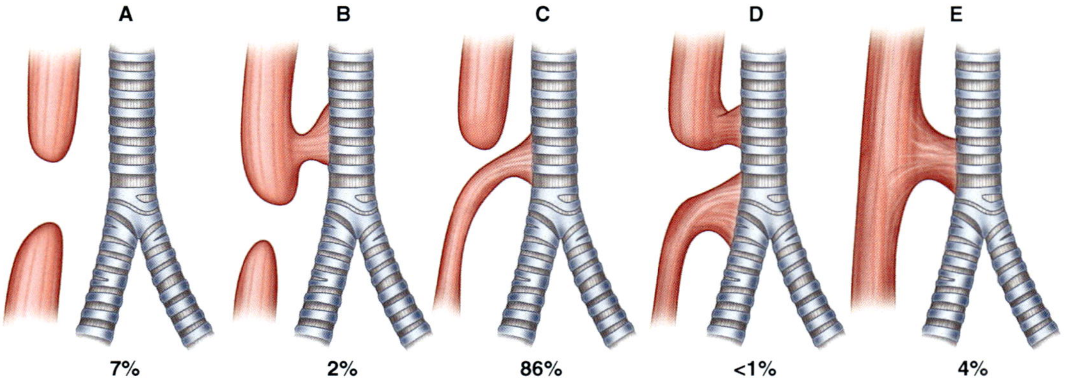

Fig. 42.10 Gross classification of esophageal atresia (Pardy et al.) [54]

Management

If diagnosed prenatally, karyotyping is recommended to diagnose chromosomal abnormalities and have a better idea of prognosis of the fetus. Delivery is also recommended at a tertiary care center, where pediatric surgery services are available [1]. A fetal magnetic resonance imaging to visualize the pouch sign had the highest sensitivity (94.7%) of EA detection. However, this is costly and usually not available in LMICs [54].

If EA/TEF is suspected, abdominal and chest x-rays with a radiopaque nasogastric tube should be done after delivery (Fig. 42.11). It will be the most informative for confirmation of EA/TEF, diagnosis of associated anomalies, and visualization of a possible duodenal atresia. A renal ultrasound, cardiac workup, and karyotyping (if not done already) should be done to assess for associated anomalies. Cardiac echocardiogram will indicate the sidedness of the aortic arch, which will determine operative approach [1].

Preoperatively, it is important to stabilize the newborn. Endotracheal intubation is avoided as positive pressure ventilation may pass through the fistula and cause severe gastric distension and injury. The proximal pouch is also suctioned with close monitoring to ensure satisfactory function of the suction tube. Intravascular access and monitoring of vital signs should be done [53]. EA/TEF should be surgically corrected within 24 h. If the patient is demonstrating respiratory compromise, emergent ligation of the TEF or gastrostomy is indicated. Ligation of the fistula allows the most efficient redirection of ventilatory flow into the airway. However, if surgical skill is limited to gastrostomy creation, this option prevents gastric overdistension and rupture. In a setting with high-level NICU care, gastrostomy creation alone with meticulous proximal pouch suction may also be considered as it maintains the thoracic cavity untouched for future repair. A patient born with isolated esophageal atresia should undergo gastrostomy tube creation with delayed repair of the EA. EA/TEF is a complicated anomaly which requires a robust neonatology and surgery team. Early transfer of patients after stabilizing surgery is recommended. Temporizing the proximal pouch secretions may be dealt with meticulous naso-esophageal tube suctioning or with creation of cervical esophagostomy ("spit" fistula). EA/TEF repair is performed through the following steps: [1].

1. A suction catheter is placed into the proximal esophageal pouch.
2. A muscle-sparing thoracotomy is made below the right scapula. (If it is a right-sided

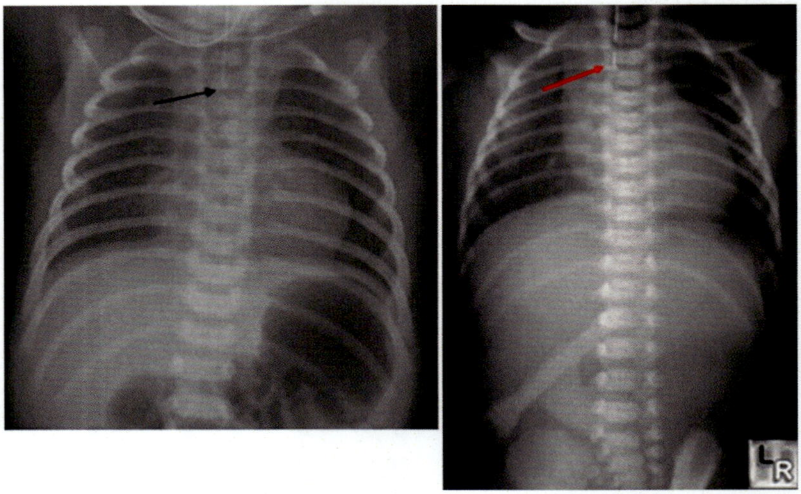

Fig. 42.11 Babygram of EA with and without TEF. Note the distal air in the photo on the left. (https://www.semanticscholar.org/paper/Oesophageal-atresia.-Beale-Lakhoo/a539b7c36552c8246b37eef4c92c9c2d9415826b/figure/1)

aortic arch, a left thoracotomy is often performed.)

3. The fourth intercostal space is opened at the superior margin of the fifth rib.
4. An extrapleural dissection is performed to identify the azygos vein. The azygos vein is often tied and divided to maximize visualization of the posterior mediastinum.
5. The tracheoesophageal fistula is then identified, isolated, and divided with a 1 mm cuff at the trachea. The cuff is sewn with a nonabsorbable suture.
6. A feeding tube is passed down to the distal esophagus to ensure its patency and to empty the stomach.
7. The upper atretic esophagus is identified as the anesthesiologist provides downward tension using the catheter.
8. A transverse incision is made at the distal end of the proximal pouch to open it.
9. A single-layer, end-to-end anastomosis is made using interrupted absorbable sutures. The posterior layer is performed first.
10. The feeding tube is guided through the anastomosis to ensure its patency and prevent back walling during creation of the anterior layer of the anastomosis, which is then safely completed.

There are numerous postoperative complications that one must consider. Anastomotic leaks occur in 15–20% of the cases. Drainage is usually contained to the extrapleural space; therefore, the neonate should be monitored via parenteral nutrition and drainage, until the leak is healed. Esophageal strictures occur in about 30–40% of the cases and are more common in patients who have had anastomotic leaks, anastomotic tension, or gastroesophageal reflux. Treatment is dilatation under general anesthesia. GER occurs in 40–65% of the patients. It can be treated clinically via dietary modification, positioning of the infant, and medications such as omeprazole. If unsuccessful, Nissen fundoplication is sometimes needed. Esophageal dysmotility is very common in these patients. Infants may experience symptoms of aspiration, dysphagia, or food bolus obstruction. Tracheomalacia is also a common finding in children with TEF, due to structural and functional weakness of the trachea leading to tracheal lumen obstruction. However it is only clinically significant in 10–20% of the patients, and the symptoms improve with age [53].

Congenital Diaphragmatic Hernia (CDH)

Epidemiology

The global prevalence of CDH is 2.3 in 10,000 births [55]. However, the hidden prenatal mortality of CDH makes its true prevalence higher. Posterolateral defects (Bochdalek hernia) make up 70–75% of the cases, 23–28%% are due to an anterior-medial defect (Morgagni hernia), and 2–7% are due to central defects [56]. A defect on the left side is more common than one on the right [1]. If it is an isolated case of CDH, survival rate is 70–80%. However, patients who require ECMO have a survival rate approximately of approximately 50% [57].

Etiology and Pathophysiology

Diaphragm development occurs between the 4th and 12th weeks of fetal development. The development of CDH is still poorly understood. The current hypothesis is the "dual-hit hypothesis," in which pulmonary hypoplasia occurs before diaphragm development. The first insult is bilateral lung hypoplasia prior to full development of the diaphragm, due to both genetic and environmental factors. The second insult only affects the lung ipsilateral to the diaphragm defect, due to chemoreceptor signaling from compression of the lung by herniated abdominal organs [57]. Lung hypoplasia is associated with smaller area for gas exchange, thickened alveolar walls, and increased interstitial tissues. The smaller cross-sectional area of the pulmonary vessels leads to vascular remodeling and hypertrophy of the muscle layer of the arteries, which can cause persistent pulmonary hypertension [57].

In cases of severe CDH, pulmonary changes can also invariably affect the cardiovascular system. Abdominal contents in the thoracic cavity can cause rotation of the heart, leading to decreased blood flow across the foramen ovale, leading to decreased filling of the left side of the heart and therefore decreased left ventricle (LV) growth. Therefore, the combination of pulmonary arterial hypertension, right ventricular hypertrophy, and LV hypoplasia can lead to severe pulmonary hypertension [57].

Risk Factors

CDH is more prevalent in male infants. Also, mothers older than 35 have a higher risk for having infants with CDH [55]. Forty percent of CDH cases are associated with chromosomal and genetic anomalies [56]. The most common chromosomal anomalies are trisomy 18, 13, and 21 (in order of prevalence) [55]. Some genetic syndromes associated with CDH are Fryns syndrome and Cornelia de Lange syndrome [56]. Pulmonary and cardiovascular anomalies are common in newborns with CDH [56].

Clinical Manifestations

CDH is usually diagnosed prenatally, via fetal ultrasound. Abdominal organs are noted herniated into the thoracic cavity [56] (Fig. 42.12). Indirect signs include polyhydramnios, mediastinal shift, or abnormal cardiac axis [56]. Severity of CDH can be determined by lung size, position of the liver and stomach, lung-to-head ratio (LHR), and presence of other congenital anomalies [58]. An LHR less than 1.0 at 24 weeks' gestation predicts a high likelihood of perinatal mortality [58].

In LMICs where fetal ultrasound is not regularly available, newborns will more commonly present postnatally with respiratory distress. The patient may have symptoms such as grunting, poor feeding, tachypnea, and cyanosis. Upon physical exam, the affected hemithorax will have decreased respiratory movement. On the affected side, upon auscultation, one may hear decreased breath sounds and audible bowel sounds. X-ray will show herniated abdominal contents into the thoracic cavity on the affected side (Fig. 42.13). If the patient presents late, there may be signs of failure to thrive and poor respiratory reserve during exercise [1]. There are very few places in LMICs where ECMO is available to rescue the infant.

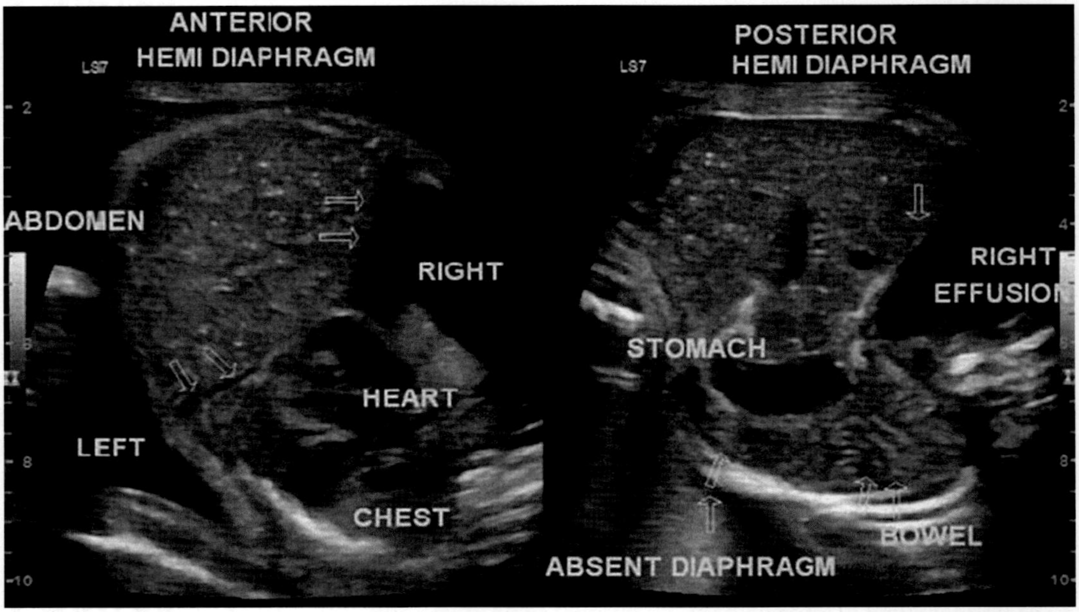

Fig. 42.12 Prenatal US image of CDH with herniation of abdominal contents into thoracic cavity (https://prod-images-static.radiopaedia.org/images/26757938/fc720f9cc37d26a755821af8f47736_big_gallery.jpeg)

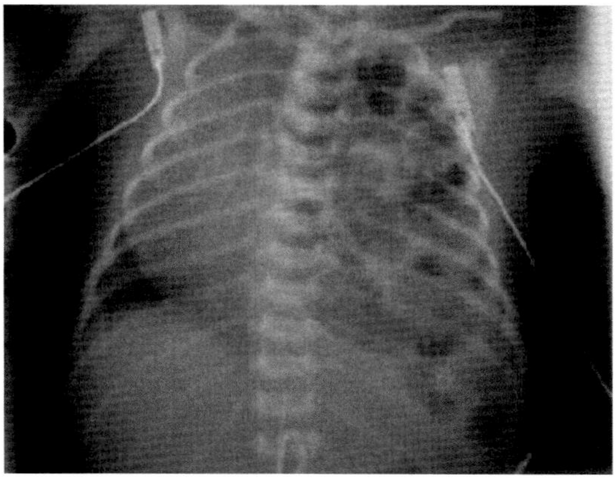

Fig. 42.13 Chest x-ray showing left CDH with herniation of intestines into thoracic cavity. https://img.medscapestatic.com/pi/meds/ckb/66/21866tn.jpg X-ray imaging of CDH

Management

If diagnosed prenatally, prenatal counseling for the mother is essential. She can be advised of the possible complications of CDH as well as congenital anomalies that may accompany this condition. Ultrasound surveillance is recommended to monitor for any prenatal complications. It is essential for patients with CDH to be delivered at a tertiary hospital with access to a NICU and pediatric surgeons [56]. The best outcomes are with a term delivery; there are no differences in survival outcomes for spontaneous vaginal delivery, induced vaginal delivery, or elective cesarean section [59].

Upon delivery, the newborn should be immediately intubated endotracheally, and abdominal contents should be decompressed via a nasogastric or orogastric tube [40]. *Permissive hypercapnia and gentle ventilation are recommended*, by maintaining preductal saturations between 80 and 95%, postductal saturations greater than 70%, and PaCO2 levels between 50 and 70 mmHg [57]. Gentle ventilation techniques are essential and should be further emphasized in hospital settings that do not have access to ECMO. Early echocardiography is necessary to assess for cardiac anomalies and complications due to CDH. Hemodynamic monitoring is essential. Providers will need to closely monitor vital signs and get peripheral intravenous access for fluid resuscitation. It may also be necessary to give vasopressors such as dopamine and dobutamine to maintain blood pressure and reduce right-to-left shunting [1].

In resource-limited settings, stabilization and gentle ventilation are crucial. Repair should be performed when the patient's cardiopulmonary function is stable [60]. The physiologic stress of surgery often causes a temporary worsening of the clinical condition that the treating team needs to be prepared to support. During repair of the CDH, which is often approached through a subcostal incision, care must be taken when reducing the intra-abdominal organs back into the abdominal cavity. The diaphragm edges should be unfurled without weakening the diaphragm. A primary closure should be completed only if it can be accomplished without tension. Otherwise, a patch (most commonly Gore-Tex) should be placed to bridge the defect. Again, *avoidance of tension during repair is crucial*. A dome or curve shape should be incorporated in the fashioning of the patch to decrease tension on the closure. This will decrease recurrence rate. If an artificial patch is not available, a muscular flap may be used to close the defect; however, the surgeon must have experience with this type of closure. If possible, the abdominal incision is closed. If intra-abdominal pressure from returned abdominal contents is too high, then a temporary abdominal closure should be fashioned to prevent abdominal compartment syndrome and respiratory compromise. Chest tubes are usually not necessary, and the patient should be monitored.

Long-term follow-up is essential in patients with CDH. Chronic lung disease, GERD, growth failure, developmental delay and behavior disorders, sensorineural hearing loss, hernia recurrence, and orthopedic deformities are common in this population. GERD is able to be managed with medical therapy alone in the majority of patients. Threshold for surgical management is higher than in children without CDH due to the adhesive disease found in the upper abdominal region after CDH repair. Recurrence occurs in about 5–50% of the cases. It is higher in patients who require patch closure. Surgical management is necessary via primary or reinforced closure [61].

Colon and Rectal Congenital Malformations

Hirschsprung's Disease

Epidemiology

It is estimated that 1 in 5000 children is diagnosed with Hirschsprung's disease (HD) across all ethnics groups, with a ratio of 4:1 for males to females [62].

Pathophysiology

HD occurs due to a congenital absence of parasympathetic ganglionic cells of the rectum and to varying distances proximal to it, causing intestinal obstruction. This occurs due to a disruption to the neural crest cell development between weeks 5 and 12 of gestation [63].

Risk Factors

HD is associated with chromosomal abnormalities, such as trisomy 21. These genetic abnormalities also are associated with other anomalies, such as gastrointestinal, central nervous system, genitourinary, musculoskeletal, cardiovascular, and craniofacial abnormalities. Increased risk has also been noted in siblings of individuals with HD [64].

Clinical Manifestations

Most HD is diagnosed at the neonate stage. Symptom associated with HD is failure to pass meconium in the first 24–48 h (60–90% of children present with this symptom). 63–91% of the children also experience abdominal distension, and 19–37% have bilious vomiting due to intestinal obstruction. Particularly when the diagnosis is delayed, some may present with Hirschsprung-associated enterocolitis (HAEC), in which patients develop fever, a distended abdomen, and foul-smelling diarrhea. *HAEC is a serious condition that may progress to toxic megacolon.* It needs to be promptly treated with rectal irrigations, broad-spectrum antibiotics, and fluid resuscitation [64].

Once there is a high suspicion for HD, imaging can be done to further investigate the condition. An upright abdominal X-ray should be done to look for signs of intestinal obstruction, such as distended bowel loops and air-fluid levels, with absence of air in the rectum [65]. Contrast enema may show a narrow rectum, a rectosigmoid ratio less than 1, and transition zone (between ganglionic and aganglionic segment of the colon due to HD) [65].

The gold standard for diagnosis is a rectal biopsy. The biopsy is done at least 1–1.5 cm proximal to the dentate line. Diagnosis is confirmed with the absence of ganglion cells in the submucosal and myenteric plexuses. Proximal biopsies are performed to assess the extent of disease. Hypertrophic nerve trunks may also be visualized, although this finding is not always present. Acetylcholinesterase enzyme histochemistry and calretinin immunohistochemistry can be used. AChE stains abnormal parasympathetic nerve fibers in the lamina propria and muscularis mucosa and therefore would be increased staining in HD. Calretinin is a vitamin D-dependent Ca-binding protein that is expressed in ganglion cells and therefore would be absent in the setting of HD [65]. *Histologic examination and diagnosis of HD require a high level of training in surgical pathology.* These specimens need to be evaluated in a lab that has experience with HD. Some specialized stains may not be available in LMICs. Diagnosis will depend on confirming the absence of ganglion cells and possibly the presence of hypertrophic nerve trunks.

Management

Initial management aims to relieve the obstruction via serial rectal washouts, using warm saline. Colostomy or ileostomy should be considered if there is no appropriate surgical skill and in particular if there is no appropriate pathology support to provide satisfactory repair and specimen interpretation. This will allow diversion of fecal stream and relief of GI obstruction and optimize interpretation of biopsy specimen.

Corrective surgery is accomplished by resecting the aganglionic segment and performing an endorectal pull-through anastomosis [66]. Either laparoscopically or with an open incision, seromuscular and full-thickness biopsies should be taken up to some distance proximal to the transition zone, as defined by imaging. This will confirm presence of ganglion cells and allow a safe anastomosis. A Swenson, Soave, or Duhamel procedure may be used. Surgeon comfort level should dictate which technique is used.

Some patients present later in childhood, often with chronic constipation. Older children may require a two-staged approach to deal with the chronically dilated colon. If rectal irrigations are not sufficient to decompress the bowel, an ileostomy may need to be performed, prior to pull-through procedure. Malnutrition must also be addressed, as it will make the anastomosis at risk of complications, such as leakage [66].

Early complications of HD surgery include anastomotic leak, rectal stenosis, ileus, and intestinal adhesive obstruction. Wound infections may also occur. If the affected and therefore resected area is long, it may lead to fluid and electrolyte losses. In the long run, children may experience stricture, postoperative enterocolitis, and abnormal bowel function [1]. It is important to inform the family that HAEC may still occur after surgery and educate them on what signs and symptoms to look for. Management again involves rectal irrigation, antibiotics, and supportive care.

Anorectal Malformations

Epidemiology

The prevalence of Anorecal Malformations (ARMs) globally is approximately 1 in 5000 births, with a slightly higher prevalence in males [67].

Pathophysiology and Risk Factors

The etiology of ARMs is unknown but is most likely caused by a combination of genetic and environmental abnormalities. Approximately 5% of ARM cases are associated with Down syndrome. Anorectal malformation may be part of the VACTERL syndrome, which is an association of vertebral, anorectal, cardiac, tracheoesophageal, renal, and limb anomalies. Genetic mutations that affect hindgut development can cause ARMs. In terms of environmental factors, some studies have shown associations between pre-pregnancy obesity and maternal asthma [68].

Clinical Manifestations

The presentation can vary depending on the site of fistulization. In males, the most common type is an imperforate anus with a rectourethral fistula. There can also be a recto-bladder, recto-urethra-prostatic, recto-urethra-bulbar, and recto-perineal fistula. In females, the most common is an imperforate anus with a recto-vestibular fistula. Recto-perineal fistula and cloaca with a short (<3 cm) or long (>3 cm) common channel may also occur [69].

During the newborn physical exam, an anus is not appreciated. However, a full newborn exam may not be performed in many cases, especially if the delivery is not done at a healthcare facility. Therefore, newborns with ARM may present with abdominal distention and failure to pass meconium. In this case, the physician should do a detailed physical examination to see if meconium is observed along the perineum, along a midline raphe or a bucket-handle deformity. In females, the posterior portion of the vestibule should be examined for a recto-vestibular fistula. Gauze can also be placed at the penis or urethral opening to see if there is meconium-tinted urine. An invertogram can also be used to see whether the infant has a blind pouch, without a fistula [1].

Management

As genitourinary defects are often associated with anorectal malformations, it is important to evaluate for these anomalies using ultrasound. This will also be important for any urologic concerns that can be addressed during time of colostomy. Plain radiographs of the sacrum and spinal ultrasound can also be done to examine vertebral anomalies. An ECHO should be performed to identify any cardiac anomalies. Finally, abdominal and chest x-rays with a nasogastric tube in place should be done, to evaluate for any tracheo-esophageal anomalies [69].

Surgical management is dependent on whether a lesion is considered low or high. A lesion is low if the meconium is in the perineum, there is a bucket-handle lesion, or there is a blind pouch less than 1 cm from the anal dimple, as seen in an invertogram. Invertograms need special consideration as they may lack accuracy in defining level. All other lesions are considered high [1].

In LMICs, a divided colostomy will be the operation of choice in all but the most specialized pediatric surgical centers. A high lesion requires a descending colostomy. The general steps are explained below: [1].

1. An oblique incision is made in the left abdomen, starting just superolateral to the pubis and extending laterally.
2. The proximal sigmoid is identified and transected.
   (a) The proximal stoma is connected to the upper GI tract and will drain stool.
   (b) The distal stoma will drain mucus material.
3. The distal colon must be irrigated thoroughly to remove meconium.
4. Both stomas are secured to the fascia using absorbable sutures.
5. Parastomal herniation is prevented by using a generous number of sutures to approximate the peritoneum, fascia, and muscle around the stoma.
6. A wide-spaced skin bridge is created between the stomas to accommodate the stoma appliance and decrease wound complications.

After the child reaches 2–3 months with adequate weight gain, a posterior sagittal anorectoplasty (PSARP) can be done. For high anorectal malformations, combined perineal and abdominal approach is often necessary. Delay may be chosen to maximize weight gain and nutrition and optimize surgical outcomes [67].

The neo-anus anastomosis will most often need dilations. Once the desired size is achieved (depending on the patient's age), the colostomy can be closed [69]. Patients after surgical management of ARMs must follow up with the surgeon regularly. The most common complication postoperatively is constipation. Therefore, laxatives and dietary changes are necessary to avoid the sequelae of constipation. Patients may also have fecal incontinence, which can be managed by giving an enema after a main meal. Urinary incontinence may also occur if there are sacral deformities or nerve damage from the operation. A surgeon-led bowel management program will optimize outcomes of these patients [69].

References

1. Ameh EA, Bickler SW, Lakhoo K, Nwomeh BC, Poenaru D. Pediatric Surgery: a comprehensive textbook for Africa. 2nd ed. Springer Nature Switzerland; 2020.
2. To T, Wajja A, Wales PW, Langer JC. Population demographic indicators associated with incidence of pyloric stenosis. Arch Pediatr Adolesc Med. 2005;159(6):520. https://doi.org/10.1001/archpedi.159.6.520.
3. Peeters B, Benninga MA, Hennekam RCM. Infantile hypertrophic pyloric stenosis—genetics and syndromes. Nat Rev Gastroenterol Hepatol. 2012;9(11):646–60. https://doi.org/10.1038/nrgastro.2012.133.
4. Pandya S, Heiss K. Pyloric stenosis in Pediatric Surgery. Surg Clin N Am. 2012;92(3):527–39. https://doi.org/10.1016/j.suc.2012.03.006.
5. Rich BS, Dolgin SE. Hypertrophic Pyloric Stenosis. :7.
6. Kimura K, Mukohara N, Nishijima E, Muraji T, Tsugawa C, Matsumoto Y. Diamond-shaped anastomosis for duodenal atresia: an experience with 44 patients over 15 years. J Pediatr Surg. 1990;25(9):977–9. https://doi.org/10.1016/0022-3468(90)90241-Z.
7. Kapfer SA, Rappold JF. Intestinal malrotation-not just the pediatric surgeon's problem. J Am Coll Surg. 2004;199(4):628–35. https://doi.org/10.1016/j.jamcollsurg.2004.04.024.
8. Petrikovsky BM. First-trimester diagnosis of duodenal atresia. Am J Obstet Gynecol. 1994;171(2):569–70. https://doi.org/10.1016/0002-9378(94)90307-7.
9. Santulli TV, Blanc WA. Congenital atresia of the intestine: pathogenesis and treatment. Ann Surg. 1961;154:939–48.
10. Kluth D, Jaeschke-Melli S, Fiegel H. The embryology of gut rotation. Semin Pediatr Surg. 2003;12(4):275–9. https://doi.org/10.1053/j.sempedsurg.2003.08.009.
11. Walker K, Badawi N, Hamid CH, et al. A population-based study of the outcome after small bowel atresia/stenosis in New South Wales and the ASustralian Capital Territory, Australia, 1992-2003. J Pediatr Surg. 2008;43(3):484–8. https://doi.org/10.1016/j.jpedsurg.2007.10.028.
12. Forrester MB, Merz RD. Population-based study of small intestinal atresia and stenosis, Hawaii, 1986–2000. Public Health. 2004;118(6):434–8. https://doi.org/10.1016/j.puhe.2003.12.017.
13. Choudhry MS, Rahman N, Boyd P, Lakhoo K. Duodenal atresia: associated anomalies, prenatal diagnosis and outcome. Pediatr Surg Int. 2009;25(8):727–30. https://doi.org/10.1007/s00383-009-2406-y.

14. Escobar MA, Ladd AP, Grosfeld JL, et al. Duodenal atresia and stenosis: long-term follow-up over 30 years. J Pediatr Surg. 2004;39(6):867–71. https://doi.org/10.1016/j.jpedsurg.2004.02.025.
15. Kucińska-Chahwan A, Posiewka A, Bijok J, Jakiel G, Roszkowski T. Clinical significance of the prenatal double bubble sign - single institution experience: double bubble sign - clinical significance. Prenat Diagn. 2015;35(11):1093–6. https://doi.org/10.1002/pd.4652.
16. Bailey PV, Tracy TF, Connors RH, Mooney DP, Lewis JE, Weber TR. Congenital duodenal obstruction: a 32-year review. J Pediatr Surg. 1993;28(1):92–5. https://doi.org/10.1016/S0022-3468(05)80364-1.
17. Werler MM, Sheehan JE, Mitchell AA. Association of vasoconstrictive exposures with risks of gastroschisis and small intestinal atresia. Epidemiology. 2003;14(3):349–54.
18. Sweeney B, Surana R, Puri P. Jejunoileal atresia and associated malformations: correlation with the timing of in utero insult. J Pediatr Surg. 2001;36(5):774–6. https://doi.org/10.1053/jpsu.2001.22958.
19. Stollman TH, Wijnen RMH, Draaisma JMT. Investigation for cystic fibrosis in infants with jejunoileal atresia in The Netherlands: a 35-year experience with 114 cases. Eur J Pediatr. 2007;166(9):989–90. https://doi.org/10.1007/s00431-006-0342-6.
20. Juang D, Snyder CL. Neonatal bowel obstruction. Surg Clin N Am. 2012;92(3):685–711. https://doi.org/10.1016/j.suc.2012.03.008.
21. Zanconato G, Msolomba R, Guarenti L, Franchi M. Antenatal care in developing countries: the need for a tailored model. Semin Fetal Neonatal Med. 2006;11(1):15–20. https://doi.org/10.1016/j.siny.2005.10.002.
22. Opportunities for African Newborns – Practical data, policy and programmatic support for newborn care in Africa. Save the Children's Resource Centre. Accessed 7 June 2022. https://resourcecentre.savethechildren.net/pdf/3381.pdf/
23. Chardot C. Biliary atresia. Orphanet J Rare Dis. 2006;1(1):28. https://doi.org/10.1186/1750-1172-1-28.
24. Miltenburg DM, Nuchtern JG, Jaksic T, Kozinetiz C, Brandt ML. Laparoscopic evaluation of the pediatric inguinal hernia—a meta-analysis. J Pediatr Surg. 1998;33(6):874–9. https://doi.org/10.1016/S0022-3468(98)90664-9.
25. Gödeke J, Muensterer O. Femoral, direct, and rare inguinal hernias in children—an update. Eur J Pediatr Surg. 2017;27(06):484–94. https://doi.org/10.1055/s-0037-1608684.
26. Parelkar SV, Oak S, Gupta R, et al. Laparoscopic inguinal hernia repair in the pediatric age group—experience with 437 children. J Pediatr Surg. 2010;45(4):789–92. https://doi.org/10.1016/j.jpedsurg.2009.08.007.
27. Yeap E, Nataraja RM, Pacilli M. Inguinal hernias in children. Australian J General Pract. 2020;49:6.
28. Schier F, Klizaite J. Rare inguinal hernia forms in children. Ped Surgery Int. 2004;20(10):748–52. https://doi.org/10.1007/s00383-004-1291-7.
29. Davenport M. ABC of general paediatric Surgery: inguinal hernia, hydrocele, and the undescended testis. *BMJ*. 1996;312(7030):564–7. https://doi.org/10.1136/bmj.312.7030.564.
30. Kelly KB, Ponsky TA. Pediatric Abdominal Wall defects. Surg Clin N Am. 2013;93(5):1255–67. https://doi.org/10.1016/j.suc.2013.06.016.
31. Pawlak M, East B, de Beaux AC. Algorithm for management of an incarcerated inguinal hernia in the emergency settings with manual reduction. Taxis, the technique and its safety. Hernia. 2021;25(5):1253–8. https://doi.org/10.1007/s10029-021-02429-1.
32. Hoballah JJ, Scott-Conner CE, Chong HS. Operative dictations in general and vascular Surgery. Springer Science+Business Media; 2017.
33. Talwar A, Talwar A, Talwar A. Multiple cases of umbilical hernias in children in rural Ghana. Lancet. 2019;394(10193):159. https://doi.org/10.1016/S0140-6736(19)31289-9.
34. Bittner JG. Incarcerated/strangulated hernia. Adv Surg. 2016;50(1):67–78. https://doi.org/10.1016/j.yasu.2016.03.006.
35. Chirdan LB, Uba AF, Kidmas AT. Incarcerated umbilical hernia in children. Eur J Pediatr Surg. 2006;16(1):45–8. https://doi.org/10.1055/s-2006-923792.
36. Division of Education of the American College of Surgeons. Pediatric Umbilical Hernia Repair. Published online April 23, 2013. Accessed May 4, 2023. https://www.facs.org/media/u53k0uhw/ped_umbilical.pdf.
37. Clark RH, Sousa J, Laughon MM, Tolia VN. Gastroschisis prevalence substantially decreased from 2009 through 2018 after a 3-fold increase from 1997 to 2008. J Pediatr Surg. 2020;55(12):2640–1. https://doi.org/10.1016/j.jpedsurg.2020.03.010.
38. Sekabira J, Hadley GP. Gastroschisis: a third world perspective. Pediatr Surg Int. 2009;25(4):327–9. https://doi.org/10.1007/s00383-009-2348-4.
39. Baerg J, Kaban G, Tonita J, Pahwa P, Reid D. Gastroschisis: a sixteen-year review. J Pediatr Surg. 2003;38(5):771–4. https://doi.org/10.1016/jpsu.2003.50164.
40. Ameh EA, Chirdan LB. Ruptured exomphalos and gastroschisis: a retrospective analysis of morbidity and mortality in Nigerian children. Pediatr Surg Int. 2000;16(1–2):23–5. https://doi.org/10.1007/s003830050006.
41. Wesonga AS, Fitzgerald TN, Kabuye R, et al. Gastroschisis in Uganda: opportunities for improved survival. J Pediatr Surg. 2016;51(11):1772–7. https://doi.org/10.1016/j.jpedsurg.2016.07.011.
42. Feldkamp ML, Carey JC, Sadler TW. Development of gastroschisis: review of hypotheses, a novel hypothesis, and implications for research. Am J Med Genet A. 2007;143A(7):639–52. https://doi.org/10.1002/ajmg.a.31578.
43. Oakes MC, Porto M, Chung JH. Advances in prenatal and perinatal diagnosis and management of gastroschisis. Semin Pediatr Surg. 2018;27(5):289–99. https://doi.org/10.1053/j.sempedsurg.2018.08.006.

44. Harper LM, Goetzinger KR, Biggio JR, Macones GA. Timing of elective delivery in gastroschisis: a decision and cost-effectiveness analysis. Ultrasound Obstet Gynecol. 2015;46(2):227–32. https://doi.org/10.1002/uog.14721.
45. Gamba P, Midrio P. Abdominal wall defects: prenatal diagnosis, newborn management, and long-term outcomes. Semin Pediatr Surg. 2014;23(5):283–90. https://doi.org/10.1053/j.sempedsurg.2014.09.009.
46. Wright NJ, Sekabira J, Ade-Ajayi N. Care of infants with gastroschisis in low-resource settings. Semin Pediatr Surg. 2018;27(5):321–6. https://doi.org/10.1053/j.sempedsurg.2018.08.004.
47. Wilson RD, Johnson MP. Congenital Abdominal Wall defects: an update. Fetal Diagn Ther. 2004;19(5):385–98. https://doi.org/10.1159/000078990.
48. Khan FA, Hashmi A, Islam S. Insights into embryology and development of omphalocele. Semin Pediatr Surg. 2019;28(2):80–3. https://doi.org/10.1053/j.sempedsurg.2019.04.003.
49. Brioude F, Kalish JM, Mussa A, et al. Clinical and molecular diagnosis, screening and management of Beckwith–Wiedemann syndrome: an international consensus statement. Nat Rev Endocrinol 2018;14(4):229–249. https://doi.org/10.1038/nrendo.2017.166.
50. Verla MA, Style CC, Olutoye OO. Prenatal diagnosis and management of omphalocele. Semin Pediatr Surg. 2019;28(2):84–8. https://doi.org/10.1053/j.sempedsurg.2019.04.007.
51. Goyal A. Oesophageal atresia and tracheo-oesophageal fistula. Arch Dis Child Fetal Neonatal Ed. 2006;91(5):F381–4. https://doi.org/10.1136/adc.2005.086157.
52. Spitz L, Kiely EM, Morecroft JA, Drake DP. Oesophageal atresia: at-risk groups for the 1990s. J Pediatr Surg. 1994;29(6):723–5. https://doi.org/10.1016/0022-3468(94)90354-9.
53. Pinheiro PFM, Silva ACS, e, Pereira RM. Current knowledge on esophageal atresia. World J Gastroenterol. 2012;18(28):3662–72. https://doi.org/10.3748/wjg.v18.i28.3662.
54. Pardy C, D'Antonio F, Khalil A, Giuliani S. Prenatal detection of esophageal atresia: a systematic review and meta-analysis. Acta Obstet Gynecol Scand. 2019;98(6):689–99. https://doi.org/10.1111/aogs.13536.
55. Paoletti M, Raffler G, Gaffi MS, Antounians L, Lauriti G, Zani A. Prevalence and risk factors for congenital diaphragmatic hernia: a global view. J Pediatr Surg. 2020;55(11):2297–307. https://doi.org/10.1016/j.jpedsurg.2020.06.022.
56. Leeuwen L, Fitzgerald DA. Congenital diaphragmatic hernia. J Paediatr Child Health. 2014;50(9):667–73. https://doi.org/10.1111/jpc.12508.
57. Chatterjee D, Ing RJ, Gien J. Update on congenital diaphragmatic hernia. Anesth Analg. 2020;131(3):808–21. https://doi.org/10.1213/ANE.0000000000004324.
58. Kovler ML, Jelin EB. Fetal intervention for congenital diaphragmatic hernia. Semin Pediatr Surg. 2019;28(4):150818. https://doi.org/10.1053/j.sempedsurg.2019.07.001.
59. Burgos CM, Frenckner B, Luco M, Harting MT, Lally PA, Lally KP. Prenatally diagnosed congenital diaphragmatic hernia: optimal mode of delivery? J Perinatol. 2017;37(2):134–8. https://doi.org/10.1038/jp.2016.221.
60. Moyer VA, Moya FR, Tibboel D, Losty PD, Nagaya M, Lally KP Cochrane Neonatal Group. Late versus early surgical correction for congenital diaphragmatic hernia in newborn infants. Cochrane Database Syst Rev. 2000;2010(5). https://doi.org/10.1002/14651858.CD001695.
61. Section on Surgery and the Committee on Fetus and Newborn. Postdischarge follow-up of infants with congenital diaphragmatic hernia. Pediatrics. 2008;121(3):627–32. https://doi.org/10.1542/peds.2007-3282.
62. Duess JW, Hofmann AD, Puri P. Prevalence of Hirschsprung's disease in premature infants: a systematic review. Pediatr Surg Int. 2014;30(8):791–5. https://doi.org/10.1007/s00383-014-3540-8.
63. Butler Tjaden NE, Trainor PA. The developmental etiology and pathogenesis of Hirschsprung disease. Transl Res. 2013;162(1):1–15. https://doi.org/10.1016/j.trsl.2013.03.001.
64. Haricharan RN, Georgeson KE. Hirschsprung disease. Semin Pediatr Surg. 2008;17(4):266–75. https://doi.org/10.1053/j.sempedsurg.2008.07.005.
65. Das K, Mohanty S. Hirschsprung disease — current diagnosis and management. Indian J Pediatr. 2017;84(8):618–23. https://doi.org/10.1007/s12098-017-2371-8.
66. Smith C, Ambartsumyan L, Kapur RP. Surgery, surgical pathology, and postoperative Management of Patients with Hirschsprung Disease. Pediatr Dev Pathol. 2020;23(1):23–39. https://doi.org/10.1177/1093526619889436.
67. Wood R, Levitt M. Anorectal malformations. Clin Colon Rectal Surg. 2018;31(02):061–70. https://doi.org/10.1055/s-0037-1609020.
68. Wang C, Li L, Cheng W. Anorectal malformation: the etiological factors. Pediatr Surg Int. 2015;31(9):795–804. https://doi.org/10.1007/s00383-015-3685-0.
69. Levitt MA, Peña A. Anorectal malformations. Orphanet J Rare Dis. 2007;2:33. https://doi.org/10.1186/1750-1172-2-33.

43 How to Manage Common Orthopedic Injuries in Low- and Middle-Income Countries

Katherine A. Rosenwasser, Nicholas C. Danford, and Joshua E. Hyman

Surgeons must be very careful when they take the knife!
Underneath their fine incisions stirs the Culprit - Life!
– Emily Dickinson

Abbreviations

AC	Acromioclavicular
CT	Computed tomography
LMICs	Low- and middle-income countries
MRI	Magnetic resonance imaging
RLS	Resource-limited setting
VAC	Vacuum-assisted closure
VTE	Venous thromboembolism

K. A. Rosenwasser (✉) · N. C. Danford
Columbia University Vagelos College of Physicians and Surgeons, New York, NY, USA
e-mail: kar2153@cumc.columbia.edu; ncd2117@cumc.columbia.edu

J. E. Hyman
Columbia University Vagelos College of Physicians and Surgeons, New York, NY, USA

Department of Orthopedic Surgery, Columbia University Medical Center, New York, NY, USA
e-mail: jh736@cumc.columbia.edu

Introduction

The purpose of this chapter is to describe common orthopedic pathologies and assist the clinician without subspecialty training in orthopedic surgery in identifying and initially treating orthopedic emergencies. The chapter also aims to educate the clinician without subspecialty training in orthopedic surgery in deciding when nonsurgical (closed) treatment can be successfully employed and by what means he or she may do so.

When treating common orthopedic injuries in a resource-limited setting (RLS), the physician should keep in mind that the standard of care in any setting, whether resource limited or not, is often non-operative. Therefore, for many diagnoses, both the patient and physician can anticipate excellent outcomes with proper non-operative management. Deciphering which injuries may be treated conservatively treated and which will require operative intervention and/or referral to a specialist with training in orthopedic surgery is the goal, albeit not always possible in a RLS. We define a RLS as any healthcare institution that does not have the financial and/or logistical capacity to procure enough material or personnel

M. A. Hardy, B. R. Hochman (eds.), *Global Surgery*, https://doi.org/10.1007/978-3-031-28127-3_43

to treat every patient. We understand that this is a broad definition. Accordingly, resource-limited settings exist along a broad spectrum, as certain institutions have access to more supplies and personnel than others in low- and middle-income countries (LMICs).

The chapter is organized into three sections: (1) general principles of closed (non-operative) fracture treatment, (2) common orthopedic emergencies, and (3) injuries to specific anatomic locations. The specific injuries are discussed as closed, isolated injuries. Patients with open fractures or those who sustain polytrauma may undergo different treatments depending on associated injuries.

General Principles of Closed Fracture Treatment

To successfully treat an orthopedic injury, the physician must understand when to immobilize a joint, when to limit weight-bearing, and for how long to do so. He or she must also know how to successfully immobilize a joint, which means knowing how to use common materials such slings, plaster, and/or fiberglass in a way that limits motion where motion should be limited and permits motion where motion should be permitted. Additionally, the provider need know how to safely apply these devices in a way that does not harm a patient's skin from pressure sores or burns. Lastly, he or she must know when to perform a closed reduction via manipulation and when a closed reduction is not necessary.

Splinting with plaster and casting with fiberglass are invaluable and necessary skills to have when treating orthopedic injuries. There are many types of splints and casts and numerous techniques for applying them. In general, *knowledge of the proper way to pad an extremity for splinting or casting is a critical safety step. Additionally, understanding the basics of the material properties of plaster and fiberglass (e.g. that the materials heat as they dry and may cause skin burns) can be the difference between helping and harming a patient.*

Each different type of splint or cast has different anatomic areas that need to be padded more than others, and each injury requires limb and/or joint positioning in specific ways. Thus, it is difficult to make prescriptions about the amount of padding needed and the correct positioning of joints. Throughout the chapter, we describe salient points of splinting and casting specific injuries as part of the discussion of a specific injury. General principles are presented in Box 43.1.

Box 43.1 General Principles of Splinting and Casting

Do:

- Apply multiple layers (three to five) of cotton padding to bony prominences.
- Use cool water for fiberglass and cool-to-room temperature water for plaster to avoid skin burns.
- Apply circumferential dressing, especially ace wrap, loosely.
- Obtain post-splinting or casting radiographs to confirm proper bony alignment, joint positioning, and material (fiberglass and plaster) placement.

Do not:

- Wrap cotton padding, elastic (ace) wrap, fiberglass, or any circumferential dressing tightly, especially in the upper extremity.
- Use warm water for plaster or fiberglass, as this may cause skin burns.

- Place any form of immobilization without understanding which joints to immobilize and which to leave free. If uncertain, ask somebody with experience in splinting and casting specific injuries.

Materials to obtain:

- Shears.
- Gloves.
- Cool water.
- Stockinette.
- Cotton padding.
- Fiberglass and/or plaster.
- Elastic bandage (ace wrap).
- Paper tape.

General steps, splinting:

- Apply cotton padding so that bony prominences are well padded, generally with three to five layers of padding.

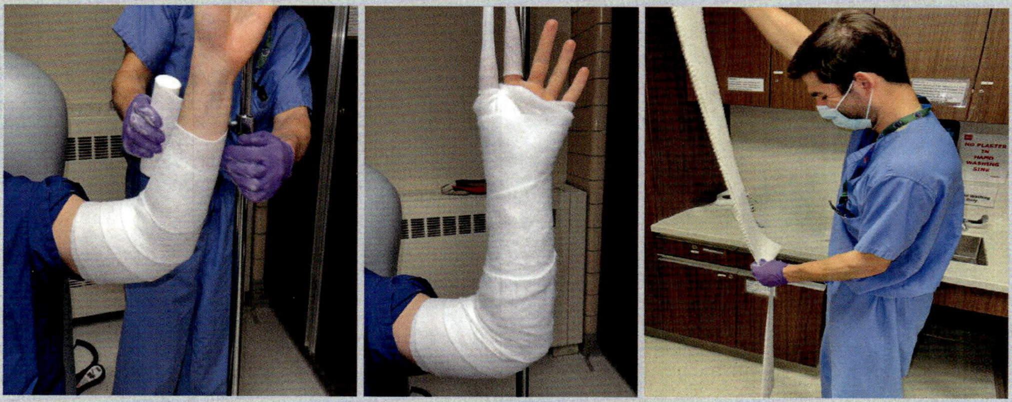

- Measure and prepare plaster by repeatedly folding plaster until there are eight to ten layers.
- Place plaster in water, squeeze water from plaster, and flatten plaster so that the layers co-laminate.
- Ensure the extremity and/or joints that are being immobilized are properly positioned.
- Apply plaster.

- Place additional roll of cotton padding over plaster to prevent adhesion between plaster and elastic wrap.

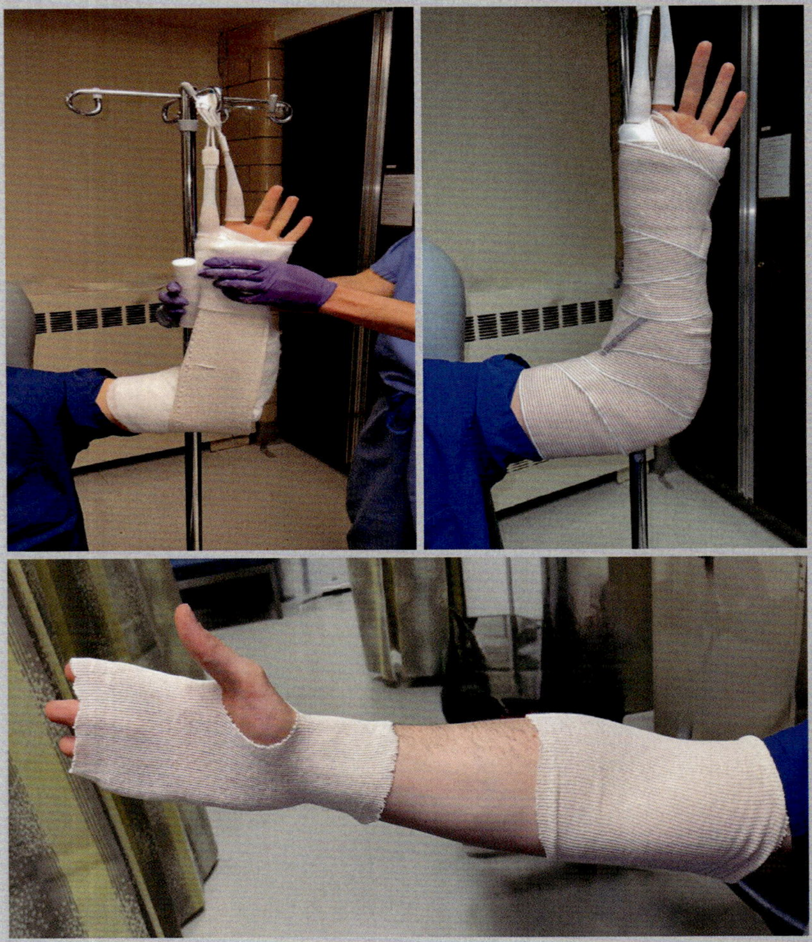

- Apply elastic wrap *without pulling tightly.*
- Allow plaster to harden while applying desired mold and/or holding splint in the desired position.

General steps, casting:

- Apply stockinette (note that this step is not necessary but prevents fraying and breakdown of cotton padding, which is useful if the cast will remain in place for a number of weeks).

- Apply cotton padding so that bony prominences are well padded, generally with three to five layers of padding.

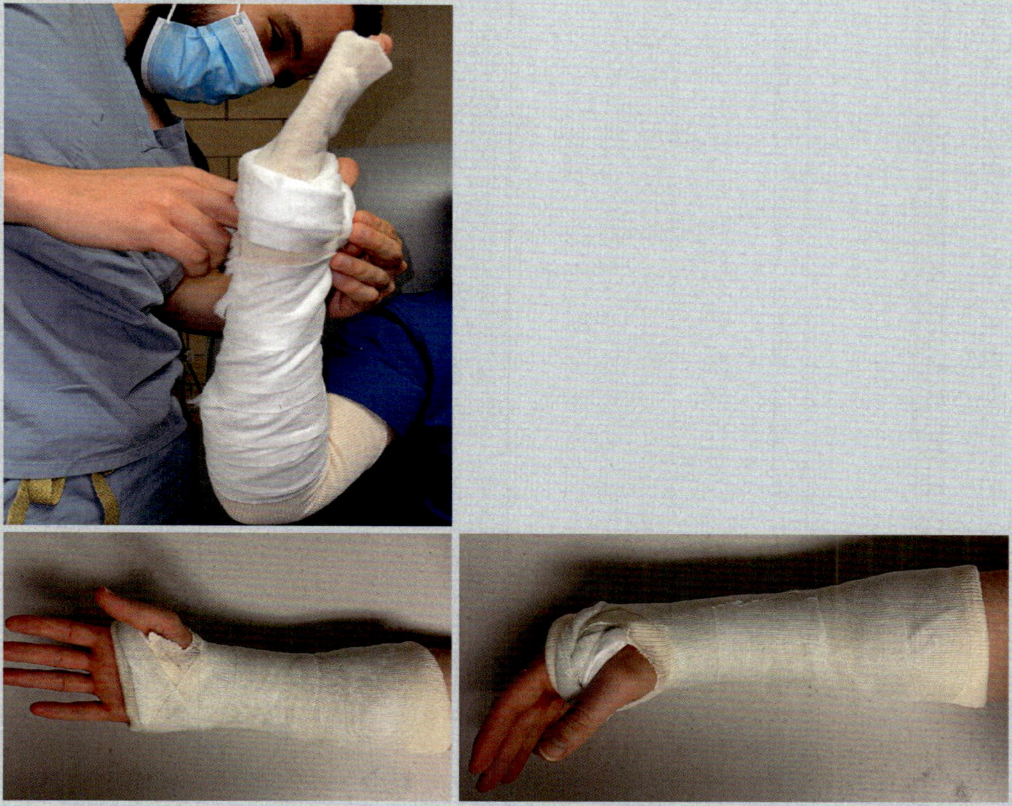

- Submerge fiberglass in cool water, and ring out excess water.
- Roll fiberglass onto the extremity so that there are no wrinkles in the fiberglass and so that it is not stretched tightly. Each roll of fiberglass should overlap the previous one by 50%.
- Apply a mold, if needed.
- Fold stockinette so that the initial fiberglass layer and cotton padding are covered proximally and distally by stockinette.
- Apply a second layer or fiberglass.

Common Orthopedic Emergencies

Differentiating between Emergency and Urgency

Certain orthopedic injuries must be treated as emergencies, meaning treatment should be rendered as soon as possible. Other injuries require urgent treatment and allow some time, usually on the order of hours to days, for proper diagnosis and/or other emergent management of concomitant pathology. Box 43.2 provides a list of common orthopedic injuries classified by emergencies and urgencies.

Box 43.2 Orthopedic Injuries That Require Emergent or Urgent Treatment

Emergent treatment (treat as soon as possible)

- Compartment syndrome.
- Vascular injury causing limb ischemia.
- Septic joint.
- Necrotizing fasciitis.
- High-pressure injection injury.
- Pelvic ring fracture associated with hemodynamic instability.
- Open fracture.

Urgent treatment (treatment can be delayed on the order of a few hours and even in certain situations days)

- Joint dislocations.
- Fractures that benefit from closed reduction (e.g., certain distal radius fractures and tibial shaft fractures).
- Surgical treatment of hip fractures.

Compartment Syndrome

Compartment syndrome is defined by an increase in pressure within a fascial compartment. It can occur in any extremity but most commonly occurs in the leg and the forearm. More rarely, it occurs in the foot, thigh, gluteal compartment, hand, and arm. Symptoms are intractable pain and later in the disease course, loss of sensation and circulation. Physical exam findings are tense compartments, pain with passive flexion and/or extension of the muscles within a given compartment, and in advanced cases, diminished pulses and pale, cool skin. Treatment is immediate fasciotomies of the involved compartments.

For compartment syndrome of the leg, we prefer a two-incision approach with a lateral incision from the fibular head to the lateral malleolus followed by release of the lateral and anterior compartments. Medially, an incision from just distal to the knee joint to the medial malleolus allows release of the superficial posterior compartment and deep posterior compartment. The deep posterior compartment is accessed and released via elevation of the soleus muscle from the tibia. The wounds are typically kept open with vacuum-assisted closure (VAC) dressing and negative pressure until the skin can be closed or a split-thickness skin graft can be applied. If VAC dressings are not available, wet to dry dressings may be placed and changed daily.

For compartment syndrome of the forearm, we also use a two-incision approach for fasciotomies of the volar (flexor), dorsal (extensor), and mobile wad compartments. The volar incision runs from just proximal to the wrist crease to just distal to the ulnar aspect of the elbow flexion crease. The dorsal incision begins in the midline dorsally over the wrist and extends to the radial aspect of the elbow, which allows release of the mobile wad in addition to the dorsal (extensor) compartment.

Open Fractures

Open fractures are defined by bone that disrupts the dermis. Open fractures are often high-energy injuries. During workup, the setting of the injury should be ascertained, as injuries that occur in certain locations such as farms are treated differently from other open fractures. On exam, bone will not always be visible. Skin damage should be noted. Fat globules exudating through the skin are a sign of open fracture because it indicates that fatty bone marrow contents are communicating with the outside world. Injuries are commonly classified based on the Gustilo-Anderson classification [1]. Intravenous antibiotics are initiated as soon as possible, ideally within 1 hour of injury. A first-generation cephalosporin is used for type I and II injuries, and an aminoglycoside such as gentamicin is added for type III injuries. Finally, for highly contaminated injuries (such as those occurring on a farm), penicillin is added for coverage of clostridial species. Fractures are debrided within 24 hours of injury and are typically stabilized at that time as well.

Hemodynamically Unstable Pelvic Ring Injuries

Pelvic ring injuries may be associated with hemodynamic instability because the massive force required to cause the injury can damage both the arterial and venous system, which in turn causes life-threatening hemorrhage. Emergency treatment depends on availability of resources and patient hemodynamic status. For a pelvic ring injury characterized by a widened pubic symphysis and hemodynamic instability, the fastest, cheapest, and most dependable emergency reduction tactic that can be lifesaving is placement of a pelvic binder (Fig. 43.1).

Septic Arthritis

Septic arthritis is an infection of a joint, most commonly a bacterial infection, but fungal infections are encountered as well. Patients present with joint pain in the absence of trauma to the joint and often have an associated fever. Patient history may include recent illness or invasive procedures (e.g., dental procedures). Patients with risk factors such as immunocompromise, diabetes mellitus, rheumatologic disease, and intravenous drug use should be identified during history taking. The most important aspects of the physical examination are inspection for joint effusion and range of motion, as patients inevitably have pain with limited range of motion. Laboratory analysis is crucial in making a diagnosis. Serum white blood count and erythrocyte sedimentation rate (ESR) are frequently elevated. ESR and C-reactive protein (CRP) are highly sensitive but not specific [2]. An arthrocentesis for analysis of synovial fluid is also critical as it allows a count of fluid white blood cell count, fluid culture, and crystal assay. Radiographs are necessary to rule out traumatic injury, foreign body, and tumors. The differential diagnosis is important because crystalline arthropathy (frequently gout) mimics septic arthritis. Crystalline arthropathy typically improves with anti-inflammatory medications, and crystals are identified on synovial fluid analysis. To prevent chondrolysis, immediate surgical debridement, either open or arthroscopically, is necessary.

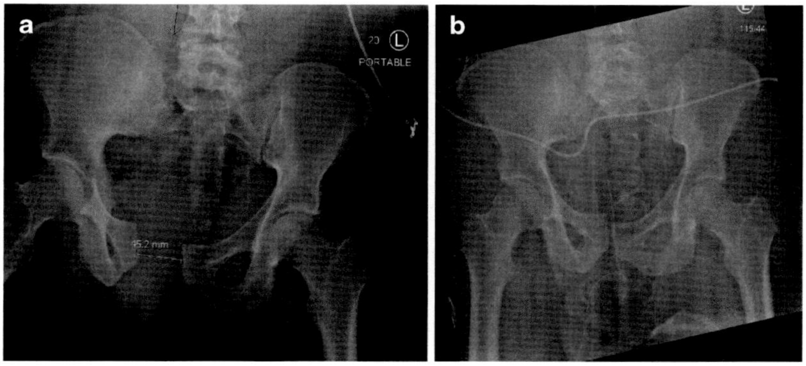

Fig. 43.1 Pelvic ring injury with associated hemodynamic instability (**a**) that improved after placement of a pelvic binder (**b**)

Injuries to Specific Anatomic Locations

A Note on Fracture Classification

Fracture classification is necessary for understanding an injury (making a diagnosis) and determining treatment. It facilitates communication and helps categorize injuries for research as well. Classifications have evolved for specific injuries. Two groups dedicated to the study and practice of orthopedic trauma, the Arbeitsgemeinschaft für Osteosynthesefragen (AO) and the Orthopedic Trauma Association (OTA), have classified every fracture of the extremity and spine, in some cases by incorporating previously used and popular classification systems [3]. For each injury in this chapter, we describe the most commonly used classifications where appropriate. In some cases, this includes the AO/OTA system and in others eponymous or other classifications. Often in clinical practice, fractures are described anatomically, with reference to which part of a bone is injured and the injury pattern.

Upper Extremity

Clavicle Fractures

Common injury patterns: Clavicle fractures are typically in either the midshaft or distal third of the clavicle and can present with varying levels of displacement. Plain radiographs are necessary for an accurate diagnosis.

Treatment options: Most closed injuries, even midshaft fractures with significant shortening, angulation, and/or comminution, can be treated with a simple sling and a period of rest. Active and passive range of motion exercises can begin at 2–3 weeks after injury. Strengthening of the extremity including the shoulder can begin at 6–8 weeks after injury, or when the patient has well-controlled pain and radiographic evidence of healing. We recommend that patients avoid contact sports for 4 months after injury. Patients tolerate residual deformity including shortening well [4]. There is significant debate which acute closed middle and distal clavicle fractures are best treated operatively (Fig. 43.2) [5–7].

Acromioclavicular Joint Injuries

Common injury patterns: Acromioclavicular (AC) joint injuries are created by any force that causes disruption to the ligamentous complex that unites the joint. Patients present after a traumatic event with tenderness over their AC joint and decreased active and passive range of motion of the shoulder. Injuries are classified based on degree and direction of radiographic displacement as well as reducibility of the joint on exam. The most common classification system is the Rockwood classification [8].

Treatment options: Non-operative treatment is indicated for closed types I through III AC joint injuries. Patients are placed in a sling, and range of motion exercises are initiated 1 week after injury. Lifting and sports are not permitted until

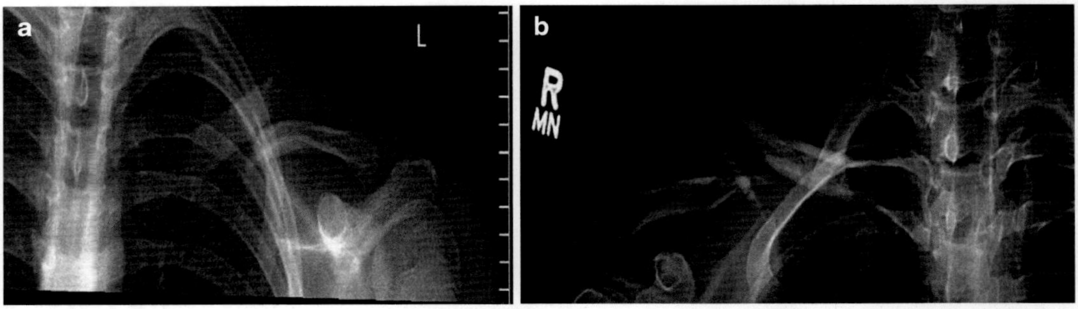

Fig. 43.2 Despite significant shortening in (**a**) and angulation and comminution in (**b**), both closed isolated fractures can be treated non-operatively

the patient has full and pain-free shoulder range of motion, which can take anywhere from 2 to 6 weeks depending on the severity of the injury. Types IV through VI AC injuries may benefit from surgical intervention. Although certain orthopedists support surgical intervention for type III injuries, the highest-quality evidence available for AC joint injuries suggests that non-operative and operative treatment have similar outcomes [9].

Glenohumeral Joint Dislocations and Fracture Dislocations

Common injury patterns: Glenohumeral joint dislocations occur most frequently when an external rotation force acts upon the abducted arm, causing the humeral head to dislocate anteriorly in relation to the glenoid. Posterior glenohumeral dislocations are less common and occur when a posteriorly directed force is applied to the adducted and internally rotated arm. To make an accurate diagnosis, radiography including an axillary or Velpeau view of the shoulder is necessary [10]. Fractures associated with traumatic glenohumeral joint dislocations may occur either on the glenoid or humeral side of the joint. Anterior inferior glenoid fractures associated with anterior dislocations are known as bony Bankart lesions. Posterior humeral head impaction fractures associated with anterior shoulder dislocations are called Hill-Sachs lesions. Proximal humerus fractures may also occur with glenohumeral joint dislocations.

Treatment options: Following closed reduction of the shoulder, non-operative treatment with a sling, early range of motion, and strengthening exercises when the patient is pain-free and has attained full shoulder range of motion can be successful for many patients. Patients who are older than 30 years of age, do not generally engage in contact sports (military or civilian sports), do not have significant associated glenoid or humeral bony defects, and have not previously experienced a dislocation event are the best candidates for non-operative management. Despite a favorable prognosis with non-operative treatment, many patients develop arthritis as a result of their injury [11]. Patients who do not meet these criteria may benefit from further orthopedic care [12]. Finally, glenohumeral joint dislocations with associated proximal humerus fractures will benefit from surgical intervention, especially if the humerus is irreducible.

Proximal Humerus Fractures

Common injury patterns: Fractures of the proximal humerus are seen in young people after high-energy traumatic events such as motor vehicle collisions or falls from height. They are also exceedingly common in elderly individuals after ground level falls. An understanding of bony anatomy of the proximal humerus is necessary for making a diagnosis and determining treatment. The bone is divided into four anatomic regions that reliably form fracture fragments: the humeral head, the greater tuberosity, the lesser tuberosity, and the humeral shaft. Fractures are classified according to the number of parts that a fracture creates, with a part defined as either greater than 1 centimeter of displacement between fracture fragments or 45° of angulation [13].

Treatment options: Treatment varies depending on displacement as well as which specific parts are part of the injury pattern. Most proximal humerus fractures without associated dislocations, especially fractures in elderly patients, can be treated non-operatively [14, 15]. This treatment protocol is performed with a sling and early active range of motion, usually beginning within 1 to 3 weeks of injury. The patient is advanced to strengthening at 8 to 12 weeks after injury depending on patient pain, range of motion, and radiographic evidence of healing. In younger patients with significantly displaced tuberosity fractures (greater than 1 centimeter), fractures with significant angulation (greater than 45°) and head split fractures may benefit from surgical intervention.

Humeral Shaft Fractures

Common injury patterns: Humeral shaft fractures occur in the diaphysis of the humerus. Physical exam, the presence of associated injuries (polytrauma), and radiographic assessment guide treatment. Fractures are classified by location in the diaphysis of proximal, middle, or distal third and by fracture pattern. Spiral, transverse, and comminuted are three of the most commonly seen patterns. Radial nerve palsies occur in 10–15% of humeral shaft fractures [16].

Treatment options: Closed, isolated injuries can be treated in a coaptation splint. For the common pattern of varus angulation, a valgus inducing force is applied upon splint application (Fig. 43.3). After one week, patients are transitioned to either a functional (Sarmiento) brace or can be maintained in a splint if bracing is not available. In this early period of 1–3 weeks after injury, patients are instructed to avoid active abduction and to avoid resting the elbow on the arm of a chair or a table as this may induce angulation at the fracture site. Range of motion exercises can begin at 6 weeks after injury. Strength training begins at 12 weeks. Patients with angulation of 20 –30 in the sagittal and coronal planes, respectively, and up to 3 cm of shortening can anticipate return of nearly normal function [17]. Closed fractures with significant angulation and shortening, fractures that occur in the polytraumatized patient or a patient with an ipsilateral forearm injury (floating elbow), and those associated with brachial plexus or vascular injuries are indicated for operative intervention.

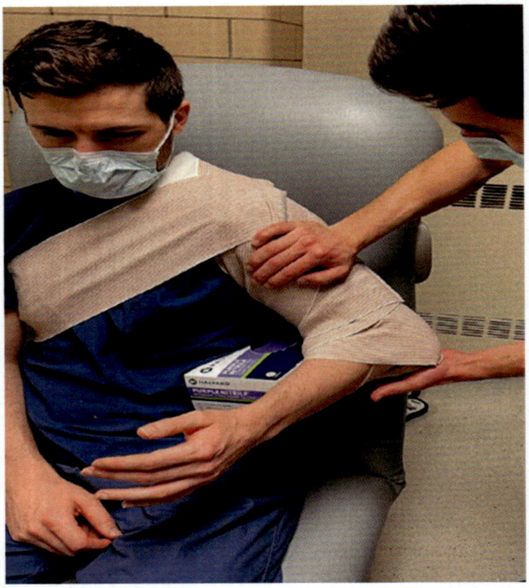

Fig. 43.3 The coaptation splint is a plaster splint that forms a "U" around the elbow and immobilizes the humerus, ending distal to the axilla medially and just distal to the sternocleidomastoid muscle laterally. The figure demonstrates the application of a valgus-inducing mold, a common maneuver for varus angulated midshaft humerus fractures

Elbow Dislocations and Fracture Dislocations

Common injury patterns: Elbow dislocations can be either simple (without associated fracture) or complex (fracture dislocations). The most common pattern is posterolateral dislocation of the radial head from its normal articulation with the capitellum of the humerus. Fracture dislocations that involve fractures of the radial head and coronoid are known as terrible triad injuries. Fractures of the proximal ulna with associated radial head dislocation are Monteggia injuries. Fractures of the olecranon with radiocapitellar instability and maintenance of an anatomic proximal radioulnar joint relationship are transolecranon fracture dislocations.

Treatment options: Simple dislocations can be treated successfully with closed reduction, a short period of rest in a long arm splint, and early range of motion that is initiated at 1 week after injury. Closed reduction is accomplished with traction and anteriorly directed pressure against the olecranon. Close follow-up is necessary to assess for persistent instability that may require further orthopedic care. Fracture dislocation variants of terrible triads, Monteggia injuries, and transolecranon fracture dislocations often require surgical intervention. These injuries are challenging to treat both operatively and non-operatively [18–20].

Olecranon Fractures

Common injury patterns: Olecranon fractures can disrupt the extensor mechanism of the elbow. As isolated injuries, they are frequently seen in middle-aged to elderly individuals after a ground level fall. Physical exam should include an assessment of the extensor mechanism. The best way to isolate this mechanism is to have the patient extend the forearm against gravity, which requires positioning the arm in full abduction at the shoulder. Radiographs demonstrate varying degrees of displacement and comminution, which helps guide treatment.

Treatment options: Nondisplaced or minimally displaced fractures are treated with a long arm splint for 1 week. The elbow becomes stiff after injury, so early passive motion is important. Active elbow extension is avoided for 6 weeks. Many orthopedists and surgeons treat displaced fractures associated with loss of ability to extend the elbow surgically. This treatment paradigm has been challenged for patients greater than 75 years of age [21].

Radial Head Fractures

Common injury patterns: When they occur as isolated injuries, radial head fractures are classified based on the amount of displacement and comminution. The examination is a critical feature of fractures of the radial head as displacement that blocks motion of the elbow joint portends a poorer prognosis with non-operative treatment. Such mechanical blocks to motion can be identified on physical exam with an intra-articular injection of local anesthetic to the elbow. Once the local anesthetic has controlled the patient's pain, the examiner can be confident that pain is not confounding assessment of range of motion. Mason described the most commonly used classification system in 1954. It is based on radiographic findings [22].

Treatment options: Mason type I fractures and type II fractures without a mechanical block to motion can be treated non-operatively with a simple sling for 1 to 3 days [23]. After this time, the patient is encouraged to discard the sling and begin active range of motion of the elbow. When pain permits, upper extremity strengthening can begin. Operative treatment is indicated for fractures that prevent elbow flexion and extension and fractures associated with elbow joint instability.

Fractures of the Diaphyseal Forearm

Common injury patterns: Fractures of the diaphysis of the radius and ulna have important implications for forearm pronosupination. Fractures in which the pathology is limited to the forearm and does not involve the elbow or the wrist are classified according to which bone is fractured (radius, ulna, or both) and by fracture pattern (transverse, comminuted, oblique, segmental). Fractures of the radius and ulna are referred to as a both bone forearm fracture. An isolated ulna fracture resulting from a direct blow to the forearm is known as a nightstick fracture.

Treatment options: Isolated injuries of the ulna including nightstick fractures with less than 50% translation and 10° of angulation are treated non-operatively with a short-arm cast or splint for 2 weeks, after which, the patient is transitioned to a brace. Weight-bearing is delayed until signs of radiographic union are present and the patient's pain is well controlled. Isolated radial shaft fractures and both bone forearm fractures are better treated operatively rather than non-operatively, as non-operative treatment leads to high rate of malunion and nonunion that cause functional deficits (Fig. 43.4) [24, 25].

Distal Radius Fractures

Common injury patterns: Distal radius fractures are exceedingly common, especially in the elderly population, for which they are the second most common fracture [26]. Fractures are often described using eponyms. For older patients, the Colles fracture is commonly seen. It is characterized by dorsal displacement of the distal fragment and apex volar angulation. Injuries to

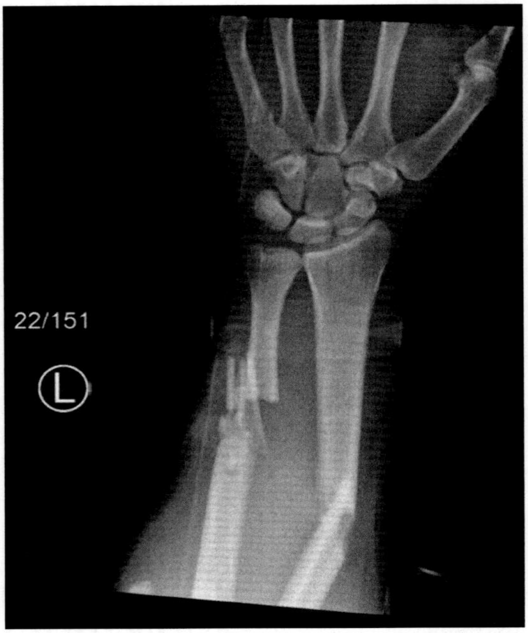

Fig. 43.4 A both bone forearm fracture that if treated non-operatively will lead to significant loss of forearm pronosupination

younger patients are best characterized according to the relationship of the fracture to the articular surface and degree of displacement. Extra-articular fractures do not involve the articular surface, and partial articular fractures involve the joint surface, but the uninvolved joint surface maintains its anatomic relationship with the more proximal aspect of the radius, and complete articular fractures are defined by fractures that disrupt the joint surface and the entirety of the bony connection between the metaphysis and the diaphysis.

Treatment options: There is extensive debate and an abundance of literature on treatment of distal radius fractures. One systematic review and meta-analysis included 70 randomized controlled trials for surgical treatment options [27]. In general, patients greater than 60 years of age can be treated with closed reduction and a sugar tong splint, short arm splint, or short arm fiberglass cast depending on physician treatment preference. We prefer a sugar tong splint to control pronosupination of the forearm during the acute treatment phase. Even patients with residual displacement have good functional outcomes [28]. Younger patients with complete or partial articular fractures with greater than 2 millimeters of articular surface displacement, greater than 3 mm of shortening, and greater than 10° of dorsal angulation (all after closed reduction) likely benefit from operative intervention [29].

Fractures of the Carpus and Metacarpals

Common injury patterns: There are a wide variety of fractures and injuries to the carpus and metacarpal bones. The most important injuries to recognize and treat are scaphoid fractures, perilunate dislocations and fracture dislocations, metacarpal base fractures including Bennett fractures, metacarpal shaft fractures, and metacarpal neck fractures.

Scaphoid fractures occur in either the distal, waist (mid-portion of the scaphoid), or proximal pole. They present with wrist pain and anatomic snuffbox tenderness as well as tenderness over the scaphoid tubercle on the volar aspect of the wrist. Computed tomography (CT) and magnetic resonance imaging (MRI) if available can be useful in making an accurate diagnosis if plain radiographs do not reveal a fracture, but history and exam raise concern for a fracture of the scaphoid [30].

Perilunate dislocations commonly occur in young people after high-energy injuries. They are characterized by disruption of wrist ligamentous and/or bony stability and resultant dislocation of the lunate from the remainder of the carpus. The dislocating force can also cause a scaphoid fracture, in which case the diagnosis is a trans-scaphoid perilunate dislocation. Patients complain of wrist pain. Plain radiographs reveal the diagnosis but can be missed in up to 25% of cases [31]. A timely diagnosis is important because the injury can be associated with acute carpal tunnel syndrome and eventual loss of median nerve function at the level of the wrist.

Metacarpal base fractures can occur in isolation or as part of a fracture dislocation of the carpal-metacarpal joint. Fractures of the base of the thumb have characteristic deforming forces and are known as either Bennett fractures if there is no comminution or Rolando fractures if there is significant comminution.

Metacarpal shaft fractures are described based on fracture pattern, with transverse and oblique fractures the most common patterns. Shaft fractures can occur alone or in combination with adjacent metacarpals. Metacarpal neck fractures occur commonly in the fifth digit. These fractures are referred to as boxer's fractures.

Treatment options: Minimally displaced scaphoid waist or distal pole fractures can be treated with 6 to 8 weeks of thumb spica splinting or casting followed by gradual return to activities of daily living and heavy lifting. Proximal pole fractures have very high rates of nonunion and are best treated surgically.

Perilunate dislocations require urgent closed reduction, which if not successful should be reduced surgically. After a successful reduction, carpal stabilization using percutaneous or open fixation methods is indicated.

Metacarpal base fracture dislocations must be reduced urgently. Metacarpal base fractures without associated dislocation can be treated non-operatively with a metacarpal mitt splint (Fig. 43.5). Certain metacarpal base fractures such as Bennett fractures can benefit from surgical treatment. Without surgical fixation, Bennett fractures often displace, and the patient will lose extension and abduction force of the thumb [32].

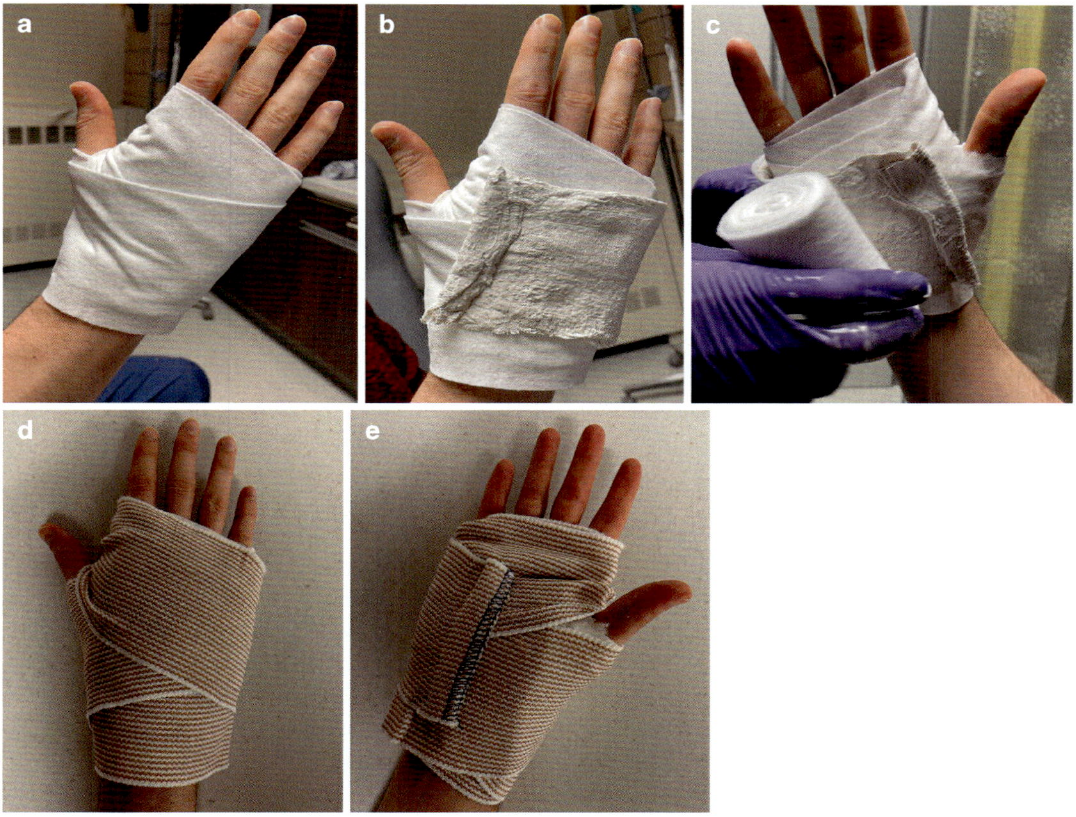

Fig. 43.5 The metacarpal mitt is a versatile splint that can treat a variety of metacarpal fractures. It can prevent finger stiffness associated with the use of other splints. (**a**) Cotton padding is applied to the hand, after which (**b**) a 4-inch plaster layer is applied keeping the metacarpal-phalangeal and wrist joints free for motion. (**c**) A layer of cotton padding prevents adhesion between the elastic wrap and plaster. The final splint with elastic wrap but not plaster covering the metacarpal-phalangeal and wrist joints is shown in (**d**) and (**e**)

Metacarpal shaft fractures without significant shortening and without adjacent metacarpal injury can be treated non-operatively with a period of immobilization and a metacarpal mitt splint. Metacarpal neck fractures, especially boxer's fractures, may heal with an apex dorsal deformity that is well tolerated by the patient [33].

Phalanx Fractures of the Hand, Phalanx Dislocations, and Nail Bed Injuries

Common injury patterns: Fractures of the proximal, middle, and distal phalanx of the hand are common. The proximal phalanx deformity for extra-articular fractures is one of apex volar angulation due to the deforming forces acting upon it. The middle phalanx deformity can be apex volar or dorsal. Distal phalanx fracturs are often associated with nail bed injuries. Fractures are described based on anatomic location of head, shaft, or base, fracture pattern, and degree of articular involvement.

Phalanx dislocations of the proximal interphalangeal joint (PIP) and distal phalangeal joint (DIP) are also common.

Any examination of the hand must include an assessment of extensor and flexor tendon competence. This is accomplished by having the patient actively flex and extend a joint. Findings are either corroborated or come into question with a test of passive tenodesis. A symmetric cascade of obligatory finger flexion should occur with wrist extension. Similarly, a cascade of finger extension should occur with passive wrist flexion.

Treatment options: Extra-articular phalanx fractures without significant angulation (less than 10°), shortening (less than 2 millimeters of shortening), and without significant rotational deformity on exam are treated with buddy taping or splinting for 2 to 3 weeks. After this time, an active and passive range of motion protocol is initiated. This is particularly important to prevent stiffness. Fractures that do not meet these criteria and fractures with a displaced articular surface may benefit from referral to an orthopedist, as a variety of fixation methods can maintain reduction until bony healing.

Distal phalanx tuft fractures with a nail bed injury can be treated non-operatively if the nail bed injury is small (less than 50% or so of the nail bed is occupied by a subungual hematoma). If the nail bed injury has disrupted the nail or contains a large subungual hematoma, the nail should be removed and the nail bed irrigated and repaired with 5–0 or 6–0 absorbable or non-absorbable sutures, after which the patient is placed on antibiotics for a week. We favor cephalexin or, for contaminated wounds, trimethoprim-sulfamethoxazole and amoxicillin-clavulanic acid for 7 days.

Simple phalanx dislocations can be closed reduced by accentuating the deformity of the dislocation, after which a force that reduces the joint is applied. For example, the PIP joint commonly dislocates dorsally. The joint can be hyperflexed, after which a volarly directed force is applied to the base of the middle phalanx. Joint stability should be assessed after reduction.

Injuries to Specific Anatomic Locations: Lower Extremity

Fractures of the Pelvis and Acetabulum

Common injury patterns: Pelvic ring fractures are associated with high rates of mortality, especially when they occur in the setting of high energy, multiple other injuries, and hemorrhage requiring resuscitation [34]. Likewise, acetabular fractures are injuries that can put a patient's life at risk if appropriate acute care is not rendered.

After a patient is stabilized, a better assessment of the fracture is made with computed tomography. Plain radiographs of the pelvis and acetabulum also allow for accurate diagnosis, but do not allow for as accurate assessment of intra-articular bodies and joint impaction and displacement.

For the non-orthopedist in a resource-limited setting, the important elements of a pelvic ring fracture to identify are pubic symphysis displacement (widening) and sacroiliac joint displacement (Fig. 43.6). Acetabular fractures must be assessed in the emergent period for hip joint dislocation, which can be diagnosed easily on plain radiographs.

Treatment options: After emergent stabilization and resuscitation (discussed in more detail in the section on orthopedic emergencies), patients with a pelvic ring injury characterized by a vertically displaced hemipelvis and acetabular fractures characterized by joint dislocation or subluxation are best placed in skeletal traction. Further workup and surgical planning then commence after consultation with an orthopedist.

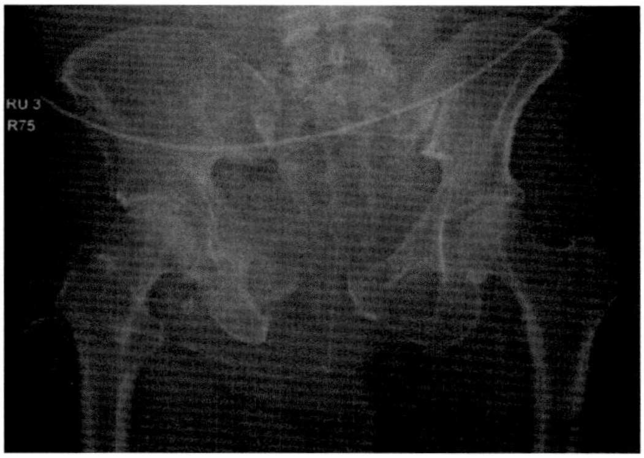

Fig. 43.6 Anteroposterior pelvic radiograph demonstrating widening of the pubic symphysis anteriorly and displacement of the sacroiliac joint posteriorly. This injury requires emergent stabilization with a pelvic sheet or binder

Femoral Neck Fractures

Common injury patterns: Femoral neck fractures are debilitating injuries that occur in any age group. Because these fractures occur within the hip joint capsule, they have poor capacity for healing, and sequelae of nonunion and/or avascular necrosis of the femoral head are common. They can be either displaced or non-displaced (Fig. 43.7).

Treatment options: Non-operative treatment of femoral neck fractures is associated with chronic pain, loss of ambulatory capacity, and, especially in the elderly population, sarcopenia from bed rest that can prevent meaningful recovery. Because of poor outcomes with non-operative treatment, femoral neck fractures should be treated operatively unless a patient is medically unfit or unsafe for surgery. There is general agreement that surgical intervention should take place within 24 h for younger patients and within 48 h for older patients. In younger patients, expeditious treatment decreases the risk of avascular necrosis, and in older patients, it is associated with a reduction in mortality [35, 36]. Timing is also determined by medical stability of a patient, and patients should be as medically optimized as rigorously as possible before proceeding to surgery.

Fig. 43.7 AP (**a**) and lateral (**b**) views of a non-displaced fracture of the left femoral neck

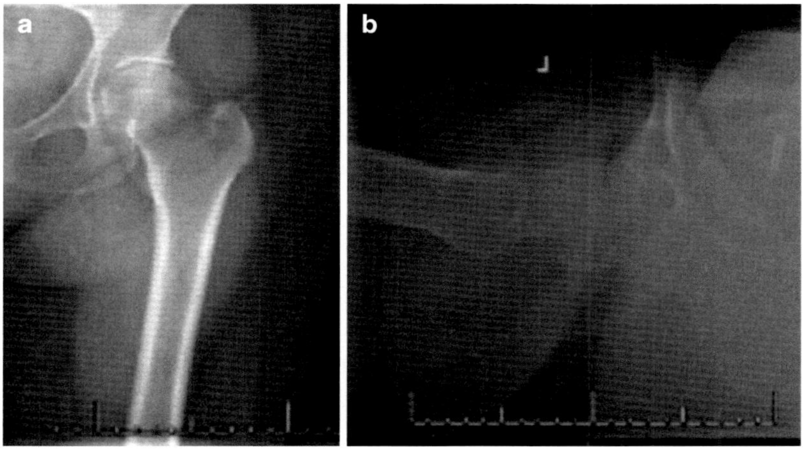

Fractures of the Intertrochanteric Region of the Femur

Common injury patterns: The intertrochanteric (IT) region of the proximal femur is extracapsular and thus receives a more robust blood supply than the intracapsular (femoral neck) area. Fractures that occur in this area typically heal with appropriate treatment. Fractures can be either stable, defined as a simple fracture line that runs through the IT region from superolateral to inferomedial and which is non- or minimally displaced, or unstable, defined as comminuted fractures, fractures that require manipulation for reduction, or fractures in which the main fracture line runs from superomedial to inferolateral. These latter fractures are called reverse obliquity intertrochanteric fractures.

Treatment options: Non-operative treatment should be avoided unless a patient is medically unfit for surgery or resources do not allow surgical stabilization. If necessary, non-operative treatment should include measures to prevent venous thromboembolism, pneumonia, and bedsores. There are a variety of surgical treatment methods that are determined by fracture pattern, patient age, and patient functional status.

Femoral Shaft Fractures

Common injury patterns: Femoral shaft fractures are described by location in the bone of proximal, middle, or distal third and by fracture pattern of transverse, oblique, spiral, comminuted, or segmental. Among other concomitant injuries, patients are at risk for an ipsilateral femoral neck fracture. Dedicated hip and pelvis radiographs can be sufficient for making the diagnosis of an ipsilateral femoral neck fracture, but a CT scan improves the clinician's ability to make the diagnosis [37].

Treatment options: Patients with femoral shaft fractures are treated in the emergency setting with skin or skeletal traction until the patient is ready to proceed to the operating room. If a patient does not have access to an operating room or if surgery will be delayed to a significant amount of time, skeletal rather than skin traction is necessary, and the patient must be assessed daily on rounds for skin especially heel pressure sores, pin site infection, and signs and symptoms of common problems that occur from prolonged bed rest such as pneumonia and VTE. We do not recommend splinting or casting of these injuries.

Closed or open reduction with intramedullary stabilization is the standard of care for femoral shaft fractures. There has been significant debate about surgical timing for femoral shaft fractures. Patients at higher risk for complications such as fat embolism and adult respiratory distress syndrome have associated lung injuries and/or are hemodynamically unstable, often gauged by blood lactate level above 2.5–4.0 mm/L and trending upward [38].

Distal Femur Fractures

Common injury patterns: Distal femur fractures occur in young people after high-energy trauma and in elderly people after low-energy trauma such as ground level falls. In elderly patients, they are associated with high rates of mortality up to 1 year after injury and in this sense can be considered similar to geriatric hip fractures [39]. They can be understood best using the AO/OTA classification of periarticular fractures, with an A type defined as an extra-articular fracture, B-type partial articular, and C-type complete articular (articular fracture with complete dissociation of the articular surface from the meta-diaphysis) [3].

Treatment options: Distal femur fractures in both the young and elderly are best treated surgically. Non-operative care should be limited to medically unfit patients or patients for whom surgery is not otherwise feasible.

Dislocations of the Knee and Traumatic Knee Instability

Common injury patterns: Dislocations of the knee joint are severe injuries associated with neurovascular damage. The tibia and/or femur can be dislocated in any direction, depending on the direction of the applied force at the time of injury. Exam and imaging should focus on identifying nerve and vascular injury. If a patient has asymmetric or weak dorsalis pedis pulses on exam or an expanding hematoma about the knee, he must be assumed to have a vascular injury until proven otherwise. Advanced imaging with CT angiography is used to diagnose vascular injury [40].

Treatment options: Immediate reduction of a knee dislocation is necessary. The patient should be sedated. Traction should then be applied to the extremity, which is often enough to complete the reduction. After reduction, an assessment of stability is completed. If the knee demonstrates persistent subluxation or dislocation on either exam or fluoroscopic examination, an external fixator that spans the knee is applied (Box 43.3).

Box 43.3 Note on External Fixation

External fixation is an important part of the armamentarium of a clinician treating orthopedic injuries. Stainless-steel pins of varying diameter depending on the bone being stabilized are inserted proximal and distal to an injury, which may be proximal and distal to a joint, for example, when using a knee-spanning external fixator to stabilize a knee dislocation. The pins are then connected by rods, which are held to one another using connecting bolts.

The following principles of external fixation should be used when applying an external fixator:

- An external fixator should ideally hold a reduction. It is used to gain anatomic length, alignment, and rotation of an injured extremity.
- Plan pin sites based on future incision for definitive surgery. Future incisions cannot go through pin sites.
- Factors that increase stability of an external fixation construct are:
  - Increased pin and/or rod diameter.
  - Pin spacing with placement both near and far from the fracture.
  - Use of additional bars.
  - Use of additional pins.
  - Placement of pins in better bone, usually diaphyseal as opposed to metaphyseal.
- Respect and understand anatomy: pin sites should be chosen so that they are in safe pin entry zones.

Bony stability is necessary for vascular repair, if needed. A brace, splint, or cast can be used for knee immobilization if the knee is stable after reduction (Fig. 43.8). Emergent treatment of knee dislocations includes consultation with a vascular or general surgeon who can assist with vessel repair, if necessary. After the patient and limb are stabilized, further workup, typically with MRI, and eventual reconstruction of damaged ligaments can take place under the care of an orthopedist.

Tibial Plateau Fractures

Common injury patterns: These common injuries span a range of pathology from minimal displacement to severe displacement associated with soft tissue injuries that preclude meaningful recovery and can necessitate amputation. The most common classification is the Schatzker classification, which is meaningful for communication, treatment planning, and prognosis [41]. Similar to knee dislocations, a thorough neurovascular exam is necessary so that limb-threatening injuries are not missed. A CT scan is often not necessary for diagnosis but is invaluable to the orthopedist for surgical planning.

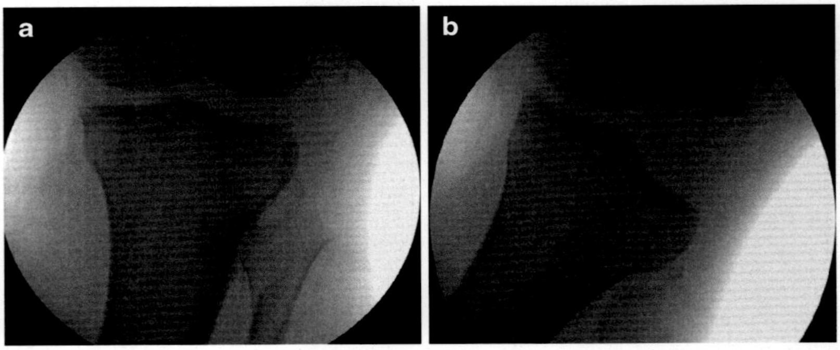

Fig. 43.8 25-year-old man after a motor vehicle collision. He had a popliteal artery injury requiring repair. After reduction of a knee dislocation (**a**), the exam under fluoroscopy revealed significant lateral joint widening on varus stress (**b**). An external fixator was applied to stabilize the knee for vascular repair

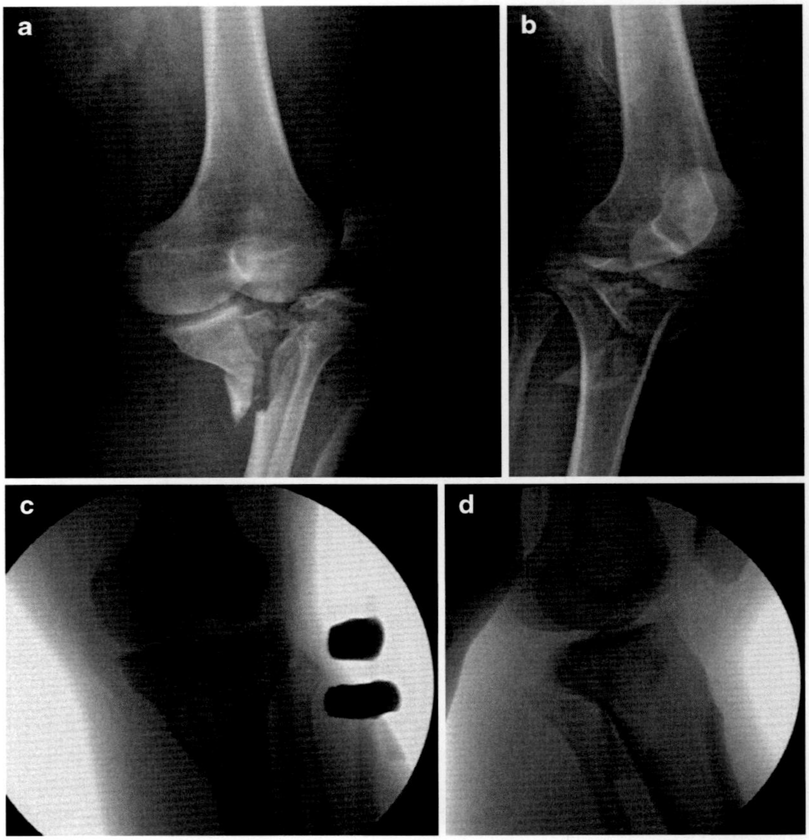

Fig. 43.9 22-year-old man after a scooter accident. A partial medial articular, Schatzker IV-type fracture is diagnosed on injury radiographs in (**a**) and (**b**). After application of an external fixator, length, rotation, and alignment of the extremity are restored in (**c**) and (**d**)

Treatment options: Low-energy, minimally displaced injuries can be treated non-operatively with a brace or cast for 6 weeks, followed by physical therapy for motion, ambulation, and strength training. High-energy injuries with significant displacement are treated with an external fixator *with the goal of restoring extremity length, rotation, and alignment*. When soft-tissue tension and/or blistering allows, surgical intervention is the standard of care for injuries associated with significant displacement (Fig. 43.9).

Tibial Shaft Fractures

Common injury patterns: Fractures of the tibial shaft occur in either the proximal, middle, or distal third of the bone and can be spiral, transverse, oblique, comminuted, or segmental. Because the anteromedial aspect of the tibia is subcutaneous, fractures of the tibia are prone to being open injuries.

Treatment options: Fractures with less than 50% translation, 5° of angulation in the coronal plane, 10° of angulation in the sagittal planes, 10° of rotational malalignment, and 1 centimeter of shortening can be treated in a long leg splint or cast for 3 weeks, after which the patient is transitioned to a functional brace and, if pain allows, made weight-bearing as tolerated.

Fractures of the Tibial Plafond (Pilon Fractures)

Common injury patterns: Fractures of the tibial plafond (pilon fractures) are defined as any fracture occurring within or near the weight-bearing surface of the tibia. The AO/OTA classification is commonly used to describe the injury. Type A fractures are extra-articular, type B partial articular, and type C complete articular fractures (Fig. 43.10).

Treatment options: Management of tibial plafond fractures in the acute setting includes stabilization with an external fixator followed by a period of soft tissue rest, after which definitive surgical stabilization takes place, with the goal of restoring the anatomy of the joint surface and length, alignment, and rotation of the metadiaphyseal region of the tibia. Outcomes after plafond fractures are poor even with surgical management, with one study showing that patient-reported outcomes were worse than not only the general population but patients who had experienced an acute myocardial infarction, pelvic fracture, or acquired immunodeficiency syndrome (AIDS) [42].

Rotational Ankle Fractures

Common injury patterns: A rotational mechanism of injury at the ankle can produce a fracture of the lateral malleolus, the medial malleolus, or the posterior malleolus or an injury at any combination of these anatomic locations. Fracture dislocations are common with rotational injuries. Soft tissue considerations about the ankle are also paramount because of the important functional role of the ankle syndesmosis, the ligamentous complex that spans and allows dynamic stabilization at the distal tibial-fibular joint.

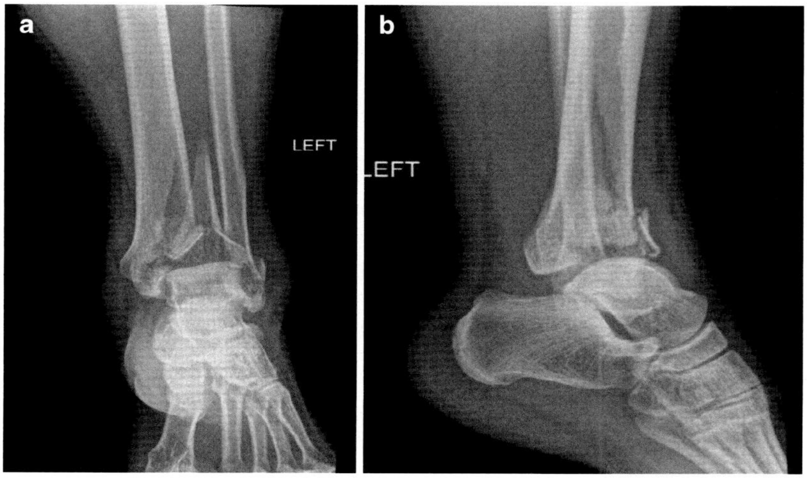

Fig. 43.10 Anteroposterior (**a**) and lateral (**b**) radiograph of the left ankle of a 43-year-old man who fell off a ladder. There is a fracture of the articular surface of the distal tibia and discontinuity between the articular surface and the metadiaphyseal region, making this an AO/OTA type C fracture

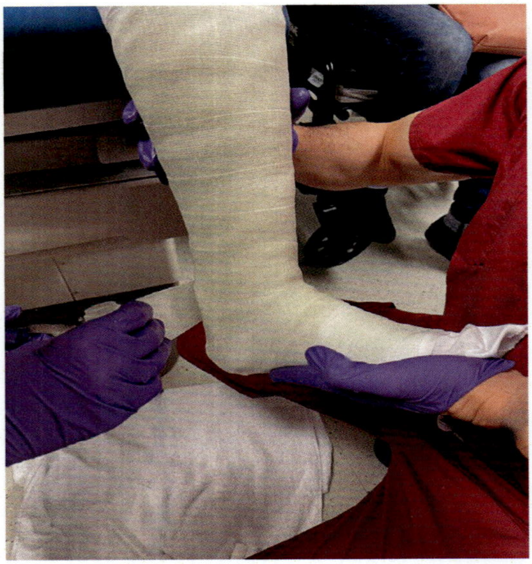

Fig. 43.11 A dorsiflexion force is applied at the ankle while applying a short leg splint. During cast application, this dorsiflexion force allows for fiberglass placement without wrinkles. After cast placement, the force is maintained to prevent the ankle from assuming its resting plantar-flexed position

Fractures are classified in many ways. The Lauge-Hansen classification is one of the most popular systems [43]. Knowing a fracture classification is as important as recognizing syndesmotic injury.

Treatment options: In the acute setting, an ankle fracture can be treated with a short leg splint or cast and a period of immobilization. Isolated lateral malleolus fractures with a stable mortise on radiographs (either weight-bearing radiographs or stress examination) can be made weight-bearing as tolerated. Dislocations should be reduced urgently. This may be accomplished with local anesthesia in the ankle joint. The ankle should be immobilized in a small amount of dorsiflexion to prevent an equinus contracture of the joint (Fig. 43.11). Referral to an orthopedist will help guide the decision between operative and non-operative treatment.

Talus and Calcaneus Fractures

Common injury patterns: Fractures of the hindfoot can be devastating injuries. Often, they occur in the setting of high-energy trauma, e.g., jumping off a building. Plain radiographs are necessary for diagnosis.

Treatment options: Emergent management consists of a short leg splint for talus fractures and a "bulky" splint with extra padding at the heel for calcaneus fractures. Certain minimally displaced fractures can be treated non-operatively with 6 to 8 weeks of non-weight-bearing, but any displacement of either fracture is best evaluated by an orthopedist.

Midfoot and Forefoot Injuries

Common injury patterns: Midfoot and forefoot injuries can occur in a variety of locations. Lisfranc fractures, dislocations, or fracture dislocations are easily missed and can lead to chronic pain and disability for a patient. This injury is characterized by disruption of the ligamentous connection between the medial cuneiform and the base of the second metatarsal. The injury occurs along a spectrum of mild ligamentous attenuation to dislocation of the entire tarsal-metatarsal joint. Because the Lisfranc ligament provides stability to the arch of the foot, if it is disrupted and not stabilized, the midfoot will lose its structural integrity and collapse.

Metatarsal fractures and fractures of the phalanges of the foot are common. Dislocations at the metatarsal-phalangeal (MTP) joint are common as well. Fractures of the proximal aspect of the fifth metatarsal receive significant attention because of the importance of differentiating between avulsion-type injuries of the base and transverse fractures just distal to the base (Jones fractures), which heal less reliably [44].

Treatment options: In the acute setting, midfoot and forefoot injuries can be treated with a short leg splint and a period of non-weight-bearing. Certain injuries such as base of the fifth metatarsal avulsion fractures can be made weight-bearing as tolerated. Lisfranc injuries, either confirmed or suspected, and Jones fractures should be referred for orthopedic management.

Injuries to Specific Anatomic Locations: Pediatric Injuries

Pediatric patients present with different fracture patterns from those commonly seen in adults. Additionally, pediatric fractures can result in growth arrest or deformity because of injury to the physis.

Distal Humerus Supracondylar Fractures

Common injury patterns: Physical exam of pediatric patients with elbow pain should include a thorough neurovascular exam with particular attention paid to radial pulse as well as potential deficits of the anterior interosseous branch of the median nerve, ulnar nerve or radial nerve, depending on fracture pattern.

Distal humerus supracondylar fractures are either extension type or flexion type, with extension type being more frequent. Plain radiographs reveal varying degrees of displacement and are categorized with the Gartland classification system [45]. Occult fractures (no visible fracture) are diagnosed based on the finding elbow pain and radiographically with the "fat pad sign" of edema posterior to the distal humerus, which displaces the fat pad that normally occupies this area.

Treatment options: Patients with an absent or weak radial pulse and a cool hand are taken emergently to the operating room for a closed reduction, after which the radial pulse and hand perfusion are reexamined. If the hand remains dysvascular, exploration of the brachial artery is undertaken. Patients with an absent or weak radial pulse but a pink (well-perfused) hand are treated based on fracture pattern and observed with serial examinations over the course of at least 24 hours. Finally, patients with a palpable radial pulse are treated based on fracture pattern, with more displaced injuries commonly treated surgically.

Occult fractures or Gartland type I injuries are treated with a long arm cast for 3 weeks, after which the cast is removed, and the patient is made weight-bearing as tolerated as long as pain is well controlled and the elbow has regained range of motion. A long arm cast should include a supracondylar mold, and the elbow should be flexed to 60° or 70°. The olecranon, ulnar head, and radial styloid must be well padded, and the fingers including the thumb should remain free for unrestricted movement. Debate exists regarding surgical versus non-surgical treatment of Gartland type II injuries [46].

Distal Humerus Lateral Condyle Fractures

Common injury patterns: Patients presenting with elbow pain and plain radiograph findings of a lateral condylar fractures of the distal humerus undergo an additional internal oblique view of the elbow. The internal oblique view helps best visualize the fracture to determine displacement.

Treatment options: Minimally displaced fractures are treated with a long arm cast for 3 weeks. Displaced fractures should be referred for orthopedic evaluation.

Both Bone Forearm Fractures and Distal Radius Fractures

Common injury patterns: Both bone forearm fractures range from minimally displaced fractures or fractures with associated plastic deformation to fractures with significant displacement. Distal radius fractures occurring about the physis are classified with the Salter-Harris classification system.

Treatment options: For both bone forearm fractures, minimally displaced fractures are treated with a long arm cast. Displaced fractures can be closed reduced in the emergency department. Intravenous sedation is usually necessary to perform a closed reduction. Reduction is maintained with a long arm cast. Adequacy of reduction is assessed radiographically. Certain injuries, especially displaced fractures in older children, are often treated surgically.

For distal radius fractures occurring in young children, a long arm cast is helpful to prevent self-discontinuation of immobilization. For distal radius fractures occurring in older children, a short arm cast is sufficient for treatment. Similar to both bone forearm fractures, displaced fractures of the distal radius can be closed reduced in the emergency department. Casting is maintained for up to 6 weeks. Serial radiographs obtained weekly for the first 2 to 3 weeks after injury ensures that if reduction is lost, appropriate treatment including potential surgery can be considered.

Femoral Shaft Fractures

Common injury patterns: Femoral shaft fractures can occur in the proximal, middle, or distal third of the femur. If there is any suspicion for non-accidental trauma, appropriate social services should be notified according to local practice.

Treatment options: Patient age dictates treatment. Patients younger than 6 months of age are treated with 3–6 weeks with a Pavlik harness. Patients between 6 months and 5 or 6 years of age undergo closed reduction and hip spica cast application. Patients older than 6 years of age and less than 50 kilograms of weight are best evaluated by an orthopedic surgeon and usually benefit from surgical stabilization. The caregivers of patients undergoing treatment for femoral shaft fractures should be educated on the possibility of leg length discrepancy that develops in the first 1 to 2 years after injury [47].

Distal Femoral Physeal Fractures

Common injury patterns: Fractures of the physis of the distal femur can be associated with neurovascular injury. If distal pulses are weak, asymmetric, or absent, additional studies such as ankle-brachial indices and CT angiogram are necessary to evaluate for injury of the popliteal artery.

Treatment options: Displaced fractures are often treated surgically. Patients and caregivers should be educated on the potential for leg-length discrepancy. As opposed to femoral shaft fractures, which can result in an injured extremity that is longer than the contralateral side, distal femur physeal fractures can result in an injured extremity that is shorter and/or angulated as compared to the contralateral side because of growth arrest at the physis [48].

Transitional Ankle Fractures

Common injury patterns: The physis of the distal tibia closes in a predictable manner, which leads to predictable injury patterns that occur at age 14 or so in girls and 16 or so in boys who sustain rotational ankle injuries. The two most common patterns are Tillaux fracture (Salter-Harris III) and triplane fracture (Salter-Harris IV). Plain radiographs are necessary as part of initial workup. A CT scan best assesses displacement of the articular surface of the ankle.

Treatment options: Minimally displaced fractures are treated with a long leg cast and non-weight-bearing for 3–6 weeks. Displaced fractures may require surgical treatment and evaluation by an orthopedist.

References

1. Kim PH, Leopold SS. In brief: Gustilo-Anderson classification. [corrected]. Clin Orthop Relat Res. 2012;470:3270–4. https://doi.org/10.1007/s11999-012-2376-6.
2. Margaretten ME, Kohlwes J, Moore D, Bent S. Does this adult patient have septic arthritis? JAMA. 2007;297:1478–88. https://doi.org/10.1001/jama.297.13.1478.
3. Meinberg EG, Agel J, Roberts CS, Karam MD, Kellam JF. Fracture and dislocation classification compendium—2018. J Orthop Trauma. 2018;32:S1. https://doi.org/10.1097/BOT.0000000000001063.
4. Goudie EB, Clement ND, Murray IR, Lawrence CR, Wilson M, Brooksbank AJ, Robinson CM (2017) The influence of shortening on clinical outcome in healed displaced midshaft clavicular fractures after nonoperative treatment. JBJS 99:1166–1172. https://doi.org/10.2106/JBJS.16.01010.
5. Hall JA, Schemitsch CE, Vicente MR, Dehghan N, Nauth A, Nowak LL, Schemitsch EH, McKee MD, Canadian Orthopaedic Trauma Society (COTS). Operative versus nonoperative treatment of acute displaced distal clavicle fractures: a

Multicenter randomized controlled Trial. J Orthop Trauma. 2021;35:660–6. https://doi.org/10.1097/BOT.0000000000002211.

6. Canadian Orthopaedic Trauma Society. Nonoperative treatment compared with plate fixation of displaced midshaft clavicular fractures. A multicenter, randomized clinical trial. J Bone Joint Surg Am. 2007;89:1–10. https://doi.org/10.2106/JBJS.F.00020.
7. Woltz S, Stegeman SA, Krijnen P, van Dijkman BA, van Thiel TPH, Schep NWL, de Rijcke PAR, Frölke JPM, Schipper IB. Plate fixation compared with non-operative treatment for displaced midshaft clavicular fractures: a Multicenter randomized controlled Trial. J Bone Joint Surg Am. 2017;99:106–12. https://doi.org/10.2106/JBJS.15.01394.
8. Gorbaty JD, Hsu JE, Gee AO. Classifications in brief: Rockwood classification of acromioclavicular joint separations. Clin Orthop Relat Res. 2017;475:283–7. https://doi.org/10.1007/s11999-016-5079-6.
9. Tamaoki MJ, Lenza M, Matsunaga FT, Belloti JC, Matsumoto MH, Faloppa F. Surgical versus conservative interventions for treating acromioclavicular dislocation of the shoulder in adults. Cochrane Database Syst Rev. 2019;10:CD007429. https://doi.org/10.1002/14651858.CD007429.pub3.
10. Rouleau DM, Hebert-Davies J, Robinson CM. Acute traumatic posterior shoulder dislocation. JAAOS - Journal of the American Academy of Orthopaedic Surgeons. 2014;22:145–52. https://doi.org/10.5435/JAAOS-22-03-145.
11. Hovelius L, Rahme H. Primary anterior dislocation of the shoulder: long-term prognosis at the age of 40 years or younger. Knee Surg Sports Traumatol Arthrosc. 2016;24:330–42. https://doi.org/10.1007/s00167-015-3980-2.
12. Burns TC, Owens BD. Management of Shoulder Instability in in-season athletes. Phys Sportsmed. 2010;38:55–60. https://doi.org/10.3810/psm.2010.10.1808.
13. Neer CS. Displaced proximal humeral fractures. I. Classification and evaluation. J Bone Joint Surg Am. 1970;52:1077–89.
14. Rangan A, Handoll H, Brealey S, Jefferson L, Keding A, Martin BC, Goodchild L, Chuang L-H, Hewitt C, Torgerson D, Trial Collaborators PROFHER. Surgical vs nonsurgical treatment of adults with displaced fractures of the proximal humerus: the PROFHER randomized clinical trial. JAMA. 2015;313:1037–47. https://doi.org/10.1001/jama.2015.1629.
15. Beks RB, Ochen Y, Frima H, Smeeing DPJ, van der Meijden O, Timmers TK, van der Velde D, van Heijl M, Leenen LPH, Groenwold RHH, Houwert RM. Operative versus nonoperative treatment of proximal humeral fractures: a systematic review, meta-analysis, and comparison of observational studies and randomized controlled trials. J Shoulder Elb Surg. 2018;27:1526–34. https://doi.org/10.1016/j.jse.2018.03.009.
16. Shao YC, Harwood P, Grotz MRW, Limb D, Giannoudis PV (2005) Radial nerve palsy associated with fractures of the shaft of the humerus. The Journal of Bone and Joint Surgery British volume 87-B:1647–1652. https://doi.org/10.1302/0301-620X.87B12.16132.
17. Rutgers M, Ring D. Treatment of diaphyseal fractures of the humerus using a functional brace. J Orthop Trauma. 2006;20:597–601. https://doi.org/10.1097/01.bot.0000249423.48074.82.
18. Luengo-Alonso G, García Lamas L, Jiménez Díaz V, Ferrero Recasens J, Porras Moreno MA, Cecilia López D. Trans-olecranon fracture dislocations: how should we treat them? Injury. 2021;52(Suppl 4):S131–6. https://doi.org/10.1016/j.injury.2021.02.058.
19. Xiao RC, Chan JJ, Cirino CM, Kim JM. Surgical Management of Complex Adult Monteggia Fractures. J Hand Surg Am. 2021;46:1006–15. https://doi.org/10.1016/j.jhsa.2021.07.023.
20. Chen NC, Ring D. Terrible triad injuries of the elbow. J Hand Surg Am. 2015;40:2297–303. https://doi.org/10.1016/j.jhsa.2015.04.039.
21. Duckworth AD, Clement ND, McEachan JE, White TO, Court-Brown CM, McQueen MM. Prospective randomised trial of non-operative versus operative management of olecranon fractures in the elderly. Bone Joint J. 2017;99-B:964–72. https://doi.org/10.1302/0301-620X.99B7.BJJ-2016-1112.R2.
22. Mason ML. Some observations on fractures of the head of the radius with a review of one hundred cases. BJS (British Journal of Surgery). 1954;42:123–32. https://doi.org/10.1002/bjs.18004217203.
23. Mulders MAM, Schep NWL, de Muinck KR-JO, Kodde IF, Hoogendoorn JM, Goslings JC, Eygendaal D. Operative vs. nonoperative treatment for Mason type 2 radial head fractures: a randomized controlled trial. J Shoulder Elb Surg. 2021;30:1670–8. https://doi.org/10.1016/j.jse.2021.02.025.
24. Kloen P, Wiggers JK, Buijze GA. Treatment of diaphyseal non-unions of the ulna and radius. Arch Orthop Trauma Surg. 2010;130:1439–45. https://doi.org/10.1007/s00402-010-1071-x.
25. Fracture of the Distal Radial Shaft MISTAKES IN MANAGEMENT *.
26. Shauver MJ, Yin H, Banerjee M, Chung KC. Current and future National Costs to Medicare for the treatment of distal radius fracture in the elderly. J Hand Surg Am. 2011;36:1282–7. https://doi.org/10.1016/j.jhsa.2011.05.017.
27. Woolnough T, Axelrod D, Bozzo A, Koziarz A, Koziarz F, Oitment C, Gyemi L, Gormley J, Gouveia K, Johal H. What is the relative effectiveness of the various surgical treatment options for distal radius fractures? A systematic review and network meta-analysis of randomized controlled trials. Clin Orthop Relat Res. 2021;479:348–62. https://doi.org/10.1097/CORR.0000000000001524.
28. Chung KC, Kim HM, Malay S, Shauver MJ, WRIST Group. Comparison of 24-month outcomes after treatment for distal radius fracture: the WRIST randomized clinical Trial. JAMA Netw Open. 2021;4:e2112710. https://doi.org/10.1001/jamanetworkopen.2021.12710.

29. Kamal RN, Shapiro LM. American Academy of orthopaedic surgeons/American Society for Surgery of the Hand clinical practice guideline summary management of distal radius fractures. J Am Acad Orthop Surg. 2022;30:e480–6. https://doi.org/10.5435/JAAOS-D-21-00719.
30. Sabbagh MD, Morsy M, Moran SL. Diagnosis and Management of Acute Scaphoid Fractures. Hand Clin. 2019;35:259–69. https://doi.org/10.1016/j.hcl.2019.03.002.
31. Herzberg G, Comtet JJ, Linscheid RL, Amadio PC, Cooney WP, Stalder J. Perilunate dislocations and fracture-dislocations: a multicenter study. J Hand Surg Am. 1993;18:768–79. https://doi.org/10.1016/0363-5023(93)90041-Z.
32. Griffiths JC. Fractures at the base of the first metacarpal bone. J Bone Joint Surg Br. 1964;46-B:712–9. https://doi.org/10.1302/0301-620X.46B4.712.
33. WESTBROOK AP, DAVIS TRC, ARMSTRONG D, BURKE FD (2008) The clinical significance of malunion of fractures of the neck and shaft of the little finger metacarpal. J Hand Surg Eur Vol 33:732–739. https://doi.org/10.1177/1753193408092497.
34. Holstein JH, Culemann U, Pohlemann T, Working Group Mortality in Pelvic Fracture Patients. What are predictors of mortality in patients with pelvic fractures? Clin Orthop Relat Res. 2012;470:2090–7. https://doi.org/10.1007/s11999-012-2276-9.
35. Chan DS. Femoral neck fractures in young patients: state of the art. J Orthop Trauma. 2019;33:S7. https://doi.org/10.1097/BOT.0000000000001366.
36. Danford NC, Logue TC, Boddapati V, Anderson MJJ, Anderson FL, Rosenwasser MP. Debate update: surgery after 48 hours of admission for geriatric hip fracture patients is associated with increase in mortality and complication rate: a study of 27,058 patients using the National Trauma Data Bank. J Orthop Trauma. 2021;35:535–41. https://doi.org/10.1097/BOT.0000000000002075.
37. Tornetta P, Kain MSH, Creevy WR. Diagnosis of femoral neck fractures in patients with a femoral shaft fracture. Improvement with a standard protocol. J Bone Joint Surg Am. 2007;89:39–43. https://doi.org/10.2106/JBJS.F.00297.
38. D'Alleyrand J-CG, O'Toole RV. The evolution of damage control orthopedics: current evidence and practical applications of early appropriate care. Orthop Clin North Am. 2013;44:499–507. https://doi.org/10.1016/j.ocl.2013.06.004.
39. Merino-Rueda LR, Rubio-Sáez I, Mills S, Rubio-Suárez JC. Mortality after distal femur fractures in the elderly. Injury. 2021;52(Suppl 4):S71–5. https://doi.org/10.1016/j.injury.2021.03.066.
40. Stannard JP, Sheils TM, Lopez-Ben RR, McGwin G, Robinson JT, Volgas DA. Vascular injuries in knee dislocations: the role of physical examination in determining the need for arteriography. J Bone Joint Surg Am. 2004;86:910–5.
41. Zeltser DW, Leopold SS. Classifications in brief: Schatzker classification of tibial plateau fractures. Clin Orthop Relat Res. 2013;471:371–4. https://doi.org/10.1007/s11999-012-2451-z.
42. Pollak AN, McCarthy ML, Bess RS, Agel J, Swiontkowski MF. Outcomes after treatment of high-energy tibial plafond fractures. JBJS. 2003;85:1893–900.
43. Tartaglione JP, Rosenbaum AJ, Abousayed M, DiPreta JA. Classifications in brief: Lauge-Hansen classification of ankle fractures. Clin Orthop Relat Res. 2015;473:3323–8. https://doi.org/10.1007/s11999-015-4306-x.
44. Metzl JA, Bowers MW, Anderson RB. Fifth metatarsal Jones fractures: diagnosis and treatment. J Am Acad Orthop Surg. 2022;30:e470–9. https://doi.org/10.5435/JAAOS-D-21-00542.
45. Alton TB, Werner SE, Gee AO. Classifications in brief: the Gartland classification of supracondylar humerus fractures. Clin Orthop Relat Res. 2015;473:738–41. https://doi.org/10.1007/s11999-014-4033-8.
46. Abzug JM, Herman MJ. Management of supracondylar humerus fractures in children: current concepts. J Am Acad Orthop Surg. 2012;20:69–77. https://doi.org/10.5435/JAAOS-20-02-069.
47. Kim TG, Park MS, Lee SH, Choi KJ, Im B-E, Kim DY, Sung KH. Leg-length discrepancy and associated risk factors after paediatric femur shaft fracture: a multicentre study. J Child Orthop. 2021;15:215–22. https://doi.org/10.1302/1863-2548.15.200252.
48. Bellamy JT, Ward LA, Fletcher ND. Evaluation of pediatric distal femoral physeal fractures and the factors impacting poor outcome requiring further corrective surgery. J Pediatr Orthop B. 2021;30:6–12. https://doi.org/10.1097/BPB.0000000000000733.

How to Care for Women's Health in Low- and Middle-Income Countries: A Quick Overview and Procedural Guide for the Surgeon

44

Reinou S. Groen, Megan Hadley, and O. K. (Bomi) Ogedengbe

Communities and countries and ultimately the world are only as strong as the health of their women.

– Michelle Obama

Abbreviations

BV	Bacterial Vaginosis
CT	*Chlamydia Trachomatis*
D&C	Dilation and Curettage
GTD	Gestational Trophoblastic Disease
HCG	Human Chorionic Gonadotropin
LMP	Last Menstrual Period
MVA	Manual Vacuum Aspiration
NG	*Neisseria Gonorrhoea*
Ob-Gyn	Obstetrics and Gynecology
PAS	Placenta Accreta Spectrum
PID	Pelvic Inflammatory Disease
PTSD	Post-Traumatic Stress Disorder
STI	Sexually Transmitted Infections
TOA	Tubo-Ovarian Abscess
US	Ultrasound

R. S. Groen (✉)
Department of Obstetrics and Gynecology, Alaska Native Medical Center, Anchorage, AK, USA
e-mail: rgroen@southcentralfoundation.com

M. Hadley
Department of Gynecology and Obstetrics, Johns Hopkins Hospital, Baltimore, MD, USA
e-mail: mhadley8@jhmi.edu

O. K. (B.) Ogedengbe
West African College of Surgeons (WACS), Lagos, Nigeria

Introduction

Women's health and maternity care are global health priorities and make up an essential part of ensuring the well-being of a population. Quality maternal and women's healthcare is important for the health and dignity for the individual and for the progress, safety, and longevity of the community. A majority of the contributing causes of maternal morbidity and mortality are preventable. Therefore, healthcare providers, clinics, and hospital systems have the opportunity to serve a pivotal role in eliminating unnecessary deaths, by providing access to lifesaving interventions. Maternity care is often a time when people choose to interact with the health system, and when it provides quality care, it will cultivate community's greater sense of trust in the system. This ultimately encourages others to engage in and seek healthcare.

Since women have traditionally many roles in the household, (job) markets, and childcare, engaging in their own health may only be feasi-

M. A. Hardy, B. R. Hochman (eds.), *Global Surgery*, https://doi.org/10.1007/978-3-031-28127-3_44

ble if healthcare meets them halfway. Therefore, the focus for women's care may start with neonatal or childcare may need to be distributed around markets and a woman's schedule of work.

Many functions of obstetrics and gynecology (ob-gyn) can be practiced by healthcare workforces other than doctors. Midwives, nurses, and community health workers have essential roles in guiding women's healthcare due to their proximity and their accessibility. A strong basic healthcare network that provides the basics of public health including vaccinations, basic antenatal care, and birth control services is necessary for the community to access further (surgical) healthcare services in an efficient and successful manner. It is therefore of utmost importance for ob-gyn personnel to clearly understand the quality of their primary services and their referral patterns to be able to increase the health of the community.

The obstetrician/gynecologist and other providers of women's healthcare also must assure a continued quality of care and control within its own work setting. In areas where the primary care is deficient, the obstetrical services suffer the most when women have been denied adequate access to care. Maternal morbidity or "near losses" should be rare with current knowledge and basic medical/surgical interventions. Analysis of any severe morbidity should include the three-delay model in which each incident is addressed according to (1) decision to search for care, (2) time of transportation and referral, and (3) delay in the healthcare system. This approach has been found highly constructive for the hospital staff for strengthening the healthcare system for very ill women. Each incident of severe morbidity will indicate some delay of care or delay in recognition, which, when evaluated, can lead to improvements in (1) public knowledge around childbearing, (2) transportation improvements, (3) correction of other aspects of access to care, and (4) evaluation of the effectiveness of the hospital. This type of review offers opportunities for continued medical education, thorough evaluation of the infrastructure, and, instead of blaming, strengthens (health)caretakers.

When women present for care, it is important first to exclude pregnancy-related morbidities and problems. It is also most important to remember that many medical or surgical problems and diseases may occur despite being pregnant. All too often, a known positive pregnancy test causes delay or even cancelation of treatments, which may not be in the best interest of the woman or the evolving pregnancy.

This chapter provides an overview of gynecologic and obstetric procedures and practices that health systems can prioritize in the development of women's health services. These services will provide women, neonates, and families with lifesaving care. This chapter is not a surgical textbook for all ob-gyn interventions that may be needed. The recommended reading section at the end provides resources to full surgical guides.

Pregnancy Dating and Pregnancy Abnormalities in the First and Second Trimester

Pregnancy determination and dating are extremely important as basic components of obstetric care. Pregnancy should always be considered during medical evaluations of women of reproductive age. The possibility of pregnancy can easily be confirmed by a urine beta-hCG testing if available; this is often sensitive enough to detect pregnancy within 7–10 days of conception.

Following confirmation of pregnancy, identifying the location of the pregnancy and determining the gestational age become the next steps in care. The standard and most common method for dating a pregnancy is by using the first day of the last menstrual period (LMP) to calculate the current gestational age. However, exact dates can be difficult to determine for many women, especially for those in whom menses is less predictable or for whom traditional calendar systems are infrequently used to keep track of cycles. Therefore, there are other methods to help confirm location and age.

The physical examination can provide additional information. During a bimanual examination, the uterus will feel globular and enlarged beginning at 6 weeks. By 12 weeks, the uterine fundus can usually be palpated above the pubic symphysis, and by 20 weeks, the uterus can be palpated at the umbilicus. After 20 weeks of gestation, fundal height, measured in centimeters from the pubic symphysis to the top of the uterine fundus, correlates approximately with gestational age in non-obese women.

In addition to the examination, when ultrasound (US) is available, it should be utilized to visualize the pregnancy location and to help establish accurate dating. A location other than in the intrauterine cavity of the uterus is called an ectopic pregnancy, which will be discussed later in this chapter. Dating in the first 14 weeks is performed by measuring the crown-rump length. This is performed by measuring the maximum length from the cranium to the caudal end of the fetal pole. If this measurement is greater than 8.4 cm, the gestational age is likely greater than 14 weeks; biometry should be utilized instead to determine accurate dating. Biometry includes averaging a series of measurements: biparietal diameter, head circumference, abdominal circumference, and femur length. The earlier in the pregnancy that dating is performed, the more accurate are the results. Once the pregnancy is confirmed, the location has been determined, and the gestational age is assessed, the final step is to determine the viability of the fetus. This is conducted by either visualizing a heartbeat on US or hearing the beat when available by Doppler or fetoscopes. Fetal heart rates between 110 and 160 are considered to be in the normal range.

Ectopic Pregnancy

Not all pregnancies implant within the intrauterine cavity. Implantation outside the uterine cavity is considered ectopic and most commonly occurs inside the fallopian tube. Women who have an ectopic pregnancy classically present with abdominal pain (often severe, may include guarding and rebound tenderness) and vaginal bleeding. In severe cases, ectopic pregnancies can present as hemodynamic instability or shock, typically from intra-abdominal hemorrhage after rupture. Ectopic pregnancy should be excluded in any woman in the reproductive age who presents with abnormal vaginal bleeding and abdominal pain. It should also be highly suspected in a woman with an IUD in place and a positive pregnancy test. On physical examination, there may be a palpable adnexal mass, and the uterus may also be enlarged in response to hormonal stimulation; the examination elicits pelvic and abdominal pain and particularly cervical motion tenderness.

Women who are hemodynamically unstable require emergent resuscitation for hemorrhagic shock, which should include large-bore IVs, fluid boluses, and blood transfusions as needed. A surgeon should imminently proceed with an exploratory laparotomy or laparoscopy if available and perform a salpingectomy if an ectopic pregnancy is found, which is a highly effective treatment (see Box 44.1). A salpingostomy can be considered in limited circumstances to preserve fertility (e.g., if the other tube is not functional). This, however, does increase the risk of subsequent ectopic pregnancies and should only be used if the woman will have access to emergency surgery in the future. In addition, a salpingostomy leads to increased blood loss.

Box 44.1 Salpingectomy/Salpingostomy

Salpingectomy

1. Two babcock clamps are placed around the tube to elevate it into view.
2. An avascular space of the mesosalpinx is identified, and a window is created.
3. Two Kelly clamps are placed lateral and medial with the tip in the created window and encompassing the most medial part of the tube as well as the fimbriated ends laterally.
4. The tube is removed from the uterus on the medial side by sharp dissection.
5. The mesosalpinx is transected.
6. Double ligation of the lateral and medial placed tissue under the Kelly clamps with an absorbable suture.
7. If there is a lot of large vasculature in the mesosalpinx, the vessels can be isolated, clamped, and ligated separately.
8. In the case of a severe adhesions or otherwise inability to remove the full tube, removal of a segment of the tube will also result in sterility.

Salpingostomy

1. Assure access to the enlarged fallopian tube.
2. Incise the fallopian tube over the distended portion, in a longitudinal manner.
3. Remove all products of conception with suction or with a blunt surgical tool. Sometimes traction–counter-traction can be used.
4. Make the surgical site hemostatic.
5. Consider closing the defect with a small 4–0 absorbable suture if indicated for hemostasis.
6. Follow-up hCG until zero prior to new conceptions; if there is no decrease or a plateau in hCG over 2 weeks, consider methotrexate treatment.

Gestational Trophoblastic Disease/ Molar Pregnancy

Gestational Trophoblastic Disease (GTD) is a term used to describe a spectrum of diseases of placental origin. Molar pregnancies are noninvasive forms of GTD that occur when pregnancies end up with an abnormal combination of genetic material from the egg and sperm. Women may present with abnormal bleeding, severe vomiting (hyperemesis), or a uterus that is larger than expected for the gestational age of the pregnancy. Sometimes, "grape-like" structures can be seen in the vagina. On US, molar pregnancies can have a classic mixed echogenic or "snowstorm" appearance. US is used for diagnosis along with higher-than-expected beta-hCG. Molar pregnancies can be classified as either partial or complete based on pathologic evaluation of the products of conception; initial management is the same for either type.

Treatment should include removal of the products from the uterine cavity by suction. Curettage is not recommended given the increased risk of uterine perforation in this scenario. Pitocin should be infused (20 units/L in 4 h) after cervical dilation and suction to prevent hemorrhage. Hysterectomy should be considered for women who experience severe hemorrhage. In case of an advanced partial molar pregnancy, there may be a (life) fetus present, which would complicate the suction procedure and may need a dilatation and extraction of the fetus vaginally or via a cesarean procedure while maintaining the utmost care not to seed any of the uterine contents into the abdomen.

RhoGAM should be administered to Rh negative women, and beta-hCG should be monitored after removal of a molar pregnancy because of the risk of malignancy (GTN). Once the beta-hCG has normalized, the risk of GTN becomes very small. If the beta-hCG does not fall to non-pregnant levels, further interventions may be required, such as chemotherapy or even hysterectomy. Women should be counseled to use contraception during monitoring of beta-hCG.

Miscarriages/Abortion Care

Miscarriage or abortion, also referred to as early pregnancy loss, should be on the differential for any reproductive-aged woman who presents with vaginal bleeding and sometimes with concurrent abdominal cramping. There is no way of telling if a miscarriage/abortion is spontaneous or induced. Loss of pregnancy, regardless of the circumstances, is a devastating time for women and needs to be met with compassionate care. Miscarriages are categorized as either threatened, missed (asymptomatic), incomplete, or complete. The determination is made based on pelvic examination of the cervical os (open vs closed) and on ultrasound examination. Regardless of type of miscarriage, all Rh-negative women should receive RhoGAM.

Threatened Painless vaginal bleeding with an USG examination that shows a viable embryo with the presence of a heartbeat inside the uterine cavity. The cervical os is closed on examination, and no fetal tissue has passed. About half of these pregnancies will continue as a viable pregnancy, and about half will progress to a miscarriage; therefore, a woman should be counseled on both possibilities and managed expectantly.

Missed A missed miscarriage will show an empty sac (≥25 mm in diameter) or an embryo (CRL ≥7 mm) without a heartbeat present on US. However, most women present with intermittent vaginal bleeding and sometimes mild cramping. The cervical os will be closed on examination, and the woman may not have many symptoms, and the uterus will be smaller in size than the expected gestational age based on her last menstrual period. Management can be either expectant with the follow-up that the miscarriage occurred, medical, or surgical (see below).

Complete A complete miscarriage will not show any remaining products of conception on US, and the endometrial strip will be thin, measuring less than ~1 cm. The cervical os will be closed on examination, and she will not have further bleeding. Further treatment is not required for a complete miscarriage.

Incomplete or Inevitable If an incomplete miscarriage is left untreated, the women will be at risk for severe anemia, sepsis, or death. Incomplete abortion may be life-threatening from severe hemorrhage. The cervical os remains open, and products of conception may be seen at the internal os. In such instances, removal of the products of conception and parenteral ergometrine or buccal misoprostol given immediately may be lifesaving.

Septic Miscarriage If a patient demonstrates signs or symptoms of infection, a septic abortion should be suspected. These can include pain, fever, foul discharge, cervical motion or uterine tenderness, or vital sign changes (hypotension, tachycardia, tachypnea). Septic abortions are responsible for 20% of maternal mortality worldwide. Broad-spectrum antibiotics and sepsis management, including fluid resuscitation, should be swiftly administered, followed in 6 h by prompt but careful uterine evacuation to remove the source of infection. Extra caution should be taken during the procedure, as these women are at high risk for uterine perforation from the effects of infection on the myometrium. Use of US guidance can reduce the risks of perforation and should be used if available. Infrequently, a laparotomy is indicated for assessment of uterine perforation or removal of the uterus if hemorrhage is uncontrolled or uterus is gangrenous.

Medical management is an option for either missed or incomplete miscarriages occurring for pregnancies up to 9 weeks, provided the woman is stable, bleeding is limited, there are no signs of infection, and follow-up care is readily available. Misoprostol 600 mcg can be administered sublingually or orally, or 800 mcg can be administered vaginally. These dosages may be repeated twice, 3 h apart, if needed. Mifepristone 200 mg orally can also be given 24 h prior to misoprostol, which increases the likelihood that the miscarriage will pass without additional intervention. However, if medical management is not effective or if the woman is not a candidate as stated above, surgical management should then be performed.

Manual Vacuum Aspiration (MVA) is the safest surgical method of evacuating an incomplete or missed miscarriage, and multiple studies have demonstrated that this method can be safely performed by trained advanced practitioners (midwives, nurse practitioners, etc.) in addition to physicians. A dose of doxycycline or a second-generation cephalosporin given within 60 minutes of the procedure decreases the risk of infection. The procedure can be performed under local anesthesia such as a paracervical block if tolerated by the patient: oral or IV sedation should also be considered to minimize pain or trauma. If the cervix is closed, it can be dilated with dilators, increasing size cannulas, or misoprostol. Misoprostol 400mcg sublingual or 600mcg PO can be used for gestational ages up to 14 weeks and should ideally be given 3 h prior to procedure. The patient should be placed in dorsal lithotomy position, and the procedure should be carried out under sterile conditions. If MVA is not available, a dilation and curettage (D&C) may be performed instead. The products of conception should then be evaluated and if possible an US done, to ensure no products were retained.

Box 44.2 How to Do a Uterine Aspiration

1. Patient should be in lithotomy position. Feel with bimanual examination the direction of the uterus, which can be straight or flexed posterior or anterior.
2. Vaginal cleaning with Betadine (or other non-alcoholic antiseptic).
3. Sterile speculum is inserted into the vagina, followed by 1% lidocaine cervical block, aiming just next to the cervix at 4 and 8 o'clock.
4. Tenaculum at 12 o'clock on the cervix to straighten out the uterus and stabilize it.
5. If products are seen in the cervical os, they can be removed with a ring forceps. The ring forceps can also be introduced carefully into the uterus to remove placenta and larger parts of the fetus as needed.
6. If dilatation is indicated, use the cervical dilators until the cannula size corresponding with the gestational age can pass. Excessive force may perforate the uterus, so caution should be taken only to pass the dilator through the internal os maximum ~5 cm deep. If the correct-sized cannula can be inserted into the uterus, you may proceed with the MVA.
7. The procedure is primarily done under surgeon's palpation, but an US could be useful to evaluate the direction of the cannula and the evaluation of the uterine cavity at the end of the procedure. When ultrasound is unavailable, one must rely on classical findings of an empty uterus including a tightening uterus around the canula and uterine grit felt with the aspirator or curette.
8. Use bimanual massage and uterotonic medications (methergine, hemabate, misoprostol, and Pitocin) if bleeding continues despite removal of all the products of conception. See "Postpartum Hemorrhage" section for details.

Common side effects from medical and surgical management of miscarriages include both pain and nausea, which should be anticipated and treated. Tetanus vaccination should be provided if booster has not been received in the past 5 years, and tetanus immunoglobulin should be administered for any (suspicion) of prior unsupervised/non-medical abortion. Underlying causes of miscarriage should also be considered, with evaluation for infection (malaria, STIs) performed for those with other clinical signs or risk factors. Often, the cause of miscarriage is not determined as most are due to chromosomal abnormalities. The risk increases with increasing maternal age.

Antenatal Care: The Basics

In antenatal care, women are educated, screened, and treated for diseases that may affect their offspring or their own fitness and are followed for the fetal growth and for their well-being. Education and screening are tailored to the women's needs, and they include information about warning signs for preterm labor, preeclampsia, and preparedness for delivery. Screening includes endemic treatable infectious diseases, like malaria, syphilis, HIV, hepatitis, and others, as well as screening for blood type (Rhesus antigen), anemia, and diabetes, if feasible.

First dating must establish a clear progression of uterine size that corresponds with the gestational age (Fig. 44.1); if this is not consistent, then there may be underlying pathology that needs to be addressed. A uterus large for gestational age may reflect a fetal problem including multiple gestations, polyhydramnios, hydrocephalus, suspected macrosomia, or gynecological problems. These include molar pregnancy, uterine fibroids, or other masses in pregnancy. Small for gestational age can relate to intrauterine growth restriction with its variety of causes.

Programs in antenatal care are frequently conducted by (public health) nurses, midwives, and local health workers, and patients may or may not benefit from US imaging.

It is of great importance for an obstetrician to have easy communication lines and easy access for referrals from the community for antenatal care, as we saw in the previous section on miscarriage and bleeding. Throughout pregnancy, the

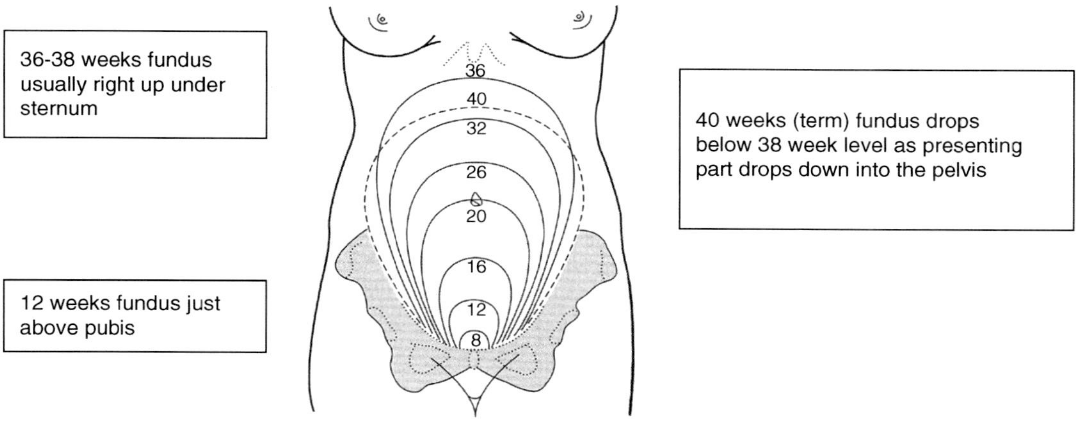

Fig. 44.1 Uterine size and gestational age.. *Source From Carcio HA, Secor RM. Advanced Health Assessment of Women: Clinical Skills and Procedures. fourth ed. New York, NY: Springer Publishing Company; 2019:136*

woman's health or fetal well-being may abruptly change. Women need access to a reliable health center where they can be triaged, treated, or quickly referred to the right level of care for their emergencies. Only with that kind of collaboration can antenatal care be effective to avert morbidity and mortality.

Vaginal Deliveries and Complication Management

Women have delivered newborns since the beginning of time, and the clinician has limited involvement even if (s)he is present during a vaginal birth. It is only at those times that things do not go as planned that there may be a need for quick, effective intervention. Intervention may be indicated for (1) arrest of dilatation in first stage of labor, (2) arrest of descent during second stage of labor, or (3) during the third stage of labor if the placenta is not delivered or a postpartum hemorrhage occurs. This part of the chapter will describe actions for those scenarios, which may be outside of nurse's/midwives' competencies.

Arrest in the first stage of labor will likely resolve with uterine stimulation, rupture of membranes, and adherence to the local protocols and timelines. A surgeon may be needed to evaluate a patient for arrest of progress despite the local protocols for stimulation and rupture of membranes, and if a cervical dilation is not complete, the only way to deliver is via cesarean delivery (see next section).

Arrest in the second stage of labor is diagnosed when the woman, despite reaching complete dilatation and pushing, does not deliver the neonate in 2–3 h; a vaginal operative delivery should be considered when there is a cephalic presentation, fully dilated cervix, and a well-engaged fetal head (the fetal head is at least 2 cm past the ischial spines). If there is no previous hands-on training of operative delivery by the provider, this should not be attempted on a live fetus. In general terms, vacuum extraction is done by placing the cup on the flexion point of the head and giving steady traction during a contraction while the woman assists with a push. With the forceps applied, again, steady traction is given while the woman pushes. When either instruments are used, assure (1) good anesthesia/comfort for the mother, (2) an empty bladder, (3) a fully dilated cervix, (4) no maternal tissue in either instrument, and (5) the right angle of traction (first down then go with the pelvic curve up). Lastly (6) if this fails, be ready to perform a cesarean delivery. On a live neonate, one should never attempt a vacuum followed by a forceps or vice versa.

Special Delivery Scenarios

Delivery of Multiples As mentioned above, a multiple gestation should be suspected with a large uterus, the feeling of multiple heads on palpation of the abdomen, or multiple heartbeats. Sonography can confirm your diagnosis. After the delivery of the first infant, clamp the cord and do *not* deliver the placenta. If the second twin is coming in cephalic presentation, delivery can continue as with the first twin; however, if there is no cephalic presentation, the feet should be grasped on an internal examination, and the baby should be delivered breech. In general, only if the first fetus is cephalic, vaginal delivery is recommended. If the first twin is breech, transverse, or any variant of this, a cesarean delivery is recommended.

Breech Delivery In a singleton breech delivery, the main course of action is to do nothing until delivery of the fetal body is complete, then assure sacrum anterior position by rotating the fetal body at the hips; arms can be delivered by swiping them over the chest anteriorly and downward starting with sliding your fingers along the scapula and then shoulder followed by the humerus, and pull only when the elbow is reached. For the head, apply suprapubic pressure rather than traction on the fetal body. In case of a head entrapment by the cervix, administer sublingual nitroglycerin; in case of (perceived) entrapment of the head by bony structures, apply suprapubic pressure, or apply piper forceps (Figs. 44.2 and 44.3).

Shoulder dystocia When a fetal head is delivered but is not followed by the fetal body, the shoulders may be impacted behind the symphysis. Such shoulder impaction is more likely to happen in a fetus large for gestational age affected by maternal gestational diabetes when the fetal

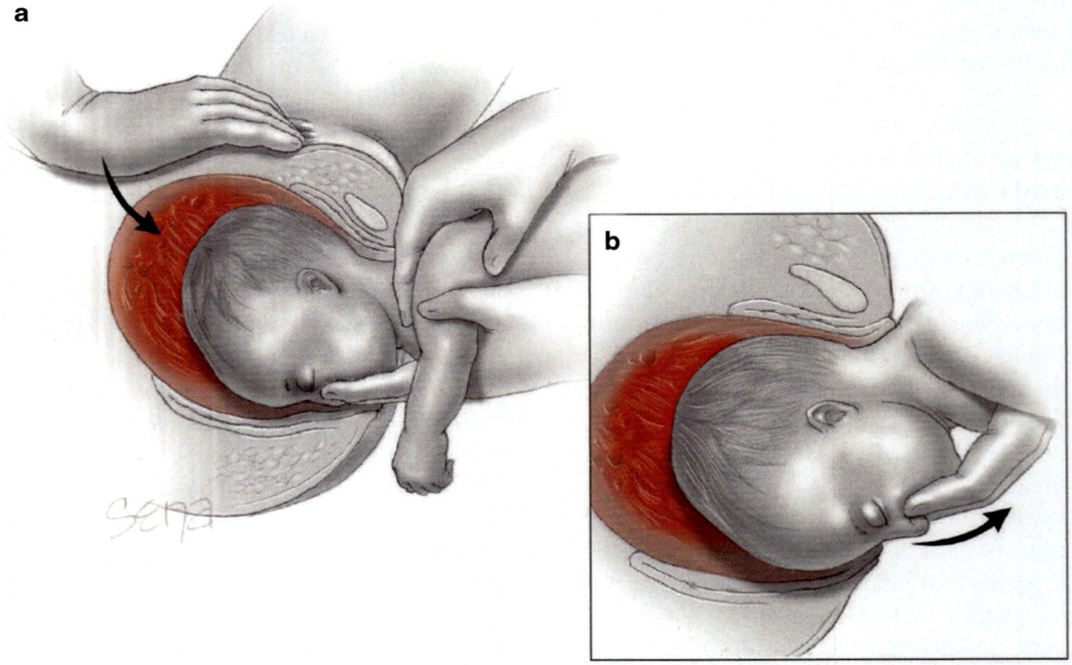

Fig. 44.2 (**a**) Delivery of the aftercoming head using the Mauriceau maneuver. Note that as the fetal head is being delivered, flexion of the head is maintained by suprapubic pressure provided by an assistant. (**b**) Pressure on the maxilla is applied simultaneously by the operator as upward and outward traction is exerted. *Source: Chap.* 28 *Breech presentation and delivery in Cunningham FG,* et al *Eds; Williams Obstetrics, 25e Edition eBook*

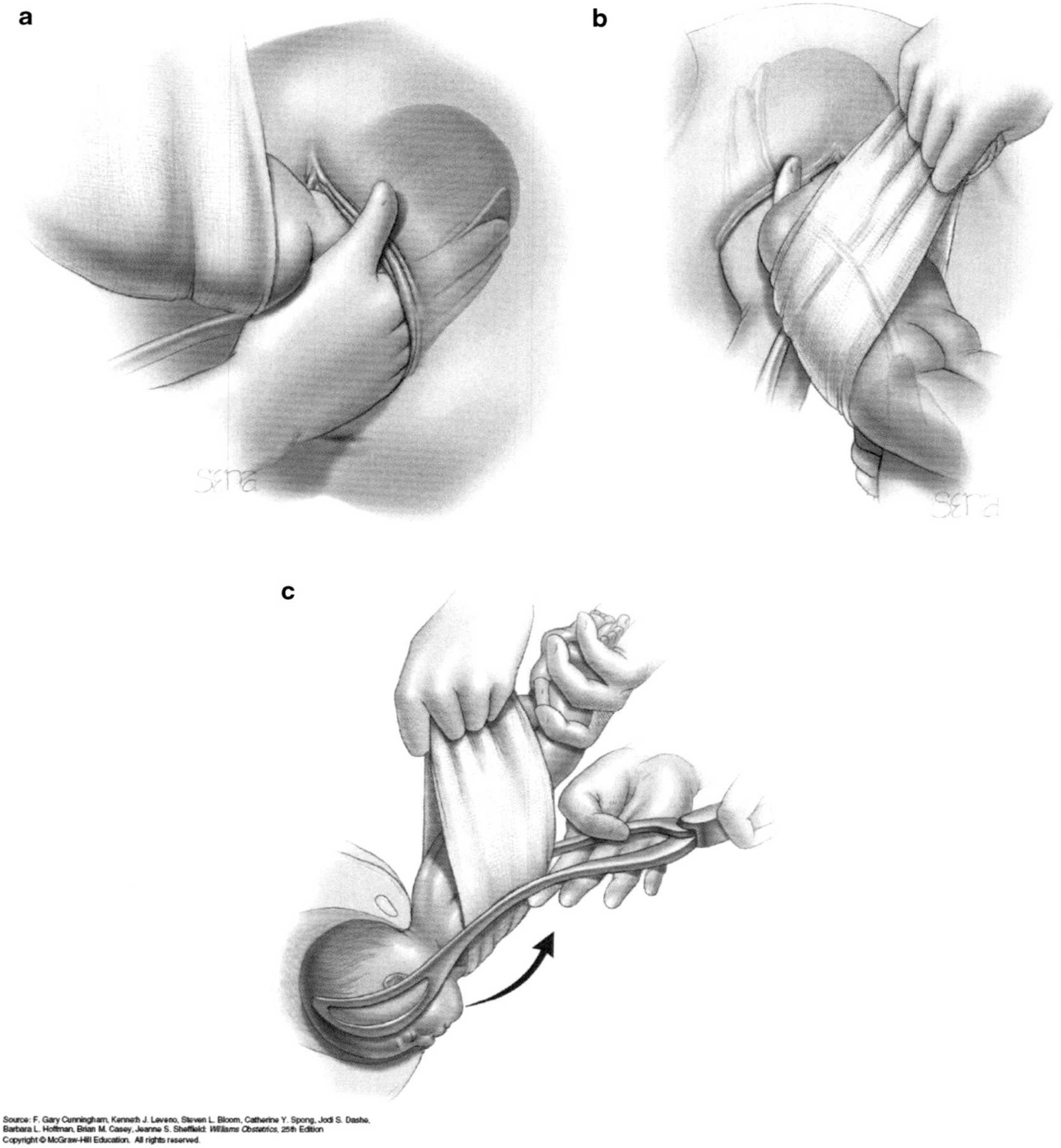

Fig. 44.3 Piper forceps for delivery of the aftercoming head. (**a**) The fetal body is held elevated using a warm towel, and the left blade of forceps is applied to the aftercoming head. (**b**) The right blade is applied with the body still elevated. (**c**) Forceps delivery of the aftercoming head. Note the direction of movement shown by the arrow. Source: Chap. 28 Breech presentation and delivery in Cunningham FG, et al., Eds. Williams Obstetrics, 25e Edition eBook

shoulders may be overdeveloped and fetal head is not the largest part of the neonate's body. There may be, therefore, a disproportion in the bony structure of the fetal shoulder gird to the pelvis of the delivering mom. This then needs to be resolved by addressing the axes of the shoulders in relation to the pelvic structure. A "how to" is provided in Box 44.3.

Box 44.3 How to Deliver the Fetal Body if there Is a Shoulder Dystocia

1. **Instruct the woman to stop pushing.** Tell the women that her baby's shoulders need to be repositioned and pushing would not assist in delivery at this time.
2. Flex maternal hips by bringing her thighs cephalad/externally; this is called the **McRoberts** position.
3. Apply **suprapubic pressure** directly above the symphysis to rotate the fetal shoulder from the fetal back to the front.
4. Attempt delivery of the **posterior arm** by entering the vagina on the maternal sacral side, and make space if needed with an episiotomy.
5. **Rubin or Woods corkscrew maneuver**: Roll the anterior or posterior fetal shoulder to the chest side, or rotate the body 180 degrees by applying pressure to the fetal shoulder.
6. **Gaskin maneuver**: Have the woman go into hand and knees, and apply downward pressure to deliver the posterior shoulder.
7. **Repeat all the above until delivered.**
8. Consider **clavicle fracture.**
9. **Zavanelli maneuver**: The fetal head is pushed back into the pelvis following the cardinal movements in reverse order (external rotation back to occiput anterior, flexion of the fetal head, and internal rotation to replay occiput in line with fetal back).

Episiotomy If the perineum of the women is impacting the delivery and fetal heart tones indicate need for expedited delivery, an episiotomy should be considered. This is not the standard for every delivery and leads to more blood loss and possible painful intercourse in the future. Closure of the episiotomy is similar to repair of a laceration.

Postpartum Complications

Laceration Repair

During birth, lacerations can occur to the cervix, vaginal wall, labia, or perineum including the anal musculature. Repair is indicated for hemostasis, functionality, and cosmesis. Key to a good repair is visualization and identification and approximation of all the separate anatomical layers. Use absorbable sutures, and close each layer separately with the finest suture available with good tension strength. Vicryl 2–0 is appropriate for most layers. Use a finer suture for the rectal mucosa.

Classification of the tear is related to the tissues involved. In a first-degree laceration, only the skin or vaginal mucosa is involved but no perineal muscles. A second-degree laceration involves the perineal body, which needs its own support in sutures for correct healing. A third-degree laceration includes the rectal sphincter, which can only be identified by a rectal examination of the tear. The sphincter muscle may have retracted and needs to be identified with allis forceps in order to be approximated. Lastly, a fourth-degree tear also includes the rectal mucosa and needless to say needs also a layered repair starting from the rectal mucosa.

Postpartum Hemorrhage

Postpartum hemorrhage is the main cause of maternal morbidity globally. This is a preventable cause of death if diagnosed and treated promptly. Only half of the women who have a postpartum hemorrhage may have preceding risk factors including large uterine distention from (1) large infant, (2) multiple gestation, or (3) large infant, (2) multiple gestation, or (3) uterine fibroids etc, or the hemorrhage follows aprolonged labor. Each healthcare facility that provides birthing services should be capable of prevention as well as addressing the immediate care needs of postpartum women who experience a hemorrhage.

Prevention of hemorrhage postpartum starts with (1) correctly assessing the labor course and timely referral if there is prolonged labor, as this leads to higher risk for postpartum hemorrhage. Secondly, after the birth of the neonate, (2) there should be prompt assessment and active management of placental delivery within 30 min. This can be in most cases accomplished with IM or IV (diluted) Pitocin, abdominal uterine massage, and controlled cord traction. If the placenta is not delivered in 30 min, a manual removal should be undertaken.

Treatment of a postpartum hemorrhage cannot be delayed as any blood loss may be detrimental to the woman. Immediate action is to provide large IV access, intravenous fluids, as well as blood products to replace the ongoing blood loss. There are four causes of postpartum hemorrhage (referred to as 4 *T*s, (1) Tissue, (2) Tone, (3) Trauma, and (4) Thrombin): (1) Retained tissue (placenta or membranes or blood clots), (2) uterine atony, (3) trauma to the birth canal, and (4) coagulopathy, usually secondary by blood loss of >25% of blood volume, rarely due to a preexisting coagulopathy. While retained tissue is identified or excluded by means of an intra-uterine exam or uterine sweep, the uterine tone needs to be addressed with uterine massage, including bimanual massage (one hand in the vaginally and one on the abdomen compressing the uterus) and with medications as indicated in Table 44.1. Trauma needs to be addressed as soon as tone is found not to be the problem, and lacerations are repaired as noted above. Trauma to the cervix can also lead to excessive blood loss as can uterine rupture lead to severe vaginal or intra-abdominal bleeding.

A hemorrhage in the setting of a miscarriage or molar pregnancy is essentially addressed in the same way as described above. In early pregnancy, however, oxytocin may be less effective since there may not be many oxytocin receptors. Special clinical scenarios include uterine inversion and placenta with abnormal adherence to the myometrium or placenta accreta spectrum (PAS). These life-threatening scenarios can be seen together. PAS is more common in women who have had uterine surgery prior to the index pregnancy. Traction on the placenta can cause a uterine inversion, although uterine inversion can also be seen without a PAS. Repositioning of the uterus in normal anatomical position is needed, and thereafter medication to increase the uterine tone is warranted. If bleeding continues, or if PAS is diagnosed, urgent surgery with a postpartum hysterectomy is most often the only way to address this serious problem and save the woman's life.

Regardless of the cause of bleeding after 500 cc of blood loss, tranexamic acid 1gram IV should be given as a single dose to reduce the risk of severe morbidity related to disseminated intravascular coagulopathy.

Postpartum Fever

Postpartum fever is also a severe cause of morbidity in women. All medical and surgical causes of fever apply to postpartum women with the

Table 44.1 Uterotonic medications

Medication	Dosage	Administration	Dose frequency	Contraindications	Side effects
Oxytocin (Pitocin)	10–80 IU	IV drip in 1 L of LR; IM as bolus	Continuous drip	None	Hyponatremia
Methylergonovine (methergine)	0.2 mg	IM; intrauterine; PO	Every 15 min–2 h (max 8 doses)	Hypertension, (pre) eclampsia	Hypertension
15-methyl prostaglandin F2 (Hemabate)	0.25 mg	IM; intrauterine	Every 15 minutes (max 8 doses)	Active cardiac, pulmonary (asthma) or hepatic/renal disease	Diarrhea, nausea
Misoprostol (Cytotec)	600–1000 mcg	PR; buccal	Single dose	None	Fever, nausea

additional burden of endometritis, mastitis, and perineal infections in case of lacerations. If endometritis cannot be excluded, broad-spectrum antibiotics should be started as soon as possible, as a lifesaving measure. Lastly, local epidemiological factors need to be considered, including malaria and tuberculosis.

Cesarean Delivery

A cesarean delivery is indicated for some obstetrical scenarios, which include fetal malpresentation (transverse lie, large infant in breech, first twin breech), cephalopelvic disproportion, placenta previa, failed operative delivery, arrest of dilation, prior vertical uterine scar, severe antepartum bleeding with signs of shock, uterine rupture, and history of more than one previous lower uterine segment cesarean delivery.

The procedure steps are presented in Box 44.4. Although this is overall a straightforward and rewarding surgical procedure, it only remains simple if one (1) stays in the lower uterine segment, (2) avoids the lateral vasculature if possible, and (3) uses traction rather than dissection upon entry.

Box 44.4 How to Perform Cesarean Delivery

1. Skin sharp: Pfannenstiel incision (quicker recovery/better cosmesis) or midline vertical (less blood loss more access to full abdomen).
2. Subcutaneous: preferably by traction to avoid damage to vasculature.
3. Fascia: open sharply in midline, and continue with scissors, or if doing a Pfannenstiel, continue with traction.
4. Separate rectus muscle bluntly if possible, or open first, and then bluntly retract.
5. Peritoneum: blunt entry if no prior surgery.
6. Enter bladder retractor to protect bladder (Foley inserted prior to the case, or have women void prior to surgery), and use a Richardson retractor or moist laps for visualization of the lower uterine segment.
7. Identify the lower uterine segment, which is below the round ligaments, a thinner muscle layer which does not show any contracting fibers.
8. Transversely open the lower uterine segment until the membranes.
9. Pierce the membranes with blunt part of an instrument or digitally, and open the uterus with caudal/cranial traction.
10. Cup hand around presenting part of the fetus in the pelvis, and lift to the hysterotomy. Deliver infant by fundal pressure, and start Pitocin IV or IM.
11. Clamp and cut the cord and hand neonate off the surgical field; deliver the placenta with uterine massage and cord traction.
12. Remove all tissue from the uterus, and clamp any acutely bleeding vessels with Atraumatic forceps/clamps.
13. Close hysterotomy with absorbable suture for hemostasis avoiding the bladder and the lateral vessels.
14. Close fascia with delayed absorbable suture, close subcutaneous suture if thicker than 2 cm, and close skin.

In certain delivery scenarios, the fetus will not be able to be delivered through the preferred lower transverse incision, and a different incision is made. Figure 44.4 shows two main types of incision. The preferred incision is the lower uterine segment incision, which does not involve the active uterine segment. A classical uterine incision, involving the active uterine segment, is higher.

Postpartum hemorrhage after a cesarean delivery or vaginal delivery may require an exploratory laparotomy and management with uterine artery ligations (Fig. 44.5) or compression sutures (Fig. 44.6) and lastly at times a hysterectomy. Hysterectomy principles for post-pregnancy uteri are similar to non-pregnancy-related hysterec-

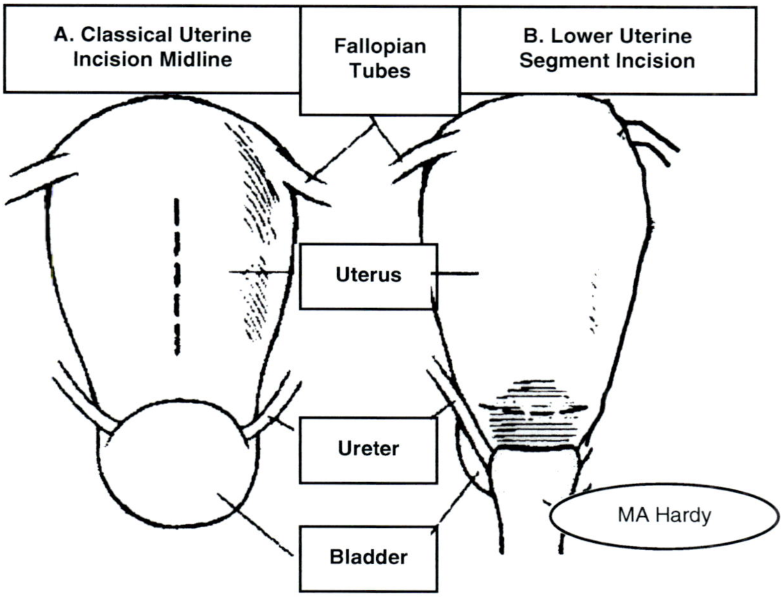

Fig. 44.4 Most frequently used uterine incision with preference for an incision in the lower uterine segment (**b**) Classical incision (**a**) has an increased risk (up to 25% chance) of rupture if patient is to undergo labor in a next pregnancy. In areas where family planning and surgical resources may be inconsistently available, it is important to avoid a classical incision unless necessary. Indications for a classical incision include a large fibroid mass of the cervix or PAS with the placenta located anteriorly. In some cesarean deliveries, the lower uterine segment is not well developed (premature delivery) or is not large enough for delivery, and extensions of the incision go into the active segment of the uterus. If the active segment is used for neonatal extraction, this part should be closed in several layers to avoid postpartum bleeding and reduce the risk of spontaneous rupture of the uterus (prior to labor contractions) and risk of future PAS

Fig. 44.5 Places for uterine artery ligation in case of postpartum hemorrhage, apply bilateral as indicated. *Source:* https://www.glowm.com/article/heading/vol-13--obstetric-emergencies--nonconservative-and-conservative-surgical-management-of-pph/id/413063#.YmXZwujMJnI *fig. 17*

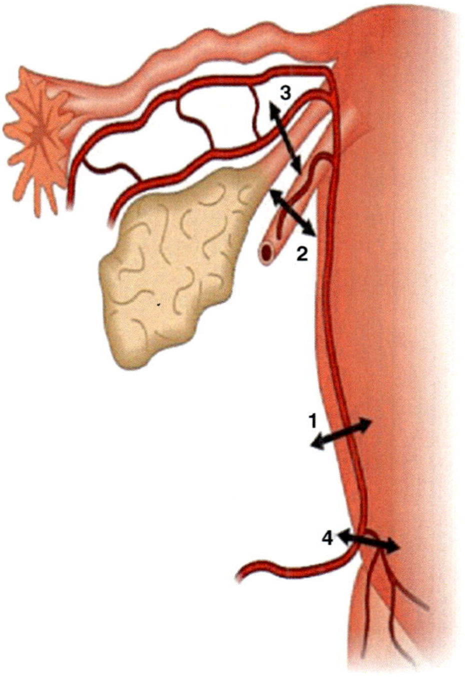

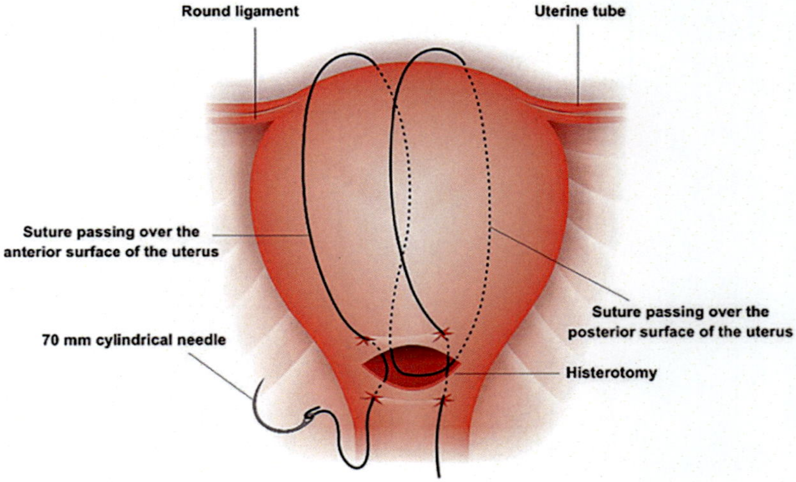

Fig. 44.6 Uterine compression sutures or B-Lynch suture for uterine atony if all other methods fail. *Source:* https://www.glowm.com/article/heading/vol-13--obstetric-emergencies--noAQ5nconservative-and-conservative-surgicalmanagement-of-pph/id/413063#.YmXZwujMJnI

tomy. Following pregnancy, the ureters are closer to the operating field, and more care needs to be taken to avoid their injury.

Family Planning and Birth Spacing

For a woman to decide when she is ready for pregnancy and childbearing is instrumental for the outcome of the pregnancy and of motherhood experience from both a maternal and neonatal perspective. This extends beyond the prosperity of the mother and the child to the full family and society. Women should have options for birth control including long-acting reversible contraceptives like intra-uterine devices and implants as well as short-term options like pills, ring, and patches (Table 44.2). Most of all, women should have relations with persons who respect their choice of birth control and comply, when asked, with barrier methods like condoms. Research shows that birth spacing leads to better health for the children; it is therefore recommended that at least 1 year separates one delivery from the next start of a pregnancy. It should preferably be 2 years in areas where infants rely on breastmilk for most of their caloric intake. There is no indication to avoid breastfeeding an infant while newly pregnant. Breast feeding itself may lead to decreased ovulations, but breastfeeding is not a reliable source of birth control.

There are few absolute contraindications to the use of birth control. Estrogen-containing birth control should be avoided in women who have a high risk of venous thrombotic events or those with aura-associated migraines, as strokes have been reported in this subset of women.

Table 44.2 Birth control options with their benefits and practicalities

Most Effective

Least Effective

Methods	Number of pregnancies expected (per 100 women)*	Use	Some Risks or Side Effects* This chart does not list all of the risks and side effects for each product.
Sterilization Surgery for Women	less than 1	Onetime procedure. Permanent.	Pain Bleeding Infection or other complications after surgery
Sterilization Surgery for Men	less than 1	Onetime procedure. Permanent.	Pain Bleeding Infection
IUD Copper	less than 1	Inserted by a healthcare provider. Lasts up to 10 years.	Cramps Heavier, longer periods Spotting between periods
IUD with Progestin	less than 1	Inserted by a healthcare provider. Lasts up to 3-5 years, depending on the type.	Irregular bleeding No periods (amenorrhea) Abdominal/pelvic pain
Implantable Rod	less than 1	Inserted by a healthcare provider. Lasts up to 3 years.	Menstrual Changes Mood swings or depressed mood Weight gain Headache Acne
Shot/Injection	6	Need a shot every 3 months.	Loss of bone density Irregular bleeding/bleeding between periods Headaches Weight gain Nervousness Dizziness Abdominal discomfort
Oral Contraceptives "The Pill" (Combined Pill)	9	Must swallow a pill every day.	Spotting/bleeding between periods Nausea Breast tenderness Headache
Oral Contraceptives "The Pill" (Extended Continuous Use Combined Pill)	9	Must swallow a pill every day.	Spotting/bleeding between periods Nausea Breast tenderness Headache
Oral Contraceptives "The Mini Pill" (Progestin Only)	9	Must swallow a pill at the same time every day.	Spotting/bleeding between periods Nausea Breast tenderness Headache
Patch	9	Put on a new patch each week for 3 weeks (21 total days). Don't put on a patch during the fourth week.	Spotting/bleeding between menstrual periods Nausea Stomach pain Breast tenderness Headache Skin irritation
Vaginal Contraceptive Ring	9	Put the ring into the vagina yourself. Keep the ring in your vagina for 3 weeks and then take it out for one week.	Vaginal discharge, discomfort in the vagina, mild irritation Headache Mood changes Nausea Breast tenderness
Diaphragm with Spermicide	12	Must use every time you have sex.	Irritation Allergic reactions Urinary tract infection
Sponge with Spermicide	12-24	Must use every time you have sex.	Irritation
Cervical Cap with Spermicide	17-23	Must use every time you have sex.	Irritation Allergic reactions Abnormal Pap test
Male Condom	18	Must use every time you have sex. Provides protection against some STDs.	Irritation Allergic reactions
Female Condom	21	Must use every time you have sex. Provides protection against some STDs.	Discomfort or pain during insertion or sex Burning sensation, rash or itching
Spermicide Alone	28	Must use every time you have sex.	Irritation Allergic reactions Urinary tract infection
OTHER CONTRACEPTION			
Emergency Contraceptives (EC): May be used if you did not use birth control or if your regular birth control fails (such as a condom breaks). It should not be used as a regular form of birth control. Emergency contraception prevents about 55 - 85% of predicted pregnancies.			
Levonorgestrel 1.5 mg (1 pill) Levonorgestrel .75 mg (2 pills)	7 out of every 8 women who would have gotten pregnant will not become pregnant after taking this EC.	Swallow the pills as soon as possible within 3 days after having unprotected sex.	Menstrual changes Lower stomach (abdominal) pain Headache Nausea Dizziness Vomiting Breast pain Tiredness
Ulipristal Acetate	6 or 7 out of every 10 women who would have gotten pregnant will not become pregnant after taking this EC.	Swallow the pills within 5 days after having unprotected sex.	Headache Nausea Abdominal pain Menstrual pain Tiredness Dizziness

Source: https://www.fda.gov/media/150299/download

Surgical Sterilization

Surgical sterilization is a very cost-effective and permanent way to prevent future pregnancies. Couples have two options: (1) vasectomy (outpatient-external procedure) and (2) salpingectomy (inpatient intra-abdominal procedure). A salpingectomy, sometimes referred to as tubal sterilization or tubal ligation, is (partial) removal of the tubes and is performed similarly to a salpingectomy used for a tubal ectopic pregnancy. A tubal removal is easily done during a cesarean delivery after the removal of the infant and the closure of the uterus. If a woman desires a tubal ligation after a vaginal birth, access to the uterus can be obtained with a small sub-umbilical incision. Tubal removal outside of pregnancy, so-called interval tubal ligation, can be performed via laparoscopy or mini-laparotomy. A small 3–4 cm Pfannenstiel incision is sufficient in a patient with a BMI of 25 or less. The actual salpingectomy is explained in Box 44.1.

We cannot stress enough the superiority of a vasectomy over a salpingectomy. The vasectomy is easier and quicker with less risk of major complications since this is an extracorporeal procedure. It can be done under local anesthesia. Although a vasectomy is a permanent solution to sterilization, it may be reversed since only a small segment of the vas deference is removed.

Hysterectomy

Indications for hysterectomy include but are not limited to abnormal uterine bleeding from adenomyosis or uterine fibroids, gestational trophoblastic disease, cervical, endometrial or ovarian cancer and postpartum hemorrhage. In general, the ovaries are left in place unless there are oncological reasons to remove them. Historical, cultural, and spiritual ideas have made hysterectomy a controversial topic in medicine. Women need to be advised that after a hysterectomy, there is no option for childbearing other than surrogate if ovaries are preserved or eggs are cryopreserved. A surgeon needs to be aware of the local (legislative/cultural) practices concerning a hysterectomy prior to performing this procedure. Since a hysterectomy may be a lifesaving, last option in certain cases of hemorrhage in pregnancy, the on-call obstetric team should communicate clearly to the full team including the patient what is needed to save the woman's life. The principles of hysterectomy are like any other organ removal; it includes (1) isolation of the structure and its vasculature, (2) avoidance of nearby organs (bladder, bowel and ureters), and (3) thorough hemostasis. The uterus consists in most cases of two tubes, one uterine body, and a cervix and all should be removed. Postpartum hysterectomy could be done supracervically, in cases where a laboring uterus does not have clear boundaries between the cervix and the vagina, to avoid injury to the ureters. A supra-cervical hysterectomy under those circumstances avoids prolonged surgery with possible complications and should be considered. Gynecologists are trained in vaginal hysterectomy, a specialized procedure and another option most frequently performed for small uteri in relation to pelvic organ prolapse.

Oophorectomy

Ovarian function goes beyond the reproductive phase, and therefore oophorectomy is only considered in cases of large masses suspicious for cancer or ovarian cancer metastases and for necrotic ovaries secondary to torsion. In all other cases, the ovary is de-torsed, mass removed by means of ovarian cystectomy, and ovary left in place after hemostasis is confirmed.

Box 44.5 How to Do a Hysterectomy Via Exploratory Laparotomy

1. Place a uterine manipulator or sponge stick/probe in the vagina for identification of the vaginal canal. For a postpartum uterus a ring forceps can be placed on the anterior and posterior part of the cervix. Place a foley catheter.
2. Enter the pelvis via Pfannenstiel or Maylard or Midline vertical incision depending on indication and size of the uterus.
3. Place two forceps on either side of the uterus on the round ligament for traction.
4. Isolate, Clamp, Cut and Tie (ICCT) the fallopian tubes and clamp and cut through the mesosalpinges.
5. ICCT the utero-ovarian ligament and ICCT the round ligament. (Care for ureters!)
6. Below the round ligament the broad ligament will split into two leaves.
7. Make sure the assistance is pushing the uterus up with the vaginal probe to identify the vagina and to ensure that the ureters are away from the lower uterine segment.
8. Continue opening up the anterior broad ligament unto the vesico-uterine reflection on both sides till ends meet, this can be done sharply as this is an avascular space.
9. Open up the posterior broad ligament towards the uterosacral ligaments. Again an avascular space.
10. ICCT the Uterine arteries. (Care for the ureters!)
11. Identify the vaginal canal with the vaginal probe and clamp from lateral to midline, cut and over sew the vaginal top while including the posterior peritoneum and sacral ligaments. Strong, absorbable sutures in figure of eight formation will do well.

Box 44.6 How to Do an Ovarian Cystectomy/Oophorectomy

1. Assure access to the pelvis.
2. Isolate the ovary of concern, de-torse ovary if an ovarian torsion is found, and blood flow restored; even a complete purple ovary may be revived if given time.
3. For ovarian cystectomy: open the ovarian cortex, and identify the ovarian cyst wall; keep the cyst wall intact, and with blunt and sharp dissection, isolate the cyst for removal. Close the ovarian cortex with small caliber absorbable suture.
4. For oophorectomy: Identify the infundibulopelvic (IP) ligament, and make a window in the broad ligament to isolate the IP away from the ureter. Clamp, cut, and tie the IP, and clamp, cut, and tie the uterine-ovarian ligament.

Office Management of Gynecological Concerns

Women may present to any medical outpatient or office for gynecological concerns. These concerns can range from abnormal vaginal discharge to pain, pelvic organ prolapse, or urinary/defecation concerns, as well as difficulty to conceive. In many cultures, these topics are not easily talked about, and it can be assumed that the problem likely has been going on longer than acknowledged, and local remedies have been tried prior to presentation. The woman may indicate her gynecological problem only at the end of her visit while stating she came for something more trivial. It is beyond this chapter to include all gynecological office management, but we will address the vaginal discharge as this is a frequent concern and of public health importance.

Vaginal Discharge and Sexually Transmitted Infections (STIs)

The vagina and the cervix excrete a clear, sometimes whitish, sour-smelling discharge and mucus, which is normal; it provides natural cleaning of the vagina. This physiological discharge may become affected by semen, douching, or use of tampons, all which makes the vagina less acidic, which in turn affects overgrowth of *Lactobacillus* leading to bacterial vaginosis (BV). Discharge for BV is grayish with a fishy smell, and evaluation of vaginal fluid under the microscope will indicate epithelial cells covered with bacteria. BV is treated with a week of metronidazole 500 mg twice daily. Yeast spores or hyphae can also be seen on a microscope. This discharge is generally white and the vaginal mucosa sometimes erythematous and can be painful and fragile. A vaginal yeast infection can generally be treated with miconazole locally but sometimes is in need for Diflucan 150 mg PO. Severe or recurrent yeast infections should lead to evaluation for diabetes.

Greenish discharge is more likely, but not necessarily *Neisseria gonorrhoeae* (NG), an STI that can cause pelvic inflammatory disease or tubo-ovarian abscesses or ureteral strictures in males. When concerned for or confirmed for NG, frequently *Chlamydia trachomatis* (CT) is also involved. CT is frequently the cause of tubal-related infertility and therefore should be treated as soon as suspected/diagnosed. Since both NG and CT can also be asymptomatic, many countries have screening programs.

Pelvic pain is a complicated medical problem but can be caused by pelvic inflammatory disease (PID) and tubo-ovarian abscess (TOA). These are infectious processes which may involve NG or CT but are often polymicrobial. PID can be treated as outpatient with 2 weeks of doxycycline/metronidazole if the patient is able to tolerate PO. In all other cases and if a TOA is suspected or confirmed with US, she should receive intravenous broad-spectrum antibiotics including anaerobic coverage.

Vaginal ulcerations may be a sign of primary syphilis, genital herpes, or granuloma inguinale or lymphogranuloma venereum or human immunodeficiency virus, for which we refer to the local diagnostic and treatment protocols.

With any STI confirmation, the treatment includes partner testing and treatment.

A Bartholin's gland cyst or infection is another common gynecological problem seen in the office. The Bartholin's glands are situated at about 4 and 8 o'clock in the beginning of the vaginal canal. These glands can get obstructed or infected. An non-infected Bartholin's cyst is not in need of any treatment unless it causes problems. A painful swollen gland is infected and needs to be drained. An I&D can suffice, and the entry point is best made behind the hymenal ring to avoid scarring and pain. In recurrent infection, a drain should be placed. For women over 50 y/o with an enlarged or infected Bartholin's cyst, malignancy should be excluded.

Sexual Violence

Rape and sexual violence are of great global concern, affecting one in three females in their lifetime worldwide. These are sexual acts that are performed without consent of the individual, which can have lasting physical, social, and emotional consequences. The surgeon should be able to provide emergency care to individuals who have been affected by sexual violence and be able to do so using a trauma-informed approach without applying judgment to the nature or severity of the claim.

A trauma-informed approach involves the ability of providers to realize the effects of trauma on individuals, families, and communities, to recognize the signs and symptoms of trauma, to respond in a safe and welcoming environment that promotes resilience and healing, and to resist interventions that result in re-traumatization. Keyways to incorporate trauma-informed care include ensuring the patient is cared for in a private setting and the provider is attentive with no distractions. People respond to trauma differently, and the response does not necessarily reflect the severity or validity of the trauma experience. A provider should be able to provide the patient with information about what to expect regarding their evaluation and care and should let the patient drive the pace and maintain control over what services they desire.

Interview of the patient should be focused on obtaining medically relevant details, and documentation should be fact-driven. An objective voice should be maintained, using language such as "patient states..." and incorporating direct quotes when necessary. A thorough physical exam should be performed with precise descriptions of any physical findings, including an oral, pelvic, or rectal examination when indicated. During the physical exam, consideration should be taken as to whether evidence collection for forensic evaluation is available in the setting and whether a trained forensic examiner is available. Emergency stabilization of the patient should always be prioritized over forensic evaluation. In addition to the physical exam, consider CT imaging or FAST ultrasound examinations if available or indicated.

Care provided should include comprehensive testing for sexually transmitted infections including HIV for any patient who has experienced sexual violence. If the patient was at risk of exposure to any bodily secretions, consider providing post-exposure prophylaxis for HIV if within 72 h of exposure. In addition, where available, emergency contraception should be offered.

Sexual violence and trauma can also result in post-traumatic stress disorder (PTSD) or other conditions affecting mental well-being. Symptoms of PTSD include intrusive thoughts, hypervigilance, sleep interruption, anxiety, agitation, or social isolation. Mental health services should be offered and provided to the patient to allow for proper identification and treatment of these symptoms.

Conclusion

In this chapter, we have outlined the most common gynecological and obstetrical clinical scenarios and procedures one may encounter. Surgeries related to birth and reproductive organs can be lifesaving and frequently are needed in an urgent fashion. Preparing for these emergencies includes being informed about the local customs and laws surrounding these procedures. Regardless of their pregnancy status, women require the same resuscitation efforts and attention for their emergencies as any other patient.

Further Reading

1. Cunningham FG, Leveno KJ, Bloom SL, Spong CY, Dashe JS, Hoffman BL, Casey BM, Sheffield JS. Williams obstetrics. 24th ed. New York: McGraw-Hill Education; 2014.
2. https://www.glowm.com/ https://www.glowm.com/resource-type/resource/textbook
3. Primary Surgery Volume One Non-Trauma from Maurice King.
4. Groen RS, Kushner AL. Obstetrics. In: Meara JG, McClain CD, Rogers SO, Mooney DP, editors. Global surgery and Anesthesia manual: providing Care in Resource-Limited Settings. Boca Raton: CRC Press; 2015. p. 219–46.
5. Mandigo M, Groen RS. Chapter 17 *Gynecology and obstetrics*. In: Adrian Park and Raymond Price, editor. Global surgery – the essentials. Springer International Publishing AG; 2017.

How to Manage Urologic Problems in Low- and Middle-Income Countries

45

Nicholas A. Romas

"Gnothi seauton" Know your own self.

– Hippocrates, "Father of medicine"

Abbreviations

BPH	Benign prostatic hyperplasia
EMB	Ethambutol
HPV	Human papilloma virus
INH	Isoniazid
PKD	Polycystic kidney disease
RMP	Rifampin
STDs	Sexually transmitted diseases
TURP	Transurethral resection of the prostate

Penis and Male Urethra [1]

Phimosis is a condition in which the contracted foreskin cannot be retracted over the glans. Chronic infection from poor hygiene is the most common cause. Most cases occur in uncircumcised males. Edema, erythema, and tenderness of the prepuce and the presence of purulent discharge usually cause the patient to seek medical attention. The initial treatment is with broad-spectrum antimicrobial drugs, and then later, circumcision may be needed [2].

Paraphimosis is the condition in which the foreskin once retracted over the glans cannot be replaced in its normal position. The condition can be treated by firmly squeezing the glans for 5 mins, and the skin can then be drawn forward over the glans. Circumcision should be administered after inflammation has subsided.

Peyronie's disease has plastic induration of the penis affecting middle-aged and older men. Patients complain of painful erections, curvature of the penis, and poor erections distal to the involved area. Examination of the penile shaft reveals a palpable dense fibrous plaque of varying sizes. Multiple plaques are sometimes seen. Spontaneous remission occurs in about 50% of cases. Medications have limited success. In recent years, a number of operative procedures have been used in refractory cases.

Priapism is an uncommon condition of prolonged erection. The disorder is idiopathic in 60% of cases, while the remaining 40% of cases are associated with a disease. There are multiple causes, but *ischemic priapism* must be consid-

N. A. Romas (✉)
Columbia University Medical Center,
New York, NY, USA
e-mail: nar1@cumc.columbia.edu

M. A. Hardy, B. R. Hochman (eds.), *Global Surgery*, https://doi.org/10.1007/978-3-031-28127-3_45

ered a urologic emergency. Epidural or spinal anesthesia can be effective. The sludged blood can then be evacuated through a large needle placed through the glans. Various shunt and fistula techniques can be performed to prevent recurrence. Impotence is the worst sequel of priapism. It is more common after prolonged priapism (several days). Early recognition (within hours) and prompt treatment offer the best opportunity to avoid impotence.

Acquired urethral stricture is common in men but rare in women. Most acquired strictures are due to infection or trauma, particularly infection from long-term use of indwelling urethral catheters. External trauma, for example, pelvic fractures, can cause severe and complex strictures. Urethral strictures are fibrotic narrowings.

Sexually Transmitted Diseases

Sexually transmitted diseases (STDs) [3] are most common in young adults between the ages of 18 and 28, as well as middle-aged, divorced individuals. It is also important to remember that STDs range among the top five risks of international travelers, along with diarrhea, hepatitis, and motor vehicle accidents. The brunt of the STD burden, both in risk and consequences, falls on women. When exposed to STD, women are more likely to become infected and are much more likely to be asymptomatic. STD can cause pelvic inflammatory disease with subsequent risks of chronic pain syndromes, ectopic pregnancy, and infertility. A urologist should have a high index of suspicion for underlying STD in women who present with recurrent UTI and in those who are symptomatic with sterile urine cultures. Up to 50% of women with signs of UTI during emergency examination had subsequent positive cultures for STD.

Genital herpes infection is caused by HSV-2 in 80–85% of cases, while HSV-1 is responsible for 15–20% of cases. Primary infection is associated with painful ulcers of the genitalia or anus and bilateral painful inguinal adenopathy in 80% of cases. Urethral lesions may cause urinary retention in women. The diagnosis should be confirmed by ruling out other ulcerative disorders and obtaining a Tzanck smear. Primary therapy consists of acyclovir or valacyclovir.

Chlamydia trachomatis is the most common bacterial STD in the United States. Men will typically experience lower urinary tract symptoms attributed to urethritis, epididymitis, or prostatitis and may notice clear or white penile discharge. Up to 85% of women may be asymptomatic until the infection has progressed to the pelvis. Specimens obtained from urethral or cervical swabs, urine, or prostatic fluids should be cultured. Treatment consists of azithromycin or doxycycline.

Lymphogranuloma venereum has initial manifestation of infection as usually a single painless ulcer on the penis, anus, or vulvovaginal area. Patients usually present with painful unilateral suppurative inguinal adenopathy that occurs 2–6 weeks after resolution of the ulcer. Perirectal or deep iliac lymph node enlargement may occur if the primary lesion arises from the cervix or rectum. Significant tissue damage may occur, leading to labial fenestration, urethral destruction, anorectal fistulas, elephantiasis of the penis, scrotum, or labia. Complement fixation or indirect fluorescence antibody titers may be necessary to confirm diagnosis. Treatment is required with doxycycline, erythromycin, or sulfisoxazole.

Primary and secondary syphilis is caused by a spirochete, *Treponema pallidum*, with incubation periods that vary between 3 and 90 days. A single clean ulcer that is usually nontender appears on the glans, corona, or perianal area in men and on the labial or anal area in women. It is typically associated with bilateral nontender inguinal adenopathy. Secondary syphilis may present up to months following the initial infection as mucocutaneous lesions and constitutional symptoms. Dark field examination of specimens obtained from primary or secondary lesions will reveal the spirochete. Penicillin and doxycycline are the preferred therapies.

Gonorrhea is caused by a gram-negative diplococcus, *Neisseria gonorrhoeae*. Men will typically experience lower urinary tract symptoms with associated mucopurulent urethral discharge.

Women may have symptoms of vaginal/pelvic discomfort and dysuria and may have abnormal vaginal discharge. Swabs taken from the urethra and the cervix or rectum should be cultured. Preferred treatment is ceftriaxone IM, but oral-dose regimens include cefixime, ciprofloxacin, and ofloxacin.

Chancroid is the most common STD worldwide and affects men more often than women. It causes a painful shaggy ulcer on the penis or vulvovaginal area. It is associated with inguinal adenopathy that is typically unilateral and with a tendency to fistulize. *Haemophilus ducreyi*, the causative organism, is difficult to culture. PCR assays have been shown to be a sensitive and specific means of detecting *Haemophilus ducreyi*. Treatment is simple azithromycin or ceftriaxone, ciprofloxacin, or erythromycin.

Trichomoniasis is caused by a protozoan, *Trichomonas vaginalis*, and is an obligate to the vagina or urethra. Men have little or no symptoms, but women may notice a foamy-white or greenish vaginal discharge and pruritus. Vaginal wet mount or urine examined microscopically reveals the flagellated organisms. Treatment consists of the administration of metronidazole.

Genital warts (condyloma acuminata) are caused by human papilloma virus (HPV) of 20 types. HPV may be associated with nonspecific symptoms such as vulvodynia, pruritus, or malodorous vaginal discharge. The diagnosis is usually made through the visualization or palpation of nontender papillomatous genital lesions. High-risk HPV are associated with invasive cancers of the penis and cervix. Cryotherapy or surgical removal along with podophyllin or trichloroacetic acid is recommended. Urethral or bladder lesions should be surgically excised. Fluorouracil (5FU) instillation may be necessary to completely eradicate papillomatous lesions.

Scabies infection is caused by the mite *Sarcoptes scabiei* and presents with elongated papules. Susceptible areas include the penile shaft and glans, finger webs, and axillary folds. Confirming the diagnosis may require microscopic evidence of the mite (or eggs). Permethrin cream or lindane lotion is applied to all areas of the body.

Scrotum (Scrotal Mass and Acute Scrotum) [4]

There are many causes of acute and chronic scrotal pathology. The emphasis will be on those that require emergency medical or surgical treatment. Appropriate evaluation of the patient with any scrotal abnormality is crucial as a delay in recognition of the offending process or administration of treatment may result in testicular loss. Diagnosis of an acute or swollen scrotum is largely dependent on a detailed history and careful examination.

Testicular torsion refers specifically to a rotation of the spermatic cord and testicle that results in venous and arterial compromise and ultimately gonadal loss. Emergency surgery is required to salvage the testis. Torsion of the testicular or epididymal appendages usually occurs between the ages of 2 and 12 years old. Torsion of the appendix testis should not be a clinical diagnosis unless the offending appendages can be palpated at the superior pole of the testis. Complete resolution of symptoms usually occurs after appendage necrosis. Diagnosis can be confirmed by ultrasonography if available.

Hydrocele, defective absorption of fluid by the tunica vaginalis, is common in adults. Connection with the peritoneal cavity can produce congenital hydrocele. Treatment in adults consists of drainage of hydrocele and resection of the tunica vaginalis. In children, an inguinal incision is needed between internal and external with high ligation of the processus vaginalis and excision of sac.

Spermatocele clinically presents as a unilateral scrotal mass, which is nontender, lying in a position superior and posterior to the testicle. They are usually small but may become large enough to clinically resemble a hydrocele. Treatment consists of surgical spermatocelectomy.

Varicocele is defined as dilated and incompetent complex of veins within the pampiniform plexus of the spermatic cord. A left-sided varicocele is found in 15% of healthy young men. In contrast, the incidence of a left varicocele in subfertile men approaches 40%. Bilateral varicoceles are uncommon in healthy men (<10%). The finding of semen abnormalities constitutes the most common indication for varicocele surgery.

Testicular tumors are incidentally discovered by the patient during palpation. The usual presentation is a painless lump, nodule, and hardness of the testicle. Treatment for testicular tumors includes radical orchiectomy and radiation with and without systemic chemotherapy (depending on the tumor's histologic composition, size, and staging).

Fournier's Gangrene

Fournier's gangrene is a urologic emergency and is a form of necrotizing fasciitis that originates in the perineum and can be widespread and life-threatening. Patients typically present with sudden onset of scrotal edema, pain, and areas of black or bluish skin. Sources of infection may include periurethral or perirectal abscesses, but often no definitive source can be determined. Treatment must resume immediately and includes aggressive antibiotic coverage in addition to wide debridement of all involved tissue. Salvage of the testicle involves placement of the testicle into an ectopic subcutaneous pouch. A scrotal pouch can be reconstructed after resolution of the infectious process.

Male Sexual Dysfunction [5]

It is estimated that more than half of men aged 40–70 years in the United States are unable to attain or maintain a penile erection. Advances in pharmacologic therapy for erectile dysfunction (ED) coupled with a better understanding of male sexual dysfunction have resulted in greater numbers of patients seeking care for sexual problems. Oral phosphodiesterase type 5 inhibitors have emerged as the preferred first-line treatment of ED worldwide. Erectile function can now be evaluated by the response to these agents at home or by intracavernous injection of vasoactive agents in the office. Patient satisfaction with penile prostheses is high. Current treatments continue to evolve.

Disorders of the Bladder [6]

Exstrophy of the bladder is a rare congenital anomaly with complete ventral defect of the urogenital sinus and the overlying skeletal system. Treatment consists of staged repair of the anomaly (see Chap. 35 – Pediatrics).

Interstitial cystitis of unknown etiology presents with urinary frequency and bladder pain. It affects men and women of all ages. Common symptoms are bladder pain worsened with bladder filling, certain food intake, and burning dysuria. Treatment with anticholinergics is frequently used to control frequency and urgency. Amitriptyline has been shown to improve symptoms including pain and frequency. Intravesical instillations of dimethyl sulfoxide (DMSO), heparin, Bacillus Calmette-Guerin, and sodium hyaluronate are also used with some benefits.

Numerous foreign objects have been found in the urethra and bladder of both men and women. Commonly reported objects are intrauterine contraceptive devices, hernia repair mesh, vaginal sling material, and bone fragments after trauma. The presence of a foreign body causes cystitis and hematuria. Cystoscopy or suprapubic removal is indicated.

Diverticula

Most vesical diverticula are acquired and are secondary to either obstruction distal to the vesical neck or to neurogenic bladder. Often the diverticulum lies just superior to the ureter and causes vesicoureteral reflux. The diverticulum is devoid of muscle and has no expulsive power. It therefore contains residual urine and may lead commonly to chronic infection. If diverticulectomy is performed, then bladder outlet obstruction must also be performed.

Vesical Fistulas

The bladder may communicate with the skin, intestinal tract, or femoral reproductive organs. The causes are as follows:

1. Primary intestinal disease, diverticulitis, colon cancer, and Crohn's disease.
2. Primary gynecologic disease, difficult labor, cancer of the cervix.
3. Trauma.

The bladder may be inadvertently injured during gynecologic or intestinal surgery, cystotomy for stones, or prostatectomy, which may lead to a persistent cutaneous fistula.

Symptoms from a vesicointestinal fistula include bladder irritability, passage of debris and gas through the urethra, and usually a change in bowel habits.

Imaging studies, CT scan, and MRI are sensitive tests for enterovesical fistula. It may show mass adjacent to the bladder and air in the bladder. Cystoscopy shows a severe localized inflammatory reaction from which bowel contents may exude.

The surgical repair of fistulas caused by benign disease or operative trauma is highly successful. Post-radiation necrosis offers a more guarded prognosis. Fistulas secondary to invading cancers present difficult problems.

Pelvic Lipomatosis [7]

The cause of pelvic lipomatosis is not known. The disorder seems to affect principally Black men in the 20–40-year age group with hypertension. There are no pathognomonic symptoms. There may be some dysuria or mild urinary obstructive symptoms. Examination may demonstrate microscopic hematuria and a distended or enlarged pear-shaped bladder. Radiological studies may show dilatation of both ureter tracts and an upward displacement and lateral compression of the bladder. In the perivesical area, x-ray reveals areas of radiolucency compatible with fatty tissue. Surgical options in patients with obstructive uropathy include ureteral stenting, percutaneous nephrostomy, ureteral reimplantation, and urinary diversion. Pelvic exploration should be approached cautiously, since there is obliteration of normal anatomic planes and increased vascularity with the fatty mass.

Urinary Stone Disease [8]

Urinary calculi are solid particles in the urinary system. Patients present with pain, nausea, vomiting, hematuria, and possibly chills and fever from secondary infection. Diagnosis is based on urinalysis and non-contrast CT scan. Treatment is with analgesics; antibiotics for infection; sometimes instrumentation to remove it, shock-wave lithotripsy if available; or endoscopic surgery.

In a patient who has passed a first Ca calculus, the likelihood of forming a second calculus is about 15% at 1 year, 40% at 5 years, and 80% at 10 years. Recovery and analysis of the calculus, measurement of calculus-forming substance in the urine, and the clinical history are needed to plan prophylaxis.

Urinary Tract Infections (UTIs) [9]

UTIs can be divided into upper tract infections, which involve the kidneys, and lower tract infections, which involve the bladder, urethra, or prostate. However, in practice, differentiating between the sites may be difficult. Bacterial UTIs can involve the urethra, prostate, bladder, or kidneys. Symptoms may be absent or include urinary frequency, urgency and dysuria, lower abdominal pain, and flank pain. Systemic symptoms and sepsis may occur with kidney infections. Diagnosis is based on analysis and culture of urine. Treatment of all forms of UTI requires antibiotics. Obstructive uropathy, anatomic abnormalities, and neuropathic GU lesions usually require surgical correction. Catheter drainage of an obstructed urinary tract aids in prompt control of UTI. Occasionally, a renal cortical abscess or perinephric abscess requires surgical drainage.

Prevention

In woman who experiences >3 UTIs per year, voiding immediately after intercourse and avoiding use of a diaphragm may be helpful. Drinking cranberry juice reduces pyuria and bacteriuria. If these techniques are unsuccessful, post-coital antibiotic may be effective.

Chronic Pyelonephritis

Chronic pyelonephritis is chronic pyogenic infection of the kidneys that occurs only in patients with major anatomic abnormalities. Symptoms include fever, malaise, and flank discomfort. Diagnosis is with urinalysis, culture, and imaging tests. Treatment is with antibiotics and correction of any structural disorders. Reflux of infected urine into the renal pelvis is the usual mechanism; other causes include obstructive uropathy, struvite calculi, and most commonly vesicoureteral reflux.

Benign Prostatic Hyperplasia [10]

Benign prostatic hyperplasia (BPH) is a nonmalignant adenomatous overgrowth of the periurethral prostate gland. Symptoms are those of bladder outlet obstruction, urinary frequency, urgency, nocturia, hesitancy, incomplete emptying, terminal dribbling, overflow incontinence, or complete urinary retention. Diagnosis is based on digital rectal examination, cystoscopy, transrectal ultrasonography, CT, and MRI. Treatment options include 5-alpha-reductase inhibitors, alphablockers, and surgery. Complete obstruction requires immediate decompression. A standard catheter is first choice but may require a stiffer catheter or one with a coude tip. If this catheter cannot be passed, flexible cystoscopy or insertion of filiforms and followers that progressively open and dilate the urinary passage. Suprapubic percutaneous decompression of the bladder may be used. For patients with mild-to-moderate obstructive symptoms, alpha-adrenergic blockers may improve voiding. The 5-alpha reductase inhibitors may reduce prostate size, improving voiding over months, especially in patients with larger (730 ml) glands. A combination of both classes of drugs is superior to monotherapy.

Surgery is performed when patients do not respond to drug therapy. Transurethral resection of the prostate (TURP) is the standard. The incidence of erectile dysfunction after TURP is between 5% and 35%, of incontinence about 1%. Larger prostates (775 g) may require open surgery. Multiple other procedures are also used, which include intraurethral stents, balloon dilatation, microwave thermotherapy, high-intensity focused ultrasound thermotherapy, laser ablation, electrovaporization, and radiofrequency vaporization.

Prostatitis [11]

Prostatitis refers to a group of disorders that presents with a combination of irritative or obstructive urinary symptoms and perineal pain. It is estimated that 35–50% of males will experience the pain and discomfort of prostatitis during some period in their lives. The quality of life of patients with chronic prostatitis is significantly worse than that experienced by patients with BPH or localized prostate cancer. Some result from bacterial infection of the prostate gland and others from a poorly understood combination of noninfectious inflammatory factors. Diagnosis is clinical, along with microscopic examination and culture of the urine samples obtained before and after prostate massage. Treatment is with a fluoroquinolone if the cause is bacterial. Nonbacterial causes are treated with warm sitz baths, muscle relaxants, and anti-inflammatory drugs.

Prostate Cancer [12]

Prostate cancer is the most prevalent non-skin cancer and the second leading cause of cancer deaths among men. The risk factors are as follows: men 65 and older (average age of men with prostate cancer is 66), family history (you are twice as likely to get prostate cancer if your dad, brother, or son had/has it), and race/ethnicity (African American men have far higher diagnosis and mortality rates for prostate cancer than the overall male population). Prostate cancer is usually adenocarcinoma. Symptoms are rare until urethral obstruction occurs. In a advanced disesese findings may include the following symptoms and signs: hematuria, symptoms of bladder obstrucition, e.g., straining, hesitancy, weak and intermittent urine stream, and even urinary retention requiring Foley catheter drainage. Bone pain may result from osteoblastic metastases to the bone (commonly pelvis, ribs, vertebral bodies). Diagnosis is suggested by digital rectal examination or prostate-specific antigen measurement and confirmed by biopsy. Transrectal ultrasound-guided needle biopsy can be done in a clinic without general anesthesia. MRI has also been very helpful. Prognosis for most patients with prostate cancer, especially when it is localized or regional, is very good; more men die with prostate cancer than of it.

Treatment is with prostatectomy, radiation therapy, and new chemotherapy agents for metastatic disease. In elderly patients, watchful waiting has been used. Researchers have explored effectiveness of a prostate cancer educational program in high-burden neighborhoods. This study showed that gathering at-risk men for discussions about prostate cancer or other health concerns may increase their prostate cancer knowledge and intention to talk to a doctor about prostate cancer screening.

Specific Infections of the Genitourinary Tract [13]

Tubercle bacilli (Mycobacterium) may invade one or more (or even all) of the organs of the genitourinary tract and cause a chronic granulomatous infection that shows the same characteristics as tuberculosis in other organs. Urinary tuberculosis is a disease of young adults (60% of patients are between ages of 20 and 40) and is more common in males than females. Proper urinalysis affords the most important clue to the diagnosis of genitourinary tuberculosis. Persistent pyuria without organisms on culture means tuberculosis until proved otherwise. Cultures for tubercle bacilli from the first morning urine are positive in a very high percentage of cases. Ultrasound and computed tomography (CT) show calcifications, renal contractions, and scars, as well as ureteral and calyceal strictures suggestive of genitourinary tuberculosis. Genitourinary tuberculosis is extrapulmonary tuberculosis. The primary treatment is medical therapy. Surgical excision of a massively infected organ, when indicated, is merely an adjunct to overall therapy. A combination of drugs is usually desirable. The following drugs are effective in combination: (1) isoniazid (INH), (2) rifampin (RMP), and (3) ethambutol (EMB). The European Association of Urology recommends 2 or 3 months of intense triple drug therapy (INH, RMP, and EMB) daily followed by 3 months of continuation therapy with INH and RMP.

Treatment of Infectious Complications

Perinephric abscess usually occurs when the kidney is destroyed, but this is rare. The abscess must be drained, and nephrotomy should be done either then or later to prevent development of a chronic draining sinus. If ureteral stricture develops on the involved side, ureteral dilatations offer a better than 50% chance of cure. The severely involved bladder may cause incompetence of the ureterovesical junction on the uninvolved side. Some form of urinary diversion may be required.

Candidiasis. Candida albicans is a yeast-like fungus that is a normal inhabitant of the respiratory and gastrointestinal tracts and the vagina. The intense use of potent modern antibiotics is apt to disturb the normal balance between normal and abnormal organisms, thus allowing fungi such as *Candida* to overwhelm an otherwise healthy organ. The patient may present with vesical irritability or symptoms and signs of pyelonephritis. The diagnosis is made by observing mycelial or yeast forms of the fungus microscopically. The diagnosis may be confirmed by culture. Treatment is with oral fluconazole, and vesical candidiasis usually responds to alkalinization of the urine with sodium bicarbonate. Candida should be treated in symptomatic patients, patients with neutropenia, renal transplant patients, and patients who will undergo urologic procedures.

Actinomycosis. Actinomycosis is a chronic granulomatous disease in which fibrosis tends to be marked and spontaneous fistulas are the rule. On rare occasions, the disease involves the kidney, bladder, or testis by hematogenous invasion from a primary site of infection. The bladder may also become diseased by direct extension from the appendix, bowel, or oviduct. The microscopic demonstration of the organisms, which are visible as yellow bodies called "sulfur granules," confirms the diagnosis. If persistently sought, these may be found in the discharge from sinuses or in the urine. Penicillin is the drug of choice, but if secondary infection is suspected, a sulfonamide is added; streptomycin is also efficacious. Surgical drainage of the abscess or, better, removal of the involved organ is usually indicated.

Schistosomiasis (bilharziasis). Schistosomiasis is caused by a blood fluke and is a disease of warm climates. In its three forms, it affects about 350 million people. *Schistosoma mansoni* is widely distributed in Africa, South and Central America, Pakistan, and India. *Schistosoma japonicum* is found in the Far East, and *Schistosoma haematobium* is limited to Africa, Saudi Arabia, Israel, Jordan, Lebanon, and Syria. Humans are infected when they come in contact with larva-infected stagnant water in canals, ditches, or irrigation fields during swimming or bathing or while farming. Penetration of the skin by the cercariae causes allergic reactions with cutaneous hyperemia and itching that are more intense in people infected for the first time. The patient complains of symptoms of malaise, fatigue, and lassitude, low-grade fever, excessive sweating, headache, and back ache. When the ova are laid in the bladder wall and begin to be extruded, the patient complains of terminal, slightly painful hematuria that is occasionally profuse. Symptoms can become progressive, characterized by increased frequency, suprapubic and back pain, profuse hematuria, pyuria, and nocturia. These are likely to occur with secondary infections, ulceration, or malignancy. Renal pain may be due to ureteral stricture, vesicoureteral reflux, or secondary stones, ulceration, or malignancy. In early uncomplicated cases, there are essentially no clinical findings. Later, a fibrosed, pitted bilharzial glans penis, a urethral stricture or fistula, or a perineal fibrous mass may be found. A suprapubic bladder mass or a swelling may be felt on abdominal exam. Rectal examination may reveal a fibrosed prostate, an enlarged seminal vesicle, or a thickened bladder base. Urinalysis usually reveals the terminal-spined dead or living ova, blood, pus cells, and bacteria. Malignant squamous cells may also be seen. A variety of immunologic methods have been used to confirm the diagnosis of schistosomiasis. Abdominal and pelvic CT may show hydronephrosis, dilated and tortuous ureters, ureteral strictures, or a small, contracted bladder. Gross irregular defects of the bladder wall may represent cancer. Praziquantel, metrifonate, and oxamniquine are the drugs of choice in treating schistosomiasis. Antibiotics are needed to overcome or control secondary infections. Treatment of the complications of schistosomiasis of the genitourinary tract makes demands on the skill of both the surgeon and the internist.

Filariasis. Filariasis is endemic in the countries bordering the Mediterranean, in South China and Japan, the West Indies, and the South Pacific islands. *Wuchereria bancrofti* is an adult nematode that invades and obstructs the lymphatics. This leads to lymphangitis and lymphadenitis. Not infrequently, inflammation occurs in the epididymis, the testis, scrotum, and spermatic cord. These structures then become edematous, boggy, and at times tender. In advanced cases, obstruction of major lymph channels may cause chyluria and elephantiasis. Diethylcarbamazine albendazole is the treatments of choice. Elephantiasis of the external genitalia may require surgical excision. In endemic areas, mosquito abatement programs must be intensively pursued.

Echinococcosis (hydatid disease). Involvement of the urogenital organs by hydatid disease is relatively rare in the United States. It is common in Australia, New Zealand, South America, Africa, Asia, the Middle East, and Europe. Livestock are the intermediate hosts, and canines, especially dogs, are the final hosts. The adult tapeworm (*Echinococcus granulosus*) inhabits the intestinal tracts of carnivorous animals. Its eggs pass out with feces and may be ingested by such animals as sheep, cattle, pigs, and occasionally humans. In humans, the liver is principally involved, but about 39% of infested humans develop echinococcosis of the kidney. If a cyst of the liver should rupture into the peritoneal cavity, the tapeworm heads may directly invade the retrovesical tissues, thus leading to the development of cysts in this area. Nephrectomy is generally the treatment of choice for renal hydatid disease. Medical treatment includes albendazole or praziquantel (before surgery). Retroperitoneal cysts are best treated by marsupialization and curettage.

Renal Cell Carcinoma [14]

Renal cell carcinoma is the most common renal cancer. Symptoms appear late and include hematuria, flank pain, and sometimes a palpable mass. Diagnosis is by CT or MRI and occasionally by biopsy. Treatment is with surgery for early disease and typically an experimental protocol followed by surgery for advanced disease. Risk factors include smoking, obesity, excess use of phenacetin, and acquired cystic kidney disease in dialysis patients.

Cancers of the renal pelvis and ureters are usually transitional cell carcinomas and occasionally squamous cell carcinoma. Symptoms include hematuria and sometimes pain. Diagnosis is by CT, cytology, and sometimes biopsy. Risk factors are the same as those for bladder cancer. Also, inhabitants of the Balkans with endemic familial nephropathy are inexplicably predisposed to develop upper tract transitional cell cancer.

Treatment is surgery. Periodic cystoscopy is indicated because renal, pelvic, and ureteral chancres tend to recur in the bladder, and such recurrence, if detected at an early stage, may be treated by fulguration, transurethral resection, or intravesical instillation. Management of metastases is the same as that for metastatic bladder cancer.

Congenital Anomalies of the Kidneys [15]

Congenital anomalies occur more frequently in the kidney than in any other organ. Some cause no difficulty but may (e.g., hypoplasia, polycystic kidney) cause impairment of renal function. It has been noted that children with gross deformity of an external ear, which is associated with ipsilateral maldevelopment of the facial bones, are apt to have a congenital abnormality of the kidney on the same side as the visible deformity. Lateral displacement of the nipples has been observed in association with bilateral renal hypoplasia.

Adult polycystic kidney disease (PKD is an autosomal dominant hereditary condition and almost always bilateral (95% of cases). The disease encountered in infants is different from that seen in adults. The former is an autosomal recessive disease in which life expectancy is short, whereas that diagnosed in adulthood is autosomal dominant. Symptoms ordinarily do not appear until age 40. Cysts of the liver, spleen, and pancreas may be noted in association with both forms. The kidneys are larger than normal and are studded with cysts of various sizes. Anemia may be noted, caused either by chronic loss of blood into the cysts, sometimes associated with pain, or, more commonly, by the hematopoietic depression accompanying uremia. Proteinuria and microscopic (if not gross) hematuria are the rule. Pyuria and bacteriuria are common. CT scanning is an excellent noninvasive technique used to establish the diagnosis of polycystic disease. The multiple thin-walled cysts filled with fluid and the large renal size make this imaging method extremely accurate (95%) for diagnosis. The patient should be put on a low-protein diet and fluids forced to 3000 ml or more per day. When the patient is in the state of absolute renal insufficiency, one should treat as for uremia. Hypertension should be controlled, and hemodialysis and/or renal transplant is indicated. There is no evidence that excision or decompression of cysts improves renal function. If a large cyst is found to be compressing the upper ureter, causing obstruction, it should be resected or aspirated. Patients with PKD should not have their cysts drained electively for fera of bleedin and/or infection.

Simple cyst of the kidney is usually unilateral and single but may be multiple and, more rarely, bilateral. It differs from polycystic kidneys both clinically and pathologically. If the cyst becomes infected, intensive antimicrobial therapy should be instituted; antimicrobial drugs have been found to attain very low concentrations in the cyst fluid. Therefore, percutaneous drainage is often required. Surgical excision of the extrarenal portion of the cyst wall and drainage are curative when percutaneous drainage fails. Yearly sonography is recommended as a method of following the cyst for changes in size, configuration, and internal consistence. CT scan may be done if changes suggest carcinoma. Most cysts cause little difficulty.

References

1. McAninch JW. Smith and Tanagho's General Urology. Edition 18. Mc Graw Hill. 2013;41:633–43.
2. Kursh ED, Ulchaker JC. Office urology: the Clinician's guide. Springer Science & Business Media; 2000.
3. Krieger JN. Smith and Tanagho's General Urology. Edition 18. Mc Graw Hill. 2013;16:238–47.
4. Cherullo EE, Ulchaker JC. Office Urology: The Clinician's Guide. Humana Press Inc. 2001;26:355–67.
5. Lue TF. Smith and Tanagho's General Urology. Edition 18. Mc Graw Hill. 2013;39:596–614.
6. Shinohara K. Smith and Tanagho's General Urology. Edition 18. Mc Graw Hill. 2013;38:583–91.
7. Pais VM. Jr., Strandhoy JW, Assimos DG. Campbell-Walsh Urology. Edition, Saunders. 2007;9:1218.
8. Stoller MD. Smith and Tanagho's General Urology. Edition 18. Mc Graw Hill. 2013;17:249–77.
9. Beers MH. The Merck Manual. Edition 18. Merck Research Laboratories. 2006;231:1968–73.
10. Beers MH. The Merck Manual. Edition 18. Merck Research Laboratories. 2006;240:2042–45.
11. Beers MH. The Merck Manual. Edition 18. Merck Research Laboratories. 2006;240:2045–47.
12. Beers MH. The Merck Manual. Edition 18. Merck Research Laboratories. 2006;241:2052–54.
13. Tanagho EA, Kane CJ. Smith and Tanagho's General Urology. Edition 18. Mc Graw Hill. 2013;15:223–35.
14. Beers MH. The Merck Manual. Edition 18. Merck Research Laboratories. 2006;241:2055–56.
15. McAninch JW. Smith and Tanagho's General Urology. Edition 18. Mc Graw Hill. 2013;23:513–22.

Corrections to: How to Establish Surgical Teaching, Guidance, and Simulation Practices in Low- and Middle-Income Countries

Shamir O. Cawich, Paul Shridath Ramphal, Marlon Mencia, Chris Dodgion, and Alazar Berhe Aregawi

Correction to:
Chapter 16 in : M. A. Hardy, B. R. Hochman (eds.), *Global Surgery*, https://doi.org/10.1007/978-3-031-28127-3_16

In the original version of the book, the first name for Dr. Aregawi had been missed out.

Hence, the author's name has been updated to Alazar Berhe Aregawi in the revised version of the book.

The updated original version of this chapter can be found at https://doi.org/10.1007/978-3-031-28127-3_16

M. A. Hardy, B. R. Hochman (eds.), *Global Surgery*, https://doi.org/10.1007/978-3-031-28127-3_46

Index

M. A. Hardy, B. R. Hochman (eds.), *Global Surgery*, https://doi.org/10.1007/978-3-031-28127-3

P